Browse's Introduction to the Symptoms and Signs of Surgical Disease

Fourth edition

Norman L. Browse Kt MD FRCS FRCP
Professor of Surgery, Emeritus, University of London, UK
Honorary Consulting Surgeon, St Thomas' Hospital, London, UK
Formerly, Chairman, London University MBBS and MS Examiners
Formerly, Member of Court of Examiners, Royal College of Surgeons of England, UK
Formerly, Member of Council and Chairman of Examinations Committee and
  Academic Board, Royal College of Surgeons of England, UK
Past-President, Royal College of Surgeons of England, UK

John Black MD FRCS
Consultant Surgeon, Worcestershire Royal Hospital, UK
Member of Council, Royal College of Surgeons of England, UK
Examiner, Intercollegiate Board in General Surgery, UK

Kevin G. Burnand MS FRCS MBBS
Professor of Vascular Surgery and Chairman of the Academic Department of Surgery
  and Anaesthesia in the Cardiovascular Divison of King's College at the St Thomas'
  Campus, London, UK
Honorary Consultant Surgeon to Guy's and St Thomas' Foundation Trust, London, UK

William E.G. Thomas MS FRCS
Consultant Surgeon and Clinical Director, Sheffield Teaching Hospitals Trust, Member
  of Council, Royal College of Surgeons of England, UK
Formerly, Member of Court of Examiners, Royal College of Surgeons of England and
  Panel of Examiners for the Intercollegiate Board in General Surgery, UK

Hodder Arnold

A MEMBER OF THE HODDER HEADLINE GROUP

First published in Great Britain in 1978
Second edition 1991
Third edition 1997

This fourth edition published in 2005 by
Hodder Education, a member of the Hodder Headline Group,
338 Euston Road, London NW1 3BH

http://www.hoddereducation.com

Distributed in the United States of America by
Oxford University Press Inc.,
198 Madison Avenue, New York, NY10016
Oxford is a registered trademark of Oxford University Press

British Library Cataloguing in Publication Data
A catalogue record for this book is available from the British Library

Library of Congress Cataloging-in-Publication Data
A catalog record for this book is available from the Library of Congress

ISBN-10 [normal]   0 340 81571 X
ISBN-13: 978 0 340 81571 7
ISBN-10 [ISE]   0 340 81579 5 (International Students' Edition, restricted territorial availability)
ISBN-13: 978 0 340 81579 3
ISBN-10 [ELST]   0 340 81580 9
ISBN-13: 978 0 340 81580 9

3 4 5 6 7 8 9 10

Commissioning Editor: Georgina Bentliff
Development Editor: Heather Smith
Project Editor: Wendy Rooke
Production Controller: Jane Lawrence
Cover Design: Amina Dudhia

Typeset in 10/12 pt Minion by Charon Tec Pvt. Ltd, Chennai, India
www.charontec.com
Printed and bound in India

What do you think about this book? Or any other Hodder Arnold title?
Please visit our website at www.hoddereducation.co.uk

We dedicate this book to all those who have supported
us thoughout our clinical careers:

Our wives,
families,
consultant colleagues,
registrars and house officers,
nurses in the wards, outpatients and operating rooms,
secretaries and laboratory staff,

ould have been

to write this book.

Contents

Preface to the First Edition

I believe that the main object of basic medical education is to train the student to talk to and to examine a patient in such a way that he can discover the full history of the patient's illness, elicit the abnormal physical signs, make a differential diagnosis and suggest likely methods of treatment. The object of further medical training is to amplify these capabilities in range and depth through practical experience and specialist training.

It is surprising, but a fact, that some students present themselves for their qualifying examination unable to take a history or to conduct a physical examination in a way that is likely to detect all the abnormal symptoms and signs. Even more are unable to interpret and integrate the facts they do elicit. I think there are two reasons for these deficiencies. First, and most important, students do not spend enough time seeing patients and practising the art of history taking and clinical examination. It is essential for them to realize at the beginning of their training that the major part of medical education is an **apprenticeship**, an old but well-proven system whereby the apprentice watches and listens to someone more experienced than himself and then tries it himself under supervision. The second reason is the lack of books which describe how to examine a patient and explain how the presence or absence of particular symptoms and signs lead the clinician to the correct diagnosis.

In this book I have attempted to describe, in detail, the relevant features of the history and physical signs of the common surgical diseases in a way which emphasizes the importance of the routine application of the techniques of history taking and examining.

The details of these techniques are fully described, and headings such as age, sex, symptoms, position, site, shape and surface are constantly repeated in an unobtrusive way. I hope that when you have finished reading the book you will have these headings so deeply imprinted in your mind that you will never forget them. If so, I will consider that the book has succeeded, for you will always take a proper history and perform a correct and complete examination.

Because the main object of the book is to emphasize the proper techniques of history taking and clinical examination, I have described only the common conditions that you are likely to see in a surgical clinic. Indeed the whole book is presented in a manner similar to that used by most teachers when they are in the presence of the patient. Special investigations and treatment are completely excluded because neither can be applied sensibly if you get the history and physical signs wrong.

To make the book useful for revision, I have put a number of the lists and classifications in special Revision Panels. The photographs are close to the relevant text but their legends contain enough information to make the picture-plus-legend a useful revision piece.

I hope this book will be more of a **teach-book** than a **text-book**, which will be read many times during your basic and higher medical training. There is a well-known saying 'A bad workman always blames his tools'. The doctor cannot make this excuse because his basic tools are his five senses. If he has not trained his senses properly in the manner described in this book and kept them finely honed by constant practice, he will practise bad medicine but he will have only himself to blame.

Norman Browse
1978

Preface to the Third Edition

The diseases and abnormalities described in this book have not changed for many thousands of years, nor have their symptoms and signs. Why then produce a third edition? The main reason is to improve and modernize the presentation of the information within the book in the belief that better presentation facilitates and improves learning.

Whereas the symptoms and signs of surgical disease have not changed in the past 20 years, methods of printing and publishing have. Computer graphics and colour printing now enable publishers to produce books of superb design, with infinite varieties of colour, at acceptable costs. The main changes in this new edition are therefore the introduction of colour into the general presentation and design, and the conversion of all 'blackboard-style' line drawings into coloured illustrations – still simple – but giving them the added impact on the memory provided by colour.

At the same time I have tried to illustrate all the clinical conditions with colour photographs – except for the few rare conditions, worthy of presentation, for which modern colour photographs are difficult to obtain. Unfortunately, the current trend is for patients to be unwilling to be photographed for illustrations to be used in books for teaching, thus making the compilation of a comprehensive library of clinical photographs far more difficult than it used to be.

I have also added a considerable number of new Revision panels, now on a blue background, as students find them particularly helpful.

To remind students of their importance, the illustrations of methods of clinical examination (mostly black-and-white photographs) are outlined in Revision Panel blue.

I hope this revised presentation will give the book a new modern appearance and that it will continue to be attractive to new readers in the same way that it has been to the gratifyingly large number of students who have acquired it for their libraries over the past 20 years.

Sir Norman Browse
1997

Preface to the Fourth Edition

The first edition of this book was written, 25 years ago, to help medical students develop their bedside clinical skills, namely, their ability to take a full clinical history and to conduct a complete clinical examination – the prime purpose of medical education.

Although the symptoms and signs of the common 'surgical' diseases have not changed for centuries, the style in which they are presented in textbooks and our understanding of the underlying pathological processes and, in some instances, their classification have. These changes have prompted the production of this fourth edition.

The past 25 years have also seen changes in the style and methods of medical education, especially in the UK, with the term 'problem-orientated medicine' purporting to describe the current popular approach. This is not a new approach. Students beginning their medical training have always been taught to begin the taking of a history by asking the patient 'What are you complaining of?'. To me, this is and always has been a problem-orientated approach.

Having asked all the questions about the patient's main complaint, together with those concerning all the other bodily systems, the student's growing knowledge of the symptoms and signs of individual diseases inevitably begins to guide them to those further questions which are likely to illuminate the cause of the main complaint. This is why it is helpful to learn the symptoms and signs of the common diseases from a book at the same time as acquiring that knowledge through growing clinical experience. This book seeks to expedite that learning.

I firmly believe that what some criticize as dogmatic teaching – following a strict ritual when taking a history and performing an examination – must remain a vital part of clinical education because it accelerates diagnosis and helps avoid errors and omissions.

Medical students know and appreciate this. The continuing success of this book indicates that it helps to fill the deficit that exists in those new courses of medical education that have mistakenly reduced the apprenticeship aspects of learning medicine.

Having retired from clinical practice, I felt it was important to ask three surgical colleagues with an approach to clinical teaching similar to my own, but who are still clinically active, to join me as editors. They have combined Chapters 2 and 3 and Chapters 13 and 15 of the third edition into single chapters (now Chapters 3 and 14) and added a new chapter on the symptoms and signs of trauma (Chapter 2).

In this edition, John Black has revised Chapters 8, 12, 13, 14, 16 and 17; Kevin Burnand has revised Chapters 1, 3, 7 and 15 and written the new Chapter 2; and William Thomas has revised Chapters 4, 5, 6, 9, 10 and 11. I have collated and edited their revisions to ensure that the book's original systematic approach and style of presentation were maintained. I am most grateful for their hard work and willing co-operation. When the fifth edition is needed, in 5–8 years' time, I know it will be in excellent hands.

I hope this edition retains its style as a ward-round 'teach-book' aimed directly at the individual student rather than a library-shelf textbook. Whenever possible, the illustrations have been kept on the same page as the relevant text, as have many of the revision panels. All are there to help you reinforce those vital items of knowledge which must be in your mind when sitting in front of a patient – not hidden somewhere in the memory of a computer.

Note. Throughout the book, whenever a particular complaint is more common in one sex, the patient has been referred to as 'he' or 'she' accordingly. If there is no sexual predominance, 'they' has been used in the singular sense.

Sir Norman Browse
2005

Acknowledgements

The advice and contributions of many surgical colleagues throughout the UK to previous editions have already been acknowledged but they are still part of the substance of this edition. Added to this group must be Dr Jane Terris, Consultant in A&E Medicine, Dr Elizabeth Graham, Consultant in Medical Ophthalmology and Mr Kieran Healey, Consultant Plastic Surgeon, all of St Thomas' Hospital, who gave valuable advice on Chapters 2 and 3, and Mr David Douglas, Consultant Orthopaedic Surgeon, Sheffield Teaching Hospitals NHS Foundation Trust, who advised on Chapter 4.

In these days of word processors and computers, much of the secretarial work has been done by the four editors themselves, at home, but we are most grateful for the secretarial assistance of Elizabeth Webb and Patricia Webb of the Academic Department of Surgery at St Thomas' Hospital.

Over the past 2 years we have received and are most grateful for the constant support given by all the editorial team of Hodder Arnold led by Georgina Bentliff.

Last, but by no means least, we thank our wives and families for accepting the disruptions to family life that the preparation of this fourth edition has imposed upon them.

History taking and clinical examination

You must be constantly alert from the moment you first see the patient, and employ your eyes, ears, nose and hands in a systematic fashion to collect information from which you can deduce the diagnosis. The ability to appreciate an unusual comment or minor abnormality, which can lead you to the correct diagnosis, only develops from the diligent and frequent practice of the routines outlined in this chapter. **Always give the patient your whole attention and never take short cuts.**

In the outpatient clinic try to see patients walk into the room, rather than finding them lying, undressed, on a couch, in a cubicle. General malaise and debility, breathlessness, cyanosis, and difficulty with particular movements are much more obvious during exercise.

It may also be helpful to see and speak to anyone who is accompanying the patient. A parent, spouse or friend can often provide valuable information about changes in health and behaviour not noticed by the patient. Remember, however, that many patients are inhibited from discussing their problems in front of a third person. It can also be difficult if the relative or friend, with the best of intentions, constantly replies on behalf of the patient. When the time comes to examine the patient, the friend or relative can be asked to leave; further questions can then be asked in private. It is helpful if a nurse is present.

Patients like to know to whom they are talking. They are probably expecting to see a specific consultant. You should **tell patients your name** and explain why you are seeing them. **It is particularly important for medical students to do this.**

Talk with patients or, better still, let them talk to you. At first, guide the conversation but do not dictate it. Treat patients as the rational, intelligent human beings they are. They know more about their complaints than you do, but they are usually unable to interpret their significance. At all stages explain what you are doing, and why you are doing it.

The patient may not be fluent in your own language and require an interpreter. When conducting an interview through an interpreter, keep your questions short and simple, and have them translated and answered one at a time. You will have to use lay terms if you are to be easily understood.

You should not use leading questions to which there is only one answer. All questions should leave the patient with a free choice of answers. You should avoid saying, 'The pain moves to the right-hand side, doesn't it?'. This is a 'leading question' because it implies that it should have moved in that direction, and an obliging patient will answer 'Yes' to please you. The patient should be asked if the pain ever moves? If the answer is 'Yes', you must then ask the supplementary question, 'Where does it go?'. Sometimes, however, patients fail to understand your question and you may have to suggest a number of possible answers, which can be confirmed or rejected.

When a patient is having difficulty communicating with you, remember that a question that you do not think is a leading one may be interpreted incorrectly by the patient if they do not realize that there is more than one answer. For example, 'Has the pain changed?' can be a bad question. There are a variety of ways in which the pain can change – severity, nature, site, etc. – but patients may be so disturbed by the intensity of the pain that they think only of its severity and forget the other features that have changed. In such situations, it often helps to include the possible answers in the question; for example, 'Has the pain moved to the top, bottom, or side of your abdomen or anywhere else?', 'Has the pain got worse, better or stayed the same?', or 'Can you walk as far, less far, or the same distance as you could a year ago?'.

The patient should provide the correct answer providing you ask the question correctly. Do not be over-concerned about the questions – worry about the answers, and accept that it will sometimes take a long time and a great deal of patience and perseverance to get a good history.

HOW TO TAKE THE HISTORY

The history should be taken in the order described below and in Revision panel 1.1. Do not write and talk to the patient at the same time; however, it is important to document dates and times and the full drug history with accuracy, which you may not remember when you have finished the examination and left the room. Brief notes are therefore essential.

Make sure you know, and always record, the patient's name, age, sex, ethnic group, marital status, occupation and address; and always record the date of the examination.

The present complaint

It is customary to ask the patient 'What are you complaining of?' and to record the answer in the patient's own words.

It is currently fashionable to talk about 'problems' rather than 'complaints'. There is no difference, but problem-orientated management sounds more sympathetic.

If you ask 'What is the matter?' the patient will probably tell you their diagnosis. It is better not to know the diagnoses made by the patient, or other doctors, because none may be correct. It is better to try to seek out the patient's complaints. These should be listed in order of severity, with a record of precisely when and how they started. Whenever possible, it should be noted why the patient is more concerned with one complaint than another.

The history of the present complaint

The full history of the main complaint or complaints must be recorded in detail, with precise dates. It is important to get right back to the beginning of the problem. For example, a patient may complain of a recent sudden attack of indigestion. If further questioning reveals that similar symptoms occurred some

years previously, their description should be included in this section.

Remaining questions about the affected system

When a patient complains of indigestion it is sensible, after recording the history of the indigestion, to ask other questions about the alimentary system because many of the replies may aid in diagnosing the main complaint.

Systematic direct questions

These are direct questions that every patient should be asked, because the answers may amplify your knowledge about the main complaint and will often reveal the presence of other disorders of which the patient was unaware, or thought irrelevant. Negative answers are just as important as positive answers.

The standard set of direct questions is described in detail below because they are so important. It is essential to know them by heart because it is very easy to forget to ask some of them. **When you have to go back to the patient to ask a forgotten question, you invariably find the answer to be very important.** The only way to memorize this list is by taking as many histories as possible and writing them out in full. All the answers to every question, whether they be positive or negative, must be recorded.

The alimentary system

Appetite Has the appetite increased, decreased, or remained unchanged? If it has decreased, is this caused by a lack of desire to eat, or is it because of apprehension as eating always causes pain?

Diet What type of food does the patient eat? Are they vegetarian? When do they eat their meals?

Weight Has the patient's weight changed? By how much? Over how long a time? Many patients never weigh themselves, but they usually notice if their clothes have got tighter or looser and friends may have told them of a change in physical appearance.

Teeth and taste Can they chew their food? Do they have their own teeth? Do they get odd tastes and sensations in their mouth? Are there any symptoms of water brash or acid brash? (This is sudden filling of

Revision panel 1.1
Synopsis of a history

Names; age and date of birth; sex; marital status; occupation; ethnic group; hospital or practice record number

Present complaints or problems (PC, CO) Preferably in the patient's own words.

History of present complaint (HPC) Include the answers to the direct questions concerning the system of the presenting complaint.

Systematic direct questions
(a) *Alimentary system and abdomen (AS)*
    Appetite. Diet. Weight. Nausea. Dysphagia. Regurgitation. Flatulence. Heartburn. Vomiting. Haematemesis. Indigestion pain. Abdominal pain. Abdominal distension. Bowel habit. Nature of stool. Rectal bleeding. Mucus. Slime. Prolapse. Incontinence. Tenesmus. Jaundice.
(b) *Respiratory system (RS)*
    Cough. Sputum. Haemoptysis. Dyspnoea. Hoarseness. Wheezing. Chest pain. Exercise tolerance.
(c) *Cardiovascular system (CVS)*
    Dyspnoea. Paroxysmal nocturnal dyspnoea. Orthopnoea. Chest pain. Palpitations. Dizziness. Ankle swelling. Limb pain. Walking distance. Colour changes in hands and feet.
(d) *Urogenital system (UGS)*
    Loin pain. Frequency of micturition including nocturnal frequency. Poor stream. Dribbling. Hesitancy. Dysuria. Urgency. Precipitancy. Painful micturition. Polyuria. Thirst. Haematuria. Iincontinence.
    In men Problems with sexual intercourse and impotence.
    In women Date of menarche or menopause. Frequency. Quantity and duration of menstruation. Vaginal discharge. Dysmenorrhoea. Dyspareunia. Previous pregnancies and their complications. Prolapse. Urinary incontinence. Breast pain. Nipple discharge. Lumps. Skin changes.
(e) *Nervous system (NS, CNS)*
    Changes of behaviour or psyche Depression. Memory loss. Delusions. Anxiety. Tremor. Syncopal attacks. Loss of consciousness. Fits. Muscle weakness. Paralysis. Sensory disturbances. Paraesthesiae. Dizziness. Changes of smell, vision or hearing. Tinnitus. Headaches.
(f) *Musculoskeletal system (MSkS)*
    Aches or pains in muscles, bones or joints. Swelling joints. Limitation of joint movements. Locking. Weakness. Disturbances of gait.

Previous history (PH) Previous illnesses. Operations or accidents. Diabetes. Rheumatic fever. Diphtheria. Bleeding tendencies. Asthma. Hay fever. Allergies. Tuberculosis. Syphilis. Gonorrhoea. Tropical diseases.

Drug history Insulin. Steroids. Anti-depressants and the contraceptive pill. Drug abuse.

Immunizations BCG. Diphtheria. Tetanus. Typhoid. Whooping cough. Measles.

Family history (FH) Causes of death of close relatives. Familial illnesses in siblings and offspring.

Social history (SH) Marital status. Sexual habits. Living accommodation. Occupation. Exposure to industrial hazards. Travel abroad. Leisure activities.

Habits Smoking. Drinking. Number of cigarettes smoked per day. Units of alcohol drunk per week.

the mouth with watery or acid-tasting fluid – saliva and gastric acid respectively.)

Swallowing If they complain of difficulty in swallowing (dysphagia), ask about the type of food that causes difficulty, the level at which the food sticks, and the duration and progression of these symptoms. Is swallowing painful?

Regurgitation This is the effortless return of food into the mouth. It is quite different from vomiting, which is associated with a powerful involuntary contraction of the abdominal wall. Do they regurgitate? What comes up? If food, is it digested or recognizable and undigested? How often does it occur and does anything, such as stooping or straining, precipitate it?

Flatulence Does the patient belch frequently? Does this relate to any other symptoms?

Heartburn Patients may not realize that this symptom comes from the alimentary tract and they may have to be asked about it directly. It is a burning sensation behind the sternum caused by the reflux of acid into the oesophagus. How often does it occur and what makes it happen, e.g. lying flat or bending over?

Vomiting How often do they vomit? Is the vomiting preceded by nausea? What is the nature and volume of the vomitus? Is it recognizable food from previous meals, digested food, clear acidic fluid or bile-stained fluid? Is the vomiting preceded by another symptom such as indigestion pain, headache or giddiness? Does it follow eating?

Haematemesis Always ask if they have ever vomited blood because it is such an important symptom. Old, altered blood looks like 'coffee grounds'. Some patients have difficulty in differentiating between vomited or regurgitated blood and coughed-up blood (haemoptysis). The latter is usually pale pink and frothy. When patients have had a haematemesis, always ask if they have had a recent nose bleed. (They may be vomiting up swallowed blood.)

Indigestion or abdominal pain Some people call all abdominal pains indigestion; the difference between a discomfort after eating and a pain after eating may be very small. Concentrate on the features of the pain, its site, time of onset, severity, nature, progression, duration, radiation, course, precipitating, exacerbating and relieving factors (see pages 7–10).

Abdominal distension Have they noticed any abdominal distension? What brought this to their attention? When did it begin and how has it progressed? Is it constant or variable? What factors are associated with any variations? Is it painful? Does it affect their breathing? Is it relieved by belching, vomiting or defaecation?

Defaecation How often does the patient defaecate? What are the physical characteristics of the stool?

- **Colour**: brown, black, pale, white or silver?
- **Consistence**: hard, soft or watery?
- **Size**: bulky, pellets, string or tape like?
- **Specific gravity**: does it float or sink?
- **Smell**?

Beware of the terms 'diarrhoea' and 'constipation'. They are lay words and mean different things to different people. These words should not be written in the notes without also recording the frequency of bowel action and the consistence of the faeces.

Rectal bleeding Has the patient ever passed any blood in the stool? Was it bright or dark? How much? Was it mixed in with or on the surface of the stool, or did it only appear after the stool had been passed?

Flatus, mucus, slime Is the patient passing more gas than usual? Has the patient ever passed mucus or pus? Is defaecation painful? When does the pain begin – before, during, after, or at times unrelated to defaecation?

Prolapse and incontinence Does anything come out of the anus on straining? Does it return spontaneously or have to be pushed back? Is the patient continent of faeces and flatus? Have they had any injuries or anal operations in the past?

Tenesmus Do they experience any urgent, painful but unproductive desire to pass stool? This is called tenesmus.

Change of skin colour Have the patient's skin or eyes ever turned yellow (jaundiced)? When? How long did it last? Were there any other accompanying symptoms such as abdominal pain or loss of appetite? Did the skin itch?

The respiratory system

Cough How often does the patient cough? Does the coughing come in bouts? Does anything, such as a change of posture, precipitate or relieve the coughing? Is it a dry or a productive cough?

Sputum What is the quantity (teaspoon, dessertspoon, etc.) and colour (white, clear or yellow) of the sputum? Some patients only produce sputum in the morning or when they are in a particular position.

Haemoptysis Has the patient ever coughed up blood? Was it frothy and pink? Were there red streaks in the mucus, or clots of blood? What quantity was produced? How often does the haemoptysis occur?

Dyspnoea Does the patient wheeze? Does he get breathless? How many stairs can he climb? How far can he walk on a level surface before the dyspnoea interferes with the exercise? Can he walk and talk at the same time? Is the dyspnoea present at rest? Is it present when sitting or made worse by lying down? (Dyspnoea on lying flat is called **orthopnoea**.) How many pillows does the patient need at night? Does the breathlessness wake them up at night – **paroxysmal nocturnal dyspnoea** – or get worse if they slip off their pillows? There are classifications that grade dyspnoea numerically, but it is better to describe the causative conditions rather than write down a number.

Is the dyspnoea induced or exacerbated by external factors such as allergy to animals, pollen or dust? Does the difficulty with breathing occur with both phases of respiration or on expiration?

Pain in the chest Ascertain the site, severity and nature of the pain. Chest pains can be continuous, pleuritic (made worse by inspiration), constricting or stabbing.

The cardiovascular system
Cardiac symptoms

Breathlessness Ask the same questions as those described above under 'Respiratory system'.

Orthopnoea and paroxysmal nocturnal dyspnoea Orthopnoea and paroxysmal nocturnal dyspnoea are the forms of dyspnoea especially associated with heart disease.

Pain Cardiac pain begins in the mid-line and is usually retrosternal but may be epigastric. It is often described as constricting or band-like. It is usually brought on by exercise or excitement. The patient should be asked if the pain radiates to the neck or to the left arm and whether it is relieved by rest.

Palpitations These are episodes of tachycardia which the patient notices as a sudden fluttering or thumping of the heart in the chest.

Ankle swelling Do the ankles or legs swell? When do they swell? What is the effect on the swelling of bedrest and/or elevation of the leg?

Dizziness, headache and blurred vision These are some of the symptoms associated with hypertension and postural hypotension.

Peripheral vascular symptoms

Does the patient get pain in the leg muscles on exercise (intermittent claudication)? Which muscles are involved? How far can the patient walk before the pain begins? Is the pain so bad that he has to stop walking? How long does the pain take to wear off? Can the same distance be walked again? Is there any pain in the limb at rest? Which part of the limb is painful? Does the pain interfere with sleep? What positions relieve the pain? What analgesic drugs give relief? Are the extremities of the limbs cold? Are there colour changes in the skin, particularly in response to a cold environment? Does the patient experience any paraesthesiae in the limb, such as tingling or numbness?

The urogenital system
Urinary tract symptoms

Pain Has there been any pain in the loin, groin or suprapubic region? What is its nature and severity? Does it radiate to the groin or scrotum?

Oedema Do any parts of the body other than the ankles swell?

Thirst Is the patient thirsty? Do they drink excessive volumes of water?

Micturition How often does the patient pass urine? Express this as a day/night ratio. How much urine is passed? Is the volume and frequency excessive (polyuria)? Is micturition painful? What is the nature and site of the pain? Is there any difficulty with micturition, such as a need to strain or to wait? Is the stream good? Can it be stopped at will? Is there any dribbling at the end of micturition? Does the bladder feel empty at the end of micturition or do they have to pass urine a second time?

Urine Has the patient ever passed blood in the urine? When and how often? Have they ever passed gas bubbles with the urine (pneumaturia)?

Symptoms of uraemia These include headache, drowsiness, visual disturbance, fits and vomiting.

Genital tract symptoms

MALE

Scrotum, penis and urethra Has the patient any pain in the penis or urethra during micturition or intercourse? Is there any difficulty with retraction of the prepuce or any urethral discharge? Has the patient noticed any swelling of the scrotum? Can he achieve an erection and ejaculation?

FEMALE

Menstruation When did menstruation begin (menarche)? When did it end (menopause)? What is the duration and quantity of the menses? Is menstruation associated with pain (dysmenorrhoea)? What is the nature and severity of the pain? Is there any abdominal pain mid-way between the periods (mittelschmerz)? Has the patient had any vaginal discharge? What is its character and amount? Has she noticed any prolapse of the vaginal wall or cervix or any urinary incontinence, especially when straining or coughing (stress incontinence)?

Pregnancies Record details of the patient's pregnancies – number, dates and complications.

Dyspareunia Is intercourse painful?

Breasts Do the breasts change during the menstrual cycle? Are they ever painful or tender? Has the patient noticed any swellings or lumps in the breasts? Did she breast-feed her children? Has there been any nipple discharge or bleeding? Has she noticed any skin changes over the breasts?

Secondary sex characteristics When did these appear?

The nervous system

Mental state Is the patient placid or nervous? Has the patient noticed any changes in their behaviour or reactions to others? Patients will often not appreciate such changes themselves and these questions may have to be asked of close relatives. Does the patient get depressed and withdrawn, or are they excitable and extroverted?

Brain and cranial nerves Does the patient ever become unconscious or have fits? What happens during a fit? **It is often necessary to ask a relative or a bystander to describe the fit.** Did the patient lie still or jerk about, bite their tongue, pass urine? Was the patient sleepy after the fit? Was there any warning (an aura) that the fit was about to develop? Has there been any subsequent change in the senses of smell, vision and hearing?

Is there a history of headache? Where is it experienced? When does it occur? Are the headaches associated with any visual symptoms?

Has the face ever become weak or paralysed? Have any of the limbs been paralysed or had pins and needles? Has there ever been any buzzing in the ears, dizziness or loss of speech? Can the patient speak clearly and use words properly?

Peripheral nerves Are any limbs or part of a limb weak or paralysed? Is there ever any loss of cutaneous sensation (anaesthesia)? Does the patient experience any paraesthesiae (tingling, 'pins and needles') in the limbs?

Musculoskeletal system

Ask if the patient suffers from pain, swelling or limitation of the movement of any joint. What precipitates or relieves these symptoms? What time of day do they occur? Are any limbs or groups of muscles weak or painful? Can he walk normally? Has he any congenital musculoskeletal deformities?

Previous history of other illnesses, accidents or operations

Record the history of those conditions which are not directly related to the present complaint. Ask specifically about tuberculosis, diabetes, rheumatic fever, allergies, asthma, tropical diseases, bleeding tendencies, diphtheria, gonorrhoea, syphilis, and the likelihood of intimate contact with carriers of the human immunodeficiency virus (HIV).

Drug history

Ask if the patient is taking any drugs. Specifically, enquire about steroids, anti-depressants, insulin, diuretics, anti-hypertensives, hormone replacement therapy and the contraceptive pill. Patients usually remember about drugs prescribed by a doctor but often forget about self-prescribed drugs they have bought at a pharmacy. Is the patient sensitive to any drugs or any topical applications such as adhesive plaster? If they are, write it in large letters on the front of the notes.

Immunizations

Most children are immunized against diphtheria, tetanus, whooping cough, measles, mumps, rubella and poliomyelitis. Ask about these, and smallpox, typhoid and tuberculosis vaccination.

Family history

Enquire about the health and age, or cause of death, of the patient's parents, grandparents, brothers and sisters, and ask about any children who have died. Draw a family tree if there is obvious familial disorder (e.g. lymphoedema). If the patient is a child, you will need information about the mother's pregnancy. Did she take any drugs during pregnancy? What was the patient's birth weight? Were there any difficulties during delivery? What was the rate of physical and mental development in early life?

Social history

Record the marital status and the type and place of dwelling. Ask about the patient's sexual life, the sex and sexual behaviour of their sexual partners and the nature of their physical relationships. Ask about the patient's occupation, paying special regard to contact with hazards such as dusts and chemicals. What are the patient's leisure activities? Has the patient travelled abroad? List the countries visited and the dates of the visits if these appear to be relevant.

Habits

Does the patient smoke? If so what – cigarettes, cigar or pipe? Record the frequency, quantity and duration of their smoking habit. Does the patient drink alcohol? Record the type and quantity consumed and the duration of the habit. Does the patient have any unusual eating habits?

HISTORY OF PAIN

We have all experienced pain. It is one of nature's ways of warning us that something is going wrong in our body. It is an unpleasant sensation of varying intensity. Pain can come from any of the body's systems but there are certain features common to all pains that should always be recorded.

Be careful in your use of the word **tenderness**. Tenderness is pain which occurs in response to a stimulus, such as pressure from the doctor's hand, or forced movement. It is possible for a patient to be lying still without pain and yet have an area of tenderness. *The patient feels pain – the doctor elicits tenderness.* But although patients usually complain of pain, they may also have observed and complain of tenderness if they happen to have pressed their fingers on a painful area or discovered a tender spot by accident. Thus tenderness can be both a symptom and a physical sign.

The history of a pain frequently betrays the diagnosis, so you must question the patient closely about each of the following features, some of which are depicted graphically in Figure 1.1.

Site

Many factors may indicate the source of the pain but the most valuable indicator is its site.

It is of no value to describe a pain as 'abdominal pain'; you must be more specific. Although patients do not describe the site of their pain in anatomical terms, they can always point to the site of maximum intensity, which you can convert into an exact description. When the pain is indistinct in nature and spread diffusely over a large area, you must describe the area in which the pain is felt and the point (indicated by the patient) of maximum discomfort. It is also worthwhile asking about the depth of the pain. Patients can often tell you whether the pain is near to the skin or deep inside.

Time and mode of onset

It may be possible to pinpoint the onset of the pain to the minute, but if this cannot be done, the part of

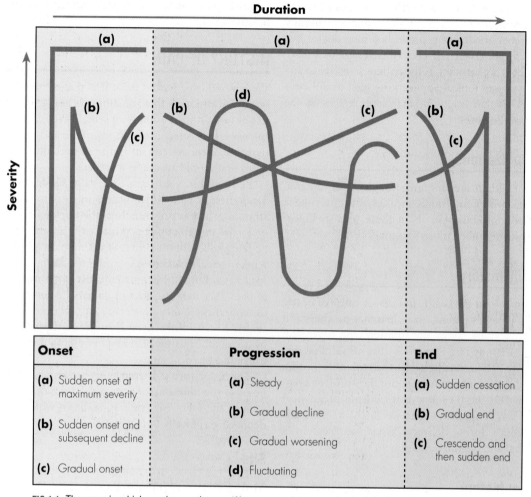

Duration

Severity

	(a)	**(a)**	**(a)**
(b)		(b)	(d)	(c)	(b)
	(c)				(c)

Onset	Progression	End
(a) Sudden onset at maximum severity	**(a)** Steady	**(a)** Sudden cessation
(b) Sudden onset and subsequent decline	**(b)** Gradual decline	**(b)** Gradual end
(c) Gradual onset	**(c)** Gradual worsening	**(c)** Crescendo and then sudden end
	(d) Fluctuating	

FIG 1.1 The ways in which a pain can change. (Always record dates and calculate time intervals.)

the day or night when the pain began should be recorded. You should record the calendar dates on which events occurred, but it is also very useful to add in brackets the time interval between each event and the current examination, because it is these intervals, not the actual dates, which are more relevant to the problems of diagnosis. For example, 'Sudden onset of severe epigastric pain on 16th September, 1973, at 11.00 a.m. (3 days ago)': but **remember that such comments are useless if you forget to record the date of the examination**. Whenever you write a note about a patient, whether it be a short progress note or a full history, make certain that you **start your notes by writing down the date**.

Ask if the pain began insidiously or suddenly.

Severity

Individuals react differently to pain. What is a severe pain to one person might be described as a dull ache by another. Consequently you must be wary of the adjectives used by a patient to describe the severity of their pain. A far better indication of severity is the effect of the pain on the patient's life. Did it stop the patient going to work? Did it make the patient go to bed? Did they try proprietary analgesics? Did they have to call their doctor? Did it wake the patient up at night, or stop them going to sleep? Was the pain better lying still or did it make the patient roll around? The answers to these questions provide a better indication of the severity of a pain than words such as mild, severe, agonizing or terrible. Your assessment of the way the patient responds to their pain, formed while you are taking the history, may profoundly affect your treatment.

Nature or character of the pain

Patients find it very difficult to describe the nature of their pain, but some of the adjectives which are commonly used, such as aching, stabbing, burning, throbbing, constricting, distending, gripping or colic, have a similar meaning to the majority of people.

Burning and **throbbing** sensations are within everyone's experience. We have all experienced a burning sensation from our skin following contact with intense heat, so when a patient spontaneously states that their pain is 'burning' in nature, it is likely to be so. We have all experienced a throbbing sensation at some time in our life, so this description is also usually accurate.

A **stabbing** pain is sudden, severe, sharp, and short-lived.

The adjective **constricting** suggests a pain that encircles the relevant part (chest, abdomen, head or limb) and compresses it from all directions. A pain that feels like an iron band tightening around the chest is typical of angina pectoris and almost diagnostic, but when patients speak of a **tightness** in their chest or limb do not immediately assume that they have a constricting pain. They may be describing a **tightness** caused by distension, which may occur in any structure that has an encircling and restricting wall, such as the bowel, bladder, an encapsulated tumour or a fascial compartment. Tension in the containing wall may cause a pain which the patient may describe as distension, tightness or a **bursting feeling**.

A **colicky pain** has two features. First, it comes and goes in a sinusoidal way. Second, it feels like a migrating constriction in the wall of a hollow tube which is attempting to force the contents of the tube forwards. It is not a word which many patients use and it is dangerous to ask them if their pain is colicky without giving an example. This is not difficult, because most of us have experienced colic during an episode of diarrhoea, and many women have suffered the colicky pains of labour. A recurring, intermittent pain is not necessarily a colic; it must also have a gripping nature.

'**Just a pain, doctor**'. Most pains have none of the features mentioned above and are described by many patients as 'a pain'. This may vary in severity from a mild discomfort or ache, to an agonizing pain that makes them think they are about to die. When a patient cannot describe the nature of their pain, do not press the point. You will only make them try to fit their pain to your suggestions and ultimately this may be misleading.

Revision panel 1.2
The features of a pain that must be elicited and recorded

Site

Time and mode of onset
Record the time and date of onset and the way the pain began – suddenly or gradually.

Duration
Record the duration of the pain.

Severity
Assess severity by its effect on the patient.

Nature/character
Aching, burning, stabbing, constricting, throbbing, distending, colic.

Radiation
Record the time and direction of any radiation of the pain; remember to ask if the nature of the pain changed at the time it moved.

Referral
Was the pain experienced anywhere else?

Progression
Describe the progression of the pain. Did it change or alter?

The end of the pain
Describe how the pain ended. Was the end spontaneous or brought about by some action by the patient or doctor?

Relieving and exacerbating factors

Cause
Note the patient's opinion of the cause of the pain.

Progression of the pain

Once it has started, a pain may progress in a variety of ways.

- It may begin at its maximum intensity and remain at this level until it disappears.
- It may increase steadily until it reaches a peak or a plateau, or conversely begin at its peak and decline slowly.
- The severity may fluctuate (see Fig. 1.1). The intensity of the pain at the peaks and troughs of the fluctuations, and the rate of development and regression of each peak, may vary. The pain may go completely between each exacerbation. The time between the peaks of an abdominal colic may indicate the likely site of a bowel obstruction (e.g. in upper small bowel obstruction, the frequency of the colic is every 1–2 minutes, in the ileum every 20 minutes). It is essential to find out how the pain has progressed and ascertain the timing of any fluctuations before its nature can be determined; for example, colic has two features – its gripping nature and its intermittent progression.

The end of the pain

A pain may end spontaneously, or as a result of some action by the patient or doctor. The end of a pain is either sudden or gradual. The way a pain ends may give a clue to the diagnosis, or indicate the development of a new problem.

Patients always think that the disappearance of their pain means that they are getting better. They are usually right, but sometimes their condition may have got worse.

Duration of the pain

The duration of a pain will be apparent from the time of its onset and end, but nevertheless it is worthwhile stating the duration of the pain in your notes. The length of any periods of exacerbation or remission should also be recorded.

Factors which relieve the pain

Patients will know if there is anything, such as position, movement, a hot-water bottle, aspirins, food,
antacids, etc., which relieves the pain. The natural response to a pain is to search for a way to relieve it. Sometimes patients try the most bizarre remedies and many convince themselves that some minor change in habit or a personal remedy has been helpful, so accept their replies to this question with caution.

Factors which exacerbate the pain

Anything that makes the pain worse is also likely to be known to the patient.

The type of stimulus that exacerbates a pain will depend on the organ from which it emanates and its cause. For example, alimentary tract pains may be made worse by eating particular types of food; musculoskeletal pains are affected by joint movements, muscle exercise and posture. It is perfectly reasonable to ask direct questions about those stimuli which you think might affect a pain if the initial description has indicated its source.

Radiation and referral

Radiation Radiation is the extension of the pain to another site whilst the initial pain persists. For example, patients with a posterior penetrating duodenal ulcer usually have a persistent pain in the epigastrium, but sometimes the pain spreads through the abdomen to the back. The extended pain usually has the same character as the initial pain.

A pain may occur in one site, disappear, and then reappear in another. This is not radiation: it is a new pain in another place.

Referred pain This is a pain which is felt at a distance from its source. For example, inflammation of the diaphragm will cause a pain which is felt at the tip of the shoulder. A referred pain is caused by the inability of the central nervous system to distinguish between visceral and somatic sensory impulses. From the patient's viewpoint, the pain is where they feel it – the fact that the source is some distant organ does not concern them.

Cause

It is worthwhile asking patients what they think is the cause of their pain. Even if they are hopelessly wrong, you will get some insight into their worries.

Sometimes a patient will be obsessed with the cause of his condition and careful questioning may reveal that he will gain or lose compensation or insurance money as the result of your opinion. Nevertheless, **always listen to the patient's views with care and tolerance**.

THE CLINICAL EXAMINATION

Each chapter of this book deals with a specific region of the body and its surgical diseases. Those methods of examination peculiar to each region are described in detail in the relevant chapter. The emphasis in this introductory chapter is on the importance of taking an exact and full history, but it would not be complete without a description of the basic plan of a physical examination, with particular reference to those regions not discussed in later chapters, such as the heart, the lungs and the nervous system. As this is a thumb-nail sketch of clinical examination, your knowledge will need to be enlarged by additional reading, but your understanding and ability to solve the practical problems of clinical examination can only be clarified by frequent bedside practice. Examine as many patients as you can. Nothing can be learnt without frequent practice. Repetition is the secret of learning. This axiom applies as much to the doctor as it does to the sportsman or the concert pianist. You will become confident of your interpretation of your visual, tactile and aural appreciation of the patient's body only by repeatedly exercising these senses.

Experienced clinicians rarely begin the routine physical examination without some suspicions about the diagnosis suggested by the history. Consequently, they often modify the impartial systematized examination described in textbooks such as this by specifically looking for signs which confirm or refute their tentative diagnoses, but when a sign is elicited that denies their suspicions they return to the textbook routine. Students must not do this. Although it is a practical and time-saving method in a busy clinic, and acceptable from someone with years of clinical experience who can pick out those patients to whom it can be applied, it is fundamentally wrong. Bad habits grow fast enough without encouragement. Unless students discipline themselves to use the standard textbook routine for every physical examination, many mistakes will inevitably

be made and, as time passes, some parts of the examination will be completely forgotten, with serious consequences.

The easiest way to ensure that you perform a complete examination is to learn the routine by heart and repeat it to yourself during the examination. Whilst looking at a lump, say to yourself, 'position, shape, size', etc. If you do not do this, you will find when you sit down to write your notes that you have forgotten to elicit some of the lump's physical features and will have to go back to re-examine the patient. Always keep to the basic pattern of looking, feeling, tapping and listening (inspection, palpation, percussion, auscultation), whatever you are examining. Whilst keeping to the routine it is, however, often best to examine first the part of body that is the source of the patient's complaint.

General assessment

The first part of the physical examination is performed when taking the history. While you are talking to the patient you can observe and later record their general demeanour, their intellectual ability and intelligence, and their attitudes to their disease, to you, to their treatment, and to society in general. These observations affect the manner in which you conduct the examination. Your instructions will need to be extremely simple if the patient is unintelligent, or coaxing and gentle if the patient is shy or embarrassed.

The patient's general mental state, his memory and use of words should be noted. There is a whole vocabulary used by the neurologists to describe various speech and communication disorders. Some of the common ones are:

- **dysarthria**: impaired speech caused by muscle weakness;
- **dysphasia or aphasia**: impaired or absent ability to speak caused by a neurological abnormality;
- **dysgraphia or agraphia**: impaired or absent ability to write;
- **dyspraxia or apraxia**: impaired or absent ability to perform purposeful movements in the absence of paralysis.

When a patient has been admitted as an emergency, especially if they have been injured, it is important to record their level of consciousness using the Glasgow Coma Scale.

You can also observe a number of physical characteristics when taking the history, such as posture, mobility, weight, colour of skin, facial appearance and general body build.

Revision panel 1.3
The Glasgow Coma Scale

		Score
Eyes	Open spontaneously	4
	Open to command	3
	Open to pain	2
	Do not open	1
Speech	Sensible/orientated	5
	Confused	4
	Inappropriate words	3
	Incomprehensible sounds	2
	None	1
Motor responses	Obeys commands	6
	Localizes stimuli	5
	Withdraws from stimuli	4
	Flexion responses	3
	Extension responses	2
	None	1
	Total	

Revision panel 1.4
Some common causes of weight loss

In the young	Malnutrition
	Diabetes
	Malabsorption
	Anorexia nervosa
	Tuberculosis
From middle age onwards	Diabetes
	Thyrotoxicosis
	Chronic hypoxia
	Chronic heart failure
	Malignant disease
	Senile cachexia
	Neglect

Hold the patient's hand and examine it

Make physical contact with the patient early in the examination by holding their hand and counting the pulse. It is very important for the patient to feel that you are willing to get physically as well as mentally close to them. The physical contact that is essential for the examination forges an intimate bond between you and the patient. It is an extraordinary privilege granted to you by the patient and must never be abused.

The features that can be observed by examining the hands are as follows.

Pulse See details on page 22.

Nails Look at the colour and shape of the nails. Spoon-shaped nails (koilonychia) are associated with anaemia; clubbing of the nails occurs in pulmonary and cardiopulmonary disease (see Fig. 5.24, page 160); and splinter haemorrhages under the nails are caused by small arterial emboli. Pits and furrows are associated with skin diseases such as psoriasis. Bitten nails may indicate nervousness and anxiety.

Temperature Observe the temperature of the hands – but remember that it will be affected by room temperature and the duration of exposure.

Moisture Are the patient's palms sweating excessively?

Colour Pallor of the skin of the hands, especially in the skin creases of the palm and in the nail beds, suggests anaemia. Reddish-blue hands occur in polycythaemia and cor pulmonale. The fingers may be stained with nicotine.

Callosities The position of any callosities may reflect the patient's occupation.

Examine the head and neck

Eyes

Look for any asymmetry of the position, size or colour of the eyes and especially any abnormality in the width of the palpebral fissures. This can be caused by **ptosis** (droopy eyelids) or **proptosis (exophthalmos)** when the eyeball is pushed forwards, pushing the lids apart (see Chapter 11, pages 292–4). The size and equality of the two pupils should be recorded (dilated, constricted or unequal).

The reaction of the pupil to light is checked by shining a bright light off and on the pupil. The pupil's reaction to accommodation is assessed by asking the patient to look into the distance and then to refocus on a finger held close to their eye.

The **eye movements** are examined by fixing the patient's head with one hand while asking them to watch your finger as it travels upwards and downwards and inwards and outwards to the full extremes of movement. Patients should be asked if they experience any double vision (**diplopia**) in any particular position. While the eye movements are being tested, the presence of any **strabismus** (**squint**) can usually be easily seen, which may be concomitant (divergent or convergent) or paralytic.

Look for the presence of **nystagmus** (oscillations of the eye characterized by a slow drift and a rapid jerk back) at the inward and outward extremes of movement.

Inspect the **lids**, **conjunctiva**, **cornea** and **lens**. Styes, Meibomian cysts, and blepharitis may inflame the lids or cause a swelling. The edges of the eyelids may be everted or inverted (**ectropion** or **entropion**) and the eye may water if the **tearduct** or **lacrimal sac** is blocked.

A painful red eye may be caused by acute conjunctivitis (when there is usually an associated discharge), acute iritis (when the anterior chamber of the eye is inflamed), acute glaucoma (which is associated with severe pain and a misty cornea), acute keratitis (from a corneal ulcer, seen as a cloudy opacity) or episcleritis.

When an elderly patient has a gradual loss of eyesight they are likely to have a cataract (which can be confirmed by finding a loss of part or the whole of the 'red-reflex' when a powerful light is shone on the pupil). Other possible causes of gradual loss of vision, such as optic nerve or retinal damage, can only be detected by inspecting the retina through an **ophthalmoscope**. This requires practice, and you should take every opportunity to use the ophthalmoscope by inspecting the retinae of all the patients you examine.

Ophthalmoscopy is best carried out in a darkened room to ensure that the pupils are dilated. The ophthalmoscope is an illuminated lens system which can be focused on the retina. Patients are asked to stare fixedly at a point on the wall behind the examiner. The instrument is switched on and held by its handle in the right hand. The examiner then places his right eye against the lens opening and his left hand on the patient's forehead above their right eye. He then looks through the aperture of the ophthalmoscope, brings the instrument very close to the patient's right pupil by placing his forehead against his left hand on the patient's forehead. The light can be watched illuminating the fundus, through the pupil, as the instrument and the patient's eye are brought close together. The approach should be slightly from the temporal side, at an angle of 10–15° to the direct line, to avoid noses colliding! When the pupils are level, this approach usually ensures that the optic nerve disc is the first part of the fundus to come into view. If the disc is not seen, a retinal artery should be followed back until the edge of the pale yellow disc is seen.

The optic disc is *cupped* by chronic glaucoma and swollen by *papilloedema* (see Fig. 2.3, page 46). Other abnormalities that can be detected by careful fundoscopy of the rest of the retina include haemorrhages and exudates (in diabetes and hypertension), retinal emboli and infarcts, and occasionally retinal detachment. At the end of the examination, the patient should be asked to look directly at the light of the ophthalmoscope in order to inspect the macula.

Ears and nose

Do not forget to look into the ears to inspect the external auditory canal and the ear-drum. Look up the nose. The ears and nose are often forgotten during routine examination but they are important, particularly if there is any possibility of disease in the head and neck.

Clinical examination of the ear requires an auroscope. This instrument directs a beam of light down a conical metal speculum which is viewed through a lens. The speculum is gently inserted into the external auditory meatus, while the ear is pulled gently upwards and backwards to straighten the external auditory canal. Wax may be present and must be removed before the tympanic membrane can be seen.

The whole of the tympanic membrane can only be seen if the angle of the speculum is altered. Normal tympanic membranes vary in colour, translucence and shape – so you should look at as many normal tympanic membranes as possible. The external auditory canal may contain wax or foreign bodies. You may see otitis externa (dermatitis), blood or pus. The tympanic membrane may be normal, torn (injury), bulging and inflamed (acute otitis media), or perforated (chronic otitis media).

Mouth

Note the colour and state of the lips. Ask to see the patient's tongue; observe its movement, symmetry and surface.

Look at the teeth and gums. Use a spatula to inspect the soft palate, tonsils and posterior wall of the oropharynx.

Neck

The important features to examine in the neck are the jugular veins, the trachea, the thyroid gland and the lymph glands.

Examine the cranial nerves

'On Old Olympus Towering Tops A Finn And German Picked Some Hops' is the most-used mnemonic for the names of the cranial nerves.

I Olfactory nerve

Ask the patient about their sense of smell. If thought to be abnormal, it can be specifically tested with bottles containing cloves, peppermint etc.

II Optic nerve

Visual acuity Visual acuity is tested with a *Snellen's chart* at a distance of 6 metres. Vision is expressed as a fraction of the normal: the smallest letter visible with comfort is 6/6; if letters twice that size are all that can be read, the vision is 6/12. The larger letter is visible to the normally sighted at 60 metre. Below this level of vision, 'counting fingers', 'hand-movements' and 'perception of light' are used to grade degrees of blindness. Near-vision is tested by a card covered with varying sizes of print.

Test the visual fields Sit directly in front of the patient, ask them to close one eye and look straight at you with the other eye. Keeping your hand midway between you and the patient, extend your arm so that your hand is beyond your own peripheral vision. Then gradually move it towards the mid-line until it appears in your visual field. If you and the patient have normal visual fields, you will both see your finger at the same time.

III Oculomotor nerve

This nerve supplies all but two of the extrinsic eye muscles, as well as the levator palpebrae superioris and the muscle of accommodation. When it fails to function, the eye turns downwards and outwards, the upper lid droops (ptosis) and the pupil becomes fixed (not responding to accommodation). Sometimes individual muscles supplied by the third nerve can be paralysed. To test the superior rectus muscle, ask the patient to 'look up'; the inferior rectus – 'look down'; the medial rectus – 'converge'; and the inferior oblique – 'look up and out'.

IV Trochlear nerve

This nerve supplies the superior oblique muscle, which turns the eye downwards and outwards. The patient cannot perform this movement if the nerve is damaged. The eye will look inwards and the patient will experience diplopia below the horizontal plane.

V Trigeminal nerve

This nerve has sensory and motor functions. It is sensory to the whole of the side of the face. The cutaneous distribution of its three sensory divisions – ophthalmic, maxillary and mandibular – is shown in Figure 1.2.

The trigeminal nerve is also the sensory nerve of the conjunctiva and the inside of the mouth. The conjunctival reflex (ophthalmic division) is lost if

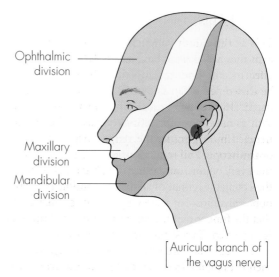

Ophthalmic division

Maxillary division

Mandibular division

[Auricular branch of the vagus nerve]

FIG 1.2 The distribution of the three sensory divisions of the trigeminal nerve.

the nerve is damaged. This is tested by touching the conjunctiva with a 'wick' of cotton or tissue paper to elicit a 'blink'. Sensation in the nose, pharynx, roof of mouth, soft palate and tonsil should also be tested. The palatal reflex (maxillary division) is elicited by placing a speculum against the palate to induce a gag reflex. The sensitivity of the tongue, lower teeth and mucous membrane over the mandible (mandibular division) is tested by touching each area with a spatula.

The taste fibres of the anterior two-thirds of the tongue travel with the lingual nerve (one of the branches of the mandibular division of the trigeminal nerve) after leaving the geniculate ganglion as the chorda tympani. Taste can be specifically tested with sweet, sour, salt and bitter substances – such as sugar, acid, salt and quinine – if this is felt to be important.

The motor fibres of the trigeminal nerve run in its mandibular division to the muscles of mastication – masseter, temporalis and the pterygoid muscles. Ask the patient to clench their teeth and feel if the masseter contracts.

VI Abducens nerve

This nerve supplies the lateral rectus muscle, which turns the eye outwards. The eye will not move when the patient attempts to look sideways and they will experience diplopia.

VII Facial nerve

This is the motor nerve to the muscles of facial expression. When a facial nerve fails to function, the affected side of the face is flabby, the eyelids cannot be closed properly, and the mouth becomes asymmetrical when the patient tries to bare their teeth. Whistling is impossible. The nucleus of the seventh nerve is in the pons varolii. Any damage to the tract or the nerve distal to the nucleus causes paralysis of the whole of one side of the face; but a lesion above the nucleus misses those fibres coming from the opposite hemisphere to the upper part of the face, so that the function of the forehead and eyelid muscles is preserved. To test the facial nerve, ask the patient to look up (the forehead should wrinkle), to close their eyes tightly (test the strength of the orbicularis oculi by trying to part the eyelids) and to show you their teeth (lips should part symmetrically).

VIII Auditory nerve

This nerve innervates the hearing mechanism in the cochlea and the position sense organs in the semicircular canals. Hearing can be tested very easily by speaking softly and asking the patient to repeat your words, or by asking them if they can hear your thumb and finger rubbing lightly together close to their ear. The deafness is called **conductive** when it is the result of an obstruction in the external meatus, tympanic membrane, middle ear cavity or ossicles of the middle ear interfering with the normal passage of airborne sounds. This is tested by striking a tuning fork and holding it next to the external auditory meatus until the patient signals that sound can no longer be heard. The base of the tuning fork is then immediately placed firmly on the mastoid process. If sound is still heard by bone conduction (a negative *Rinne's test*), the patient has a conductive deafness. If the tuning fork is placed on the centre of the forehead, an ear with a conduction deafness will appreciate a louder sound. This is *Weber's test*.

When there is **nerve perception deafness**, any sound that can be heard will be loudest in the better ear, and louder when the tuning fork is placed by the ear than when it is placed on the bone, i.e. good bone conduction = a normal cochlea and auditory nerve, whereas poor bone conduction = a defective cochlea and auditory nerve.

The sensitivity of the vestibular apparatus is tested by assessing the response to syringing the external meatus with warm and cold water. This is called the *caloric test*. These tests should only be done under careful supervision in the ENT department.

IX Glossopharyngeal nerve

This nerve is the sensory nerve of the posterior third of the tongue. It supplies the taste receptors and the sensory endings of the mucous membrane of the pharynx.

It is also motor to the middle constrictor muscle of the pharynx.

The sensory integrity of this nerve can be tested by stroking the back of the oropharynx to evoke a pharyngeal gag reflex.

X Vagus nerve

This is the motor nerve of the soft palate, pharynx and larynx, and the sensory nerve of the heart, lungs and gastrointestinal tract. When patients are asked to open their mouths wide and say 'Aarrh', the soft palate should arch upwards symmetrically. If one side of the palate is paralysed, it will not move and the uvula will be pulled over towards the functioning side. Loss of function of the recurrent laryngeal nerves (branches of the vagus) should be suspected if there is a change in the patient's voice or an inability to cough. The vocal cords must be examined with a laryngeal mirror to confirm the diagnosis.

XI Spinal accessory nerve

This nerve supplies the trapezius and sterno-mastoid muscles. The function of these muscles is tested by asking the patient to shrug their shoulders and to press the point of their chin downwards against your hand.

XII Hypoglossal nerve

This is the motor nerve of the tongue. When one hypoglossal nerve is paralysed, the tongue will deviate

---

Revision panel 1.5
Common causes of pleuritic pain

Pleurisy
Pneumonia
Pulmonary infarction (thromboembolic)
Neoplasia (primary and secondary)
Fractured ribs
Muscle strains/prolapsed intervertebral disc
Herpes zoster
Bornholm disease (Coxsackie virus)
Don't forget pathology below the diaphragm,
e.g. ruptured spleen, Curtis–Fitz–Hugh syndrome (see Chapter 15)

Revision panel 1.6
Common causes of haemoptysis

Pneumonia
Carcinoma of the bronchus
Chronic bronchitis
Pulmonary tuberculosis
Pulmonary infarction (thromboembolic)
Bronchiectasis

---

to that side when the patient tries to push it forwards. The weak side will also be wasted (see Fig. 10.14, page 261).

Examine the chest wall and lungs

Inspection

The colour and respiratory rate of the patient indicate the adequacy of ventilation. Cyanosis caused by cardiopulmonary disease is most easily appreciated by inspecting the inner aspect of the lips. Cyanosis of the nail beds and the tip of the nose and ears may be caused by a peripheral or central abnormality. Patients may be polycythaemic rather than cyanotic if the peripheral tissues are a deep reddish-purple colour and their face is red and plethoric. Cyanosis is difficult to detect in anaemic patients.

Count the rate of respiration and notice the rhythm. A fluctuating respiratory rate and volume, with periods of apnoea interspersed between episodes of tachypnoea, is called *Cheyne–Stokes* or periodic respiration. It is caused by variations in the sensitivity of the respiratory centre to normal stimuli, and occurs commonly in patients with heart failure and following severe cerebrovascular accidents.

Notice if respiration seems to require voluntary effort and compare the durations of inspiration and expiration. Watch the chest during inspiration to see if there is any inward movement of the intercostal spaces (**paradoxical movement**). This is usually caused by obstruction to the inflow of air into the lungs, but in an injured patient may indicate instability of a segment of the chest wall (e.g. two sets of fractures).

Record any abnormality in the shape of the chest. The two common deformities are funnel chest (pectus excavatum) and pigeon chest (pectus carinatum) (see Fig. 8.29, page 235).

Palpation

Trachea Check the position of the trachea at the suprasternal notch.

Chest expansion Spread your hands around the chest so that your thumbs just meet in the mid-line. Ask the patient to take a deep breath. Your thumbs should be dragged apart to a distance roughly equivalent to half the chest expansion. When the expansion is asymmetrical it will be felt and seen.

Chest expansion is the difference between the circumference of the chest at full inspiration and full expiration, measured at the level of the nipples.

Apex beat The apex beat is the lowest and most lateral point at which you can feel the cardiac impulse. It will move laterally if the heart enlarges but may also move medially or laterally if the mediastinum shifts. The mediastinum (and the trachea) will move to one side if it is pulled over by a collapsed, contracting lung or pushed over by air or fluid in the opposite pleural cavity.

Tactile vocal fremitus (Fig. 1.4, page 18) Place your whole hand firmly on the chest and ask the patient to say '99'. The vibrations that you can feel with your hand are called the vocal fremitus. Compare the strength of these vibrations on either side of the chest, front and back, and over the apical, middle and basal zones of the lung. To feel vocal fremitus the sound waves must be conducted through the air in the bronchi, bronchioles and alveoli to the chest wall. A blocked bronchus or a layer of fluid or air between the visceral and parietal layers of the pleura (a pleural effusion) will suppress the conduction of the sound waves and reduces the intensity of the palpable fremitus. A stiffening of the lung tissue with patent air passages, which occurs in very early pneumonia, increases conduction through the lung, and tactile vocal fremitus is increased.

Palpate both axillae.

Percussion

The whole of the surface of both lungs must be percussed. The surface markings of the lungs are shown in Figure 1.3. Place one hand flat on the chest wall, keeping the finger you intend to strike straight and firmly applied to the underlying skin. Tap the centre of the middle phalanx of this finger with the tip of the middle finger of the other hand. Listen carefully to the sound and compare it with the sound produced by percussing the same area on the other side of the chest.

The two areas most often forgotten when percussing the chest are the lateral zones high in the axillae and the anterior aspect of the apices behind the clavicles. Percuss the latter area by striking the clavicle directly with the percussing finger.

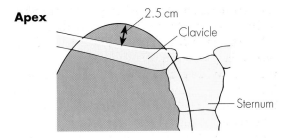

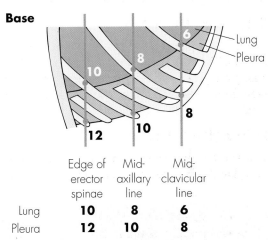

	Edge of erector spinae	Mid-axillary line	Mid-clavicular line
Lung	10	8	6
Pleura	12	10	8

FIG 1.3 The surface markings of the lung and pleura.

The normal chest gives a resonant sound when percussed; a sound which is, to some extent, felt by the percussing finger as well as being heard. Anything solid in the pleural space or in the substance of the lungs decreases the resonance and makes the sound dull. Any extra air, whether in the pleural space (a pneumothorax) or in the lung substance (an emphysematous bulla or multiple bullae), makes the sound more resonant (hyper-resonance) (page 19).

In the presence of a large pneumothorax, a ringing resonance can be heard with a stethoscope when the percussion is performed by tapping a coin held against the chest wall with a second coin.

Auscultation

The normal sounds of breathing can be heard all over the chest except over the heart and spine (page 20). They consist of an inspiratory sound followed immediately by a shorter, softer, expiratory sound. There is **no gap** between the two phases. This pattern

TACTILE VOCAL FREMITIS

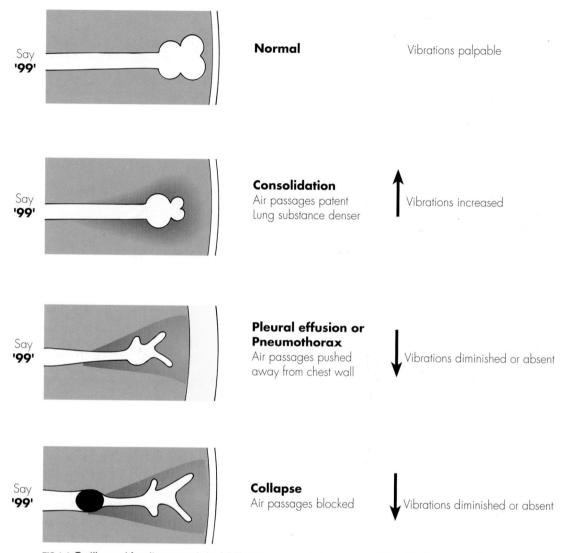

| Say '99' | **Normal** | Vibrations palpable |

| Say '99' | **Consolidation**
Air passages patent
Lung substance denser | ↑ Vibrations increased |

| Say '99' | **Pleural effusion or Pneumothorax**
Air passages pushed away from chest wall | ↓ Vibrations diminished or absent |

| Say '99' | **Collapse**
Air passages blocked | ↓ Vibrations diminished or absent |

FIG 1.4 Tactile vocal fremitus can only be felt if there are patent air passages right out to the chest wall.

is known as **vesicular breathing** and is caused by the movement of air in and out of the smaller bronchioles and alveoli – a rustling noise similar to that of gas being blown down plastic tubing.

The sound of air moving in the larger bronchioles and main bronchi is heard when the periphery of the lung has been solidified by pneumonia or collapse (atelectasis). This sound is harsher and louder than the low rustle of vesicular breathing. The inspiratory and expiratory phases are of equal length and separated by a short, silent gap. This is

called **bronchial breathing**. The quality of the sound and the presence of the gap are the two distinguishing features.

The pitch of bronchial breathing may be high or low. The high-pitched variety is sometimes called **tubular** bronchial breathing. The low-pitched variety, which sounds like the noise produced by blowing across the mouth of a jar, is called **amphoric** bronchial breathing. Amphoric sounds are heard when air is passing in and out of a cavity in the lung such as a tuberculous cavity.

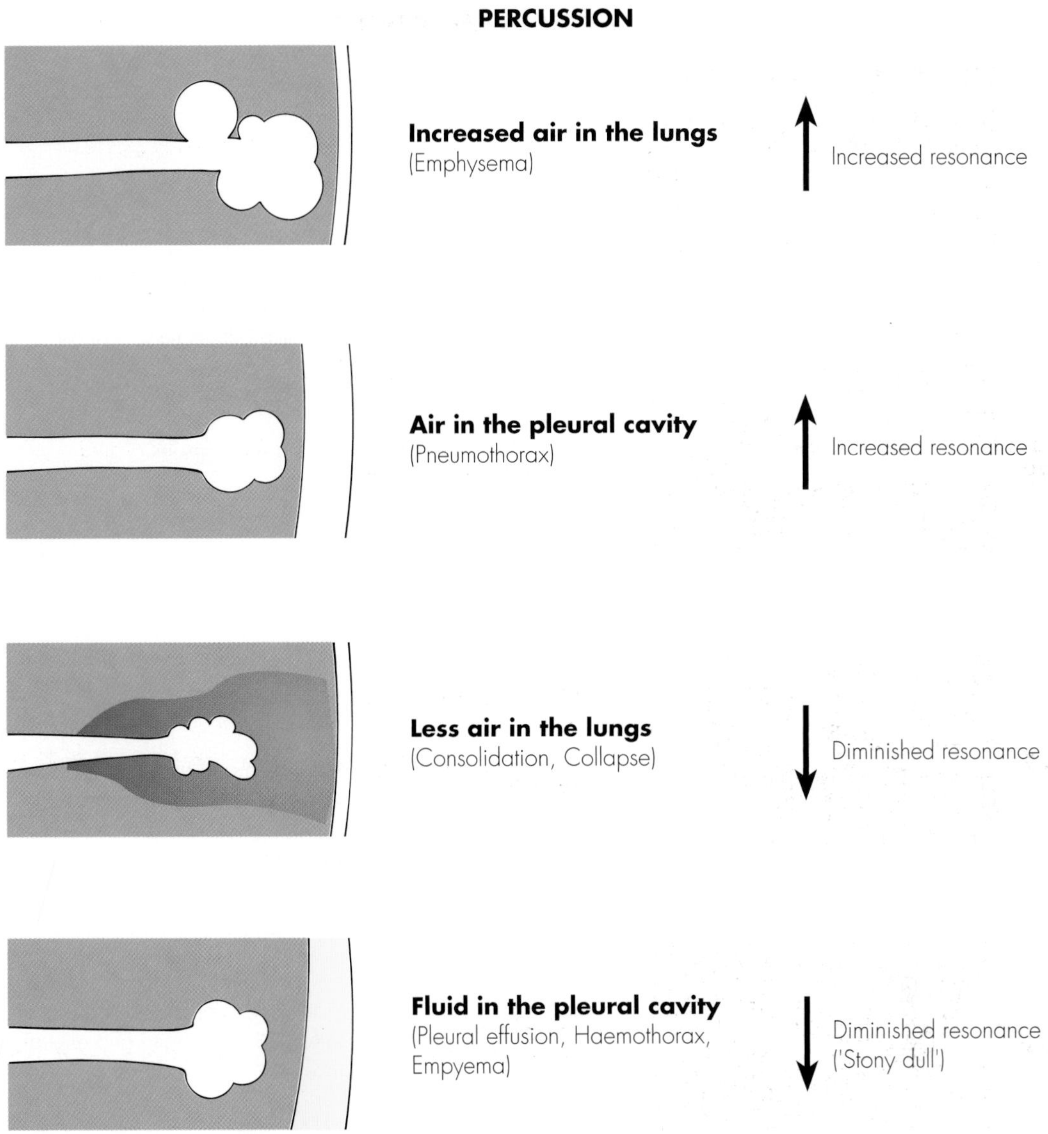

PERCUSSION

Increased air in the lungs
(Emphysema)

Increased resonance

Air in the pleural cavity
(Pneumothorax)

Increased resonance

Less air in the lungs
(Consolidation, Collapse)

Diminished resonance

Fluid in the pleural cavity
(Pleural effusion, Haemothorax,
Empyema)

Diminished resonance
('Stony dull')

FIG 1.5 The causes of changes in lung resonance.

There is a type of breath sound mid-way between vesicular and bronchial breathing, known as **bronchovesicular** breathing. In this variety the inspiratory and expiratory sounds are of equal length and slightly harsher than those of vesicular breathing, but there is **no gap between the two phases**. Bronchovesicular breathing is often heard in normal people over the anterior aspect of the upper lobes, where there are large bronchi near the surface of the lung, and must not be mistaken for bronchial breathing.

Absent sounds

Breath sounds are abolished or diminished by any process which reduces the normal conduction of sound through the lung substance and chest wall. The two common causes are bronchial obstruction (producing collapse of the distal part of the lung) and pleural effusion or pneumothorax.

When the lung alveoli are full of fluid, exudate or pus (consolidation) but the air passages remain patent, the thickened lung transmits the sound

BREATH SOUNDS

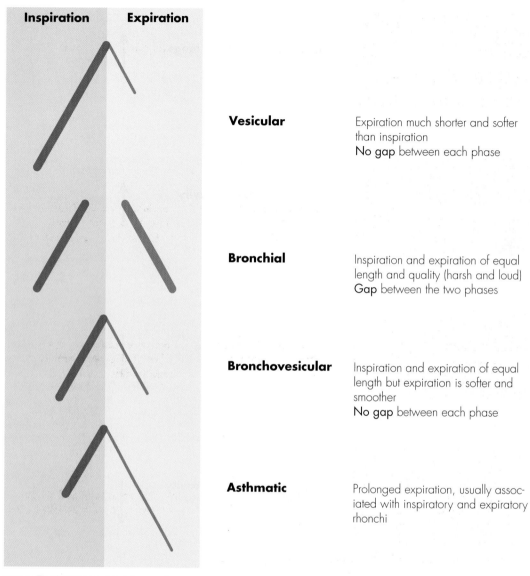

Inspiration	Expiration		
		Vesicular	Expiration much shorter and softer than inspiration **No gap** between each phase
		Bronchial	Inspiration and expiration of equal length and quality (harsh and loud) **Gap** between the two phases
		Bronchovesicular	Inspiration and expiration of equal length but expiration is softer and smoother **No gap** between each phase
		Asthmatic	Prolonged expiration, usually associated with inspiratory and expiratory rhonchi

FIG 1.6 The four types of breath sound.

from the larger bronchi. Thus bronchial breathing is heard over an area of consolidated lung. There are, however, no breath sounds over an area of collapsed lung.

Added sounds

There are three varieties of added sounds: rhonchi, râles and crepitations. These are often referred to as wheezes, coarse crackles and fine crackles by the younger generation of pulmonary physicians.

Rhonchi/wheezes These are the whistling noises made by air passing through narrowed air passages. They are commonly heard in patients with asthma or chronic bronchitis. Their pitch depends upon the velocity of airflow and the diameter of the bronchioles from which they originate. They are unmistakable.

EFFECT OF LUNG DISEASE ON THE BREATH SOUNDS

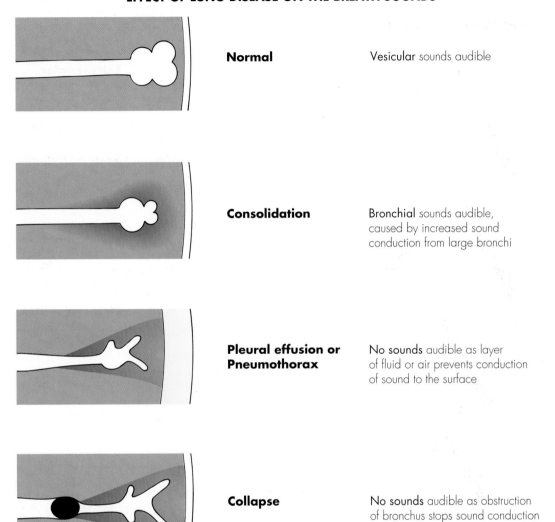

Normal

Vesicular sounds audible

Consolidation

Bronchial sounds audible, caused by increased sound conduction from large bronchi

Pleural effusion or Pneumothorax

No sounds audible as layer of fluid or air prevents conduction of sound to the surface

Collapse

No sounds audible as obstruction of bronchus stops sound conduction

FIG 1.7 The causes of abnormal breath sounds.

Râles/coarse crackles These are the coarse bubbling noises caused by air passing through bronchioles containing water, mucus or pus. The sound is identical to that made by air bubbling through water. Moving the fluid may abolish the noise, so ask the patient to take a deep breath and cough, and then listen again. If the bubbling sounds disappear, they must have been râles because crepitations cannot be abolished in this way.

Crepitations/fine crackles These are fine crackling sounds similar to the noise heard when you hold a few hairs close to your ear and roll them between your thumb and index finger. They are thought to be produced as the alveoli and their ducts pop open to allow air to enter when there is interstitial oedema. Crepitations are heard over areas of consolidation, such as pneumonia, and often provide important evidence of left ventricular failure. They are not abolished by coughing.

Some authorities do not distinguish râles from crepitations and use the all-embracing term **moist sounds** for either variety.

Pleural rub The visceral and parietal layers of the pleura normally slide easily over one another but, if the pleura is inflamed, the roughened pleural surfaces rubbing together produce a noise which is similar to the sound heard when a finger is pressed hard onto a pane of glass and then slid across it. It is a mixture of grating and squeaking sounds. A pleural rub can only be heard when the chest is moving, i.e. during inspiration or expiration. The patient usually complains of pleuritic pain over an area where there is an audible rub.

Examine the heart and circulation

Much will have been learnt about the circulation from your initial observations of the patient's colour and breathing. It is common practice to feel the pulse when you take the patient's hand at the beginning of the examination. Any abnormalities detected at this stage require reassessment by further careful palpation.

The pulse

The following features should be observed and recorded.

The rate Express the rate in beats/minute. Do not count the pulse for 5 seconds and multiply by 12; always count for 15 seconds or longer if the beat feels irregular.

The rhythm The pulse beat may be regular or irregular. When the pulse is irregular it may have a regular recurring pattern or be totally irregular. The latter is sometimes called an **irregularly irregular** pulse and indicates **atrial fibrillation**. Some common varieties of irregular pulse are shown in Figure 1.8.

The volume The examining fingers can appreciate the expansion of the artery with each beat and consequently get an impression of the amount of blood passing through the artery. Patients with a high cardiac output have a strong pulse. Patients in haemorrhagic (hypovolaemic) shock have a weak, thin, 'thready' pulse.

The nature of the pressure wave Every pressure wave has definable characteristics such as the rate of increase and decrease of pressure and the height of the pressure (see Fig. 1.9).

A steep rise followed by a rapid fall, with a large pulse pressure (high peak), is called a **collapsing**

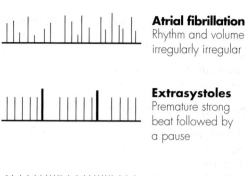

Atrial fibrillation
Rhythm and volume irregularly irregular

Extrasystoles
Premature strong beat followed by a pause

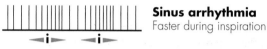

Sinus arrhythmia
Faster during inspiration

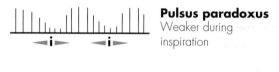

Pulsus paradoxus
Weaker during inspiration

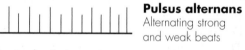

Pulsus alternans
Alternating strong and weak beats

(**i** = inspiration)

FIG 1.8 Common variations of the rhythm and volume of the pulse.

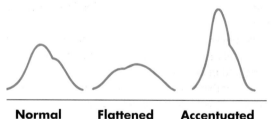

Normal	**Flattened**	**Accentuated**
The dicrotic notch is not normally palpable	Slow rise and fall, called **anacrotic**, caused by aortic stenosis	Rapid rise and fall, called a **water-hammer pulse**, caused by aortic incompetence and patent ductus arteriosus

FIG 1.9 Variations of the pulse wave.

or **water-hammer pulse** and is typical of **aortic regurgitation**. Conversely, a tight **aortic stenosis** causes a slow rise and fall.

The shape of the pulse wave can be appreciated more easily over the carotid than the radial artery.

The nature of the artery It is relatively easy to estimate the diameter of the radial artery and guess the thickness of its wall, but the presence or absence of thickening of the radial artery gives no indication of the thickness of other vessels in the body.

Measure the blood pressure

The blood pressure is usually measured in the brachial artery with a sphygmomanometer. The cuff, which must fit snugly and be at least 10 cm wide (a narrow cuff gives false readings), should be firmly wrapped around the middle of the upper arm and inflated above the systolic pressure (250 mmHg). It should then be slowly deflated until the commencement of blood flow below the cuff is detected by listening over the brachial artery at the elbow with a stethoscope or palpating the pulse at the wrist. The pressure at this point is the systolic blood pressure.

(The sounds which indicate the commencement of flow in the brachial artery below the cuff are caused by turbulent blood flow. They were first described by Korotkoff and are known as *Korotkoff sounds*.)

The cuff pressure is further reduced until the Korotkoff sounds suddenly diminish or, more often, disappear. This is the diastolic pressure.

It is worth repeating both measurements on several occasions with the patient sitting and lying down and again at the end of the examination when the patient is less worried.

Whenever there is the possibility of disease of the aorta and its branches, the blood pressure should be measured in both arms.

Remember that the readings from a very fat arm will be falsely high by as much as 10 mmHg.

Inspect the head and neck again

You will already have looked at the patient's skin, face and general demeanour. Look again for the signs particularly indicative of cardiovascular disease – **cyanosis**, **plethora** and **dyspnoea**.

Xanthomata These are grey-yellow plaques of lipid in the skin. They often occur in the skin of the upper eyelid (see Fig 3.47, page 103). Their presence may indicate an abnormal lipid metabolism such as hyperlipidaemia, but they may occur in patients with normal blood lipids.

Arcus senilis This is a white ring at the junction of the iris and sclera (see Fig. 8.14, page 227). It is said to be more common in people with advanced arteriosclerosis, but in practice is not a reliable indicator of the presence of vascular disease (see Chapter 8, page 226). It may indicate the presence of a hyperlipoproteinaemia if present in a patient under the age of 40 years.

The jugular venous pressure The pressure in the great veins is slightly greater than the pressure in the right atrium. The pressure in the right atrium is one of the most important influences of cardiac activity. An increase in the right atrial pressure increases cardiac output by stimulating an increase of cardiac contractility and rate. The right atrial pressure therefore 'drives' the heart. The pressure in the right atrium can be estimated clinically from the pressure in the internal jugular veins. In a normal person, reclining at 45°, the great veins in the neck are collapsed. There should be no visible venous pulsations above the level of the manubrio-sternal joint, which, when the patient is reclining at 45°, is at the same level as the mid-point of the clavicles (see Fig. 1.10).

The right atrial pressure is raised if there are visible pulsations in the internal jugular veins when the patient is reclining at 45°. The vertical distance between the upper limit of the venous distension and the level of the clavicle should be estimated by eye and expressed and recorded in centimetres.

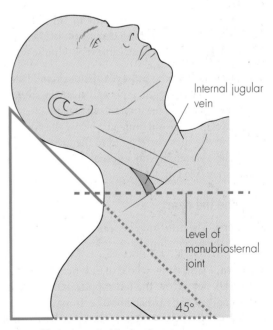

Internal jugular vein

Level of manubriosternal joint

45°

FIG 1.10 Measurement of the jugular venous pressure.

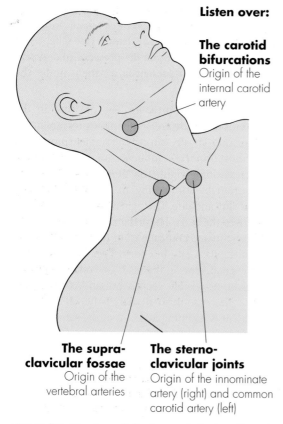

Listen over:

The carotid bifurcations
Origin of the internal carotid artery

The supra-clavicular fossae
Origin of the vertebral arteries

The sterno-clavicular joints
Origin of the innominate artery (right) and common carotid artery (left)

FIG 1.11 The sites of auscultation for vascular bruits on the neck.

Obstruction of the great veins in the superior mediastinum will also cause distension of the neck veins, but there will not be a visible venous pulse wave.

Neck arteries Feel the pulses in the neck and listen along their whole length, especially over the sterno-clavicular joints, in the supraclavicular fossae, and at the level of the hyoid bone just below the angle of the jaw. These sites correspond to the origins of the subclavian, vertebral and internal carotid arteries, respectively (see Fig. 1.11).

Examine the heart

Inspection The heart may be seen to be beating rapidly or to be heaving up the chest wall with each beat.

Palpation Place your whole hand firmly on the chest wall, just below the left nipple, and ascertain the strength of the cardiac impulse. It may be weak, normal or heaving in nature. The apex beat is the lowest and most lateral point at which the cardiac

impulse can be felt. It should be in the fifth intercostal space, near the mid-clavicular line (an imaginary vertical line which passes through the middle of the clavicle). The apex beat moves laterally and may be felt as far out as the mid-axillary line if the heart is enlarged. It may also be possible to feel vibrations, called **thrills**, which correspond to audible heart murmurs. Thrills may be felt during systole, diastole or throughout the whole cardiac cycle.

Remember to palpate the back of the chest. Thrills from abnormalities of the aorta, such as a patent ductus arteriosus or a coarctation of the aorta, are conducted posteriorly as well as anteriorly.

It is advisable to feel the femoral pulses at this stage.

Percussion The area of cardiac dullness should be delineated by percussion.

Auscultation The whole of the anterior aspect of the heart must be examined with the stethoscope, but the areas where the sounds from the four valves are best heard are shown in Figure 1.12.

Aortic area
Right second costochondral junction

Pulmonary area
Left second interspace

Lean the patient forwards and also listen along the **left** side of the sternum

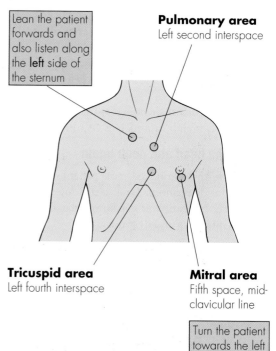

Tricuspid area
Left fourth interspace

Mitral area
Fifth space, mid-clavicular line

Turn the patient towards the left

FIG 1.12 Areas of cardiac auscultation.

Begin by listening at the apex of the heart – the mitral area. Identify the first and second heart sounds. The heart sounds are traditionally described as sounding like the words lub-dub; that is to say, the first sound is slightly longer and softer than the second sound. As this is not always the case, it is wise to confirm that the sound you believe to be the first sound corresponds to the beginning of the cardiac impulse or coincides with the subclavian or carotid pulse. Having decided which sound is which, listen carefully to the second sound. It may be sharper and shorter than usual – almost a click – or it may be split. A double, or split, second sound occurs when the aortic and pulmonary valves close asynchronously. A double sound can be heard when the sounds are 0.2 or more seconds apart and indicates pulmonary hypertension.

Next, listen carefully to the intervals between the two main sounds, and between diastole and systole, for any additional heart sounds or murmurs.

Murmurs are caused by turbulent flow and the vibration of parts of the heart. They may vary in nature from a low-pitched rumble to a high-toned swish. Try to decide whether the murmur occupies the whole or part of diastole or systole and whether its intensity changes.

Think of the way you are going to record your findings (see Fig. 1.13), two blocks for the main heart sounds (M1 and A2) and a zig-zag line for the murmur. Imagine your drawing as you listen to the sound and you will find it easier to define the timing of the murmur. A detailed description of the many heart sounds and their interpretation is beyond the scope of this book. The student must read a textbook of cardiology, but Figure 1.13 illustrates the common types of murmur and their likely causes.

The exercise just described must be repeated over the other three areas where the aortic, pulmonary and tricuspid valve sounds are best heard.

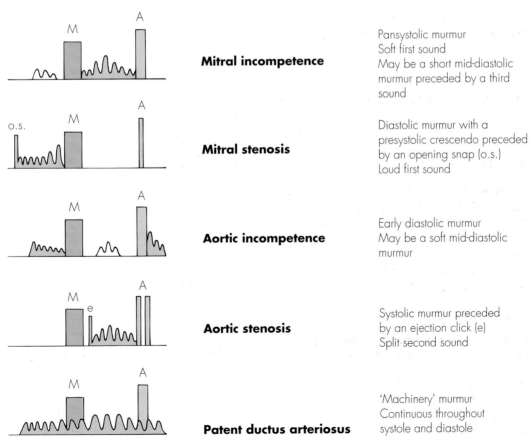

Mitral incompetence
Pansystolic murmur
Soft first sound
May be a short mid-diastolic murmur preceded by a third sound

Mitral stenosis
Diastolic murmur with a presystolic crescendo preceded by an opening snap (o.s.)
Loud first sound

Aortic incompetence
Early diastolic murmur
May be a soft mid-diastolic murmur

Aortic stenosis
Systolic murmur preceded by an ejection click (e)
Split second sound

Patent ductus arteriosus
'Machinery' murmur
Continuous throughout systole and diastole

FIG 1.13 The sounds of some common cardiac abnormalities (M = 1st heart sound, A = 2nd heart sound).

Some murmurs will be audible in more than one area. The site of maximum intensity of a murmur usually indicates its site of origin. Find this by 'inching' the stethoscope over the chest wall between the areas. The same technique should be used to assess whether murmurs in the aortic area are conducted into or coming from the neck.

The sounds at the apex, from the mitral valve, can be made louder by asking the patient to turn over onto their left side; the aortic valve sounds can be amplified by asking the patient to lean forwards.

Always listen to the heart sounds at the back of the chest. The murmur of a patent ductus or coarctation can often be heard over the aorta, posteriorly, just to the left of the mid-line.

Test for oedema

Oedema commonly appears first in the feet and ankles, but may be more apparent in the sacral and buttock regions if the patient has been bedridden for some time. Cardiac oedema is very soft, 'pits' easily and often gives the skin a pale, waxy, transparent appearance.

Revision panel 1.7
Common causes of ankle swelling

Dependency/immobility
Pregnancy
Heart failure
Low plasma proteins
Chronic venous insufficiency
Deep vein thrombosis
Lymphatic insufficiency
Chronic renal failure (nephrotic syndrome)

Revision panel 1.8
Classification of muscle strength

5	Normal
4	Weak but can overcome gentle resistance
3	Cannot overcome gentle resistance but can overcome gravity
2	Cannot overcome gravity but muscle contracts
1	Barely perceptible muscle contractions
0	No contractions

Examine the abdomen

Examination of the abdomen is described in detail in Chapter 16. It has been put there in the hope that you will read it whenever you refer to other parts of the chapter. A large amount of the surgical disease presenting to a surgical clinic is intra-abdominal and so a good technique for abdominal examination is essential.

Examination of the abdomen follows the standard pattern.

- **Inspection** for asymmetry, distension, masses, visible peristalsis and skin discolouration.
- **Palpation** for superficial and deep tenderness, the normal viscera (liver, spleen and kidneys) and any abnormal masses.
- **Percussion** of the liver and splenic areas and any other masses.
- **Auscultation** for bowel sounds and vascular bruits.
- **Rectal examination and vaginal examination.**

There are four things that are easy to forget, so do them before you start general palpation.

1. Palpate the supraclavicular lymph glands.
2. Palpate the hernial orifices.
3. Feel the femoral pulses.
4. Examine the genitalia.

Two further things which often get forgotten are auscultation and the rectal examination, but you must leave these to the end.

Examine the limbs

There are four main tissues to be examined in a limb: the bones and joints, the muscles and soft tissues, the arteries and veins, and the nerves. The first three are often involved in surgical disease and their examination is described in Chapters 4 and 7. Only the examination of the peripheral nerves is described here.

Examine the peripheral nerves

The nerves in the limbs serve three functions: motor, sensory and reflex. Examine each of these functions in turn.

Motor nerve function

Voluntary movement Ask the patient to move each joint in all directions, as far as possible. This will demonstrate any loss of voluntary muscle function and the presence of any musculoskeletal abnormalities, such as arthritis or muscle contractures, which limit movement.

Strength of the muscles Check in a systematic way the strength of the muscles which move each joint. Strength is assessed by asking the patient to move the joint against a resistance, or by asking them to keep the joint fixed while you try to move it. The latter is the simplest method because the patient only needs to be instructed to keep the limb still.

It is customary to grade muscle strength as follows:

5: normal
4: moderate, but not full strength
3: can work against gravity but not against a greater resistance
2: cannot work against gravity but the muscles contract
1: barely perceptible contractions
0: complete paralysis.

It is, however, better to describe the strength of the muscles than use a numerical code.

The segments of the spinal cord and the nerves which control each joint are listed in Revision panel 1.9.

Sensory nerve function

The peripheral nerves transmit the sensations of light touch, deep touch and pressure, pain, temperature, vibration sense, position sense, and muscular coordination.

The appreciation of light touch This is tested with a wisp of cotton wool.

Revision panel 1.9
The nerves and spinal segments which innervate the major muscle groups

Muscle groups		Spinal segments	Nerves
Shoulder	Flexion	C5, 6	Nerve to pectoralis major, circumflex nerve
	Extension	C5, 6	
	Abduction	C5, 6	Subscapular nerve
			Circumflex nerve
Elbow	Flexion	C5, 6	Musculocutaneous nerve
	Extension	C6, 7, 8	Radial nerve
Wrist	Flexion	C6, 7, 8	Median nerve and ulnar nerve
	Extension	C6, 7, 8	Radial nerve
Intrinsic hand muscles		C8, T1	Median nerve and ulnar nerve
Hip	Flexion	L2, 3, 4	Lumbar and femoral nerves
	Extension	L5, S1, 2	Inferior gluteal nerve
	Abduction	L4, 5, S1	Superior gluteal nerve
	Adduction	L2, 3, 4	Obturator nerve
	Rotation	L5, S1, 2	
Knee	Flexion	L4, 5, S1, 2	Sciatic nerve
	Extension	L2, 3, 4	Femoral nerve
Ankle	Flexion	L5, S1, 2	Medial popliteal + posterior tibial nerves
	Extension	L4, 5, S1	Anterior tibial nerve
Foot	Inversion	L4, 5	Anterior + posterior tibial nerves
	Eversion	L5, S1	Musculocutaneous nerve

Make sure that the patient cannot see you when you touch them, and touch the limb in a random manner. Move from the normal to the abnormal when mapping out an area of hypo-aesthesia. The important dermatomes are shown in Figure 1.14.

THE IMPORTANT DERMATOMES
(the others can be estimated if you remember these)

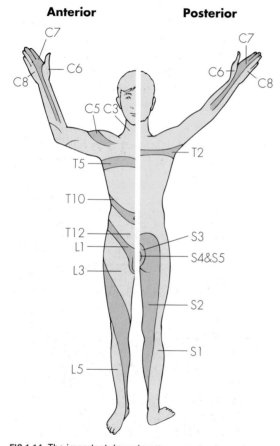

FIG 1.14 The important dermatomes.

Revision panel 1.10
The segments involved in the common stretch reflexes

Biceps jerk	C5, 6
Triceps jerk	C6, 7
Finger jerk	C8
Knee jerk	L2, 3, 4
Ankle jerk	S1, 2

Deep touch and pressure sensation This is tested by pressing firmly on the skin with a blunt object. It is unlikely to be abnormal if the response to light touch is normal.

Pain The best test of pain sensibility is the response to a pinprick. A new sterile needle must be used for each patient to avoid transmitting infection such as hepatitis. The patient must be asked whether the needle feels 'sharp' or 'blunt'.

Temperature Ask the patient to differentiate between a hot and a cold object. The simplest method is to use two test tubes, one filled with hot and the other with cold water.

Vibration sense Strike a tuning fork firmly. Place its base on a bony protuberance, such as the malleolus at the ankle, and ask the patient to describe the sensation they can feel. A description of a 'buzzing' or 'vibrating' sensation indicates normal vibration sense. Do not put these words into the patient's mind by using them in a leading question.

Position sense The proprioceptive nerve endings in a joint tell the brain about the joint's spatial orientation. Test this ability by moving the great toe or thumb into different positions of flexion or extension and ask the patient to identify them. It is easier to ask patients to state the direction in which the digit is pointing (e.g. up or down) than to use unfamiliar anatomical terms. The patient must keep their eyes shut.

Muscle coordination Test the coordination of the upper limbs by asking the patient to touch your upheld finger with their index finger and then to touch the tip of their nose. You will also be testing joint position sense if you ask them to do this a second time with their eyes shut. Coordination in the lower limbs is tested by asking the patient to slide the heel of one foot up and down the shin of the other leg. This should also be done with the eyes open and then shut.

Reflex function

The limb reflexes are all stretch reflexes and test the integrity of the spinal segments, and the motor and sensory nerves which innervate the muscles being stretched.

To stimulate a good stretch reflex you must stretch the muscle's tendon suddenly by striking it with a rubber hammer. A weak reflex can be reinforced by asking patients to clench their teeth or to interlock their fingers and try to pull them apart.

Clonus The increase in muscle tone that occurs with an upper motor neurone lesion increases the susceptibility of the tendons to the stretch reflex. Sudden and persistent stretching can cause repeated contractions known as **clonus**.

The plantar reflex Scraping the lateral aspect of the sole of the foot causes a withdrawal reflex and flexion of the great toe. If the toe extends, there is an upper motor neurone lesion. This reflex involves the L5, S1 and S2 spinal segments.

Abdominal reflexes Stroking the upper and lower abdomen causes the rectus abdominis muscle to contract. This tests the T8, 9 and 10, and T11 and 12 segments, respectively.

Cremasteric reflex Stroking the inner side of the thigh makes the cremaster contract, testing the L1 segment.

Test the urine, faeces and sputum

It is important to note the colour and smell of the urine before using the modern simple dipstick methods for testing it for sugar, blood, acetone and protein. Do not forget to measure the specific gravity of the urine and to inspect any precipitate under the microscope.

Look at the faeces if the patient complains that they are abnormal.

Look at the sputum.

HISTORY AND EXAMINATION OF A LUMP

History

Most patients with a lump feel it frequently and should be able to tell you about the history of its clinical features. Therefore you should seek answers to the following questions.

1. **When was the lump first noticed?**
   It is important to be precise with dates and terminology. Do not write 'the lump first

appeared 6 months ago', when you mean 'the lump was first noticed 6 months ago'. Many lumps may exist for months, even years, before the patient notices them.

2. **What made the patient notice the lump?**
   There are three common answers to this question:
   'I felt or saw it when washing'.
   'I had a pain and found the lump when I felt the painful area'.
   'Someone else noticed it and told me about it'.
   The presence or absence of pain is important, particularly if it is the presenting feature. In very general terms, pain is usually associated with inflammation, not neoplastic change. Most

---

Revision panel 1.11
The examination of a lump or ulcer

Local examination
  Site
  Size
  Shape
  Surface
  Depth
  Colour
  Temperature
  Tenderness
  Edge
  Composition:
  ■ consistence ⎫
  ■ fluctuation ⎪
  ■ fluid thrill   ⎬ Solid, fluid or gas
  ■ translucence ⎪
  ■ resonance
  ■ pulsatility ⎫
  ■ compressibility ⎬ Vascular
  ■ bruit ⎭
  Reducibility
  Relations to surrounding structures – mobility/fixity
  Regional lymph glands
  State of local tissues:
  ■ arteries
  ■ nerves
  ■ bones and joints
General examination

patients expect cancer to be painful – and do themselves irreparable harm by ignoring a lump just because it does not hurt them.

3. **What are the symptoms of the lump?**
The lump may be painful and if it is, you must take a careful history of the pain, as described earlier in this chapter. The characteristic feature of pain associated with acute infection is its throbbing nature.

A lump may be disfiguring or interfere with movement, respiration or swallowing. Describe the history of each symptom carefully.

4. **Has the lump changed since it was first noticed?**
This is where you use the patient's own knowledge of their physical signs. The feature that they notice is the size of the lump. They should be able to tell you if it has got bigger, smaller, or has fluctuated in size and when they noticed a change in size. They may also have appreciated other changes in the nature of the lump that they can tell you about. They may also have noticed tenderness, which may have altered in any of the ways that a pain may change.

5. **Does the lump ever disappear?**
A lump may disappear on lying down, or during exercise, and yet be irreducible at the time of your examination. The patient should always be asked if the lump ever goes away, because this physical characteristic is peculiar to only a few types of lump.

6. **Has the patient ever had any other lumps?**
You must ask this question because it might not have occurred to the patient that there could be any connection between their present lump and a previous lump, or even a coexisting one.

7. **What does the patient think caused the lump?**
Lumps occasionally follow injuries or systemic illnesses known only to the patient.

Examination

Site/position The location of a lump must be described in exact anatomical terms, using distances measured from bony points. Do not guess distances; use a tape measure.

Colour and texture of overlying skin The skin over a lump may be discoloured and become smooth and shiny or thick and rough.

Shape Remember that lumps have three dimensions. You cannot have a circular lump because a circle is a plane figure. Many lumps are not regular spheres, or hemispheres, but have an asymmetrical outline. In these circumstances, it is permissible to use descriptive terms such as pear shaped or kidney shaped.

Size Once the shape is established, it is possible to measure its various dimensions. Again, remember that all solid objects have at least three dimensions: width, length and height or depth. Asymmetrical lumps will need more measurements to describe them accurately; sometimes a diagram will clarify your written description.

Surface The first feature of the lump that you will notice when you feel it will be its surface. It may be smooth or irregular. An irregular surface may be covered with smooth bumps, rather like cobblestones, which can be called bosselated; or be irregular or rough.

There may be a mixture of surfaces if the lump is large.

Temperature Is the lump hot or of normal temperature? Assess the skin temperature with the dorsal surfaces of your fingers, because they are usually dry (free of sweat) and cool.

Revision panel 1.12
The history of a lump or an ulcer

Duration
When was it first noticed?

First symptom
What brought it to the patient's notice?

Other symptoms
What symptoms does it cause?

Progression
How has it changed since it was first noticed?

Persistence
Has it ever disappeared or healed?

Multiplicity
Has (or had) the patient any other lumps or ulcers?

Cause
What does the patient think caused it?

Tenderness Is the lump tender? Which parts are tender? Always try to feel the non-tender part before feeling the tender area, and watch the patient's face for signs of discomfort as you palpate.

Edge The edge of a lump may be clearly defined or indistinct. It may have a definite pattern.

Composition Any lump must be composed of one or more of the following:

■ calcified tissues such as bone, which make it hard;
■ tightly packed cells, which make it solid;
■ extravascular fluid, such as urine, serum, cerebrospinal fluid (CSF), synovial fluid or extravascular blood, which make the lump cystic;
■ gas;
■ intravascular blood.

The physical signs which help you decide the composition of a lump are: consistence, fluctuation, fluid thrill, translucence, resonance, pulsatility, compressibility and bruits.

Consistence The consistence of a lump may vary from very soft to very hard. As it is difficult to describe hardness, it is common practice to compare the consistence of a lump to well-known objects. A simple scale for consistence is as follows:

■ **Stony hard**: not indentable – usually bone or calcification.
■ **Firm**: hard but not as hard as bone.
■ **Rubbery**: but slightly squashable, similar to a rubber ball.
■ **Spongy**: soft and very squashable, but still with some resilience.
■ **Soft**: squashable and no resilience.

The consistence of a lump depends not only upon its structure but also on the tension within it. Some fluid-filled lumps are hard, some solid lumps are soft; therefore, the final decision about composition of a lump (i.e. whether it is fluid or solid) rarely depends solely upon an assessment of the consistence. Other features such as those peculiar to fluid may be more important.

Fluctuation Pressure on one side of a fluid-filled cavity makes all the other surfaces protrude. This is because an increase of pressure within a cavity is transmitted equally and at right-angles to all parts of its wall. When you press on one aspect of a solid lump, it may or may not bulge out in another direction, but it will not bulge outwards in every other direction.

Fluctuation can only be elicited by feeling at least two other areas of the lump whilst pressing on a third. The lump fluctuates and contains fluid if two areas on opposite aspects of the lump bulge out when a third area is pressed in. This examination is best carried out in two places, the second at right-angles to the first.

Fluid thrill A percussion wave is easily conducted across a large fluid collection (cyst) but not across a solid mass. The presence of a fluid thrill is detected by tapping one side of the lump and feeling the transmitted vibration when it reaches the other side. A percussion wave can be transmitted along its wall if a swelling is large. This is prevented by placing the edge of the patient's or an assistant's hand on the lump mid-way between the percussing and palpating hands.

Percussion waves cannot be felt across small lumps because the wave moves so quickly that the time gap cannot be appreciated or distinguished from the mechanical shaking of the tissue caused by the percussion. The presence of a fluid thrill is a diagnostic and extremely valuable physical sign.

Translucence (transillumination) Light will pass easily through clear fluid but not through solid tissues. A lump that transilluminates must contain water, serum, lymph or plasma, or highly refractile fat. Blood and other opaque fluids do not transmit light. Transillumination requires a bright pinpoint light source and a darkened room. The light should be placed on one side of the lump, not directly on top of it. Transillumination is present when the light can be seen in an area distant from the site in contact with the light source.

Attempts at transillumination with a poor-quality flashlight in a bright room are bound to fail and mislead.

Resonance Solid and fluid-filled lumps sound dull when percussed. A gas-filled lump sounds hollow and resonant.

Pulsatility Lumps may pulsate because they are near to an artery and are moved by its pulsations. Always let your hand rest still for a few seconds on every lump to discover if it is pulsating. When a lump pulsates you must find out whether the pulsations are being **transmitted** to the lump from elsewhere or are caused by the **expansion** of the lump. Place a finger (or fingers if large) of each hand on opposite sides of the lump and feel if they are pushed outwards and upwards. When they are, the lump has an *expansile* pulsation. When they are pushed in the same direction (usually upwards), the lump has a *transmitted* pulsation.

The two common causes of expansile pulsation are aneurysms and very vascular tumours.

Compressibility Some fluid-filled lumps can be compressed until they disappear. When the compressing hand is removed the lump re-forms. This finding is a common feature of vascular malformations and fluid collections which can be pushed back into a cavity or cistern. Compressibility should not be confused with reducibility (see below). A lump which is reducible – such as a hernia – can be pushed away into another place but will often not reappear spontaneously without the stimulus of coughing or gravity.

Bruits Always listen to a lump. Vascular lumps that contain an arteriovenous fistula may have a systolic bruit. Hernaie containing bowel may have audible bowel sounds.

Reducibility You should always see if a lump is reducible (disappears) by gently compressing it. A reducible lump will be felt to get smaller and then to move into another place as it is compressed. It may disappear quite suddenly after appropriate pressure has been applied. If you ask the patient to cough, the lump may return, expanding as it does so. This is called a cough impulse and is a feature of herniae and some vascular lumps. The reduction can be maintained by pressing over the point at which the lump finally disappeared. In many ways the differences between compressibility (see above) and reducibility are semantic.

Relations to surrounding structures By careful palpation, it is usually possible to decide which structure contains the lump, and what its relation is to overlying and deeper structures. The attachment of skin and other superficial structures to a lump can easily be determined because both are accessible to the examiner and any limitation of their movement easily felt. The lump should be gently moved while the skin is inspected for movement or puckering.

Attachment to deeper structures is more difficult to determine. Underlying muscles must be tensed to see if this reduces the mobility of an overlying lump or makes it easier or less easy to feel. The former indicates that the lump is attached to the fascia covering the superficial surface of the muscle or to the muscle itself; the latter that the lump is within or deep to the muscles. Lumps that are attached to bone move very little. Lumps that are attached to or arising from vessels or nerves may be moved from side to side across the length of the vessel or nerve, but not up and down along their length. Lumps in the abdomen that are freely mobile usually arise from the intestine, its mesentery or the omentum.

State of the regional lymph glands Never forget to palpate the lymph glands that would normally receive lymph from the region occupied by the lump. The skin, muscles and bones of the limbs and trunk drain to the axillary and inguinal glands; the head and neck to the cervical glands; and the intra-abdominal structures to the pre-aortic and para-aortic glands.

State of the local tissues It is important to examine the overlying and nearby skin, subcutaneous tissues, muscles and bones, and the local circulation and nerve supply of adjacent tissues. This is more relevant when examining an ulcer; but some lumps are associated with a local vascular or neurological abnormality, or cause an abnormality of these systems, so this part of the examination must not be forgotten.

General examination It is often tempting to examine only the lump about which the patient is complaining. This will cause you to make innumerable misdiagnoses. **You must always examine the whole patient.**

HISTORY AND EXAMINATION OF AN ULCER

An ulcer is a solution (break) of the continuity of an epithelium (i.e. an epithelial deficit, not a wound). Unless it is painless and in an inaccessible part of the body, patients notice ulcers from the moment they begin, and will know a great deal about their clinical features.

History

The questions to be asked concerning an ulcer follow a pattern similar to those for a lump.

1. **When was the ulcer first noticed?**
   Ask the patient when the ulcer began and whether it could have been present for some time before it was noticed. The latter often occurs with neurotrophic ulcers on the sole of the foot.
2. **What drew the patient's attention to the ulcer?**
   The commonest reason is pain. Occasionally, the presenting feature is bleeding, or a purulent discharge, which may be foul smelling.
3. **What are the symptoms of the ulcer?**
   The ulcer may be painful. It may interfere with daily activities such as walking, eating or defaecation. Record the history of each symptom.
4. **How has the ulcer changed since it first appeared?**
   The patient's observations about changes in size, shape, discharge and pain are likely to be detailed and accurate. If the ulcer has healed and broken down, record the features of each episode.
5. **Has the patient ever had a similar ulcer on the same site, or elsewhere?**
   Obtain a complete history of any previous ulcer.
6. **What does the patient think caused the ulcer?**
   Most patients believe they know the cause of their ulcer, and are often right. In many cases it is trauma. When possible, the severity and type of injury should be assessed. A large ulcer following a minor injury suggests that the skin was abnormal before the injury.

Examination

The examination of an ulcer follows the same pattern as the examination of a lump. When an ulcer has an irregular shape that is difficult to describe, draw it on your notes and add the dimensions. When an exact record of size and shape is needed, place a thin sheet of sterile transparent plastic sheet over the ulcer and trace around its edge with a felt-tipped pen.

After recording the site, size and shape of the ulcer, you must examine the base (surface), edge, depth, discharge and surrounding tissues, the state of the local lymph glands and local tissues, and complete the general examination.

Base

The base, or floor, of an ulcer usually consists of slough or granulation tissue (capillaries, collagen, fibroblasts, bacteria and inflammatory cells), but recognizable structures such as tendon or bone may be visible. The nature of the floor occasionally gives some indication of the cause of the ulcer.

- Solid brown or grey dead tissue indicates full-thickness skin death.
- Syphilitic ulcers have a slough that looks like a yellow-grey wash-leather.
- Tuberculous ulcers have a base of bluish unhealthy granulation tissue.
- Ischaemic ulcers often contain poor granulation tissue, and tendons and other structures may lie bare in their base.

The redness of the granulation tissue reflects the underlying vascularity and indicates the ability of the ulcer to heal. Healing epidermis is seen as a pale layer extending in over the granulation tissue from the edge of the ulcer.

Edge

There are five types of edge (see Fig. 1.15).

A flat, gently sloping edge This indicates that the ulcer is shallow and this type of ulcer is usually

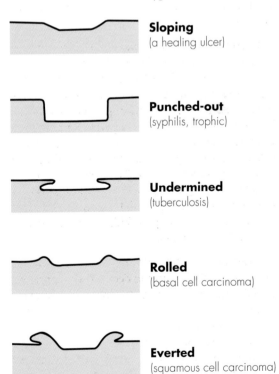

Sloping
(a healing ulcer)

Punched-out
(syphilis, trophic)

Undermined
(tuberculosis)

Rolled
(basal cell carcinoma)

Everted
(squamous cell carcinoma)

FIG 1.15 The varieties of ulcer edge.

superficial, often only half-way through the skin. Venous ulcers usually have this type of edge, but so do many other types of ulcer. The new skin growing in around the edge of a healing ulcer is pale pink and almost transparent.

A square-cut or punched-out edge This follows the rapid death and loss of the whole thickness of the skin without much attempt at repair of the defect. This form of ulcer is most often seen in the foot where pressure has occurred on an insensitive piece of skin, i.e. a trophic ulcer secondary to a neurological defect. The classic textbook example of a punched-out ulcer is the ulcer of tertiary syphilis, but these lesions are rare today in Europe. Most of the punched-out ulcers that are now seen are caused by the neuropathy of diabetes and peripheral arterial ischaemia or, outside Europe and North America, leprosy.

An undermined edge When an infection in an ulcer affects the subcutaneous tissues more than the skin, the edge becomes undermined. This type of ulcer is commonly seen in the buttock as a result of pressure necrosis, because the subcutaneous fat is more susceptible to pressure than the skin; but the classic textbook example is the tuberculous ulcer – which is now uncommon in Europe and North America.

A rolled edge This develops when there is slow growth of tissue in the edge of the ulcer. The edge looks like the heaped-up mound around an ancient Roman earthwork. A rolled edge is typical, and almost diagnostic, of a basal cell carcinoma (rodent ulcer). The edge is usually pale pink or white, with clumps and clusters of cells visible through the paper-thin superficial covering of squamous cells. Telangiectases are commonly seen in the pearly edge.

An everted edge This develops when the tissue in the edge of the ulcer is growing so rapidly that it spills out of the ulcer to overlap the normal skin. An everted edge is typical of a carcinoma and is seen in all those organs where carcinomata occur – the skin, in the bowel, in the bladder and in the respiratory tract.

Depth

Record the depth of the ulcer in millimetres, and anatomically by describing the structures it has penetrated or reached.

Discharge

The discharge from an ulcer may be serous, sanguinous, serosanguinous or purulent. There may be a considerable quantity of discharge which is easily visible, or it may only be apparent from inspection of the patient's dressings, and you may not be able to see the features of the ulcer at all if it is covered with coagulated discharge (a scab). This may have to be removed to examine the ulcer properly. **Students should not do this without the permission of the doctor in charge of the patient.**

Relations

Describe the relations of the ulcer to its surrounding tissues, particularly those deep to it. It is important to know if the ulcer is adherent or invading deep structures such as tendons, periosteum and bone – which may indicate the presence of osteomyelitis.

The local lymph glands must be carefully examined. They may be enlarged because of secondary infection or secondary tumour deposits and they may be tender.

State of the local tissues

Pay particular attention to the local blood supply and innervation of the adjacent skin. Many ulcers in the lower limbs are secondary to vascular and neurological disease. There may also be evidence of previous ulcers that have healed.

General examination

This is very important because many systemic diseases as well as many skin diseases present with skin lesions and ulcers. Examine the whole patient with care, looking especially at their hands and facies, which can supply important clues to the diagnosis.

2

The symptoms, signs and emergency management of major injuries

This is the only chapter in this book that contains advice about management. To describe the relatively small number of symptoms and signs that accompany the failure of the body's life-supporting systems without describing how, in emergency circumstances, these system failures should be treated from the moment the signs of failure are observed would be pointless. Furthermore, medical students, even in their early years of learning the basic clinical symptoms and signs of disease, are expected by the general public to know how to administer emergency first-aid measures to an injured patient.

The physical signs produced by injury are usually more evident and immediately significant than their history, *especially if the patient is unconscious*. Obtaining the history of the type of injury and the possible forces involved, including information on the injured person's habits, such as drug or alcohol addictions, from the patient, family members, friends, onlookers or first-aiders who witnessed the event is always helpful but must not interfere with the initial rapid clinical assessment and resuscitation.

Worldwide adoption of the principles enunciated in the Advanced Trauma Life Support course (ATLS) has established the value of a standardized approach to trauma assessment and management, especially in patients who have sustained injuries to more than one of their systems. This chapter follows the ATLS approach.

Some injured patients are brought directly to the accident and emergency department by ambulance, some severely injured patients may be brought in by private vehicles, or even walk into hospital, others may be given treatment at the site of the event. Even when an initial assessment has been made at the site

of the event, it must be repeated in the hospital. When ambulance staff are involved, they may radio ahead and warn of their casualty's likely injuries, a measure that allows the trauma team to be alerted and immediately available. Patients presumed to have sustained major injuries should be taken straight to the resuscitation area for their primary hospital survey.

Even patients thought to have minor injuries should be carefully assessed by an experienced nurse or doctor as soon as possible, as apparently stable patients may have sustained serious injuries, which may have passed undetected during the initial assessment, especially when an influx of many injured patients overwhelms local resources.

THE PRIMARY SURVEY AND MANAGEMENT AT THE SITE OF THE EVENT: FIRST-AID

This is carried out under the three easily remembered headings of **A**, **B**, **C**, i.e.:

- **A**irway
- **B**reathing
- **C**irculation.

This approach is particularly important when assessing patients with multiple injuries.

Airway

The signs of an obstructed airway are **cyanosis** (blue), **apnoea** (not breathing) and **stridor** (a rasping noise on respiration).

It is essential to protect and secure an adequate airway. The lungs cannot oxygenate the blood if the airway is obstructed by the jaw and tongue falling back, swollen soft tissues, direct damage to the upper airway, false teeth, vomitus or blood.

The airway of unconscious patients lying on their back often becomes obstructed by their own intra-oral soft tissues, but before they are rolled into the supine or semi-prone position, or the neck extended, always consider, and if possible exclude, an associated cervical spinal injury

All patients found to be unconscious after an injury must be assumed to have an associated injury of their cervical spine because abrupt or careless turning may further dislocate or sublux a cervical vertebra and injure the spinal cord when no injury existed, or turn partial cord damage into a complete transection. The neck should therefore be immobilized in all unconscious injured patients by longitudinal, manual support, the application of a hard collar and the use of stabilizing sand bags and tape before turning the patient onto their side, until clinical examination and radiographs have excluded unstable fractures of the cervical spine.

Compromises are inevitable if an immobilizing collar is not available at the site of injury. The presence of two first-aiders may allow one to support the neck while the other assesses and manually clears the airway, feels the neck and jaws, and assesses the respiratory effort by palpating the chest during respiration.

Airway obstruction is often relieved by lifting the jaw upwards, but may only be relieved by inserting a finger in the mouth and pulling the jaw or palate forward, especially when the obstruction is associated with a fractured maxilla or mandible.

An oropharyngeal or nasopharyngeal airway should be inserted as soon as possible, and then, in an unconscious patient, replaced by an endotracheal tube, inserted by an experience anaesthetist, because the absence of a gag reflex in an unconscious patient makes aspiration of saliva, vomitus or blood into the lungs a major hazard.

Breathing

If the patient remains cyanosed or apnoeic after the airway has been cleared, mouth-to-mouth resuscitation should be started immediately. This is easier and safer (from risks of cross-infections) if a Brook's airway, a facemask, an Ambu bag and oxygen are available. Mouth-to-mouth ventilation combined with external cardiac massage may, however, be life saving in patients who have undergone a short period of respiratory arrest.

There are few indications for heroic attempts at inserting home-made 'tracheostomy' devices at the scene of the accident. The patients are probably better served by a rapid transfer to hospital by experienced ambulance staff who have been trained in resuscitation techniques.

Circulation

It is absurd to concentrate on the detailed drills of assessment of the airway and breathing if the patient obviously has a normal airway and no neck injuries but is losing vast amounts of blood – even to the point of literally bleeding to death. Severe external bleeding at the scene of the accident requires manual compression directly over the wound or pressure proximal to the point of bleeding, where the feeding artery can be compressed against an underlying bony point.

Tourniquets should only be used to stop distal limb bleeding. They rarely work efficiently and often exacerbate bleeding by obstructing the venous outflow, while failing to occlude the arterial inflow.

An effective tourniquet makes the whole limb ischaemic and will cause permanent muscle and nerve damage if it is kept in place for more than 1.5 to 2 hours. Tourniquets can also theoretically cause re-perfusion problems when released – metabolic acidosis, myoglobulinuria and hypercalcaemia. Nevertheless a tourniquet can sometimes be life saving if it is applied at the correct pressure to a mangled bleeding limb for a short period. **The time of application must be carefully recorded and passed on to ambulance and medical staff.**

Direct manual pressure, provided it is achieving its desired effect (i.e. stopping or reducing the blood loss), is usually preferable to a tourniquet. This can be very tiring because it must be maintained until the patient reaches the hospital's accident and emergency department.

General first-aid advice

First-aiders should ensure that there is no immediate danger to themselves before approaching a casualty.

Many injured patients are best served by leaving them where they are until experienced help arrives, provided the environment is not continuing to damage or threaten them. Provided the injured patient has a strong pulse, is breathing normally and is not overtly bleeding, this is invariably the correct course of action. Patients should only be moved if there is a risk of further injury from leaving them where they are, e.g. inside a burning car.

It is, of course, important to obtain help as soon as possible so that there is always someone available to stay with the patient to monitor their pulse and breathing and provide moral support. The widespread availability of mobile phones has improved the first-aider's ability to summon help.

Under no circumstances should an injured patient be given anything to eat or drink.

THE PRIMARY SURVEY IN THE ACCIDENT AND EMERGENCY DEPARTMENT

All patients who are unconscious or suspected of having multiple or serious injuries should be admitted directly to the resuscitation area of the accident and emergency department. While medical students are rarely required to have an active role in the management of acute trauma, the opportunity to witness assessment and resuscitation in this setting is extremely valuable, as the principles of the process are relevant to many other areas of medical practice.

The clinical assessment (history and examination) and resuscitation must occur simultaneously if lives are to be saved, hence the inclusion of treatment in this chapter.

The routine A, B, C assessment must be repeated whatever happened before the hospital admission.

Airway

The neck must be protected by a collar and immobilized fully using sand bags and tape. An anaesthetist should assess the need for better control of the airway.

Look for the signs of inadequate oxygenation

Respiratory distress, apnoea, cyanosis, loss of consciousness and the presence of **major facial, neck or chest injuries that might obstruct the airway** may all indicate the need for endotracheal or nasogastric intubation once the neck has been stabilized.

Look for the signs of inadequate ventilation

The chest should be uncovered and palpated to assess **respiratory movements**. Confirm the presence of **air entry** into the lungs with a stethoscope.

The neck and jaws should be palpated to check for deformity. Insert a finger into the mouth to extract any foreign bodies and to check for jaw fractures. Occasionally severe damage to the upper airways or trachea makes intubation impossible. An emergency tracheostomy is indicated if the patient is deeply cyanosed or apnoeic and an endotracheal tube cannot be inserted safely.

Breathing

Assess the condition and function of the thoracic cage

Once you are certain that the airway is patent, assess the adequacy of ventilation by inspecting, palpating, percussing and listening to the chest for **symmetry, movement, dullness** and **breath sounds**. Patients with multiple injuries or chest problems causing hypoxia should be given high-flow oxygen through a closed circuit oxygen mask from the moment of their arrival in the accident and emergency department. An oxygen saturation monitor placed on an extremity is a valuable means of assessing the effectiveness of the patient's ventilation.

Inspection and palpation

The presence of **open wounds** or **flail segments** in the chest indicates the need for a chest drain and positive-pressure ventilation. A flail segment occurs when several ribs are fractured in two places. The flail segments sink inwards during inspiration. **Bruising** over the chest indicates that rib fractures are likely, and the presence of **surgical emphysema** suggests that the pleura has been breached. Surgical emphysema presents as a crackling sensation in the subcutaneous tissues. A 'sucking' chest wound may be present.

Percussion

A **tension pneumothorax** must be suspected if breathing is difficult, the **trachea is deviated** to the contralateral side and if there is decreased air entry over the affected lung. Although the clinical diagnosis will have to be confirmed with a chest radiograph, a chest drain should be inserted on the evidence of the clinical signs if the patient is unstable. **Bilateral tension pneumothoraces** are very rare, but cause severe cardiac and respiratory compromise, manifest as **cyanosis, severe air hunger, a weak pulse** and **hypotension**.

Remember that, with bilateral pneumothoraces, the trachea remains central but air entry is poor into both lungs. The rapid insertion of chest drains which are connected to under-water seal drainage bottles relieves the situation.

A large **haemothorax** also causes respiratory and circulatory problems, manifest as **reduced breath sounds** and a **dull percussion** note combined with **reduced vocal fremitus** and **vocal resonance**. The diagnosis should be confirmed with an erect or decubitus chest radiograph, but a chest drain may occasionally have to be inserted as an emergency measure on the basis of the clinical signs.

A large amount of blood draining from a chest may destabilize the patient and need urgent replacement into the circulation (see below), so intravenous lines should be inserted into both antecubital fossae before a haemothorax is drained. The chest drain may occasionally need to be clamped to prevent massive continuing blood loss. Lost blood should be replaced with a crystalloid solution at first, but subsequently with blood as soon as this is available (see below).

The blood pressure must be carefully and continuously monitored to confirm the adequacy of any blood volume replacement.

Flail segments rarely cause major problems initially but are indicative of a severe **underlying lung injury**. Both these problems are treated by endotracheal incubation and positive-pressure ventilation, but it must be remembered that this can cause a tension pneumothorax and may also make an existing tension pneumothorax worse. This complication should be suspected if the anaesthetist notices an increasing resistance to ventilation, a decreasing oxygen saturation and signs of circulatory embarrassment. Decreasing air entry and breath sounds indicate the need for chest drainage.

Circulation

Restoration of the circulation may take precedence over the airway and ventilation if the patient is breathing satisfactorily. It can be assessed simultaneously with the airway and breathing if an experienced anaesthetist is available to manage ventilation.

There are two major causes of circulatory embarrassment – cardiac damage/tamponade and haemorrhage. The former is rare but life threatening and easily missed. It must therefore be briefly considered in all patients with major injuries, especially in those with penetrating injuries of the chest.

Cardiac tamponade

Cardiac tamponade occurs when large quantities of blood collect within the pericardial cavity, around the heart, and embarrass its action. This reduces the cardiac output, producing a **weak pulse** and **hypotension**. The condition should be suspected if the **jugular venous pressure is markedly elevated and rises rather than falls with inspiration** (*Kussmaul's sign*); however, jugular venous distention may not occur in a patient who has lost a large quantity of blood.

Pulsus paradoxus, when the pulse volume decreases on inspiration rather than increasing, may be present. The heart sounds are usually muffled and poorly heard.

Chest radiographs may show an enlarged cardiac shadow. An echocardiogram will confirm the diagnosis.

The patient's condition may be stabilized by aspirating the blood from the pericardial sac using echocardiography and electrocardiography to ensure correct placement of the needle and catheter before definitive surgery is undertaken.

Revealed haemorrhage

Visible arterial bleeding presents as **a pulsating stream of bright red blood** coming from an open wound, whereas **venous bleeding is dark and continuous**. Arterial haemorrhage from an open wound can usually be controlled by direct digital pressure or proximal arterial compression. Sterile vascular clamps can be applied directly to bleeding arteries for temporary control before definitive surgery if these simple measures fail.

Venous bleeding always responds to simple pressure and may be made worse by the application of a tourniquet.

Revealed bleeding should always be assessed and controlled as soon as possible. There is no point in pouring fluid and blood into the circulation through intravenous catheters when an equal amount is rapidly escaping.

Concealed (internal) haemorrhage

Concealed haemorrhage is much harder to diagnose and therefore must be suspected in all patients with multiple or serious injuries. It always accompanies major fractures of long bones and fractures of the pelvis. It must, if possible, be rapidly diagnosed and treated, as it is an important, potentially irreversible, cause of death in an injured patient.

Clinical signs of haemorrhage

The diagnosis is based on finding the signs of hypovolaemic shock – **a pale, anxious, sweaty patient** with **cold extremities**, a **rapid, thready pulse, tachypnoea** and **hypotension**. These signs occur when the body redistributes the circulation in an attempt to maintain the blood flow to the vital organs (heart and brain). Other organs, such as the skin, intestine and kidneys, become inadequately perfused and poorly oxygenated. This homeostatic response is brought about by the sympathetic nervous system causing a tachycardia and vasoconstriction in the extremities. The skin becomes cool and clammy. The systolic blood pressure is usually maintained at first, but the pulse pressure (the pressure difference between systolic and diastolic pressures) may be reduced by a rise in the diastolic pressure. The rate of respiration increases to try to improve oxygenation.

Patients who arrive in the accident and emergency department without overt haemorrhage but who exhibit these signs have almost certainly lost 1–2 litres of blood. It is important to remember that young, fit patients can often tolerate considerable blood loss before they develop, often very suddenly, any signs of hypovolaemic shock, whereas elderly patients, especially those on beta-blockers or digitalis, tolerate quite small amounts of blood loss less well.

All seriously injured patients must have their pulse rate, blood pressure, respiratory rate, level of consciousness and tissue oxygenation monitored continuously. Patients with an associated head injury must be monitored using the Glasgow Coma Scale (see Revision panel 1.3, page 12). A urinary catheter and the measurement of central venous pressure provide additional valuable information for monitoring resuscitation when there are signs of hypovolaemia. An intra-arterial pressure line is also very useful for continuously monitoring the blood pressure, and allows easy sampling of arterial blood for blood gas and acid/base measurement.

Once blood loss is suspected, the patient must be given immediate fluid replacement through two wide-bore cannulae inserted into the veins of the cubital fossae. Fluid can be given faster through a central venous catheter if this has been inserted for monitoring purposes and is not contra-indicated by the presence of neck and chest injuries. One to two litres of crystalloid (normal saline) or colloid should be given *after* sending a sample of the patient's blood for grouping and cross-matching. For patients with clear signs of shock, request at least 4 units of blood.

Patients who fail to respond to the rapid restoration of their blood volume in the absence of cardiac or major respiratory problems, e.g. tamponade or tension pneumothorax, probably have severe continuing blood loss. In these circumstances the blood transfusion should be started while making a rapid assessment of the potential sites of concealed blood loss. The most common are the pleural or abdominal cavities. Fractures of the pelvis can also cause catastrophic blood loss.

The retroperitoneum can contain litres of blood with few external physical signs.

A rapid clinical examination looking for chest dullness, abdominal distension and abdominal tenderness (if the patient is conscious) should be followed by chest radiography, insertion of chest drains and computerized tomography (CT) scanning of the torso or peritoneal lavage where indicated. Properly warmed Group O Rh-negative blood or, as a last resort, uncross-matched blood can be given if the situation is dire. The patient should be transferred to an operating suite once the site of blood loss has been established.

Echocardiographs and electrocardiographs (ECGs) can be helpful if cardiac injury or coincidental cardiac disease is suspected. The ECG leads should be kept connected to a monitor for the detection of any dysrhythmias. A cardiac contusional injury should be suspected if there is widespread ST segment elevation or depression. Very occasionally, an emergency thoracotomy in the accident and emergency department may be required to relieve a tamponade, to suture a penetrating wound of the heart or to clamp the hilum of the lung or the descending aorta to prevent massive blood loss.

These heroic attempts are seldom successful. Rapid transfer to an operating theatre with trained staff, proper instruments and adequate lighting increases the chances of success.

THE SECONDARY SURVEY

Many injured patients do not deteriorate catastrophically. The majority stabilize rapidly after being resuscitated with intravenous fluids. This favourable response provides time to carry out a full secondary survey to assess other systems and body parts which may have been injured and to assess the general fitness of the patient. It is important to continue monitoring the patient while the secondary survey is being carried out to detect any further or new bleeding or chest problems.

The whole patient must be examined from the top of the head to the toes. Other blood tests, investigations and diagnostic procedures should be undertaken as necessary after the secondary survey is complete. Adequate analgesia may be needed before beginning the secondary survey, especially in fully conscious patients in whom the primary survey and resuscitation have been quickly completed.

History

A detailed history should be taken from a stable, conscious patient at this stage. It is helpful to ask the patient what they remember of the accident and useful if they can describe what happened. The mechanism of the injury and the possible physical forces involved often give a useful indication of the site and severity of the damage. Knowledge about the height of a fall, the speed of a car, the use of guns or knives, the presence of an explosion or fire and the use of protection devices such as seat belts or airbags is often helpful. If the patient is unconscious, obtain the observations and views of family, friends, bystanders or paramedics.

Pain, dysfunction and malfunction

The conscious patient should be asked if they have any localized areas of pain or malfunction, which may indicate particular areas or systems that require more detailed examination.

Conscious patients must also be asked if they had experienced any loss of consciousness during or after the injurious event. Their cognitive function should be quickly tested by asking a few questions about who they are, where they live and their occupation. The history from a third party of a lucid interval is also helpful if the patient is unconscious.

General and previous history

Take a full history of previous illnesses, operations, drugs and allergies (see Chapter 1). The patient's general fitness, occupation, tobacco and alcohol usage should be recorded following a full systematic enquiry.

Record the time that the patient last ate or drank. This is very important if the patient is to have a general anaesthetic.

General examination of a conscious patient

The head

Scalp The scalp must be inspected and palpated for lacerations, swellings, bony depression and distortion.

Orbits Palpate the margins of the orbits for depressions or irregularities.

Eyes Examine the eyes for pupil size, reaction and red-reflex. Test the eye movements and visual acuity (see Chapter 1).

Occasionally a corneal injury may lead to loss of the anterior chamber and prolapse of the iris, with an obvious collection of blood behind the cornea.

The presence of a large **subconjunctival haemorrhage** (see Fig. 8.17, page 229) that spreads to the full extent of the conjunctival attachment suggests that there is a fracture of the base of the skull. **Panda eyes** (black circumorbital haematomata around one or both eyes) (see Figs 2.1 and 8.17, pages 42 and 229) also suggest the presence of a skull base fracture or a fracture of the upper jaw. **Diplopia**, especially on looking up, is indicative of a blow-out fracture of the floor of the orbit, which often allows the eyeball to sink inwards, giving the upper face an asymmetrical appearance.

Signs of intracranial haemorrhage

A **fixed dilated pupil** which fails to respond to light indicates third nerve compression, by a contralateral

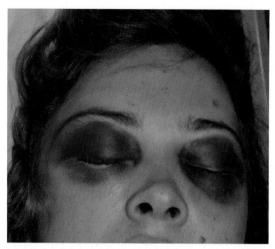

FIG 2.1 'Panda eyes'. Extensive peri-orbital extravasation of blood from a fracture of the base of the skull.

extradural haemorrhage or a direct injury to the optic nerve. Deterioration of the patient's score on the Glasgow Coma Scale – which quantifies eye opening, verbal response and motor response – and/or agitation indicate increasing cerebral compression. The patient is in 'coma' if their Glasgow Coma Score is less than 8.

Loss of upwards gaze, other cranial nerve pareses or developing contralateral hemiplegia are indicative of a cerebral haemorrhage.

Observations should also be made on the patient's mental state, including whether they are agitated or confused. A rising blood pressure, a falling pulse and slowing of respiration suggest **coning**, a condition in which the swollen brain is forced down through the medullary foramen, with subsequent loss of all vital functions. An urgent CT scan should be obtained.

The face Major facial injuries often cause considerable orbital oedema, but it is very important to retract the lids carefully, using two people if necessary, to look for any of the features described above. The cheek bones should also be palpated for a **'step'** and any asymmetry noted. Fractures of the zygoma and blow-out fractures of the orbit have to be confirmed by radiographs, but loss of sensation over the cheek from damage to the infra-orbital nerve strongly suggests a fracture of the cheek bones. Instability of the maxillary zygomatic process (a LeFort-type fracture) is tested by inserting a gloved

finger or thumb into the mouth and attempting to pull the upper jaw complex forward from the base of the skull. A fracture is present if rocking occurs. This needs to be done with care, as forceful rocking may cause a massive pharyngeal bleed, which can only be controlled by pushing the whole bony facial complex backwards to compress the bleeding vessels.

The lower jaw and its stability on the temporo-mandibular joints must also be assessed. Malocclusion and an open-bite deformity suggest a fractured jaw, as does numbness of the lower lip.

Carefully palpate and inspect the mouth, teeth and gums and record the number of missing or damaged teeth. Missing teeth indicate the need for a chest X-ray, if this has not already been performed, to exclude the possibility that they have been inhaled and are lodged in the lung.

The nose, face and ears The nose should be palpated to exclude a fracture and detect the presence of any bloody or clear fluid discharge of cerebrospinal fluid which would suggest the presence of a fracture in the anterior cranial fossa (often associated with panda eyes and an extensive subconjunctival haemorrhage).

The facial muscles (VIIth cranial nerve) and auditory acuity should be tested.

Blood or fluid coming from the ear suggests the presence of a posterior fossa fracture. The tympanic membrane must be examined with an auroscope. Bruising behind the ear (*Battle's sign*) (see Fig. 2.2) suggests a fracture in the posterior cranial fossa. Skull radiographs, specific facial views and CT scans are usually required to assess these injuries.

The neck The importance of not causing or exacerbating any spinal cord damage, especially during airway assessment, endotracheal incubation or moving the patient, is now well recognized. A full radiological assessment of the cervical spine should be carried out as soon as the patient is relatively stable if there are any concerns that the spine may have been damaged.

Pain and **local tenderness** are suggestive of a cervical fracture, but there may be few, if any, physical signs, and further assessment may have to be delayed until the condition of the cervical spine has been established. If the spine is normal, the neck can be carefully palpated for bruising and deformity

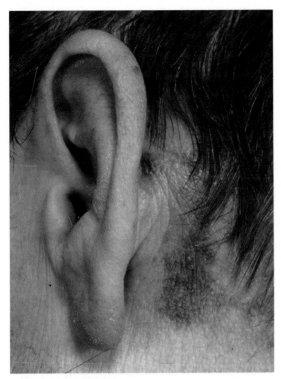

FIG 2.2 Battle's sign. Bruising behind the ear suggests a fracture in the posterior cranial fossa.

and inspected for any penetrating wounds. The position of the trachea in relation to the manubriosternal notch should be assessed to see if it is central.

Gentle palpation should detect the presence of any subcutaneous **surgical emphysema** in the neck or supraclavicular fossae.

Penetrating descending wounds of the root of the neck can be very dangerous, as they may cause damage to the supra-aortic blood vessels – the carotid, vertebral and subclavian arteries – as well as to the trachea, larynx, pharynx and oesophagus. Major structures within the upper chest can also be damaged. The presence of neurological signs or ischaemia of the upper limb suggests a major arterial injury, as does a rapidly expanding haematoma or a machinery murmur. Neck wounds should be explored in the operating theatre.

The clavicle should be palpated along its course. Severe **compound clavicular injuries** are often associated with injuries to the subclavian or axillary vessels, the brachial plexus and the apex of the lung.

Examine the vascular supply and peripheral nerves of both upper limbs to exclude these possibilities.

The chest Although the chest was quickly assessed as part of the primary survey, it should now be carefully re-examined by inspection, palpation, percussion and auscultation to detect any minor signs that may have been missed at the time of the initial examination and treatment when speedy resuscitation was essential. New signs may have developed and subtle signs may have been missed.

Test again for rib fractures. A careful inspection may detect a small flail segment. The chest should be 'sprung' by compressing it with both hands, anteroposteriorly and from side to side, and then quickly releasing. Pain on compression or release indicates the likelihood of rib fractures or costal cartilage separation from the ribs or sternum. Both can then be more accurately localized by detailed palpation. It should be remembered that rib fractures are often associated with injuries to the great vessels, lungs, spleen or liver.

The sternum must also be inspected and palpated. Sternal fractures are often associated with cardiac injuries.

Check again for the presence of a **haemothorax, pneumothorax** and **cardiac tamponade**, taking particular care to look for small pneumothoraces and an increase in the width of the mediastinum, which may be the only indication of an aortic dissection. A chest radiograph should always be obtained if there is any question of a chest injury. CT chest scans are even more accurate in detecting minor abnormalities and rib fractures.

The abdomen The primary survey of the abdomen usually detects the signs of major intra-abdominal haemorrhage, but a secondary survey is essential to pick up continuing severe haemorrhage or further bleeding following the restoration of a normal blood pressure.

Increasing **abdominal distension, tenderness** and **guarding** are all significant signs, especially when associated with a rising pulse and other signs of hypovolaemia.

The bowel sounds may or may not be abolished by free blood or bowel contents in the peritoneal cavity.

Skin bruising over the abdomen, penetrating wounds and associated rib fractures all indicate the possibility of abdominal organ damage. When doubt persists, ultrasound, CT scanning or peritoneal lavage may be indicated. A CT scan is very useful if there is an associated pelvic fracture.

Blood coming from the external urethral meatus or frank haematuria suggests kidney, bladder or urethral damage. Rectal and vaginal examination can confirm a high-riding and boggy prostate or associated vaginal injuries. The presence of these injuries must always be excluded before allowing catheterization by inexperienced junior staff or nurses. It may be preferable to insert a suprapubic catheter if palpation or percussion detects a large bladder, especially if the prostate feels abnormal or blood has been seen coming from the urethra.

Pelvic fractures are commonly associated with severe shock and with tenderness on springing the pelvis by pressing back on both iliac crests and releasing.

The upper and lower limbs All surfaces of the limbs must be fully inspected and the presence of bruising, lacerations, instability and deformity carefully noted. All the major bones should be carefully palpated along their full length to detect any bony deformity and swelling that were not appreciated by the inspection. The only indication of an undiagnosed, undisplaced fracture may be the detection of a localized point of tenderness. Major fractures are almost always associated with some deformity together with swelling from the associated bleeding.

The circulation Signs of hypovolaemic shock are common. The radial and pedal pulses should be felt and compared. The presence of equal symmetrical pulses indicates that a major vascular injury in the limbs is unlikely (see Chapter 7). Unfortunately, the peripheral pulses are often difficult to feel in a shocked, cold patient with severe limb bruising and concomitant fractures. When the pulses cannot be felt in an adequately resuscitated patient, it is helpful to measure the arterial pressure with a Doppler flow detector (see Chapter 7). Persisting pallor, especially if it only affects one limb, is a sign of severe ischaemia. The presence of a compartment syndrome must always be considered when there are combined bony and vascular injuries. This condition may also follow the successful surgical re-vascularization of an injured limb. Compartment syndromes begin with pain, tenderness and swelling over the anterior shin or calf muscles. The swelling can exacerbate the

ischaemia, obliterate the pulses and lead to muscle and nerve death if left untreated.

The nerves The peripheral nerves must be fully examined in both the upper and lower limbs if the patient is conscious. Test power, tone, coordination, sensation and the reflexes. Test the movement of joints controlled by the major muscle groups. Test sensation by the response to light touch and pinprick. Always test and document the peripheral nerves beyond any laceration. A more detailed neurological examination should be carried out if abnormal neurological signs are detected, or if the patient is unconscious (see below).

The back (thoraco-lumbar spine) The discovery of paralysis or weakness of several muscles may be the first indication of a spinal cord injury. The patient must then be carefully immobilized and 'log rolled' by a team of staff to allow examination of the spine. Log rolling allows turning of the patient in a coordinated manner that keeps the spine immobilized at all times. Detailed radiographs and even CT scans may be required if a spinal fracture or spinal cord injury is suspected. Palpation down the back over the spinous processes may detect a boggy swelling, deformity or a 'step' in the regularity of the spinous processes. While the patient is on their side, take the opportunity to inspect and palpate the back of the head, neck, torso and limbs to exclude any major injuries to this surface of the body which may have passed unnoticed at the initial survey. A rectal examination should be performed at this stage and peri-anal sensation, motor function and sphincter tone and the bulbo-cavernosus reflex tested.

The secondary survey in the unconscious patient

The secondary survey in an unconscious patient should begin with a reappraisal of the Glasgow Coma Scale to discover if the level of consciousness has changed from the initial assessment. This is important, as the whole purpose of resuscitation and assessment is to rectify factors such as hypotension or hypoxia that could cause neurological deterioration while trying to detect the presence of an intracranial haemorrhage, which can usually be treated effectively. Any suggestion of a 'lucid interval' – a period of consciousness after the injury before the patient became unconscious – is an important sign of a developing intracranial haematoma. Monitoring of the Glasgow Coma Scale must be carried out at frequent intervals in comatosed patients with a score of 8 or less. Patients must be frequently asked to open their eyes and move their limbs. If they do not respond, apply a painful stimulus by pressing hard on the bone of the upper orbit or the manubrium sterni. An ability to **localize pain** is accepted if the patient moves one or other hand to try to push away the painful stimulus, whereas flexion or, worse still, extension of the upper limbs indicates a severe brain injury.

Verbal responses are impossible to assess in patients who are anaesthetized, intubated or have suffered severe facial injuries. It must also be remembered that some head-injured patients may be mentally defective, some may have taken an overdose of drugs or alcohol, and some be unable to understand your language.

A detailed neurological examination should be carried out to discover if there are any focal neurological signs indicative of brain injury or an expanding intracranial haematoma. This should start with the examination of the size, symmetry and reaction to light of the pupils. If the brain is shifted to one side by an expanding haematoma, the **ipsilateral third nerve** becomes compressed against the rigid free edge of the tentorium cerebelli. At first this causes slight **constriction of the pupil**, but then, later, **dilatation** and eventually a **failure to respond to a bright light** being shone directly into it.

If left untreated, the haematoma will continue to expand and force the brain down through the tentorium and into the foramen magnum. The **contralateral pupil** then becomes **dilated** and **unreactive**. Eventually compression of the medulla causes **bradycardia**, a **rising blood pressure** and **depressed respiration**.

Do not forget that optic nerve injuries, previous eye disorders and drugs can also cause the pupil to be unresponsive.

Neurological examination of the limb should concentrate on detecting any evidence of hemiplegia. Unilateral paralysis, increased muscle tone, brisk reflexes and upgoing plantar reflexes on the contralateral side of the injury all indicate that a haematoma is present.

Intracranial haematomata outside of the substance of the brain develop in two sites.

- **Extradural haematomata** are usually the result of haemorrhage from the middle meningeal artery. This is often caused by a linear temporo-parietal fracture of the skull. Patients are often briefly knocked unconscious or dazed by the initial injury, but then regain consciousness (the lucid interval) before becoming drowsy and eventually losing consciousness. As the intracranial pressure rises, patients may complain of a **headache**, **blurred vision** and **vomiting**. At this time, the localizing signs described above begin to develop.

  It must be remembered that some patients develop an extradural haematoma without a lucid interval and without the classic progression of neurological signs. The certain indicator of deterioration is a progressive reduction of their Glasgow Coma Scale score. A CT scan will confirm the diagnosis.

- **Subdural haematomata** can be classified as either acute or chronic.

  Acute subdural haematomata are invariable associated with major brain injury when torn vessels on the surface of the brain continue to bleed into the subdural space. Patients are usually deeply unconscious and develop neurological localizing signs. It is very difficult to differentiate an acute subdural haematoma from an intracerebral haemorrhage, cerebral oedema or diffuse axonic injury. A CT scan of the head is essential.

  Chronic subdural haematomata usually occur in elderly patients after a minor injury which tears a vein on the surface of the brain that bleeds slowly but persistently for days or weeks. They are also common in alcoholics and patients on anti-coagulants. Patients often present with fluctuating levels of consciousness, worsening over several days or weeks. The raised intracranial pressure may cause **headache**, **vomiting**, **blurred vision** (papilloedema) (Fig. 2.3), **personality change** and **drowsiness**. Pupil changes and some neurological localizing signs are usually present. The diagnosis is confirmed by a CT scan of the brain.

Brain death

A number of patients with severe head injuries develop brain death or a persistent vegetative state. In brain death the brain stem is irreversibly damaged.

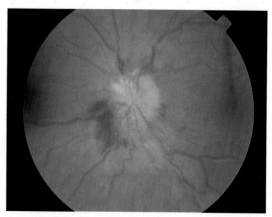

FIG 2.3 Papilloedema, a diagnostic sign of a chronically raised intracranial pressure most often caused by a space-occupying intracranial tumour or a chronic subdural haematoma. (Courtesy of Dr E Graham.)

In a vegetative state the brain survives but there is severe cortical damage. Patients with a persistent vegetative state can survive on or off a ventilator for many years. Recovery can occur after several months, but becomes increasingly unlikely as the months pass, especially if there are localizing or generalized signs of brain injury.

A number of criteria must be fulfilled to confirm brain death. Patients must be normothermic and off all drugs. Brain-dead patients are apnoeic and deeply comatosed. They have no pupillary response to light and the corneal reflexes are absent. They have no response to pain or to movement of the endotracheal tube when off all sedation. The final test is to look for the presence of a caloric vestibulo-ocular response.

The external auditory meatus is syringed with ice-cold water, which normally causes nystagmus. When this does not occur, brain death is confirmed and relatives must be appropriately counselled. Brain-dead patients are the main source of organs for transplantation.

Assessment of multiple casualties

All hospitals should have a major accident plan in which the roles of accident and emergency doctors, other medical staff, nurses, theatres, telephone staff, managers and press liaison officers are all clearly defined. These plans should be tested from time to time to assess their effectiveness and encourage familiarity. Each patient must be carefully assessed by the techniques described above into dead, immediate life-threatening injuries, those with major injuries and those who can be called the 'walking wounded'.

Scoring systems

There are a number of scoring systems which have been developed to try to improve management and outcome of patients who have been injured. These allow the results of individual centres to be compared against one and other. The **Revised Trauma Score** is probably the best measure. It allows an audit of outcome against expected recovery or likely death. Any variation from the expected outcome should be critically examined to discover if earlier diagnosis or more efficient resuscitation or treatment would have achieved a better result.

3

The skin and subcutaneous tissues

The skin is the organ that controls body temperature and fluid balance as a consequence of its barrier function (impeding water loss) and sweat glands, which are capable of increasing or decreasing the loss of water and electrolytes and body heat.

The skin consists of two layers: the epidermis, derived from ectoderm, and the dermis, derived from the mesoderm.

The epidermis

The epidermis is a stratified squamous epithelium composed of four layers:

- basal cells
- prickle cells
- granular cells
- keratin (horny layer).

Keratin, which consists of dead epidermal cells, acts as a protective coat. Increased mitoses occur in the basal layer if the keratin layer is lost, so greater amounts of keratin are produced in response to friction or pressure.

Melanoblasts, derived from the neural ectoderm of the anterior horn cells, migrate into the basal layers of the epidermis. They produce the pigment melanin in response to a number of stimuli and transfer this to the nearby keratinocytes through their dendritic processes.

Langerhans cells are also present in the epidermis and are part of the monocyte macrophage system, which processes antigen.

Merkel cells are mechano-receptors present in the epidermis.

Hair and **nails** are derived from modified keratin by invagination of the epidermis.

The dermis

The dermis is made up of collagen bundles and various proteoglycans which form a supporting framework for blood vessels, lymphatics, nerves, sebaceous glands, sweat glands and hair follicles. The dermis also contains **histiocytes** and **mast cells**, which can act as antigen-presenting cells and are part of the reticulo-endothelial system.

The dermis is subdivided into the capillary dermis and the deeper reticular dermis which sits on the deep fascia.

THE DIAGNOSIS OF SKIN CONDITIONS

There are many skin problems that require surgical treatment and form an important part of general surgical practice. This chapter concentrates on the common skin problems that are likely to be seen in a surgical clinic.

It is difficult to draw up a set of simple diagnostic pathways suitable for all skin lesions because they have such varied features. For example, a basal cell carcinoma can be a raised nodule, a flat plaque or an ulcer, and can be skin coloured, pearly white, brown or pink. It is therefore better to learn the physical features of each skin lesion, and the best way to do this is by examining as many as you can. The diagnosis of skin lesions relies heavily on careful inspection and pattern recognition. Tactile and auditory skills are less important.

When you are familiar with the physical features of the common skin lesions, do not use your knowledge to indulge in the game of 'spot diagnosis' – instant diagnosis after one brief glance. This is dangerous and likely to lead to mistakes. Always examine every skin blemish fully before making a diagnosis, however familiar the lesion.

Lesions in the skin have two basic distinguishing features: their colour and their relationship to, and effect on, the overlying epidermis. The overlying epidermis is likely to be raised and look abnormal if the abnormal tissue is in the superficial part of the dermis. An ulcer will develop if a localized area of the epidermis is destroyed. Alternatively, the overlying epidermis may be stretched but otherwise normal if there is an abnormality deep in the dermis.

It is possible, therefore, to subdivide all skin lesions into three categories:

- those with an intact but abnormal epidermis,
- those in which an area of the overlying epidermis is destroyed (ulcers),
- those covered with a normal epidermis.

Revision panel 3.1
The features of the history and examination of a lump or skin lesion that must be elicited

History
    Age
    Sex, ethnic group, occupation
    First local symptom
    Other symptoms
    Duration of symptoms
    Development of symptoms
    Persistence of symptoms
    Multiple or single lesions
    Systemic symptoms (direct questions)
    Possible cause
    Family history
    Social history
Local examination
    Site
    Shape
    Size
    Colour
    Temperature
    Tenderness
    Surface
    Edge
    Ulcer (*edge*: base, depth, discharge, surrounding tissues)
    Composition/contents:
        Consistence
        Fluctuation
        Resonance
        Fluid thrill
        Transluscence
        Pulsatility
        Compressibility
        Bruit
    Reducibility
    Relations to surrounding structures
    Lymph drainage
    State of local tissues (arteries, nerves, bones and joints)
General examination

Revision panel 3.2
The terms used to describe skin pathology

Macule	A localized change in colour of the skin which is not elevated (or palpable) or freckled
Papule	A small solid elevation, flat topped, conical, round, polyhedral, follicular (hairs), smooth or scaly
Vesicle	A small collection of fluid between the dermis and epidermis (a blister)
Bulla	A collection of fluid larger than a vesicle, under the epidermis
Wheal	A transient elevation of the skin caused by oedema
Cyst	A tumour that contains fluid
Naevus	A lesion present from birth, composed of mature structures normally found in the skin but present in excess or in an abnormal disposition. The term 'naevus' is also used to describe lesions composed of naevus cells, as in melanocytic or pigmented naevi
Papilloma	A benign overgrowth of epithelial tissue
Tumour	Literally, a swelling; commonly but inaccurately used to mean a malignant swelling
Hamartoma	An overgrowth of one or more cell types that are normal constituents of the organ in which they arise; the commonest examples are haemangiomata, lymphangiomata and neurofibromata
Ulcer	An area of solution of an epithelial surface

In the last of these, the bulk of the pathology is likely to be in the subcutaneous tissues, and even though it may be derived from a skin structure (e.g. a sebaceous gland), it is usually classified as a subcutaneous lesion.

The colour of skin lesions may be helpful in making a diagnosis. Skin lesions may be black, brown, yellow, red, or normal skin colour.

The following classification, based on the condition of the overlying epidermis and its colour, gives some idea of the multitude of lesions that you must learn to recognize.

Epidermis intact but abnormal

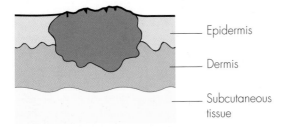

FIG 3.1 Epidermis intact but abnormal.

- **Black**
  Gangrenous skin
  Early pyoderma gangrenosum
  Early anthrax pustule
- **Brown**
  Freckles
  Seborrhoeic keratosis
  Moles of all varieties
  Malignant melanoma
  Pigmented basal or squamous cell carcinoma
  Café au lait patch
  Pigmentation following a bruise, thrombophlebitis, or venous hypertension (the epidermis may be normal in these conditions)
- **Greyish-brown**
  Wart
  Seborrhoeic keratosis
  Keratoacanthoma
- **Yellow-white**
  Xanthoma
  Lymphangioma
  Pustules of furunculosis and hidradenitis, subcutaneous calcinosis
- **Red-blue**
  Strawberry naevus

Port-wine stain
Spider naevus
Campbell de Morgan spot
Telangiectases
Pyogenic granuloma
- **Skin colour**
  Papilloma
  Early basal and squamous cell carcinoma
  Keloid scar
  Keratoacanthoma

Destruction of the overlying epidermis: ulceration

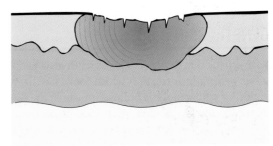

FIG 3.2 Destruction of the overlying epidermis – ulceration.

- **Sloping edge** A venous, ischaemic, trophic, neuropathic ulcer.
- **Punched-out edge** Ischaemic, trophic, or syphilitic ulcer.
- **Undermined edge** Chronic infection (tuberculosis, carbuncle), pressure sore.
- **Rolled or everted edge** Malignant ulceration.

Overlying epidermis normal

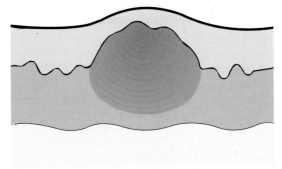

FIG 3.3 Overlying epidermis normal.

Although these lesions may have arisen from a skin structure, their mass is beneath the skin and does not affect its structure. They are usually classified as subcutaneous conditions.

Throughout this book each disease is described using the standard plan of history taking and examination presented in Chapter 1. These headings appear regularly because repetition is the secret of learning. Revise the plan of history taking and clinical examination set out in Revision panel 3.1.

CONGENITAL SKIN DISORDERS

These may be genetic or non-genetic. The latter are more common and mostly hamartomata, i.e. tumour-like malformations in which there is an overgrowth of normal tissues arranged in an irregular fashion.

GENETIC SKIN DISORDERS

Rare genetic skin disorders such as **ichthyosis** (a disorder of keratin formation which looks like lizard scales) or **epidermolysis bullosa** (in which the skin develops massive blisters after friction or minor trauma) are only likely to be encountered in a specialist dermatology clinic, whereas inherited neurofibromatosis is not rare.

Von Recklinhausen's disease
(Multiple neurofibromatosis)

This is an autosomal dominant condition in which multiple neurofibromata are present at birth and increase in number. Patients may have just a few tumours or multiple tumours over the whole body surface. The tumours are benign and contain a mixture of neural (ectodermal) and fibrous (mesodermal) tissue. The condition is associated with a number of

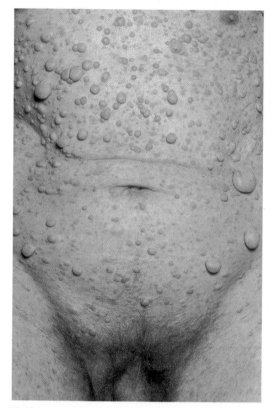

Multiple neurofibromatosis. The patient did not have a café au lait patch within the area of this photograph.

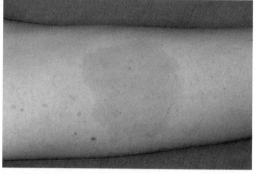

A café au lait patch on the forearm.

FIG 3.4 VON RECKLINHAUSEN'S DISEASE.

Revision panel 3.3
Congenital skin disorders

Genetic	Alopecia
	Ichthyosis vulgaris
	Epidermolysis bullosa
	Neurofibromatosis
	Plantar keratosis
Non-genetic	Hamartomata (e.g. capillary haemangiomata, lymphangiomata, venous angiomata)
	Dermoid cysts

related abnormalities, such as:

- fibro-epithelial **skin tags**,
- patches of light-brown discolouration of the skin (**café au lait patches**),
- neuromata on major nerves, especially the acoustic nerve (**acoustic neuroma**) and the sensory roots of the spinal nerves (**dumb-bell neuroma**),
- 5 per cent of neuromata undergo malignant change to a **neurofibrosarcoma**,
- **phaeochromocytoma** of the adrenal gland commonly coexist.

History

Most of the neurofibromata are present at birth but they increase in size and number during life. One of the patient's parents and half of their brothers and sisters are affected, as the disease is inherited through a dominant gene.

Examination

The patient is covered with nodules of all sizes, from minute lumps a few millimetres across to large subcutaneous nodules. Some are in the skin, some are tethered to it and some become pedunculated. The nodules vary in consistence from soft to firm, but each is distinct. They are often slightly pink. Careful examination of the skin nearly always reveals irregular patches of pale-brown pigmentation. The pigment is melanin and the patches are known as café au lait patches. They are a diagnostic feature of von Recklinghausen's disease.

The blood pressure should be measured as a coexisting phaeochromocytoma may cause hypertension. Neurological abnormalities are also common. It is important to test hearing and to examine the spinal nerves to exclude the presence of major nerve malfunction caused by neuromata on the acoustic and spinal nerves.

NON-GENETIC SKIN DISORDERS

Almost all of the following conditions are hamartomata.

Benign papilloma

A benign papilloma of the skin is a simple overgrowth of all layers of the skin. The word papilloma suggests that this lesion is a benign neoplasm, but this

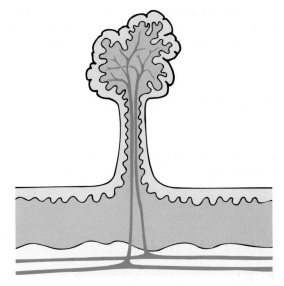

FIG 3.5 A papilloma is an overgrowth of all layers of the skin with a central vascular core.

is not the case; it is a hamartoma, and is better called a skin tag.

History

Age Papillomata can appear at any age. A few are congenital.

Symptoms The commonest complaint is that the pedunculated swelling catches on clothes or rubs against another part of the body. It can become red and swollen and ulcerate, or even infarct if it is injured. The skin that forms a papilloma contains sweat glands, hair follicles and sebaceous glands. All of these structures can become infected and make the papilloma swollen and tender. The swelling can look like a carcinoma if the granulation tissue that forms in response to the infection becomes exuberant.

Examination

Site Papillomata occur anywhere on the skin.

Shape and size Their shape can vary from a smooth, raised plaque to a papilliferous, pedunculated polyp. Their size is equally variable.

Colour They are the colour of normal skin.

Composition Papillomata are soft, solid and not compressible.

Lymph glands The regional lymph glands should not be enlarged.

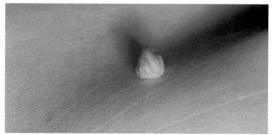

A smooth papilloma with a narrow pedicle, almost a fibrolipomatous polyp.

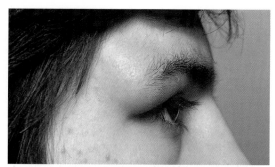

A right external angular dermoid cyst, so called because it lies beneath the outer end of the eyebrow over the external angular protuberance of the skull. This is a congenital dermoid cyst.

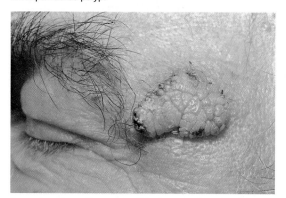

A sessile polyp with excess epithelium covering the clefts and corrugations.

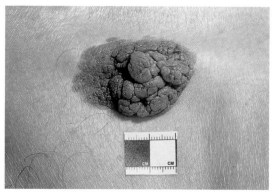

A deeply pigmented papilloma.

FIG 3.6 PAPILLOMATA.

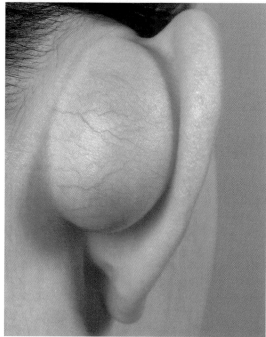

A dermoid cyst behind the ear. A congenital postauricular dermoid cyst.

FIG 3.7 DERMOID CYSTS.

Local tissues The adjacent local tissues should be normal.

Congenital dermoid cysts

A dermoid cyst is a cyst that is deep to the skin and lined by skin. There are two ways in which a piece of skin can become trapped deep to the normal skin: as an accident during antenatal development, and following an injury, which implants some skin into the subcutaneous tissue. Dermoid cysts are therefore congenital or acquired.

History

Duration The cyst may have been noticed at birth but it usually becomes obvious a few years later when it begins to distend.

Symptoms The principal 'symptom' is parental distress at the cosmetic disfigurement because most congenital dermoid cysts occur in the head and neck. Parents may also be concerned about the diagnosis. Dermoid cysts rarely become large enough to cause any serious mechanical disability and rarely become infected.

Multiplicity Congenital dermoid cysts are not usually multiple.

Examination

Site Congenital dermoid cysts are formed in intra-uterine life when the skin dermatomes fuse. They therefore occur at any point in the mid-line of the trunk, but are particularly common in the neck and face, along the lines of fusion of the ophthalmic and maxillary facial processes, and at the inner and outer ends of the upper eyebrow.

Shape and size They are usually ovoid or spherical and 1–2 cm in diameter.

Surface Their surface is smooth.

Composition Cysts on the face often feel soft, not tense and hard. They fluctuate, but will only transilluminate if they happen to contain clear fluid, instead of the usual thick, opaque mixture of sebum, sweat and desquamated epithelial cells. Large cysts conduct a fluid thrill and are dull to percussion. They are not pulsatile, compressible or reducible.

Relations Dermoid cysts lie deep to the skin, in the subcutaneous tissue. Unlike sebaceous cysts, they are not attached to the skin – or to the underlying structures.

HAEMANGIOMATA/LYMPHANGIOMATA
(See also Chapter 7)

There are many forms of cutaneous haemangioma, such as strawberry naevus, port-wine stain, spider naevus, vin rosé patch, and Campbell de Morgan spot. All are various shades of pink or red but each one has distinctive features. Once you have seen these lesions, you will always be able to recognize them. Many blanch on pressure.

Strawberry naevus

The name is an accurate description because this bright-red 'tumour', which sticks out from the surface

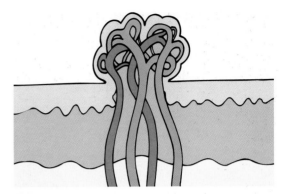

FIG 3.8 A strawberry naevus is an intradermal and subdermal collection of dilated blood vessels.

of the skin, looks just like a strawberry. The term 'naevus' is correctly used because strawberry naevi are present at birth. They are congenital intradermal haemangiomata.

History

Age Strawberry naevi are present at birth.

Sex They are equally distributed.

Duration They often regress spontaneously, a few months or years after birth.

Symptoms The child is almost always brought to the clinic by its parent because the red lump is disfiguring or a nuisance. Naevi that are rubbed or knocked may ulcerate and bleed. When they are on the buttocks they get wet and infected. More than one strawberry naevus may be present.

Examination

Site Strawberry naevi can occur on any part of the body but are most common on the head and neck.

Shape and size They protrude from the skin surface. Small naevi are sessile hemispheres, but as they grow they can become pedunculated.

Strawberry naevi are usually 1–2 cm in diameter, but they can become quite large (5–10 cm).

Surface Their surface is irregular, but covered with a smooth, pitted epithelium. There may be small areas of ulceration covered with scabs.

Colour They are either bright or dark red.

Consistence The strawberry naevus is soft and compressible but **not pulsatile**. Gentle sustained

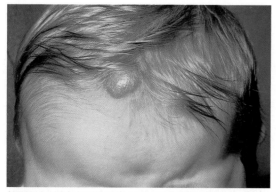

A large sessile strawberry naevus on the forehead.

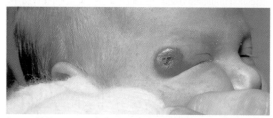

A regressing cavernous haemangioma.

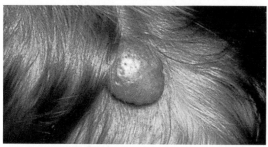

A close-up view of a strawberry naevus on the forehead showing the smooth epithelial covering and little pits which, with the red colour, make the lesion look like a strawberry.

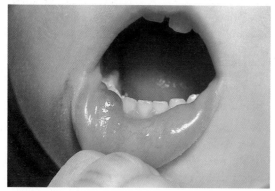

A haemangioma on the inside of the lower lip. These lesions are similar to strawberry naevi of the skin but are smooth and usually dark purple in colour.

FIG 3.9 HAEMANGIOMATA.

pressure squeezes most of the blood out of the 'tumour', leaving it collapsed, crinkled and colourless. The rate of refilling depends upon the number of feeding arteries.

Relations They are confined to the skin and are freely mobile over the deep tissues.

Lymph drainage The regional lymph glands should not be enlarged.

Surrounding tissues The blood supply of the surrounding skin is absolutely normal. This congenital condition is not associated with any other congenital vascular abnormality.

Port-wine stain

This is an extensive intradermal haemangioma, which is mostly made up of small venules and capillaries. It discolours the skin, giving it a deep purple-red colour; hence its name.

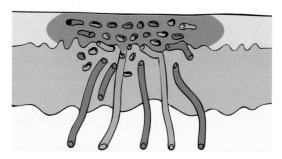

FIG 3.10 A port-wine stain is a collection of dilated venules and capillaries just below the epidermis.

History

Age Port-wine stains are present at birth and thereafter do not change in size relative to the size of the rest of the body, but their colour may alter.

Symptoms The distress these stains cause the patient's parents and the subsequent disfigurement noticed by the patient are entirely related to their colour and position. As they are often on the face, they are very noticeable. Occasionally, small vessels within the stain become prominent and bleed.

The port-wine stain may be part of a more extensive vascular deformity.

Examination

Site Port-wine stains are common on the face and at the junctions between the limbs and the trunk,

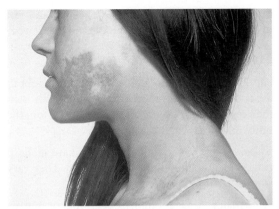

An extensive port-wine stain of the lower face and neck.

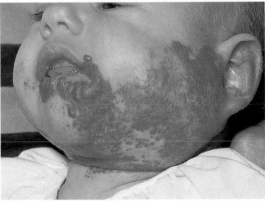

A mixture of strawberry and port-wine-stain naevi of the face, which is beginning to regress.

FIG 3.11 HAEMANGIOMATA.

i.e. the shoulders, neck and buttocks. Sometimes they seem to be confined to a single dermatome, especially when they are part of a generalized vascular deformity, but there are never any associated neurological abnormalities.

Shape and size Both are very variable.

Surface This is usually smooth, but vessels can be prominent and many bleed.

Colour Their distinctive feature is their deep purple-red colour. There may be paler areas at the edge of the patch. The colour can be diminished by local pressure, but pressure rarely returns the skin to its normal colour because all the blood vessels within the patch are abnormal.

Surrounding tissues There may be some dilated subcutaneous veins beneath and around the lesion. The sensory innervation of the stain is normal.

Venous angiomata

Venous angiomata are usually situated in the deeper levels of the subcutaneous tissues and can extend into muscles or joints (see Chapter 7), but there are usually some distended veins in the skin over the surface of the subcutaneous soft mass. These veins are usually irregularly aranged but empty with pressure. It is always wise to listen for a bruit, see below.

Spider naevi

A spider naevus consists of a solitary dilated skin arteriole feeding a number of small branches which leave it in a radial manner. It is an acquired condition and may be associated with a generalized disease.

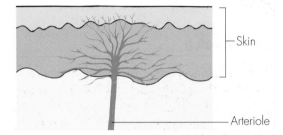

FIG 3.12 A spider naevus is a solitary dilated arteriole with visible radiating branches.

History

Spider naevi are not noticed by the patient except when they are in a prominent position on the face. They cause no symptoms. They are multiple and tend to increase in number over the years. It is important to enquire about the patient's consumption of alcohol because they may be associated with chronic liver disease.

Examination

Site Spider naevi appear on the upper half of the trunk, the face and the arms. It has been observed that this is the area of drainage of the superior vena cava, but it is doubtful if this is a significant observation.

Shape and size It looks like a little red spider. The central arteriole is 0.5–1.0 mm in diameter. The radiating vessels spread for a varying distance, usually 1–2 mm.

Colour The central arteriole is bright red and the vessels radiating from it are of a similar colour but not so red or so noticeable.

Temperature Spider naevi do not cause a change of skin temperature and are not tender.

Compressibility Spider naevi fade completely when compressed with the finger or, preferably, a glass slide, and refill as soon as the pressure is released. Compression of the central arteriole with the head of a pin makes the radiating 'legs' fade.

Local tissues There should be no other abnormalities of the local circulation.

General examination The general examination is important because spider naevi may be associated with serious diseases such as hepatic cirrhosis, tumours destroying the liver, and oestrogen-producing tumours.

Vin rosé patch

This is a congenital intradermal vascular abnormality in which mild dilatation of the vessels in the sub-papillary dermal plexus gives the skin a pale-pink colour. It is often associated with other vascular abnormalities such as extensive haemangiomata, giant limbs caused by arteriovenous fistulae (see Chapter 7) and lymphoedema.

A vin rosé patch can occur anywhere and causes no symptoms. It is not dark enough to be disfiguring and the patient has commonly accepted its presence as a minor birthmark and forgotten about it.

Campbell de Morgan spot

This lesion is a bright-red, clearly defined spot caused by a collection of dilated capillaries fed by a single or small cluster of arterioles. The cause of these spots is unknown and they are not associated with any other disease.

History

Age Campbell de Morgan spots increase in number with age. They are uncommon in people under the age of 45 years.

Duration They appear suddenly, usually one at a time, but sometimes a cluster of spots will appear in one area of the skin.

Symptoms They are not painful or tender, and not disfiguring unless they are multiple and extensive.

Examination

Site Campbell de Morgan spots appear on both aspects of the trunk, more on the upper half than the lower half. They occasionally appear on the limbs and rarely on the face.

Shape and size They are circular and have a sharp edge, which is sometimes slightly raised. They vary from 1 to 3 mm in diameter.

Colour They have a uniform deep-red or purple colour which makes them look like drops of dark-red paint or sealing wax just under the epidermis. This is their diagnostic feature.

Compressibility Although they are a collection of dilated capillaries, they do not always empty when compressed, but always fade slightly.

Lymphangioma circumscriptum

This is a circumscribed cluster of many small dilated lymph sacs in the skin and subcutaneous tissues which do *not* connect into the normal lymph system. The aetiology of these blind sacs is unexplained but, as they are congenital, it is likely that they are clusters of lymph sacs that failed to join into the lymph system during its development. Large, translucent lymph cysts confined to the subcutaneous tissues are called cystic hygromata (see page 281).

History

Sex Lymphangiomata are present at birth but may not be noticed until the skin vesicles appear a few years later. They are equally common in boys and girls.

Symptoms They are usually noticed by the child's parents, who consult the doctor because they are concerned about the 'lump' and the disfigurement it causes. Occasionally, the skin vesicles contain clotted blood, which turns them brown. Sometimes the vesicles leak clear fluid. When very prominent, the vesicles can be rubbed by clothes and may get infected and painful.

Development As the years pass, the subcutaneous cysts enlarge and become prominent and the number and extent of the skin vesicles increases.

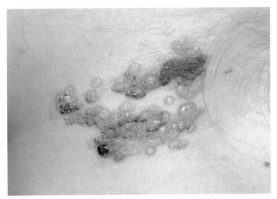

In this small, localized lesion, many of the vesicles are red, black or brown because they contain old blood.

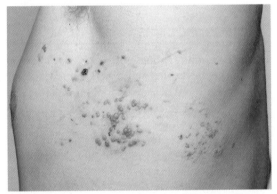

This extensive lesion spreads across the whole of the side of the chest just below the axilla. The swelling deep to the posterior part of the lesion is caused by the subcutaneous cysts.

FIG 3.13 LYMPHANGIOMATA CIRCUMSCRIPTUM.

Examination

Site Lymphangiomata circumscriptum are found at the junction of the limbs and the neck with the trunk, i.e. around the shoulder, axilla, buttock and groin.

Shape and size They may present as a single or multiple lumps.

A large area of skin may be involved – the whole of the buttock or shoulder may be abnormal – but most lymphangiomata are 5–20 cm across when they present for treatment.

Surface Their surface is smooth but their edge is often ill-defined and indistinct.

Colour The skin vesicles contain clear fluid which looks watery or yellow. Blood in the vesicles turns them red-brown or even black.

Overlying skin The subcutaneous cysts make the abnormal area bulge slightly, but the edges of this swelling are indistinct. The skin contains vesicles of varying sizes and colour, ranging from 0.5 to 3 or 4 mm in diameter.

Composition The whole lesion is soft and spongy. If the swelling is composed of multiple cysts, it will not fluctuate. If the swelling contains one or two large cysts, fluctuation, a fluid thrill and translucence will all be present.

The mass is not compressible. The dark-red or brown vesicles do not fade with pressure.

Lymph drainage The local lymph glands are usually normal unless the cysts have been infected.

Arteriovenous fistulae

These may cause a swelling in the skin or subcutaneous tissues, which may have a vascular appearance (see Chapter 7). The veins are also often distended but careful inspection may reveal pulsation, which is confined by palpation. Arteriovenous fistulae are not compressible but should have a loud machinery murmur situated over them providing that they have a high flow.

ACQUIRED DERMATOLOGICAL CONDITIONS

CONDITIONS OF THE SKIN CAUSED BY TRAUMA

Keloid and hypertrophic scars

An incised wound heals in three stages. First, the gap in the tissue is filled by blood and fibrin. This is then replaced by collagen and fibrous tissue which knit the tissues together. Finally, the fibrous tissue is organized to give the wound its maximum strength. This process, which is called healing by primary intention, is remarkably well controlled. Most surgical scars in the skin are thin lines containing the minimum amount of scar tissue. Sometimes, however,

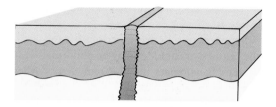

Normal scar

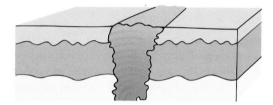

Hypertrophic scar

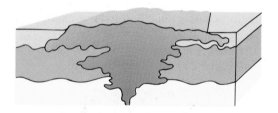

Keloid scar

FIG 3.14 Normal, hypertrophic and keloid scars.

the fibrous tissue response is excessive and the result is a hypertrophic or keloid scar.

In a **hypertrophic scar** there is an excessive amount of fibrous tissue but it is confined to the scar; i.e. it is between the skin edges. Hypertrophic scars are quite common, particularly if there has been some extra stimulus to fibrous tissue formation during healing, such as infection or excessive tension, both of which are common complications of scars crossing skin creases. Hypertrophic scars only enlarge for 2–3 months.

In a **keloid scar** the hypertrophy and overgrowth of the fibrous tissue extend beyond the original wound into normal tissues. This means that the scar has some of the characteristics of a locally malignant neoplasm. The tendency to produce keloid scars is a congenital trait, common in Negroes. Some tribes exploit the trait for the production of decorative scars on the face and trunk. Keloid scars continue to enlarge for 6–12 months after the initial injury. This is almost certainly the result of a local release of fibroblast growth factors, which are unsuppressed.

As a keloid scar grows, it can become exceedingly unsightly, is often tender to the touch and may itch. Although the cosmetic disfigurement of a hypertrophic scar may be as great as that of a keloid scar, it is important to try to distinguish the two abnormalities because hypertrophic scars do not recur after they have been excised if the causative factors are eliminated, whereas keloid scars will recur unless special measures are taken.

Callosities and corns

These conditions are known to everyone. They are areas of skin thickening and hyperkeratosis secondary to pressure and repeated minor trauma (see also Chapter 6). If the thickened skin is pushed inwards by constant pressure, e.g. on the sole of the foot or on the dorsum of the toes, it becomes painful and is known as a corn. Corns and callosities often occur over bunions and deformed toes.

History

Age Corns and callosities are more common in the elderly, not because their skin growth changes but because changes of the skeleton cause redistribution and maldistribution of weight bearing.

Symptoms Callosities may get rubbed and sore but are not usually painful. Corns are painful when pressed, because they are narrow and deep and may impinge upon deep structures.

Examination

A **callosity** is a raised, thickened patch of greyish-brown hyperkeratotic skin over an area of excessive wear and tear. Callosities are therefore common on the hands and feet, and their site varies with the patient's occupation and skeletal structure.

As they exercise a protective function, they are best left alone; but the diagnosis can be confirmed by carefully paring away the top layer of roughened skin to expose homogeneous, shiny, translucent layers of dead skin beneath.

A **corn** is a similar but smaller lesion that is pushed into the skin, thus forming a palpable nodule

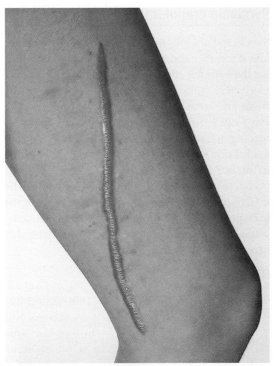

A hypertrophic scar on the medial side of the thigh following the excision of a large lipoma.

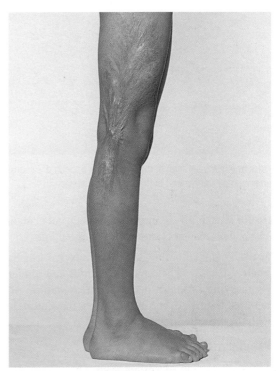

Hypertrophic scars after a burn.

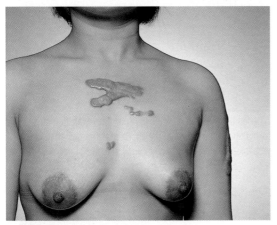

Keloid scars after tribal marking.

FIG 3.15 HYPERTROPHIC AND KELOID SCARS.

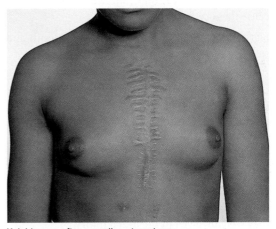

Keloid scars after a median sternotomy.

with a central yellow-white core of dead cornified epidermal cells. Corns are found on the soles of the feet, the tips of the toes and over the dorsal surface of the interphalangeal joints.

The main differential diagnosis is the **plantar wart** (verruca). These two lesions can be distinguished by paring away the top layers of skin with a knife to expose either the corn's core of dead translucent tissue, or the verruca's soft filiform processes.

Acquired implantation dermoid cysts

History

These cysts develop when a piece of skin survives after being forcibly implanted into the subcutaneous

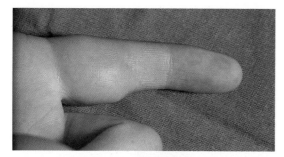

FIG 3.16 An implantation dermoid cyst that appeared 2 years after a small stab wound at the base of the finger.

tissues by an injury – often a small, deep cut or stab. The patient may not remember the initial injury.

Symptoms Implantation dermoid cysts are usually small and tense. They may be painful and tender because they usually occur in areas subject to repeated trauma. Cysts on the fingers may interfere with the grip and touch.

Examination

Site Implantation dermoid cysts are commonly found beneath skin liable to be injured, such as that of the fingers. Surprisingly, surgical incisions rarely cause these cysts.

Shape and size The cysts are spherical, smooth and small, about 0.5–1.0 cm in diameter.

Composition Implantation dermoid cysts feel hard and tense, sometimes stony hard. Their small size makes detection of their cystic nature – fluctuation and fluid thrill – almost impossible. The deduction that they are cystic usually depends solely on their shape.

Relations The overlying skin is often scarred. The cyst may be tethered to the deep aspect of the scar or even be within it. The deeper structures should be normal and the cyst freely mobile over them unless they were involved in the initial injury.

Lymph drainage The regional lymph glands should be normal.

Complications Implantation dermoid cysts rarely become infected.

Differential diagnosis The sebaceous cyst is commonly confused with the implantation dermoid cyst. The history of an old injury and the presence of a scar closely related to the cyst are the most significant diagnostic features.

Pyogenic granuloma

Small capillary loops develop in a healing wound to knit it together and provide sustenance and support for the covering epithelium. In the base of a healing ulcer these capillary loops form a layer of bright-red tissue known as granulation tissue. When the capillary loops grow too vigorously, they may form a protruding mass of tissue which becomes covered with epithelium. It is called a pyogenic granuloma because its surface is often ulcerated and infected, but it is probably neither pyogenic nor granulomatous. The infection is a secondary event and probably not the initiating stimulus. They are simply rapidly growing, sessile or pedunculated clusters of capillaries that become covered with epithelium.

History

Age Pyogenic granulomata are uncommon in children.

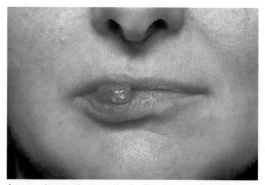

A pyogenic granuloma on the lip. This lump grew in 6 days following a minor injury to the lip. By the time this photograph was taken, the lump was covered with epithelium.

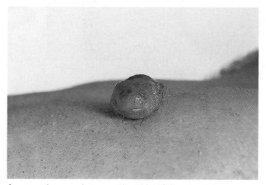

A pyogenic granuloma on the skin of the chest that appeared 4 days after a deep scratch.

FIG 3.17 PYOGENIC GRANULOMATA.

Symptoms There may be a history of a minor injury, usually a cut or scratch, but the patient cannot always remember the initial injury. Pyogenic granulomata sometimes occur in response to a chronic infection such as occurs in a paronychia.

The patient complains of a rapidly growing lump on the skin, which bleeds easily and discharges a serous or purulent fluid. So rapid is the growth of the lump (it may double in size in a few days) that most patients think it is a tumour. When it is completely covered with epithelium, the bleeding, weeping and pain stop.

Examination

Site Pyogenic granulomata are most common on those parts of the body likely to be injured, such as the hands and face.

Shape and size They begin as a hemispherical nodule which grows upwards and outwards. The lump is rarely more than 1 cm across because beyond this size the blood supply becomes inadequate. Growth from a few millimetres to full size can occur in a few days.

Surface Before the surface is epithelialized, it has a covering of dried blood or plasma. It may bleed when rubbed.

Colour At first they have the bright-red colour of healthy granulation tissue, but as they get bigger and less vascular they fade to a pale pink. When they become covered with epithelium, they turn pink or white.

Tenderness Although they are not painful, they are sometimes slightly tender.

Composition Pyogenic granulomata are soft.

Relations They are usually confined to the skin.

Complications They bleed easily when knocked. Very rough handling may break a pyogenic granuloma off at its base. The base rarely bleeds very much. The granuloma may reform in the next few days, or the bare area epithelialize normally.

Natural history Once the granulations have become completely covered with epithelium, the nodule begins to shrink, but it rarely goes completely.

Differential diagnosis The important conditions to exclude are squamous carcinoma, non-pigmented melanoma and, in some parts of the world, Kaposi's sarcoma. A history of trauma and the very rapid growth are the peculiar features of a pyogenic granuloma, but an excisional biopsy is often needed to confirm the diagnosis.

Fat necrosis

Necrotic fat becomes hard and fibrous. If the necrotic mass of fat is close to the skin, the skin becomes tethered or fixed to it and in-drawn.

In the breast, which is an organ that is frequently knocked and bruised, fat necrosis may be mistaken for a carcinoma. The buttock is also a common site of fat necrosis, particularly in patients who have frequent subcutaneous injections, such as diabetics.

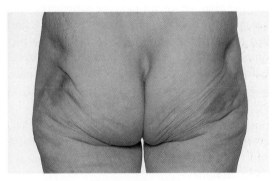

FIG 3.18 Fat necrosis of the buttock fat caused by repeated injections of insulin. Note the tethering, indrawing and pigmentation of the skin. Beneath these areas were hard, indistinct lumps of necrotic fat.

Ulcers

An ulcer is a solution of the continuity of an epithelial surface. Ulcers follow traumatic removal, or death and desquamation by disease, of the whole or part of an epithelium, and most occur in the lower limb.

Ulcers are discussed in this section on trauma because trauma is often the final cause of the skin breakdown, although there are many underlying causes that make the skin susceptible to injury and impede subsequent healing.

The features of an ulcer that must be examined and recorded are as follows.

The edge

The edge of an ulcer is the most important feature because it is the junction between healthy and diseased tissue and takes a characteristic form according to the underlying disease. There are five common types of ulcer edge (Fig. 3.19).

Sloping edge The edge slopes gently from the normal skin to the base of the ulcer. It is pale pink and consists of new, healthy epithelium growing in over the base of the ulcer. Healing ulcers have a sloping edge. The best examples are healing, traumatic and ischaemic venous ulcers.

Punched-out edge This edge drops down at right-angles to the skin surface to make the ulcer look as if it has been cut out of the skin with a punch. It indicates a localized, usually full-thickness, area of skin loss surrounded by healthy tissue. The best examples of this type of ulcer are the **deep trophic ulcer** and the ulcer left after a patch of gangrenous skin has sloughed. The condition causing the ulcer is limited to the ulcer and much less severe in the surrounding tissues, but sufficient to prevent healing. Ischaemic and syphilitic ulcers have this type of edge.

Undermined edge The disease causing this type of ulcer spreads in and destroys the subcutaneous tissues faster than it destroys the overlying skin. The overhanging skin is usually reddish-blue, friable and unhealthy. Tuberculous ulcers are usually undermined.

Rolled edge A rolled ulcer edge develops when an invasive cellular disease becomes necrotic at its centre but grows quite quickly at its periphery, so that it

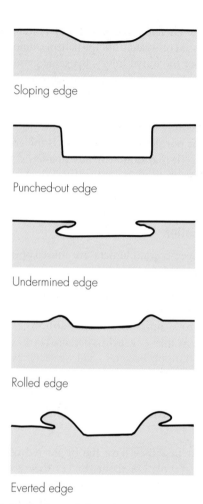

Sloping edge

Punched-out edge

Undermined edge

Rolled edge

Everted edge

FIG 3.19 The five types of ulcer edge.

rises above the surface of the skin. A rolled-edge ulcer is typical of a basal cell carcinoma. 'Rolled' is a poor description, but it is the best we have. The edge of this type of ulcer looks like the circular mound of earth found around an ancient fortification.

Everted edge When an ulcer is caused by a fast-growing infiltrating cellular disease, the growing portion at the edge of the ulcer heaps up and, in its malignant exuberance, spills over the normal skin to produce an everted edge. This appearance is typical of the squamous cell carcinoma and the ulcerated adenocarcinoma.

The base

The base of the ulcer should be examined carefully. It may be necessary to remove the slough before this can be done.

Revision panel 3.4 **Causes of ulceration of the skin of the lower limb**	
Venous	60% (half varicose and half post-thrombotic)
Ischaemia	20% (one-quarter have an associated venous cause)
Collagen disease	5% (rheumatoid and systemic lupus erythematosus)
Neuropathic	2%
Traumatic	1%
Neoplastic	1%
Many rare causes	5%
Unknown	10%

The base is likely to consist of three types of tissue.

Granulation tissue This is a red sheet of delicate capillary loops and fibroblasts covered by a thin layer of fibrin or plasma. It is the first stage of the healing process.

Dead tissue This is called a slough. When a slough separates, it may expose healthy tissues, which then become covered with granulation tissue or tissue becoming involved in the ischaemic process.

Tumour The base of a squamous cell carcinoma is the malignant tissue itself. It may be slightly vascular or necrotic but does not develop healthy granulation tissue.

Discharge

The discharge from an ulcer may be serous or serosanguinous, purulent, offensive, copious, or so slight that it dries into a scab. It should be cultured to ascertain the nature of any infecting organisms.

Venous ulcers

Venous ulcers are found in the lower medial third of the lower limb. Their site is a diagnostic feature. They are described in detail in Chapter 7.

Ischaemic ulcers

Arterial insufficiency is usually manifest at the ends of the limbs. It is rare to see ulcers caused by arterial disease at the base of the limbs or on the trunk. Ischaemic ulcers are described in detail in Chapter 7.

Trophic ulcers

A trophic ulcer is an ulcer which has developed as the result of the patient's insensitivity to repeated trauma. These ulcers are commonly associated with those forms of neurological disease which cause loss of the appreciation of pain and light touch in weight-bearing areas (see Chapter 7).

Neoplastic ulcers

The ulcers caused by basal and squamous cell carcinomata are described in detail later in this chapter.

When metastases from distant or underlying cancers appear in the skin, they may ulcerate and have features similar to those of a primary carcinomatous ulcer – an everted edge and a proliferating base.

Burns

The skin can be burnt by heat, irradiation, electrical or chemical noxious stimuli. A 'heat' burn is usually caused by direct flames, an explosion, contact with a hot object, steam or hot fluid. Burns caused by steam or hot water are called scalds. Most burns are the result of accidental household injuries, but previously rare causes such as self-immolation and torture are becoming more common.

Prophylaxis The fitting of household fire alarms and the use of non-flammable fabrics and fittings and sprinkler systems are all designed to try to reduce the incidence of household and place of work burns. Poor electrical wiring and gas leaks are potentially avoidable but continue to be a common cause of major burn injuries. Children and the elderly are particularly at risk: the young fail to recognize the hazard and the elderly are often unable to avoid it as a consequence of immobility and frailty. Education and safeguards are the best form of defence in these age groups.

First-aid Wherever possible, burnt parts should be immersed in cold water. This is easy after a scald of the hand but impractical if the whole body has been burnt. Chemicals should be washed off, and hot and damaged clothing removed.

Assessment and resuscitation As in a major injury, these two must proceed simultaneously. Intravenous access and fluid replacement are essential in any patient who has a sizeable burn, and cannulae should be placed in large veins in an area of unburnt skin. The size and depth of the burn must be carefully assessed. The burn size is measured as a percentage of total body area using the 'Rule of nines' (see Fig. 3.20). For a child, this must be modified – the head and neck being scored as 18 per cent and the lower limbs downgraded from 18 per cent to 12 per cent.

The depth of a burn used to be subdivided into six degrees, but nowadays the depth is usually categorized as being **partial** or **full thickness**.

Partial-thickness burns are further subdivided into **superficial** and **deep dermal** burns. The former are often blistered and very painful, while the latter are often pale with decreased sensation.

Full-thickness burns usually have subcutaneous fat visible in their base and are insensate.

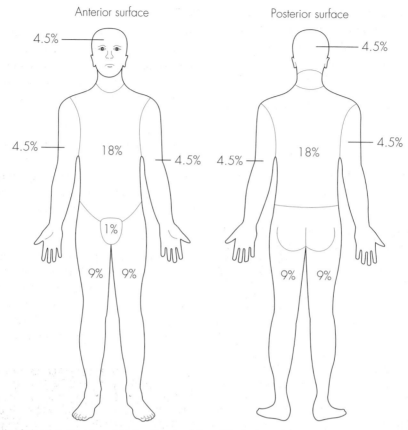

Anterior surface

Posterior surface

FIG 3.20 The 'Rule of nines' method for calculating the proportion of the body surface that has been burnt, viz. 9% for the head, 9% for each arm, 18% for each leg, 18% for the front and 18% for the back of the trunk.

A number of formulae exist for the calculation of the patient's early fluid requirement based on the extent and depth of the burn and the patient's age. These are beyond the scope of this book but it must be stressed that early and adequate fluid replacement is the most important initial treatment.

Clinical features

Pain The main problem is pain, especially in patients with superficial burns.

Skin sensation Sensation must be carefully tested whenever a full-thickness burn is suspected, and re-tested 24 hours later, when it may be easier to determine.

The airway It is important to assess the face, mouth and airways, as inhalation injury of their lining commonly accompanies extensive burns. Burns around the mouth, nose and lips should provide a high index of suspicion. The buccal mucous membrane and tongue must be inspected for mucosal burns.

Breathing Special attention must be paid to any circumferential burns of the neck or chest, as these may constrict breathing. The occurrence of stridor or a difficulty with breathing is an indication for intra-tracheal intubation and ventilation, especially if the patient is unconscious.

Circulation In addition to monitoring the airways, the state of the circulation must be repeatedly assessed, as burns are associated with massive losses of electrolytes and protein from their surface, and red cell damage or destruction.

The pulse, blood pressure, central venous pressure, urine output and haematocrit must be carefully monitored in all patients with major burns. Failure to maintain an adequate circulation may be followed by renal failure and eventually multi-organ failure. The latter is the complication that often follows septicaemia from secondary infection in and around the burns.

Circumferential burns of the limbs or digits may cause peripheral ischaemia.

Depigmentation This is a rare problem that can occur in black races after extensive scarring and burns.

Electrical burns

Most electrical burns come from faulty home appliances or the careless touching of electrodes. High-voltage burns, such as lightening strikes, with subsequent survival are uncommon because the depolarization usually causes severe cardiac arrhythmias and cardiac arrest.

A severe local burn develops at the point of entry, and adjacent nerves and muscles are often damaged. Deep tissue damage can lead to metabolic derangements, compartment syndromes, arterial and venous thrombosis and even visceral damage if the entry point is over the torso.

Radiation injury

The initial skin injury caused by radiation often resembles a standard thermal burn. The clinical evidence of the commonly associated lung and bowel damage and bone marrow depression appears later. Many patients exposed to high doses of radiation die from pulmonary complications or aplastic anaemia,

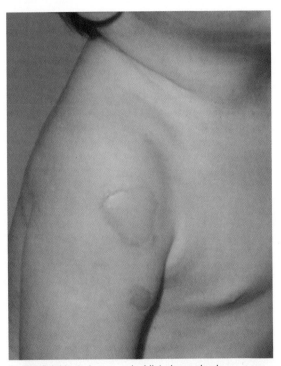

A superficial burn: hyperaemia, blistering and pain.

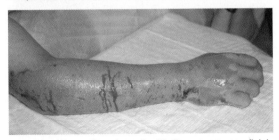

A partial-thickness burn: loss of epithelium, some superficial capillary bleeding and a few pale patches which may turn out to be deeper areas of destruction.

FIG 3.21 BURNS.

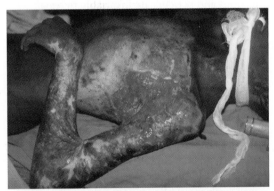

A mixture of partial-thickness and full-thickness burns.

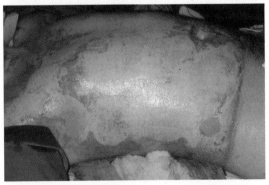

An extensive scald, probably mostly a partial-thickness burn.

and those who survive the early systemic effects may die later from radiation-induced malignant change in organs such as the thyroid gland.

Chemical burns

Most chemical burns are caused by contact with acids or alkalis; a few are caused by phosphorus and phenols. Chemical burns of the skin can be avoided by wearing protective clothing and washing off the contaminant as quickly as possible. They produce the same clinical appearance as full-thickness and partial-thickness thermal burns.

The *oral ingestion* of corrosive chemicals may destroy the lining of the oesophagus and cause life-threatening complications and serious long-term morbidity.

INFECTIONS OF THE SKIN

Skin and subcutaneous infections are common, especially when the skin is breached. The cardinal signs of rubor, calor, dolor, tumor are usually present in all infections and patients are invariably pyrexial.

BACTERIAL INFECTIONS

Impetigo

This is now a relatively rare condition. It is a staphylococcal infection that causes blistering of the hands and face. Vesicles form and rupture and are covered with a honey-coloured crust. They may form circinate or gyriform patterns. Fresh blisters form daily and may develop inflammatory halos. A microbiological swab should be sent for culture. Patients are usually referred to dermatology clinics.

Furunculosis
(boils)

Furuncles and boils are caused by infection entering a hair follicle. The infection first produces pus and then a central core of necrotic tissue.

When the lesion contains only pus it is called a furuncle; when it contains a solid core it is called a boil.

Boils are often multiple and associated with general debility, or an underlying disease such as diabetes. They can occur on any part of the body but are common in the skin of the head and neck, axillae and groins. They begin as a hard, red, tender area, which gradually enlarges and causes a throbbing pain. Eventually the tissue in the centre of the infected area dies and forms a thick yellow slough that will not separate from the adjacent tissue until it is surrounded by pus. When this happens the lump becomes fluctuant, the centre of the covering skin sloughs and the pus and necrotic core are discharged.

Hidradenitis suppurativa

Whereas boils are infections in the hair follicles, hidradenitis is an infection of the apocrine sweat glands. It is most often seen in the axillae and groins of Caucasians living in tropical countries.

The patient presents with multiple tender swellings in the axillae or groins, which enlarge and then discharge pus. The condition is made worse if there is an underlying systemic disease, such as diabetes. The site and the chronic recurring nature of this condition make it unpleasant and disabling.

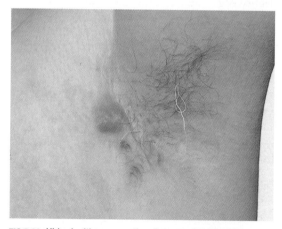

FIG 3.22 Hidradenitis suppurativa. One set of infected apocrine glands has already been excised from this man's left axilla, but another cluster has become red, swollen and tender.

Erysipelas and cellulitis

Erysipelas is an infection in the skin and subcutaneous tissues by a pathogenic *Streptococcus*. Whereas the *Staphylococcus* commonly causes a localized infection and pus formation, the *Streptococcus* spreads easily through the skin and produces a diffuse cellulitis. The erythrotoxins produced by the *Streptococcus* make the infected area red, hot, tender and oedematous. Oedema of the reddened skin gives the involved area a raised border – a diagnostic clinical appearance. The patient has a high temperature, tachycardia and general debility. Streptococcal infections rarely form thick pus.

Careful examination may reveal a source of entry for the organism, such as a small cut or a scratch. Erysipelas is especially common when there is pre-existing oedema caused by venous or lymphatic insufficiency.

Infection of the skin and subcutaneous tissues caused by other organisms, without the bright-red discolouration of the skin and the raised border, is called cellulitis. A patch of cellulitis may necrose and suppurate.

Erysipeloid

This is a Gram-positive coccal infection that is present in shellfish, meat and poultry. It commonly affects fishermen, fishmongers and butchers. It occurs in the hands, usually as a purple/red papule with a well-defined edge, and may spread to other fingers.

Anthrax

This is a spore-forming, highly resistant bacterium which is found in animal carriers and is present in wood, hide and bones. It causes a black, malignant-looking sore on the skin and patients may die rapidly from pulmonary complications.

Tuberculosis

Tuberculosis of the skin is a rarity. Primary tuberculosis of the skin produces a persistent ulcer with undermined edges. This is more commonly seen now in an unhealed BCG vaccination site. The associated lymph glands are enlarged and may suppurate.

Lupus vulgaris

This is the well-recognized cutaneous form of tuberculosis which often affects the head and neck of children. The skin is red, telangiectatic and scaly. When it is compressed with a glass slide it appears to be composed of pale yellow-brownish nodules (apple jelly). It is a slowly progressive lesion which causes massive scarring.

Syphilis

Syphilis is rare in the United Kingdom, although its incidence has slightly increased in recent years.

The **primary** sore, or **chancre**, is acquired by sexual intercourse, biting or kissing and develops between 3 and 6 weeks after inoculation. The common sites for chancres are the penis and the vulva, but they can occur on the cervix, lips, fingers, nipple or anus. A chancre is usually a 1 cm or less solid papular ulcer with an indurated base which can be lifted up like a button in the skin. Approximately 1 week after its appearance, one or more of the regional lymph glands become enlarged. Affected glands are not painful and feel rubbery. They are called **bubos**.

The **secondary stage** develops 5–6 weeks later if the primary condition is not treated. This is the result of organisms disseminating through the bloodstream. A widespread polymorphic rash develops which is not itchy and consists of macules, papules and scaly lesions. Patients often complain of **malaise, headaches** and **limb pains** when the rash begins. At first the macules are pink or copper-coloured and oval in shape with an ill-defined edge. They are widely distributed on the trunk, limbs, palms of the hands and soles of the feet. The papules have similar characteristics. The picture becomes more varied if the condition progresses untreated. The papules become florid and scaly and appear in groups, often with an annular pattern, which makes them look almost like psoriasis. This is associated with a generalized **lymphadenopathy**. **Enlargement** of the **epitrochlear lymph glands** is said to be characteristic.

Superficial erosions develop in the buccal mucosa. These may appear as tender, red patches. When they are covered by adherent mucus, they are likened to **snail tracks. It is, therefore, always important to look in the mouth and fold back the lips.**

Flat, moist plaques which are purple in colour may appear in the peri-anal and vulval skin, at the angle of the mouth and in any of the skin flexures (e.g. armpits and groins). These are called **condylomata lata**.

A patchy **loss of hair** often occurs in the late stages of syphilis, which gives patients a 'moth-eaten' appearance.

Tertiary syphilis begins 2–10 years after the initial infection. Serpiginous or arculate nodules may develop which are either scaly or ulcerated. These leave central scars which may be mistaken for lupus vulgaris (see above), though the latter is usually much more chronic in its development.

Gummata can also develop at this stage. They start as a small nodule in the subcutis but then enlarge and become red before ulcerating. The ulcer associated with gumma is discreet, **punched out** (see above) and characteristically has a **wash-leather** slough in its base.

Palmar hyperkeratosis is a rare association.

Leukoplakia of the mouth and tongue is another manifestation of the tertiary stage of syphilis. The epithelium appears thickened and white. This condition is potentially pre-malignant. Aortic aneurysms and tabes dorsalis are other important complications of the tertiary stage.

General paralysis of the insane eventually develops and is the **quaternary** (final stage) of syphilis.

Congenital syphilis is almost extinct in the home-born population of the UK because of routine serological screening in pregnancy. Affected children develop a bullous eruption on their palms and soles a few days after birth. The liver enlarges and they develop 'snuffles' from severe nasal discharge which obstructs the breathing. The bridge of the nose eventually 'caves in'. The long bones develop osteochondritis and periostitis, causing deformity.

Diagnosis The diagnosis of primary syphilis is usually made by scarifying the chancre, transferring the resultant discharge onto a microscope slide and examining it with **dark-ground** illumination for the presence of spirochaetes. There are a number of serological tests that are useful for detecting the present or prior infection.

Leprosy
(Hansen's disease)

This is increasingly appearing in all parts of the world because of the ease of air travel and shifts of large populations to seek asylum. It must always be considered in a patient from a tropical country presenting with an unusual rash. It is spread by prolonged contact.

The **'tuberculoid'** form is most commonly seen in the UK. The skin usually contains sharply defined asymmetrical areas of hypo-pigmentation with dry, scaly surfaces. Alternatively, there may be infiltrated, raised, hyperpigmented plaques with sharply

demarcated erythematous edges. These may resemble viteligo, but differ in that some pigment remains. These plaques or patches are insensate.

The **ulnar**, **peroneal** and **greater auricular nerves** are commonly thickened and easily palpable. Foot drop and ulnar palsy are common. Eventually, the insensate fingers are damaged by repeated trauma and disappear.

Patients with **lepromatous leprosy** have no resistance to the spread of organisms. The early skin lesions are small, ill-defined, erythematous macules which have a smooth and shiny surface. These become infiltrated to form plaques and nodules, especially in the face and pinnae. The polyneuritis described above is a late manifestation of this form of disease.

Diagnosis The diagnosis is made by biopsy and nasal scrapings, when the microbacteria may be seen within the granulomata consisting of epithelioid cells surrounding histiocytes and lymphocytes.

VIRAL INFECTIONS
Viral warts

Warts are papilliferous patches of overgrown hyperkeratotic skin whose growth has been stimulated by the human papilloma virus.

History

Age Warts occur at any age but are most common in children, adolescents and young adults.

Duration They grow to their full size in a few weeks, but may be present for months or years before a patient complains about them. Patients have usually made their own diagnosis and decided that there was no cause for concern.

Symptoms Warts are disfiguring. Multiple warts on the fingers can interfere with fine movements. They are only painful if they are rubbed or become infected.

Progression Once present, they may persist unchanged for many years or regress and disappear spontaneously. 'Kiss lesions' may appear on adjacent areas of skin that make frequent contact. Warts occur in crops and may come and go spontaneously.

Family history Other members of the family may have warts.

Examination

Site Warts are commonly found on the hands, but they may appear on other exposed areas that are frequently touched by the hands, such as the face, arms and knees.

Shape and size They arise as flat-topped, angular, smooth or hemispherical macules which are less than 1 cm in diameter.

Surface Their surface is rough and hyperkeratotic, and often covered with fine filiform excrescences.

Colour Warts are greyish-brown.

Composition Warts are firm and not compressible.

Lymph drainage The regional lymph glands should not be enlarged.

Differential diagnosis Squamous papilloma, molluscum contagiosum and condylomata lata are other conditions that may be considered in the differential diagnosis.

Plantar warts

Warts on the soles of the feet are fundamentally the same as any other wart, but they have a different appearance because they are pushed into the skin. They must be differentiated from callosities and corns (see description in Chapter 6, page 169).

Molluscum contagiosum

Discrete, pearly, rounded nodules with umbilicated centres are indicative of this infection. They are usually grouped in one area of the trunk. They release a white exudate when squeezed, which contains the virus.

Herpes simplex

This is the commonest skin virus. More than 60 per cent of the population are infected and remain carriers throughout their lives. The primary infection often passes unnoticed, but it may cause a severe gingivo-stomatitis with fever and local lymphadenopathy. The mouth often contains a crop of 'aphthous' ulcers. Vesicles may be present over the face, neck and even the eyes. The attack subsides in 10–14 days, but the virus remains latent in the epithelial cells of the buccal and nasal mucosa. The micro-organisms may proliferate again in response to a noxious stimulus such as a fever, sunlight, pneumonia or immune suppression.

History

Patients usually complain of a painful localized sore on their lip which develops blisters that discharge and then crust over.

Examination

Site Most lesions occur at the mucocutaneous junctions, particularly on the lips and angle of the mouth, but they may appear on the nail clefts, trunk, genitalia, cheeks and natal cleft.

Shape and size A burning, uncomfortable papule develops which is usually oval or elliptical. It is slightly raised and very tender.

Surface The papular surface is smooth at first but becomes covered in a crop of small vesicles which break to leave a crust. This heals in 7–10 days and the skin returns to normal.

Lymph drainage The draining lymph glands are rarely enlarged.

Herpes zoster

This skin rash is thought to be caused by reactivation of the chickenpox virus, which can lie dormant

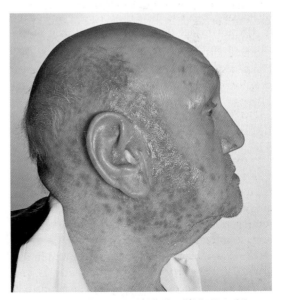

FIG 3.23 Shingles (herpes zoster) in the distribution of the mandibular nerve.

for many years in the anterior horn cells of the spinal cord.

History

Age It usually occurs after the age of 45 years.

Onset It can develop within a week of re-exposure to the varicella virus. Reactivation can be the result of tuberculosis or tumour.

Symptoms Pain occurs over the distribution of the nerve roots involved *before* the rash develops.

Examination

Site The rash can occur in any cutaneous dermatome or dermatomes. It appears in a continuous line or as patches throughout these segments. The trigeminal nerve may be involved, and if the virus enters the ophthalmic branch, the eye will be affected.

Rash Initially, there is a raised patch of erythema which rapidly becomes covered with a cluster of umbilicated vesicles. These quickly become infected and haemorrhagic before necrotic crusts form. There may be severe photophobia, with a red, watering eye if the ophthalmic division of the trigeminal nerve is involved.

Resolution The pain improves as the rash clears. The rash starts to disappear after about 10 days but, in some patients, severe cutaneous necrosis can leave disfiguring scars and there may be persisting pain.

Do not forget that herpes zoster may be the cause of severe abdominal pain before the rash develops and the diagnosis is clear.

FUNGAL INFECTIONS

Candida
(moniliasis)

This is a normal component of the body's flora and is present in the skin, mouth, vagina and gut of us all. Clinical problems only develop when there is a reduction in the normal defence mechanism which leads to infection.

Moniliasis may present in a number of different ways.

The buccal mucosa and tongue of infants or adults on prolonged courses of antibiotics may become covered in white spots or plaques.

Flexural intertrigo

Scattered soft macules may appear in the skin flexures, especially in the submammary areas and axillae of obese women. Patients with these problems should be checked for coexisting diabetes.

Balanitis

Monilial balanitis can be a problem in uncircumcized men.

Chronic paronychia

Housewives, nurses and barmaids who frequently immerse their hands for prolonged periods have an increased risk of developing this problem. The prolonged immersion causes the quick to separate from the nail plate, which allows the fungus to gain access from its reservoir in the gastrointestinal tract or vagina. Established infection causes a painful red swelling at the base of the nail. If the nail is damaged or invaded by the fungus, it becomes thickened, opaque and soft.

The differential diagnosis of a chronic paronychia includes herpetic paronychia, bacterial paronychia, collagen diseases and Buerger's disease.

Tinea pedis
(athlete's foot)

This is a common skin infection caused by one of three fungi which may be found in many surgical patients. Damage to the protective barrier function of the skin caused by athlete's foot may predispose to the entry of bacteria which can cause cellulitis, especially in patients with chronic lymphoedema.

History

Age and sex Tinea pedis has a high incidence in fit, young male athletes and swimmers who pick it up in showers and communal baths.

Symptoms Patients usually complain of itching, maceration and fissure formation in the inter-digital spaces of the toes, most often in the space between the fourth and fifth toes. One foot is usually more affected than the other. It often improves in winter and worsens in summer. The sole of the foot may also develop vesicles and itching and the palms may also develop the rash. Lymphangitis and cellulitis may develop (see above).

Examination

Site **Always** inspect between the toes.

Rash Maceration, odour and fissure formation with desquamation may be present. These may spread onto the dorsum of the foot. Asymmetry is characteristic. A vesicular eruption with bullae may be present on the soles of the feet and the palms of the hands. The nails may become distorted, white and soft. The fungus may spread to the limbs and trunk, especially the groins, where annular or ring lesions may develop.

INFESTATIONS

Scabies

This is the result of invasion of the epidermis by the *Acarus* scabies mite. The adult female is about 0.5 mm in length and is only just visible to the naked eye. The male is half this size. The fertilized female moves over the warm body until it finds a place to burrow through the horny layer of the skin. The female remains here for the rest of her life, laying two or three eggs per day for several weeks. These hatch in 3–4 days and the larvae leave the burrow and enter the hair follicles to mature. The adult mites then escape onto the skin, where mating occurs. This cycle then begins again, roughly every fortnight. Sixty per cent of burrows are on the hands and wrists, the remainder being on the soles of the feet, the genitalia, the axillae, the elbows and the buttocks.

History

In a patient who has never had scabies, an erythematous rash develops around the burrows 1 month after infestation, followed by a generalized urticarial reaction. The skin then begins to itch, especially at night. Other family members are often affected.

Examination

An urticarial rash is usually present, which in adults consists of wheals developing mostly on the trunk and limbs. Vesiculation may be present on the hands and limbs, which may become eczematous or infected.

Confirmation of diagnosis The diagnosis is confirmed by finding burrows. A magnifying lens, a good light and a sterile needle are required. The mite is visible at the anterior end of the burrow as a white oval with a black dot at its front. The needle is inserted into the burrow, which is opened up, and the mite adheres to the tip of the needle. The mite is then put on a microscope slide and inked around, and the diagnosis is confirmed. The differential diagnosis includes other causes of generalized itching.

Pediculosis capitis

Infestation with head lice is common in school children. Severe infestation causes intolerable itching and there is often secondary infection and enlarged cervical lymph glands.

Nits are present on the shafts of the hairs.

BENIGN TUMOURS AND BENIGN SKIN LUMPS

Seborrhoeic keratosis

This lesion is also called a senile wart, seborrhoeic wart, verruca senilis or basal cell papilloma. It is a benign overgrowth of the basal layer of the epidermis containing excess small, dark-staining basal cells, which raise it above the level of the normal epidermis and give it a semi-transparent, oily appearance.

History

Age Senile warts occur in both sexes but, as the name implies, they become more common with advancing years. Most people over the age of 70 years have got one or two of these lesions.

Duration They are slow growing, beginning as a minute patch which gradually increases in area. Patients do not notice the early changes in the skin

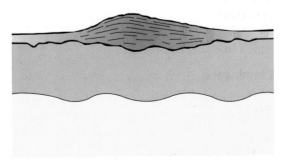

FIG 3.24 A seborrhoeic keratosis. The plaque consists of an excess number of basal cells and will peel off.

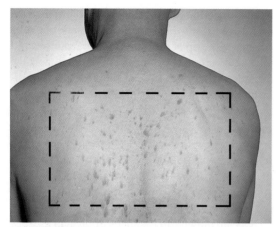

A patient whose back was covered with seborrhoeic keratoses.

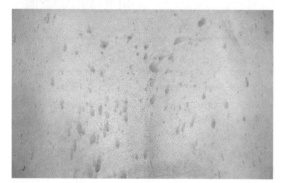

The area outlined in the upper panel is enlarged here.

FIG 3.25

and have invariably had the lesion for months or years before complaining about it.

Symptoms As the lesion gets bigger, it becomes disfiguring and may start to catch on clothes. It seldom bleeds but may get infected. Sometimes there is sufficient melanin in the lesion to make the patient think it is a mole.

Progression Senile warts gradually increase in area, but not in thickness. They can suddenly fall off, uncovering a pale-pink patch of skin.

Examination

Site Seborrhoeic keratoses occur on any part of the skin except those areas subjected to regular abrasion, such as the palms of the hands and the soles of the feet. The majority are found on the back of the trunk.

Shape and size They form a raised plateau of hypertrophic, slightly greasy skin, with a square-cut and distinct edge. They vary in size from a few millimetres to 2–3 cm in diameter.

Surface They have a rough, sometimes papilliferous, surface.

Colour Their colour varies from normal skin colour through pale yellow to dark brown, depending on the thickness of the epithelium and the quantity of melanin in the underlying skin.

Bleeding into a senile keratosis caused by trauma makes the lesion swell and turn brown – changes that may be confused with malignant change in a melanoma.

An infected keratosis also becomes swollen and tender and can be confused with a pyogenic granuloma or squamous cell carcinoma.

Consistence Senile warts are a little harder and stiffer than normal skin. The surrounding tissues are healthy, but there may be other seborrhoeic warts nearby. They have a greasy, soapy feel.

Special diagnostic feature Because seborrhoeic keratoses are patches of thick squamous epithelium, they can be picked off. They feel 'stuck on'. If you are sure of the diagnosis, you may try to pick off the edge of the plaque with blunt forceps.

When a seborrhoeic wart peels off, it leaves a patch of pale-pink skin and one or two fine surface capillaries that bleed slightly. No other skin lesion behaves like this.

Never pick hard at the edge of any lesion for fear of damaging it. Interfering in this way with a malignant tumour may hasten its local spread.

Sebaceous cysts

The skin is kept soft and oily by the sebum secreted by the sebaceous glands. The mouths of these glands open into the hair follicles. If the mouth of the gland becomes blocked, it distends with its own secretion and ultimately becomes a sebaceous cyst. Sebaceous cysts in the scalp are more correctly called **pilar** or **trichilemmal** cysts, as they arise from infundibular parts of hair follicles and have no function.

History

Age Sebaceous cysts occur in all age groups, but as they are slow growing they rarely present before adolescence. Sometimes they appear suddenly during adolescence because the skin gland secretions

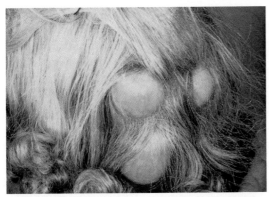

Three sebaceous cysts on the scalp. Note that you cannot see a punctum, a common finding.

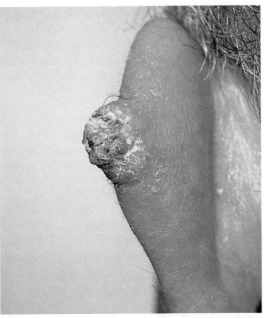

A sebaceous horn on the ear. The 'horn' is simply the hardened sebaceous material (epithelial cells and sebum) extruding from the cyst.

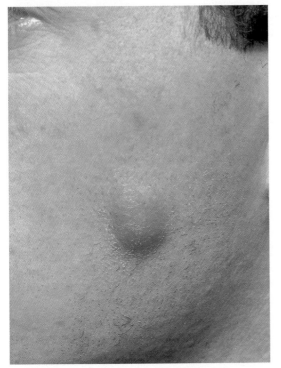

A small sebaceous cyst on the skin. The slight erythema is the residue of a recent infection in the cyst.

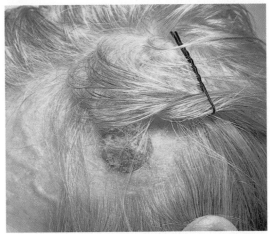

Cock's peculiar tumour. This is a mass of granulation tissue protruding from the base of a previously infected and ruptured sebaceous cyst.

FIG 3.26 SEBACEOUS CYSTS.

change at puberty, but most sebaceous cysts present in early adulthood and middle age.

Duration Sebaceous cysts are slow growing and have usually been present for some years before the patient asks a surgeon to remove them.

Symptoms Sebaceous cysts are most frequently found on the scalp, and the commonest complaint is of a lump that gets scratched when the patient is combing their hair. Such scratches may get infected. When infection develops in a cyst, it enlarges rapidly and becomes acutely painful.

A slow discharge of sebum from a wide punctum sometimes hardens to form a **sebaceous horn**.

Infection of the cyst wall and the surrounding tissues produces a boggy, painful, discharging swelling known as **Cock's peculiar tumour**. This only happens if an infected cyst is neglected.

Development Sebaceous cysts usually enlarge with time, but the increase in size is accelerated if the cyst becomes infected. Sometimes a cyst will discharge its contents through its punctum and then regress or even disappear.

Multiplicity Sebaceous cysts are often multiple.

Examination

Site Most sebaceous cysts are found in the hairy parts of the body. The scalp, scrotum, neck, shoulders and back are the common sites, but they can occur wherever there are sebaceous glands. There are no sebaceous glands on the palms of the hands and soles of the feet.

Shape and size Most sebaceous cysts are tense and spherical. Even on the scalp, where there is the unyielding skull beneath them, they remain spherical by bulging outwards and stretching the overlying skin.

They can vary from a few millimetres to 4–5 cm in diameter, but most patients seek advice before they become very large.

Surface The surface of a sebaceous cyst is smooth.

Edge The edge is well defined and easy to feel, as it is usually lying in subcutaneous fat.

Colour The skin over the cysts is usually normal.

Tenderness Uncomplicated sebaceous cysts are not tender. Pain and tenderness indicate infection.

Temperature The temperature of the skin over a cyst is normal except when the cyst is inflamed.

Composition Most sebaceous cysts feel hard and solid. Occasionally they are so tense that it is not possible to elicit fluctuation, especially if there is no firm underlying tissue to press them against. On the scalp the resistance of the underlying skull aids detection of fluctuation. They do not transilluminate because they are full of sebum.

Relations They arise from a skin structure but lie in the subcutaneous tissues, although they are attached to skin. Their point of discharge is usually along a hair follicle and, as the cyst grows, this point of fixation is often pulled inwards to become a small punctum. Only one-half of the cysts that you will see will have a visible punctum, but when it is present it is a useful diagnostic sign. Even if there is no punctum, all sebaceous cysts are attached to the skin. The area of attachment may be quite small but it prevents the cyst moving independently of the skin. Sebaceous cysts are not attached deeply.

Lymph drainage The local lymph glands should not be enlarged.

Cock's peculiar tumour

This eponym is still used by surgeons for sentimental and aesthetic reasons – it is a nice name. Cock's peculiar tumour is an infected, open, granulating, oedematous sebaceous cyst. It looks angry, sore and malignant and is often mistaken for a squamous cell carcinoma of the scalp. Granulation tissue arising from the lining of the cyst heaps up and bursts through onto the skin, giving the lesion an everted edge. The infection in the cyst wall and surrounding tissues makes the whole area oedematous, red and tender. The regional lymph glands may be enlarged.

The history usually betrays the diagnosis. The patient will tell of a long-standing lump which became painful and discharged pus spontaneously or was treated by an inadequate incision.

Sebaceous horn

A sebaceous horn arises from a sebaceous cyst.

The sebum in a sebaceous cyst may slowly exude from a large central punctum and dry and harden into a conical spike. This is a sebaceous horn. Normally the friction from clothes, and soap and water, removes the secretions of the gland as soon as they appear. A horn can only grow if the patient fails to wash the skin over the cyst. The tendency to form a horn is greater if there is a wide opening into the cyst.

Sebaceous horns can be broken off or pulled out of the cyst, because they have no intrinsic living structure.

PIGMENTED NAEVI
(Moles)

The word mole is a lay term used to describe a brown spot or blemish on the skin. The brown pigment is melanin. There are three ways in which an excess of melanin may be produced to colour the skin brown.

1. There may be a normal number of melanocytes, in their normal position, each producing an excess quantity of melanin. The lesion produced by this abnormality is called a **freckle** or **ephelis**. It is not called a mole because it does not contain an increased number of melanocytes.
2. There may be an increased number of melanocytes, in their normal position, each producing normal quantities of melanin. The lesion produced by this abnormality is called a **lentigo**.
3. There may be an increased number of melanocytes, in abnormal clusters at the dermo-epidermal junction, producing normal or excess quantities of melanin. The lesion produced by this abnormality is called a **mole** or **pigmented naevus**.

A mole becomes a **malignant melanoma** if the melanocytes invade adjacent tissues or show signs of abnormal and excessive multiplication. It is called a **dysplastic naevus** if there is no invasion but some nuclear abnormalities.

Because the three benign pathological entities described above often have similar macroscopic features, it is safest to be non-committal and call all benign melanin-producing lesions **moles** or **pigmented naevi** and malignant melanin-producing lesions **malignant melanoma**.

Pathology

Whereas the clinical appearance of pigmented naevi is infinitely variable and almost unclassifiable, moles can be defined according to their microscopic appearance (see Fig. 3.27). Melanocytes are normally found in small numbers among the cells of the basal layer of the epidermis. If they proliferate, they first cluster in this layer and then migrate into the dermis. The mature adult mole consists of clusters of melanocytes in the dermis and is therefore called an **intradermal naevus**. An intradermal naevus can be flat or raised, smooth or warty, and hairy or non-hairy. Most of the moles on the arms, face and trunk are of this variety. They hardly ever turn malignant.

If the growth and movement of the melanocytes stop before they have all migrated into the dermis, there will be clusters of cells at various stages of maturity in the epidermis and the dermis. This lesion is called a **compound cellular naevus**.

If the melanocytes remain close to the junction between the epidermis and dermis, the naevus is called a **junctional naevus**. Junctional naevi are immature and unstable and can turn malignant. The majority of malignant melanomata begin in junctional moles. Many of the moles on the palms of the hands, the soles of the feet and the external genitalia are of the junctional variety.

Melanocytes which have never reached the epidermis and therefore lie in the deep dermis or subcutaneous tissues may still proliferate and produce excess melanin. The resulting lesion has a blue appearance and is called a **blue naevus**.

The only practical clinical approach is to excise any mole that is suspected of undergoing malignant change.

History

Age Except for albinos, everyone has a few moles at birth, but the number increases during life. It has been estimated that most Caucasians have 15–20 moles. During childhood and adolescence, these may become more pigmented or completely regress. When enlarging and getting darker, a mole on a child may be clinically and histologically difficult to distinguish from a malignant melanoma, but true malignant change is uncommon before puberty.

Ethnic group Moles are more common in Caucasians living in hot countries, such as Australia, because the skin is exposed to more ultraviolet light. Moles occur in Negroes, particularly in the less pigmented areas such as the soles of feet and palms of the hands, but are rare.

Symptoms Moles rarely cause any serious symptoms. They may be disfiguring, protrude above the skin surface and catch on clothes. Itching or bleeding suggests the possibility that malignant change has occurred (see below).

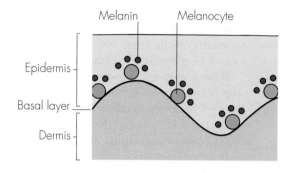

Melanin — Melanocyte

Epidermis

Basal layer

Dermis

Normal skin

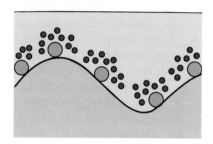

Freckle (ephelis)
Normal number of melanocytes, in normal position, producing excess melanin

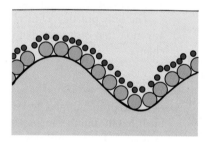

Lentigo
Excess melanocytes, in normal position, producing normal amount of melanin

Pigmented naevus/mole Excess melanocytes, in clusters, variable but usually excess melanin production

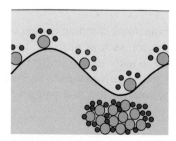

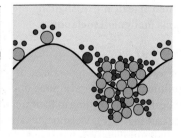

Intradermal naevus   **Compound naevus**   **Junctional naevus**

FIG 3.27 The histological varieties of pigmented spots and blemishes.

Examination

Site Moles can occur on any part of the skin, but are most common on the limbs, face, neck and trunk.

Size Most moles are 1–3 mm in diameter.

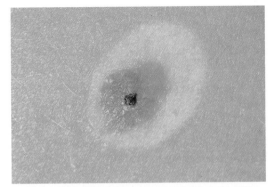

A 'halo' mole. This mole is regressing. It has faded and the skin around it has become de-pigmented.

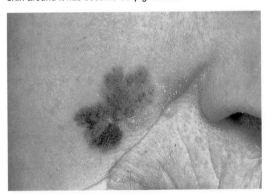

Hutchinson's lentigo on the face.

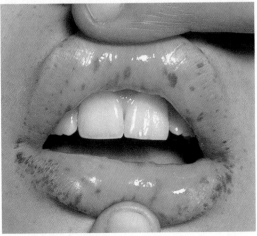

The circumoral pigmented naevi of Peutz–Jeghers syndrome.

FIG 3.28 VARIOUS PIGMENTED NAEVI.

Colour Their colour varies from light brown to black. **Amelanotic naevi** do occur, but without their pigment they are unlikely to be recognized. The colour does not fade with pressure.

Pigmented naevi may regress. A mole surrounded by a white halo of regression is known as a **halo naevus**.

Composition Moles usually have a soft consistence and are indistinguishable, by palpation, from the surrounding tissues.

Lymph glands The local lymph glands should not be enlarged.

Shape and surface There are four clinical varieties of mole.

- **Hairy mole** is a common variety. It is flat, or very slightly raised above the level of the surrounding skin, with a smooth or slightly warty epidermal covering, and has hairs growing from its surface. The presence of hairs means that the mole also contains sebaceous glands that can become infected and cause changes such as swelling and tenderness, which may be indistinguishable from malignant change. Hairy moles are always intradermal naevi.
- **Non-hairy or smooth mole** is also a common variety. The epithelium is smooth and not elevated. The brown pigment looks as if it is deep in the skin – deeper than that of the hairy mole – but this is just an optical illusion. There is no hair growing from its surface. Non-hairy moles may be intradermal, junctional or compound naevi.
- **Blue naevus** is a mole deep in the dermis. The thick overlying layers of dermis and epidermis mask the brown colour of the melanin and make it look blue. The overlying skin is often smooth and shiny. This is an uncommon type of mole, more often seen in children. It usually occurs on the face, the dorsum of the hands and feet, and the buttock.
- **Lentigo** is an area of pigmentation that appears in late adult life and is prone to undergo malignant change (see page 88).

There are two other varieties of melanotic skin pigmentation – the **café au lait** patch, and the circumoral moles of the **Peutz–Jeghers syndrome**.

The café au lait patch is an area of pale-brown pigmentation, present at birth and often associated with neurofibromatosis and sometimes with phaeo-chromocytoma. The pale-brown, milk-coffee colour is a reflection of the small amount of melanin in the lesion. Histologically these patches can be freck-les or lentigo. They do not undergo malignant change.

The Peutz–Jeghers syndrome (primarily multi-ple polyposis of the mucosa of the stomach and small intestine) is associated with multiple small moles on the skin of the face, particularly around the mouth, on the lips and in the buccal mucous membrane. Histologically these are patches of lentigo. They do not turn malignant.

BENIGN SUBCUTANEOUS SWELLINGS

Lipoma

A lipoma is a cluster of fat cells which have become over-active and so distended with fat that they have become palpable lumps. They are never malignant. Liposarcomata, which often develop in the retroperi-toneal tissues (see page 424), arise de novo.

History

Age Lipomata occur at all ages but are not common in children.

Duration They have usually been present, growing slowly, for months or years before being noticed. They rarely regress.

Symptoms Most patients present because they have noticed a lump and want to know what it is. The lump may be unsightly or interfere with movement, especially if it becomes pedunculated.

Multiplicity Patients often have many lipomata, or have had others excised in the past. Multiple con-tiguous lipomata cause enlargement and distortion of the subcutaneous tissues. This condition is called **lipomatosis**. It usually occurs in the buttocks and sometimes in the neck.

Multiple lipomatosis (Dercum's disease) is a con-dition in which the limbs and sometimes the trunk are covered with lipomata of all shapes and sizes. These can be painful and may contain angiomatous elements and therefore be **angiolipomata**.

Examination

Site Lipomata are most common in the subcuta-neous tissues of the upper limbs, chest, neck and shoulders, but they can occur anywhere.

Colour The skin that overlies the lump is normal and the veins crossing the lipoma may be visible as faint blue streaks.

Tenderness Lipomata are not usually tender, but angiolipomata are.

Temperature The temperature of the overlying skin is normal.

Shape and size Lipomata are usually spherical, but subcutaneous lipomata which develop between the skin and the deep fascia are usually discoid or hemi-spherical. Most lipomata are **lobulated**, as fat in the body is in the form of lobules. The lobules can be seen and felt on the surface and at the edge of the lump.

Lipomata come in all sizes.

Surface The surface feels smooth, but firm pressure reveals the depressions between the lobules. The lobules become more prominent with firm palpa-tion or gentle squeezing because the increased pres-sure within the lipoma makes each lobule bulge out between the fine strands of fibrous tissue that sur-round it.

Edge The edge is not circular but a series of irregu-lar curves corresponding to each lobule. Because the edge is soft, compressible and sometimes quite thin, it slips away from the examining finger. This has been described as the '*slip sign*'. It is not a very useful or a diagnostic feature. Evidence of lobulation on the surface and at the edge is the most significant physical sign.

Composition Most lipomata contain a soft but solid jelly-like fat if they are cut open immediately after removal. Small lipomata feel soft but do not fluctu-ate. Because lipomata are soft, they give the impres-sion of fluctuating, but careful examination reveals that they are just yielding to pressure and spreading out in all directions. They do not become more tense and prominent in the plane at right-angles to the palpating finger. The larger the lipoma, the more it will appear to fluctuate, but fat at body temperature is solid, not liquid.

Lipomata do not transilluminate in that they do not transmit light from a torch shone beside them,

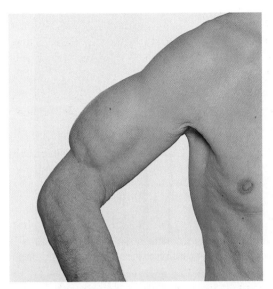

A lipoma in the subcutaneous tissues of the upper arm. Note the lobulation.

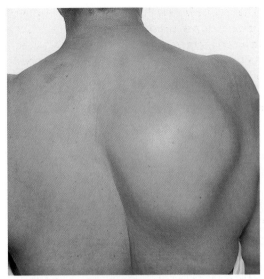

A large lipoma overlying the scapula.

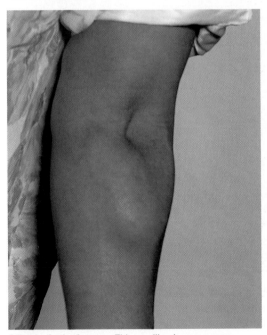

A lipoma in the forearm. This swelling became more prominent and fixed when the forearm muscles were contracted, showing that it was superficial to the muscle but attached to its fascia.

FIG 3.29 LIPOMATA.

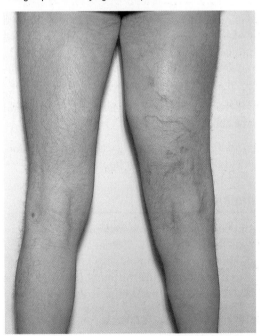

A large lipoma in the inner aspect of the upper right thigh which became less distinct when the hamstring muscles were contracted, showing that it was deep to the muscles. Note the distended veins caused by compression of the superficial femoral vein by the mass.

but they may light up if torchlight is shone directly across them. They do not have a fluid thrill and they do not reduce or pulsate.

The physical signs of pseudo-fluctuation and transillumination make them appear cystic, a false impression which emphasizes the diagnostic importance of finding lobulation.

Relations Lipomata may arise within deep structures, such as muscles. These lipomata are fixed deeply

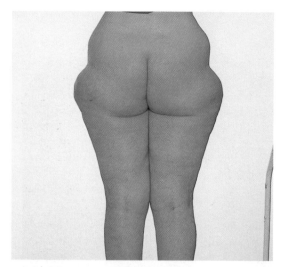

FIG 3.30 Diffuse lipomatosis over both hips.

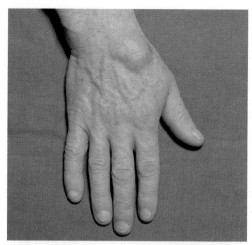

A soft multilocular ganglion on the back of the wrist.

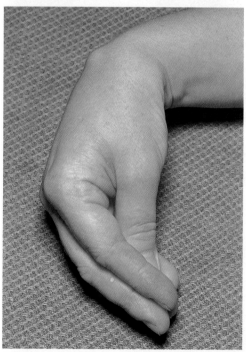

A small, tense ganglion on the back of the wrist which was only clearly visible and palpable when the wrist was flexed.

FIG 3.31 GANGLIA.

and may become more prominent if they are pushed out of the muscle, or disappear if they are drawn into the muscle when it contracts.

Subcutaneous lipomata are not attached superficially or deeply and can be moved in all directions.

Lymph drainage The regional lymph glands should not be enlarged.

Local tissues The surrounding tissues should be normal, but there may be other lipomata nearby.

Ganglion

A ganglion is a cystic, myxomatous degeneration of fibrous tissue. Ganglia can occur anywhere in the body, but they are common where there is a lot of fibrous tissue, i.e. around the joints. Ganglia are not pockets of synovium protruding from joints.

History

Age The majority present between the ages of 20 and 60 years and they are rare in children.

Duration They grow slowly over months or years.

Symptoms A ganglion is not painful. Most patients seek advice because they wish to know the diagnosis or because the lump is disfiguring. Some ganglia slip away between neighbouring bones, so giving the false impression that they are reducing into the joint, but a true ganglion should not connect with or empty into a joint. Ganglia may be injured and rupture into the subcutaneous tissues and not reappear.

Examination

Site Most ganglia are found near joint capsules and tendon sheaths, but they can occur anywhere.

Ninety per cent arise on the dorsal and ventral surfaces of the wrist joint and hand.

Shape and size　Ganglia are spherical. Some are multilocular and feel like a collection of cysts.

They come in all sizes. Small ganglia (0.5–1.0 cm) tend to be tense and spherical. Large ones, which can be up to 5–6 cm across, are flattened and soft.

Surface　They have a smooth surface.

Composition　Ganglia feel solid but their consistence can vary from soft to hard. The gelatinous material within them is very viscous, but most ganglia fluctuate, provided they are not very small or very tense. They usually transilluminate brilliantly.

Reducibility　A ganglion may slip away between deeper structures when pressed, giving the false impression that its contents have reduced into the joint.

Relations　Ganglia are usually attached to the fibrous tissue from which they originate. They are not attached to the overlying skin, which should be freely mobile over them. The mobility of a ganglion depends on the extent and nature of its deep attachment. When the tissue of origin is part of a joint capsule, tendon sheath or intramuscular septum, the ganglion becomes less mobile when these structures are made tense. Therefore remember to palpate ganglia in all positions of the underlying joint and with the surrounding muscles relaxed and tense.

Differential diagnosis　The three common swellings found close to joints are bursae, cystic protrusions of the synovial cavity of arthritic joints, and ganglia. The first two are usually soft; the ganglion is tense. With the first and third, the joint is normal.

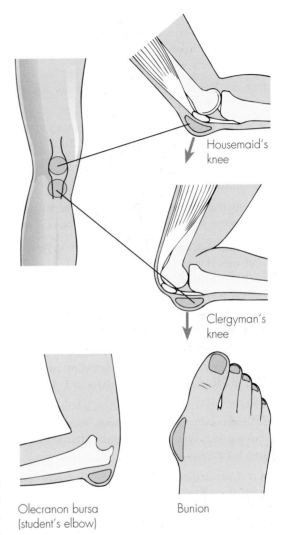

Housemaid's knee

Clergyman's knee

Olecranon bursa (student's elbow)

Bunion

FIG 3.32 The common adventitious bursae.

Subcutaneous bursae

Bursae are fluid-filled cavities, lined with a flattened endothelium similar to synovium, that develop between tendons, bones and skin to allow easier movement between them. There are a considerable number of bursae that are always present and described in anatomical textbooks, but others may develop wherever there is friction between two layers of tissue. These are called **adventitious bursae**.

History

Age　Bursae are uncommon in the young unless they have a skeletal deformity. They usually appear in middle and later life as a result of prolonged friction between skin and bone, associated with the patient's occupation or with a deformity produced by injury or arthritis.

Symptoms　Pain and an enlarging swelling at the site of repeated trauma are the common presenting symptoms. A severe throbbing pain and a rapid increase in size indicate the presence of infection.

When the bursa is an occupational hazard – such as housemaid's knee – it may stop the patient working.

Development　The growth of the swelling is usually rapid, even though the bursa has probably been present in its normal, almost empty, state for many years. A sudden increase in the quantity of fluid in the bursa that makes it enlarge is usually secondary to minor infection or trauma.

Multiplicity Bursae are often symmetrical, e.g. on both knees or elbows.

Cause The patient often knows the cause of the swelling (prolonged friction or a skeletal deformity) and may have had a similar complaint before.

Examination

Site Subcutaneous bursae occur where there is friction between skin and bone. The common sites are:

- between skin and olecranon – student's elbow,
- between skin and patella – housemaid's knee,
- between skin and patellar ligament – clergyman's knee,
- between skin and head of first metatarsal – bunion.

Shape and size Bursae are usually circular in outline with an indistinct edge, but their depth, or thickness, can vary from a few millimetres to 3–4 cm.

Surface The texture of the surface of a bursa is difficult to assess because it is intimately attached to the overlying skin. When the skin is not attached to the bursa, the surface feels smooth.

Colour They are covered with skin that has been repeatedly rubbed and worn, so it is always thickened, shiny, white and cracked.

Tenderness Bursae are only tender if they are very tense or inflamed. When they become inflamed, the overlying skin turns red and hot.

Composition Bursae contain a clear viscous fluid, similar to synovial fluid, that gives them a soft or spongy consistence. They fluctuate, transilluminate and may have a fluid thrill. These signs may be difficult to elicit if the wall of the bursa is thick or the quantity of fluid small.

Relations As a subcutaneous bursa develops between two moving tissue planes to reduce the amount of friction between them, the deep and superficial surfaces of a bursa are usually firmly attached to the two tissues it separates, so that the friction occurs between the lubricated inside surfaces of the bursa. This makes the bursa immobile and the walls impalpable.

State of local tissues The bones and joints beneath the bursa must be carefully examined because a bursa may have developed to ease the movement of the skin over a skeletal abnormality such as an exostosis or deformed joint. The overlying skin is often horny and cracked.

Complications Bursae can become inflamed by repeated trauma and by conditions which cause inflammation of synovial surfaces, such as rheumatoid arthritis and gout. They also get infected from organisms circulating in the bloodstream.

General examination Even though the patient complains of one lump, examine the same spot on the other limb because it is quite likely that they have symmetrical lesions. Also look for other skeletal abnormalities and joint diseases.

Keratoacanthoma
(Adenoma sebaceum, molluscum pseudo-carcinomatosum)

This is a self-limiting overgrowth and subsequent spontaneous regression of hair follicle cells. Because it grows rapidly, it is often mistaken for a squamous cell carcinoma.

History

Keratoacanthomata occur in adults, who complain of a rapidly growing lump in the skin. They are not painful, but can be very unsightly. The lump takes 2–4 weeks to grow and 2–3 months to regress. The

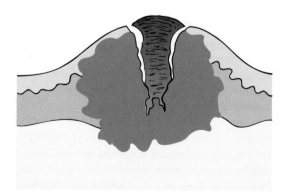

FIG 3.33 A keratoacanthoma is an overgrowth of hair follicle cells which produce a central plug of keratin. When the plug separates, the lesion usually undergoes spontaneous regression.

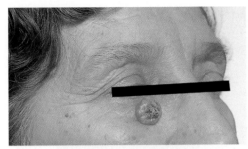

A large keratoacanthoma on the face.

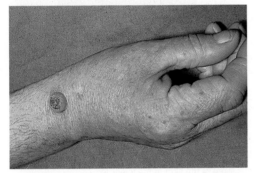

A keratoacanthoma on the wrist. The slough is just beginning to separate.

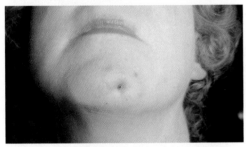

The end result if the lesion is not excised – a deep, puckered scar.

FIG 3.34 KERATOACANTHOMATA.

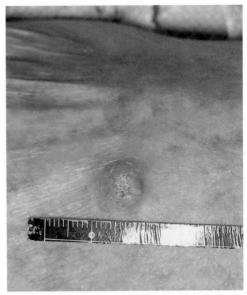

A keratoacanthoma that is beginning to collapse, the slough having separated.

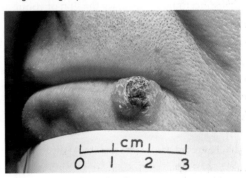

A close-up view of the slough.

cause is unknown. It may be a self-limiting benign neoplasm or an unusual response to a viral infection.

Examination

Site Keratoacanthomata are often found on the face but they can occur anywhere where there are sebaceous glands. They are usually solitary.

Shape and size The lump is hemispherical or conical and looks like a volcano when the central slough appears and the surrounding skin retracts.

The nodule is usually 1–2 cm in diameter by the time the centre of the lump begins to necrose.

Consistence The bulk of the lesion is firm and rubbery, but the central core is hard.

Colour The lump has a normal skin colour, but the necrotic centre is brown or black.

Relations The lump is confined to the skin and is freely mobile over the subcutaneous tissues.

Lymph drainage The local lymph glands should not be enlarged.

Natural history The central core eventually separates and the lump collapses, leaving a deep indrawn scar. In spite of this self-limiting natural history, keratoacanthomata are usually excised to confirm the diagnosis.

Differential diagnosis A keratoacanthoma must be differentiated from a squamous cell carcinoma. The latter grows more slowly and eventually becomes an ulcer. The diagnosis is confirmed by a pathologist after an excisional biopsy.

Hystiocytoma
(Dermatofibroma, sclerosing angioma)

This is a benign neoplasm of the fibroblasts of the dermis. Its name is derived from the many histiocytes that are present between the fibroblasts. The overlying epidermis is normal. It has also been suggested that this may be an haemangioma with a marked desmoplastic response.

History

Age Histiocytomata appear on the skin of young and middle-aged adults.

Sex Both sexes are equally affected.

Symptoms The patient complains of a slow-growing lump on the skin. The rate of growth is so slow that the lump may take years to reach a size sufficient to excite the patient's curiosity or get in the way of clothing.

There are no associated general symptoms.

Examination

Site Histiocytomata can occur anywhere, but are slightly more common on the skin of the limbs.

Shape As they grow, they form a hemispherical lump which then flattens into a thick disc. The edges of the disc may overhang its base.

Size Most patients complain of these tumours when they are 1–2 cm across, but they can grow to a considerable size if they are neglected.

Surface The skin covering the lump is often loose and slightly crinkled, even though it is inseparable from the lump.

Colour They are covered by normal-coloured epidermis, which may contain sufficient haemosiderin to give them a brown colour and therefore the appearance of a mole.

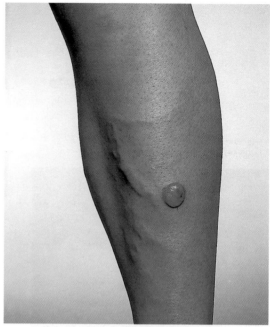

A histiocytoma of the skin of the lower leg.

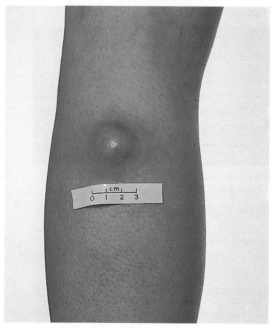

A large histiocytoma on the calf.

FIG 3.35 HISTIOCYTOMATA.

Tenderness They are not tender.

Composition These tumours usually have a rubbery or spongy consistence. They do not fluctuate or transilluminate.

Relations They are in the skin, separate from and freely mobile over the deep tissues.

Lymph drainage The local lymph glands should not be enlarged.

State of local tissues The surrounding tissues are normal.

The lymph glands

The lymph glands which receive lymph from the skin and the limbs lie in the subcutaneous tissues of the groins and axillae. The epitrochlear lymph gland in the arm and the popliteal lymph gland in the leg are present in most adults and may enlarge before the axillary or groin glands when there is disease in the hand or foot.

Lymph glands are enlarged and made tender by inflammatory conditions, and enlarged by infiltration with metastatic and primary tumours.

The diagnosis of axillary and inguinal lymphadenopathy depends as much on the site of the swellings as on the presence of multiple firm lumps in the subcutaneous tissues.

It is difficult to misdiagnose axillary or inguinal lymphadenopathy, but enlargement of the cervical lymph glands can be difficult to diagnose and is discussed in Chapter 11.

When examining the lymph glands, it is important to examine all sites containing lymph glands which might be palpable, i.e. the neck, both axillae, both groins and the abdomen.

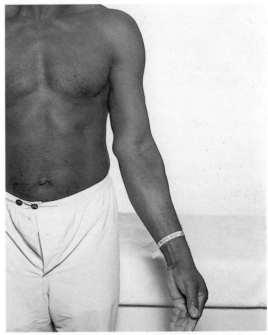

An enlarged epitrochlear lymph gland. The patient had a non-Hodgkin's lymphoma.

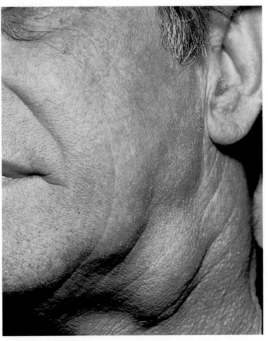

Multiple enlarged upper cervical lymph glands. The patient had a carcinoma of the nasopharynx.

FIG 3.36 LYMPH GLANDS.

Revision panel 3.5
The causes of enlargement of lymph glands

Infection
 Non-specific
 Glandular fever
 Tuberculosis
 Syphilis
 Lymphogranuloma
Metastatic tumour
Primary reticuloses
 Lymphoma
 Lymphosarcoma
 Reticulosarcoma
Sarcoidosis

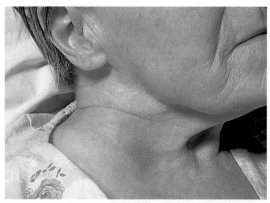

An enlarged right supraclavicular lymph gland. The patient had a carcinoma of the right breast.

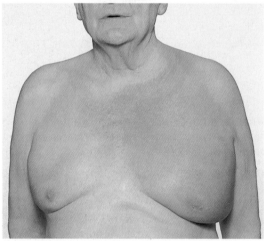

Enlarged left supraclavicular and axillary lymph glands causing oedema of the arm and chest wall. The patient had a lymphosarcoma.

FIG 3.36 continued

The size and shape of the glands should be recorded. Enlarged glands may be solitary or multiple; clearly defined, indistinct or 'matted' together; hard, rubbery or soft; tender or painless.

Whenever a lymph gland is found to be enlarged, the area of tissue it drains should be carefully examined.

TUMOURS OF THE SKIN APPENDAGES

These arise from the sebaceous glands, sweat glands, apocrine glands and hair gland cells. Most are benign and have exotic names. Five to ten per cent are malignant.

Sebaceous gland tumours

These include the **naevus sebaceous of Jadassohn**, **sebaceous adenoma** and **sebaceous carcinoma**, which is rare. They are all solitary subcutaneous tumours that are either soft and warty, or firm.

Sweat gland tumours

These include the **eccrine poroma**, the **spiradenoma** and the **acrospiroma**. These all present as solitary subcutaneous lumps, which can be reddish-pink, red-blue or stain coloured.

Syringomata also arise from the sweat glands and present as multiple flesh-coloured or yellow papules on the faces of women. **Cylindromata** (turban tumours) are rare tumours that arise from the sweat glands of the head and scalp. They present as solitary or multiple, pink, spherical or slightly flattened nodules, which may coalesce to look like a turban, hence the common name. They are soft with an ill-defined edge.

The apocrine gland tumours

These include the **apocrine hydrocystoma** and the **syringocystadenoma papilliferum**.

The hair gland tumours

These include the **trichofolliculoma**, the **trichoepithelioma**, the **trichilemmoma** and the **pilomatrixoma**. All arise as subcutaneous pink, brown or red/white nodules at different parts of the body.

Sporadic neurofibroma

Multiple familial neurofibromatosis (Von Recklinghausen's disease) is discussed on page 50.

Sporadic neurofibromata are benign tumours which contain a mixture of neural (ectodermal) and fibrous (mesodermal) elements. They are often multiple.

The tumours that are derived from nerve sheaths (the **neurilemmoma**, also known as schwannoma), are very rare.

History

Age Neurofibromata can appear at any age but usually present in adult life.

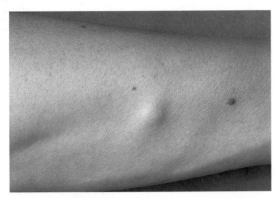

FIG 3.37 A neurofibroma on the leg of a patient with five other similar lesions.

Symptoms Most neurofibromata cause no discomfort and are rarely big enough to be disfiguring. If they are related to a nerve trunk, they may be tender and the patient may get tingling sensations in the distribution of the affected nerve.

Multiplicity Neurofibromata are often multiple.

Examination

Site They can occur anywhere in the skin and sub-cutaneous tissues. The forearms seem to be most often affected, perhaps because they are the part of the body most frequently palpated by the patient.

Shape and size Neurofibromata are usually fusiform, with their long axes lying along the length of the limb. They are rarely more than a few centimetres in length.

Composition They have the consistence of firm rubber and are dull to percussion.

Relations The surrounding structures are normal. Subcutaneous neurofibromata are mobile within the subcutaneous tissues but move most freely in a direction at right-angles to the course of the nerve to which they are connected.

Plexiform neurofibroma

Although this is a very rare condition, it is mentioned because it is one of those conditions that cause considerable diagnostic confusion if the doctor has never heard of it.

It is an excessive overgrowth of neural tissue in the subcutaneous layers which gives the tissues a swollen

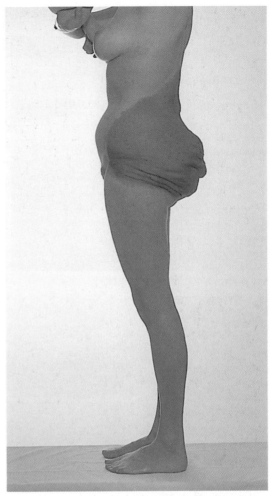

FIG 3.38 A very dark brown area of pigmentation over an extensive mixed plexiform neurofibroma and haemangioma.

and oedematous appearance. It is sometimes called elephantiasis **neurofibromatosis**. It is often misdiagnosed as lymphoedema, but the lymphatics are normal. Remember it when presented with a child with an apparent overgrowth of the soft tissues of the hand or foot. The diagnosis can only be made by the pathologist.

PRE-MALIGNANT SKIN LESIONS

Solar keratosis

Prolonged exposure of the skin to sunlight can cause areas of hyperkeratosis of the skin, which may undergo malignant change.

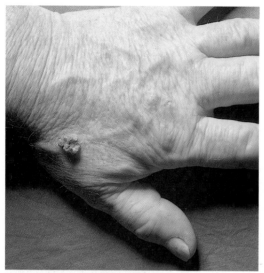

A solar keratosis on the back of the hand.

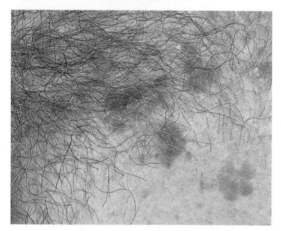

Bowen's disease on the skin of the chest.

FIG 3.39 PRE-CANCEROUS CONDITIONS OF THE SKIN.

History

The patient notices the gradual appearance of thickened patches of skin, which are not painful but can become unsightly.

Natural history Solar keratoses grow slowly and the patients, usually elderly men who have worked out of doors for many years, ignore them. These lesions must be watched carefully for any change in size or appearance.

Examination

Site Solar keratoses are commonly found on the backs of the fingers and hands, on the face and on the rim of the ears.

Shape and size Beneath their horny surface layer there is a raised plaque of skin which may vary in diameter from a few millimetres to 1 cm and protrude above the skin surface. The whole of the strip of skin along the rim of the pinna may be affected.

Colour The thickened patches of skin have a yellow-grey or red-brown colour.

Composition The keratinous layer is very hard and clearly part of the underlying skin.

Relations Solar keratoses are confined to the skin. If a nodule or patch is tethered to the underlying structures, it has turned into a squamous carcinoma and is infiltrating deeply.

Lymph drainage The local lymph glands should not be enlarged. If they are, one of the keratoses has probably become a squamous cell carcinoma.

Bowen's disease

This also is a pre-cancerous lesion. It presents as a cluster of flat, pink, papular patches which are covered with crusts. The patches and the adjacent skin have a pale-brown, thickened appearance. Patients usually believe they have a patch of eczema.

When the crusts are removed, the papules can be seen to have a wet, oozy, slightly bloody, papilliferous surface.

When in any doubt about a chronic skin lesion, it is wise to carry out a biopsy.

Hutchinson's lentigo

This eponym is used to describe a large area of pigmentation which commonly appears and slowly enlarges on the face and neck in late (after the age of 60) adult life. The surface is smooth but there may be raised, rough nodules, which correspond to areas of junctional activity and become the sites of malignant change, alongside pale areas of regression. Because the background pigmentation is so dark, areas of malignant change causing an increase in pigmentation but no thickening may pass unnoticed.

It is worth using the eponym to remind you that this mole is different from other moles because of two special features: its late development and its high incidence of malignant change. Some pathologists believe that this variety is pre-malignant or actually malignant from the start, an example of malignant change 'in situ'.

MALIGNANT DISEASES OF THE SKIN

Basal cell carcinoma
(Rodent ulcer)

This is a locally invasive carcinoma of the basal layer of the epidermis. It does not metastasize, but can infiltrate adjacent tissues. It is common in exposed skin, especially in countries where there is a high incidence of ultraviolet irradiation, i.e. bright sunlight.

History

Age The incidence of basal cell carcinoma increases with age because it is related to the duration of exposure of the skin to ultraviolet light.

Geography It is more common in countries that have much bright sunlight. (eg Australia)

Ethnic group Basal cell carcinomata are rare in dark-skinned races.

Sex Males are affected more often than females.

Duration Basal cell carcinomata grow very slowly and have usually been present for months or years before the patient seeks advice.

Symptoms The principal complaint is of a **persistent nodule** or an **ulcer with a central scab** that repeatedly falls off and then re-forms. The lesion grows slowly but eventually becomes disfiguring and annoying. It may itch. It may cause pain and, if it is neglected, becomes a deep infected ulcer. A large, neglected ulcer destroying one side of the face is now rare.

Development The lesion grows very slowly and may have been present for months or years before the patient complains about it. This long history gives the patient a false impression that the lesion is benign and unimportant.

Persistence Some basal cell carcinomata spread radially through the skin, leaving a central scar.

Multiplicity Basal cell carcinomata are often multiple.

Predisposing factors Skin that has been treated with arsenic, once a common ingredient of skin ointments, is liable to develop basal cell carcinomata.

Examination

Site Basal cell carcinomata are commonly found on the face above a line drawn from the angle of the mouth to the lobe of the ear. This does not mean that they do not occur in other sites; all skin is susceptible, particularly the skin of the scalp, neck, arms and hands.

Size Most patients complain of the nodule or ulcer when it is quite small, but basal cell carcinomata can grow to a considerable size if they are neglected. A few grow outwards from the skin to become a fungating mass on the skin surface, but the majority erode deeply, destroying the underlying tissues and forming a deep cavity – hence the name 'rodent'.

Shape Some of the many macroscopic appearances of basal cell carcinomata are shown in Figure 3.41. Only two are true ulcers, so it is better to use the term 'basal cell carcinoma', not 'rodent ulcer'. The

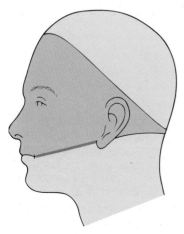

FIG 3.40 Basal cell carcinomata commonly appear in the shaded area.

> Revision panel 3.6
> **The clinical appearances of basal cell carcinomata**
>
> Nodule
> 'Cystic' (a large, seemingly transparent nodule)
> Ulcer
> Deeply eroding ulcer: the 'rodent' ulcer
> Pigmented nodule
> Geographical (advancing edge, healing centre)

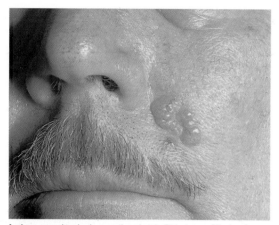

A slow-growing lesion on the cheek. This type of lesion is difficult to see and often ignored by the patient, who notices only a small scab (which periodically appears and then falls off) at the centre of a slightly thickened area of the skin.

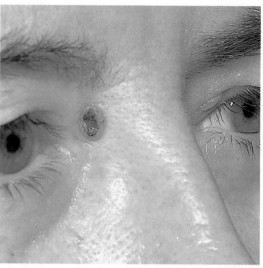

A pigmented basal cell carcinoma.

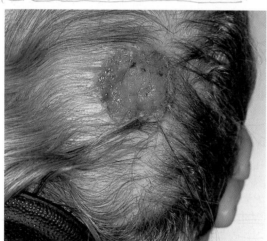

A raised, wet, weeping basal cell carcinoma that was thought by the patient to be a patch of eczema.

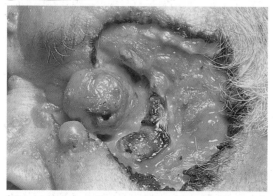

A true 'rodent ulcer'. The basal cell carcinoma has destroyed the orbit and the eye.

FIG 3.41 BASAL CELL CARCINOMATA.

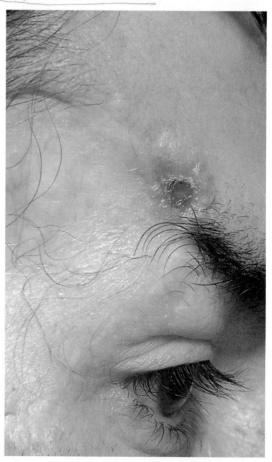

A recurrent basal cell carcinoma at the edge of a skin graft placed to cover the skin defect of a previous excision 7 years earlier.

tumour always starts as a nodule. When the central epithelium dies, the resulting ulcer develops a rolled edge. This means that the edge is raised up and rounded but not everted. If the centre of the tumour does not necrose and ulcerate, the nodule can become quite large and look like a cyst. It is not cystic, however, because it is solid and non-fluctuant, but the term 'cystic rodent ulcer' is unfortunately sometimes used to describe this appearance.

Colour The raised portion of the lesion – that is to say, its edge if it is annular, or its centre if it is a nodule – is smooth, glistening and slightly transparent. This gives the impression that there are pearl-white nodules of tissue just below the epidermis. These nodules also give the ulcerating variety its typical 'rolled edge'.

The whole lesion may be coloured brown by excess melanin.

Surface The surface of the nodular variety is covered by fine, distinct blood vessels, which may give it a pink hue.

Edge When the nodule first ulcerates, the rolled edge is circular, but as the malignant cells spread, the shape of the ulcer becomes irregular. The raised edge may be the only clue to the diagnosis if the ulcer heals. An irregular raised edge around a flat white scar is sometimes called a 'geographical' or

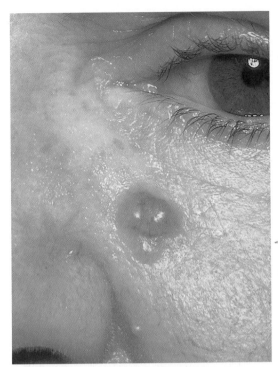

An early nodule just below the eye. These nodules are sometimes mistakenly thought to be cystic.

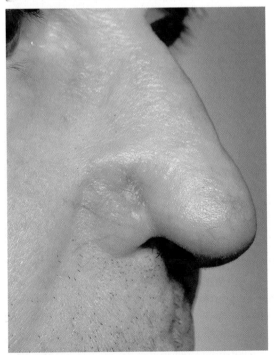

A lesion with a deep, scarred centre without a noticeably raised edge.

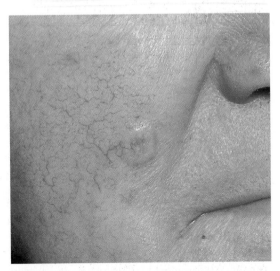

A nodular lesion spreading outwards and leaving a collapsed, scarred centre.

FIG 3.41 continued

'forest fire' basal cell carcinoma. When the ulcer erodes into deeper structures, the edge becomes more prominent and florid but not everted.

Base The base of a small rodent ulcer is covered with a coat of dried serum and epithelial cells and will bleed slightly if this layer is picked off.

The base of deeply eroding ulcers consists of fat, bone, muscle, or even the eye, all covered with poor-quality granulation tissue.

Depth Long-standing ulcers may erode deep into the face, destroying skin and bone and exposing the nasal cavity, air sinuses and even the eye, hence the name 'rodent' because the tissues look as if they have been gnawed by a rat.

Such extensive lesions are uncommon. Most basal cell carcinomata are superficial and confined to the skin.

Lymph drainage The local lymph glands should not be enlarged.

Relations A small tumour is confined to the skin and is freely movable over the deep structures. Fixation of the ulcer indicates that it has invaded deeply.

Important differential diagnoses A rodent ulcer can resemble a **squamous cell carcinoma**. The long history and the rolled edge are the clinical features that indicate its basal cell origin. A **keratoacanthoma** (see page 82) just beginning to slough at its centre can also look like an early rodent ulcer but the short history and the deep slough should suggest the correct diagnosis.

In every instance, the final diagnosis must be made by the pathologist. Sweat gland tumours and malignant melanomata are other differentiated diagnoses that should be considered.

Squamous cell carcinoma
(Epithelioma)

This is a carcinoma of the cells of the epidermis that normally migrate out towards the surface to form the superficial keratinous squamous layer. The tumour cells infiltrate the epidermis, the dermis and adjacent tissues. Microscopic examination reveals tongues of tumour cells spreading in all directions, and clusters of cells with concentric rings of flattened squamous cells at their centre. These onion-like clumps of cells are often called 'epithelial pearls', but are only seen under the microscope.

History

Age The incidence of squamous carcinoma of the skin increases with age.

Causes Prolonged exposure to sunlight, solar keratoses, Bowen's disease, certain chemicals and irradiation and the presence of old scarring, particularly following burns, or chronic ulcers are associated with an increased incidence of squamous carcinomata. Cancer of the scrotal skin was once common in chimney sweeps, and still occurs in engineers whose clothes become soaked in oil.

Duration The ulcerating tumour has usually been growing steadily for 1 or 2 months before the patient complains of it. If it is in an inaccessible part, such as in the middle of the back, it may grow quite large before being noticed.

Symptoms The patient complains of a lump, or of bleeding and discharge from an ulcer. Bleeding is more common with squamous cell than basal cell carcinomata. The tumour may become painful if it invades deep structures.

Occasionally patients notice enlarged lymph glands and are unaware of the primary tumour.

There are no systemic effects while the tumour is confined to the skin. Dissemination of tumour cells throughout the body is a late event.

Development The ulcer or nodule enlarges steadily and inexorably. The edges of a squamous cell carcinomatous ulcer become more prominent and florid.

Multiplicity There may be multiple tumours in skin affected by exposure to ultraviolet light, such as the scalp, or chemicals, such as the hands and arms.

Examination

Site Squamous cell carcinomata can occur on any part of the skin, but are more common on the exposed skin of the head and neck, hands, forearms and upper trunk. They also develop in skin subjected to repeated chemical or mechanical irritation.

Colour The everted edge of a carcinomatous ulcer is usually a dark red-brown colour because it is very vascular. The whole ulcer may be covered with old coagulated blood or serum.

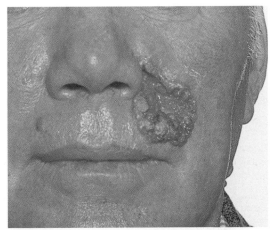

An ulcer, on the face, with an everted edge and a necrotic base.

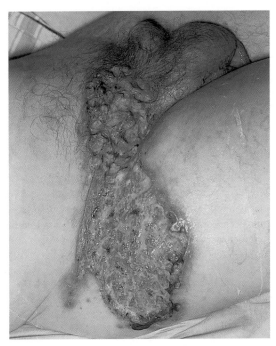

An extensive squamous cell carcinoma of the skin of the groin and scrotum.

FIG 3.42 SQUAMOUS CELL CARCINOMATA.

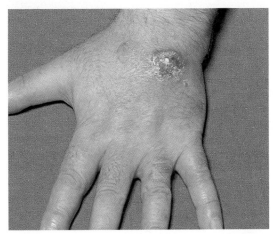

An ulcer, on the hand, whose edge is not yet everted but is raised and almost everted on the proximal side.

Tenderness The ulcer is not usually tender.

Shape and size Squamous carcinomata begin as small nodules on the skin. As they enlarge, the centre becomes necrotic, sloughs, and the nodule turns into an ulcer, which is initially circular with prominent everted edges, but can become any shape as it enlarges.

Edge Squamous cell carcinomata have an everted edge because the excessive tissue growth raises it above and over the normal skin surface.

Base The base of the ulcer consists of necrotic tumour covered with serum and blood. There is usually some granulation tissue, but this tends to be pale and unhealthy. Deep tissues may be exposed.

Depth The depth of the ulcer is affected by the nature of the underlying tissues and the virulence of the tumour. Soft tissues are easily invaded and when they slough they leave a deep ulcer.

Discharge The discharge can be copious, bloody, purulent and foul smelling. This is often the patient's most depressing and debilitating symptom.

Relations The relations to nearby tissues will vary according to the extent of the malignant infiltration. If the ulcer is immobile, the tumour has spread beyond the skin and subcutaneous tissues into deeper structures – tendon, bone and muscle.

Local lymph glands The local lymph glands are often enlarged, but this does not always mean that they contain tumour. In about one-third of patients with palpable lymph glands, the lymphadenopathy is caused by infection, which subsides after excision of the ulcer. Nevertheless it should be assumed that palpable lymph glands contain metastases.

Local tissues The surrounding tissues may be oedematous and thickened, and subcutaneous spread may involve nearby nerves. Invasion of local blood vessels can cause thrombosis and tissue ischaemia. These events are features of the late stages of the disease.

Complications Infection and bleeding are the common complications. If the ulcer erodes into a large blood vessel, the bleeding can be massive and fatal.

General examination All the lymph glands between the primary lesion and the great veins in the neck should be examined. Distant metastases are uncommon, but a pleural effusion and hepatomegaly are indicative of systemic spread.

Differential diagnosis This includes tumours of the skin appendages, cutaneous secondary deposits, basal cell carcinoma, keratoacanthoma, malignant melanoma, solar keratosis, pyogenic granuloma and an infected seborrhoeic wart.

Marjolin's ulcer
(Squamous cell carcinoma)

Marjolin's ulcer is an eponym reserved for a squamous carcinoma that arises in a long-standing benign ulcer or scar. The commonest ulcer to become malignant is a long-standing venous ulcer. The scar that is most often associated with malignant change is the scar of an old burn.

These carcinomata are very similar to an idiopathic squamous carcinoma, except that they may not be so florid. Their edge is not always raised and everted, and other features may be masked by the pre-existing chronic ulceration or scarring.

Unusual nodules or changes in a chronic ulcer or a scar should be viewed with suspicion, especially if they increase in size and develop a very smelly discharge.

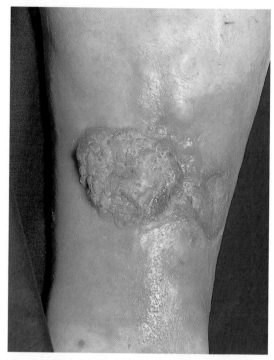

FIG 3.43 A Marjolin's ulcer. The pigmentation and scarring caused by long-standing venous hypertension and ulceration can be seen around the patch of hyperplastic neoplastic tissue.

Revision panel 3.7		
The diagnostic features of the four common surgical skin lesions		
	Duration of growth	**Physical features**
Squamous cell carcinoma	Few months	Occasional bleeding
		Nodule or ulcer with everted edge
Basal cell carcinoma	Many months or years	Nodule or ulcer with rolled edge and permanent scab
Keratoacanthoma	Few weeks	Nodule with central hard necrotic core
		No bleeding
		Spontaneous regression
Pyogenic granuloma	Few days	Soft red nodule that becomes covered with epithelium
		Bleeds easily

Malignant melanoma

Because of the confusion which has arisen from using the word 'melanoma' to describe a benign lesion and 'malignant melanoma' to describe a malignant one, use the terms mole or pigmented naevus for benign lesions and malignant melanoma for malignant lesions.

As the melanocyte originates from the neural crest and so is neuro-ectodermal in origin, it could be argued that malignant change in melanocytes should be called a carcinoma. Terms such as 'melanocarcinoma' or even 'melanosarcoma' only add to the confusion. It is therefore best to use the well-established descriptive term 'malignant melanoma'.

Cardinal symptoms of malignant change in a mole

- **Change in surface**. One of the earliest signs associated with malignant change is loss of the normal skin markings (creases) over the mole. The skin may also become rough and scaly.
- **Itching**. This is an early and significant symptom, often associated with a pale-pink halo around the mole.
- **Increase in size, shape or thickness**. The patient usually complains that a long-standing mole, or a recently developed brown spot, has grown steadily over a period of a few weeks or months. The mole or part of the mole may become wider and thicker, often changing from a flat plaque to a nodule. Alternatively the mole may simply change in outline.
- **Change in colour**. Malignant melanocytes usually produce more melanin, so the mole gets darker. The colour change is often patchy, with some areas becoming almost black, others turning blue-purple with the increased vascularity, and some areas not changing at all. Very occasionally the malignant melanocytes do not produce melanin, so that the new growth is colourless.
- **Bleeding**. As the tumour cells multiply, the overlying epithelium becomes anoxic and either ulcerates spontaneously or breaks down after a very minor injury. Bleeding is slight and a late sign.
- **Evidence of local or distant spread**. The pigment produced by the malignant melanocytes may spread diffusely into the surrounding skin to produce a brown halo around the primary lesion. The malignant cells may also spread through the skin in the intradermal lymphatics. When they stop migrating and multiply, they become small intradermal nodules. Small nodules around the primary lesion are called **satellite nodules**. Occasionally patients notice enlarged lymph glands in the groin or axilla.

Not all malignant melanomata arise in pre-existing pigmented naevi. All the changes listed above can develop in a lesion that appeared quite quickly a few weeks or months previously.

History

Age Malignant melanoma is very rare before puberty, although it has been reported in children. Most cases occur in patients aged 20–30 years or more.

Sex Malignant melanoma occurs equally in both sexes, but is found more often in the lower limbs in women and on the trunk in men.

Ethnic group Malignant melanoma is common in Caucasians and rare in Negroes. People with fair complexions, red hair and a tendency to freckle are more susceptible.

Cause Melanocytes are stimulated by ultraviolet light. White-skinned people living in those parts of the world that enjoy abundant sunlight, such as Australia and the west coast of America, have a high incidence

---

Revision panel 3.8
The changes which suggest that a mole has turned malignant

Loss of normal surface markings
(e.g. skin creases)
Change in size, shape or thickness
Change in colour
Itching
Bleeding/ulceration
Halo
    Pink (inflammatory reaction) – early
    Brown (pigment) – late
Satellite nodules

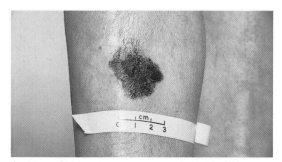

A superficial spreading melanoma. The lesion is thin, with an irregular edge and varying degrees of pigmentation.

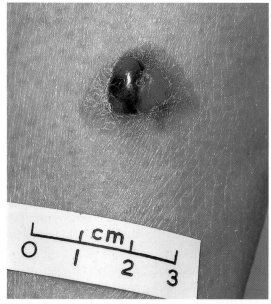

A nodular melanoma arising in a long-standing benign mole (pigmented naevus).

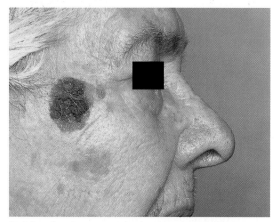

Nodules of malignant melanoma arising in a patch of Hutchinson's lentigo which had been present for many years.

FIG 3.44 MALIGNANT MELANOMATA.

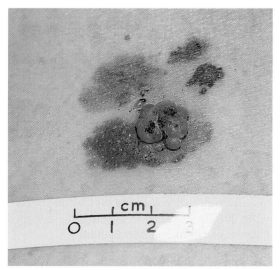

A superficial spreading melanoma with an amelanotic nodular area. The nodule had appeared within the previous month and had itched and bled.

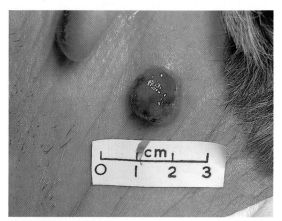

A large nodular melanoma which arose in previously normal skin.

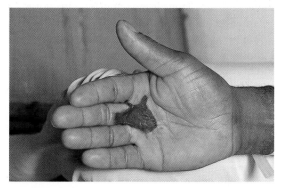

A malignant melanoma in the palm of the hand of a black-skinned manual worker.

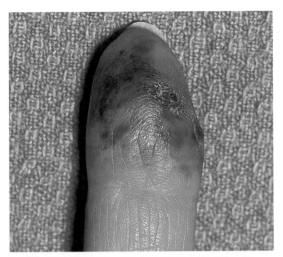

An ulcerated melanoma on the tip of the middle finger. The ulceration and lack of pigmentation caused the referring physician to think it was a chronic pulp space infection.

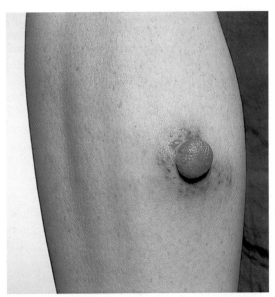

Satellite nodules of tumour cells around a nodular melanoma.

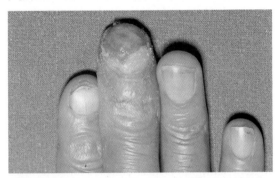

An acral lentiginous melanoma of the tip of the index finger.

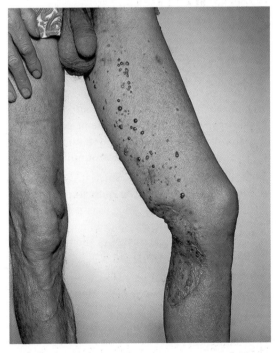

Multiple metastatic nodules of melanoma that appeared 4 years after the primary lesion (which was behind the knee) had been excised.

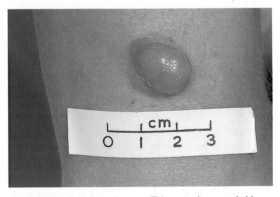

A nodular amelanotic melanoma. This arose in normal skin and was at first thought to be a histiocytoma.

FIG 3.44 continued

of malignant melanoma. Those who work out of doors in these regions, especially those with a history of repeated episodes of sunburn, are particularly susceptible.

Symptoms The cardinal features have already been described. The common reasons for seeking medical advice are a change of size or colour, bleeding, and the appearance of a brown halo or satellite nodules. It is usually the cosmetic disfigurement caused by an enlarging mole that brings the patient to the doctor, but more than 25 per cent arise de novo, i.e. in normal skin rather than in a pre-existing lesion. Malignant melanomata often itch but are not painful.

Sometimes the patient has observed the changes described above, but if the mole is on the sole of the foot or the back of the trunk where it cannot be seen, the patient may present with lymph gland enlargement or symptoms caused by distant metastases, such as weight loss, dyspnoea or jaundice.

Multiplicity Multiple malignant melanomata are very rare, but there are often multiple secondary nodules around a primary lesion Two concurrent primary lesions are very uncommon.

Examination

Site The majority of malignant melanomata are found on the limbs, head, neck and trunk. They are uncommon on the palms of the hands and the soles of the feet (except in African Negroes). They may arise in the subungual tissues, at the mucocutaneous junction and in the mouth and the anal margin.

Shape and size When first noticed, the area of malignant change is usually quite small (0.5–2 cm in diameter), but the mole in which the change has begun may be of any size. When a malignant melanoma is neglected it becomes a large, florid tumour, protruding from and overlapping the surrounding skin.

Surface When the tumour is small it is covered by smooth epithelium. When the epithelium dies, from ischaemic necrosis, the resulting ulcer is covered with a crust of blood and serum. Bleeding and subacute infection may make the surface of the tumour wet, soft and boggy.

Colour Malignant melanomata may be any colour from a pale pinkish-brown to black. If they have a rich blood supply, they develop a purple hue. Variations in the colour are common, some areas being very black and others pale.

Temperature and tenderness A malignant melanoma is no warmer than the surrounding skin, in spite of its vascularity and cellular activity, and is not tender.

Composition The primary tumour has a firm consistence. Small satellite nodules feel hard.

Relations The malignant tissue is within the skin and moves with it.

Lymph drainage The local lymph glands may be enlarged.

Surrounding tissues There may be a halo of brown pigment in the skin around the tumour and satellite nodules in the skin and subcutaneous tissue between the primary tumour and the nearest lymph glands. It is important to feel all the subcutaneous tissues along the course of the lymphatics that drain the lesion, as nodules of melanoma may be palpable.

Clinical types

Although the above description indicates that a malignant melanoma may have many forms, there are four common clinical types.

- **Superficial spreading melanoma** is the most common variety. It may occur on any part of the body, is usually palpable but thin, with an irregular edge and a variegated colour.
- **Nodular melanoma** is thick and protrudes above the skin. It has a smooth surface and a regular outline, and may arise de novo. It may become ulcerated and then often bleeds.
- **Lentigo maligna melanoma** is a malignant melanoma arising in a patch of Hutchinson's lentigo. The malignant areas are thicker than the surrounding pigmented skin, usually darker in colour, but seldom ulcerate.
- **Acral lentiginous melanoma** is a rare type of malignant melanoma but important to remember because it is often misdiagnosed as a chronic paronychia or a subungual haematoma. It presents as an irregular, expanding area of brown or black pigmentation on the palm, the sole or beneath a nail.

General examination Malignant melanoma spreads via the lymphatics to the regional lymph glands. It may then spread in the bloodstream to the lungs, liver and brain. Pleural effusions, hepatomegaly, jaundice and neurological abnormalities are indications of distant metastases. Blood-borne secondary deposits in the skin and subcutaneous tissues are not uncommon.

Mycosis fungoides

This is a rare skin lymphoma but it occasionally presents in a surgical clinic. It begins as a patch of thickening and reddening of the skin which enlarges into a plaque above the surrounding skin and then ulcerates. The lesions may be multiple. It is often associated with a generalized lymphoma.

Kaposi's sarcoma

Kaposi's sarcoma is a cutaneous sarcoma which, before the appearance of human immunodeficiency virus (HIV) infection, was a rare sporadic condition in Europe, but not uncommon and endemic in sub-Saharan Africa, particularly Zaire and Western Uganda.

The variety not associated with HIV infection runs a slow, indolent course and is only very rarely associated with spread to the intestine or generalized malignant lymphoma.

The variety associated with HIV infection and acquired immunodeficiency syndrome (AIDS) runs an aggressive course and is usually associated with systemic tumour infiltration of lymph glands, intestine, mucous membranes, lungs and other organs.

History

The patients complain of the presence of painless nodules or plaques in and beneath the skin, which often appear first in the legs. There are likely to be a multitude of systemic symptoms if the patient has AIDS.

Examination

The nodules are red, hemispherical and painless. They lie in the subcutaneous tissues, but the overlying skin is often red, adherent to and involved in the disease process. The overlying skin may break down into an ulcer.

OTHER COMMON SKIN CONDITIONS OFTEN SEEN IN SURGICAL PATIENTS

Hyperhidrosis

All skin contains sweat glands. If these glands secrete an excessive quantity of sweat (hyperhidrosis), the skin becomes soggy, white and moist.

Hyperhidrosis of the hands is a distressing condition. The sweat may drip off the fingers, and everything the patient touches gets wet.

Axillary hyperhidrosis is also embarrassing because the adjacent clothes become saturated with sweat and offensive.

Eczema/dermatitis

This is a red, weepy, vesicular rash which usually has an immune cause. There are constitutional 'endogenous' factors in all patients with eczema, but 'exogenous' sensitizing factors are also very important. The condition may be inherited, when it is often associated with hay fever and asthma. It can also be initiated by an allergy, drugs or infection, or physical problems such as an injury, scratching or varicose veins.

Drug eruptions

A whole variety of different types of rash can occur in response to drugs, including maculopapular rashes, eczema, purpura, urticaria and generalized desquamation. Occasionally patients develop severe malaise, pyrexia and generalized lymphadenopathy. A drug eruption must be considered in any patient who develops a rash (see Revision panel 3.9).

Urticaria

This used to be called **hives** and is the development of allergic wheals in the skin in response to a noxious stimulus. The condition is caused by degranulation of mast cells, which release histamine. In some patients the cause proves impossible to identify and these cases are called idiopathic. Nettle stings, jelly-fish stings and insect bites are recognized causes, as are morphine and atropine.

The term **angioneurotic oedema** is used to describe swelling of the tongue, eyelids, lips and larynx,

---

Revision panel 3.9
Common causes of drug eruption

Antibiotics
Barbiturates
Non-steroidal anti-inflammatory drugs
Diuretics
Chlorpromazine

which comes on intermittently and for which there is no known cause. Occasionally a family history is present indicating a genetic factor.

Acne and sycosis barbae

These are conditions in which the ducts of the sebaceous glands become blocked by over-activity. They may then become inflamed and secondarily infected. The condition causes comedos (blackheads) and blind cysts, which may turn into sebaceous cysts. Severe scarring may result. The condition declines after the age of 20.

Psoriasis

This condition occurs in 1–2 per cent of the Caucasian population, usually beginning between the ages of 5 and 25. About a third of those affected have a family history of the condition. It tends to improve in summer and during pregnancy. It presents as sharply demarcated, red, raised, oval plaques mainly situated over the elbows, knees and scalp. The plaques have a silver, scaly surface and the pattern of distribution varies widely. Psoriasis is often associated with an arthritis of the hands, which has to be distinguished from rheumatoid arthritis. A quarter of those affected develop pits in the nails, which are often thick, opaque, discoloured and break easily. It may occur in the flexures of the groin and axillae, where moist conditions prevent scaling.

Pityriasis rosacea

This is the commonest cause of a slightly itchy skin rash in a young person. It usually starts with a single red, oval, scaly macule, which often arises over the lower abdomen or shoulder. Three or four days later, a characteristic rash appears over the trunk, consisting of both macules and papules. The rash does not involve the skin below the upper thighs and arms and has a 'vest and pants' distribution. The long axes of the macules are arranged along the line of skin cleavage (Langer's lines). They typically have a fawn centre with a pink surround. Scaling is often present at the junction with normal skin. The rash usually clears completely in 6–12 weeks. The differential diagnosis includes drug sensitivity, tinea pedis, guttate psoriasis and secondary syphilis.

Lichen planus

This develops on the wrists as an itchy rash before spreading to the trunk and legs. Papules are present on the wrist, forearms, trunk and shins. The rash may be widespread or may remain localized to the wrist and shins. The papules are usually highly characteristic. They are flat topped, shiny, purple and often polygonal in shape. They are often umbilicated and appear in scratch marks (the *Koebner phenonomen*). They may become warty and form larger plaques, which can coalesce. Delicate, white striae, annular lesions or white dots may be present on the buccal mucosa, tongue or inside of the lips. Oral ulceration may develop but this is not painful. The condition invariably affects adults, and the face and scalp are almost never involved. Its course is very variable but it usually lasts 3–6 months.

SUBCUTANEOUS INFECTIONS

Subcutaneous abscess

Abscesses in the subcutaneous tissue are common and usually follow implantation of bacteria by a penetrating injury, or infection in a haematoma.

The common infecting organism is *Staphylococcus aureus*, but almost any organism can cause an abscess if the local conditions are favourable to its growth. An abscess is a pocket of pus (dead cells, exudate and bacteria) surrounded by granulation tissue.

History

Age Subcutaneous abscesses occur in all ages and both sexes.

Hygiene Poor social conditions and bodily hygiene will increase the chances of an infection following a minor injury such as a pinprick.

Symptoms The principal complaint is of a throbbing pain which gets steadily worse and keeps the patient awake at night.

The patient notices an area of thickening and tenderness at the site of the pain, which slowly turns into a hard mass.

The mass may discharge spontaneously, with relief of the symptoms, before the patient comes to the doctor.

Previous history Patients who are debilitated, diabetic or drug addicts may have had previous abscesses because of the debility caused by their underlying disease and frequent injections.

Habits Enquire about the drug-taking habits of the patient if you have cause to think that the abscess has followed a self-administered injection.

Examination

The four classical signs of an abscess (the *signs of Celsus*) are tumour, rubor, calor and dolor (swelling, redness, heat and pain).

Site Areas subjected to trauma are more susceptible. The hands are common sites for subcutaneous infection (see page 162).

Injections are usually given into the buttock or thigh, so these are also common sites for abscesses.

Self-administered injections by drug addicts are usually given into the veins in the cubital fossa and groin.

Shape and size The initial change is the development of a patch of induration. As the pus forms, this patch turns into a definite mass which is basically spherical.

The mass may become large and lose its spherical shape if the pus begins to spread through the subcutaneous tissues.

Surface The inner surface of an abscess is a layer of granulation tissue which is inseparable from the indurated inflamed tissues around it. Thus an abscess does not have a definable outer surface, even though its contents may be easy to feel.

Colour The overlying skin is red.

Temperature The skin over an abscess is hot.

Tenderness Abscesses become increasingly tender as the tension in the pocket of pus increases.

Edge The edge is not palpable, as the induration and oedema gradually merge into the normal tissues.

Composition In the early stages an abscess feels hard and solid. As the pus forms, the centre of the area becomes soft and, if it is not too tender to press, **fluctuant**. It is dull to percussion and not reducible.

Relations The skin over a subcutaneous abscess is invariably involved in the inflammatory process, so it is red, oedematous and fixed to the underlying mass.

If the pus points towards the skin, the skin becomes white and then black as it dies and sloughs away. When the dead skin separates, the pus can escape from the abscess. Deep fixation depends upon the size and direction of spread of the abscess.

Local lymph glands The lymph glands which receive lymph from the infected area are likely to be enlarged and tender. They may even become abscesses themselves.

Local tissues The local tissues should be normal, apart from those close to the abscess which are involved in the inflammation. There may be scars from previous abscesses.

General examination A large abscess can cause considerable systemic disturbance. The patient looks pale and ill but may be sweating and having rigors and episodes of flushing. The temperature and pulse are elevated.

Carbuncle

A carbuncle is a spreading necrotizing infection in the subcutaneous tissues, with pus and slough formation, similar to the changes that occur in a boil, but with many points of discharge through holes in the skin that appear when patches of necrotic skin slough. The subcutaneous tissue necrosis is much more extensive than the reddened area of overlying skin.

Sinuses and fistulae

Sinus

A sinus is a tract lined by granulation tissue which connects a cavity (usually an old abscess) with an epithelial surface. A sinus produces a serous or purulent discharge and fails to close if:

- the cavity is inadequately drained,
- it is caused by a specific chronic infection (e.g. actinomycosis, tuberculosis, syphilis),
- a foreign body (e.g. stitch material) is present at the bottom of the sinus,
- the cavity has epithelialized,
- the cavity has undergone malignant change,
- the surrounding tissues have poor vascularity or have been irradiated.

Sinuses commonly follow surgical wound infections and necrosis of tumours.

Sinus   Fistula

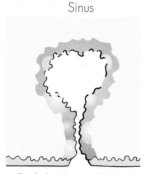
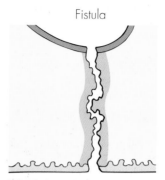

A sinus is a connection between a cavity lined with granulation tissue and an epithelial surface.

A fistula is a connection between two epithelial-lined surfaces.

FIG 3.45 THE DIFFERENCE BETWEEN A SINUS AND A FISTULA.

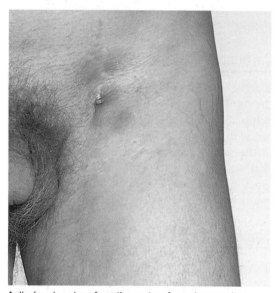
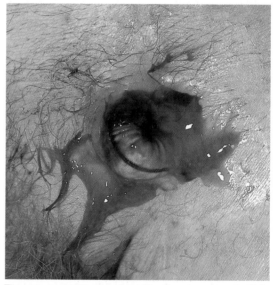

A discharging sinus from the centre of a groin wound.

The same wound 3 weeks later. The sinus has opened widely to reveal its cause – an infected Dacron arterial graft.

FIG 3.46 A SINUS AND ITS CAUSE.

Revision panel 3.10
The causes of a chronic abscess or persistent sinus

Inadequate drainage
Specific chronic infection, e.g. tuberculosis
Foreign body, e.g. a stitch
Epithelialization of the cavity
Malignant change in the wall of the cavity

Fistula

A fistula is a pathological connection between two epithelial surfaces. For example, it is possible to have a fistula between the bowel and the skin, the bowel and another loop of bowel, or the bowel and the bladder.

Fistulae are usually lined with granulation tissue but they can become epithelialized. They form when a chronic abscess bursts in two directions connecting two epithelial surfaces. They persist if they have to transmit the contents of one of the epithelial-lined cavities to the other if the former's normal outflow is obstructed.

They do not resolve until the cause of the abscess is eradicated (see above for the factors which delay abscess closure) or the obstruction to the emptying of the viscus is removed.

The common fistulae seen in surgical practice are between the anal canal and the peri-anal skin and the bowel.

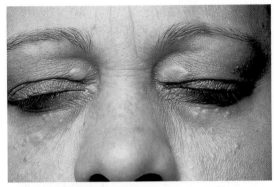

Xanthoma of the upper eyelid.

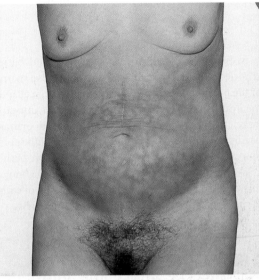

Erythema ab igne caused by the repeated application of a hot-water bottle to relieve abdominal pain.

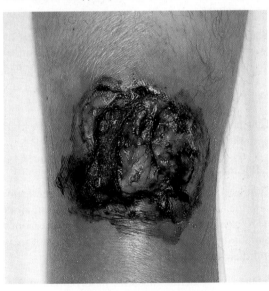

Infected necrosis (gangrene) of the skin following local trauma in a patient taking steroids.

FIG 3.47 SOME MORE SKIN LESIONS.

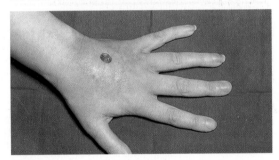

An injection ulcer on the back of the hand.

4

Muscles, tendons, bones and joints

It is essential that all doctors have a sound basic knowledge of orthopaedic disease, because so many of the patients who come to the general surgical and medical clinics have abnormalities of their musculoskeletal system. As the primary concern in orthopaedic conditions is often function, you must be able to examine the muscles, bones and joints properly, assessing function as well as any structural abnormality. This chapter describes the examination of each of these structures and some of the common abnormalities and diseases that affect them.

A GENERAL PLAN FOR EXAMINING THE MUSCLES, BONES AND JOINTS OF A LIMB

The basic approach can be broken down into five components:

- inspection
- palpation
- movement
- percussion and/or auscultation when indicated
- special tests as appropriate.

Although moving the limb would normally be part of inspection and palpation, it is such an important part of the examination that it is presented as a separate exercise and, as percussion, auscultation and special tests are not relevant to all joints or bones, the basic plan becomes inspection, palpation and movement, or in simple English:

- look
- feel
- move.

Always begin by looking at both limbs, front and back, and examining the good limb first.

Always ask the patient to perform active movement before you perform passive movements.

Inspection and movement should be performed with the patient supine and standing.

Inspection

Skin Is the skin discoloured, erythematous or oedematous? Is there any bruising that may suggest trauma? Look for scars and sinuses. Are there any abnormal or asymmetrical skin creases? Is there any localized bony tenderness suggestive of the presence of a fracture?

Shape Is there any swelling and, if so, is it diffuse or localized? Is there any deformity or postural alteration in shape and, if so, is it confined to a joint (Fig. 4.1) or is it more generalized? (Fig. 4.2) Is there any muscle wasting?

Length Compare the length of each part of the limb with the other side, at this stage by eye.

Palpation

Skin Feel the temperature of the skin. Is there any oedema – local or dependent? Feel any scars or areas of thickening and find their relation to the bones and joints. Is any part of the limb tender, and if so, is it diffuse or localized?

Shape Try to define the cause of any swelling, e.g. swelling confined to a joint may be an effusion, haemarthrosis, pyarthrosis, thickening of the synovium or localized masses related to the muscle or bone. Note the relation of any swelling to underlying or neighbouring anatomical structures and elicit all its physical characteristics, described on pages 29–32.

Record on a diagram any abnormality or degrees of deformity of alignment.

Length Measure the real length of each limb and of each bone and the apparent length of the limb (see page 114).

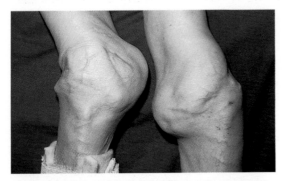

FIG 4.1 The grossly deformed knees that are the results of neuropathic joints.

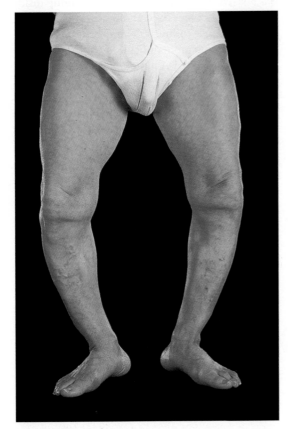

FIG 4.2 Marked deformity of the lower limbs associated with rickets.

Movement

Active Ask the patient to move each joint through its full range of movements and show you any trick or abnormal movements. Watch the limb working: standing, walking, lifting, etc.

Passive Move all the joints of the limb through their full range. Complete loss of all movement of a joint implies either surgical arthrodesis or fibrous or bony ankylosis as a result of some pathological process such as infection. Note any restriction to movement or fixed deformity which may result from contraction of the joint capsule, muscles or tendons. Locking or limitation may also occur as a result of interposition of soft tissues, bone or loose bodies. Record as accurately as possible the range of movements in degrees (e.g. 45° of flexion or 120° of extension).

Test the strength of each movement against resistance (see 'Muscle strength', page 107). Look for any clicks or crepitations in the joint on movement. Test for abnormal movements by testing the integrity of the ligaments of each joint.

Other tests

It is essential to examine the structures that keep the limb alive and make it work – the arteries and nerves.

Arteries Palpate all the pulses. Note the temperature and colour of the limb (see page 175).

Nerves Test the motor, sensory and reflex innervation of the limb.

Motor You will already have obtained some information on the ability of the muscles to contract during your examination of movement and strength. If there is any weakness, work out which muscles are affected and their nerve root innervation.

Sensory Check the appreciation of light touch, pinprick, temperature changes, deep pain, vibration sense and position sense. When applicable, record the Medical Research Council (MRC) grading of loss of sensation and its subsequent recovery or deterioration:

- **S0**: absent sensation in the area supplied by the affected nerve,
- **S1**: return of deep cutaneous pain,
- **S2**: return of some superficial pain and tactile sensibility,
- **S3**: return of superficial pain and tactile sensibility without over-reaction,
- **S3+**: return of two-point discrimination,
- **S4**: normal sensation.

Reflexes Test all the limb's reflexes, and if diminished or altered in any way, seek to identify the nerve root innervation.

SOFT TISSUES

MUSCLES AND MUSCLE DISEASE

Examination of a muscle

If a muscle appears to contain a definite lump, begin by examining the lump to ascertain its physical characteristics, as described in Chapter 1. If there is doubt about the relationship of a lump to the whole muscle, it is better to examine the muscle first and the lump second.

Inspection

Observe the shape of the muscle at rest. Note any wasting, hypertrophy or irregularity of shape caused by a lump, or displacement of the muscle. Always compare the abnormal muscle with the normal muscle of the other limb.

Observe the shape of the muscle *when it is contracting*. Alterations in shape that appear when the muscle is contracting are caused either by a lump being concealed or made more obvious by the contracting muscle, or by knotting-up or parting of ruptured muscle fibres.

Look at the neighbouring bones and joints.

Palpation

Feel the muscle at rest. Place the limb in a comfortable position so that the muscle is relaxed. Assess the texture of the muscle.

Try to decide whether any abnormality is caused by a localized swelling or an abnormal muscle. Elicit all the features of any lump that you find.

Feel the muscle when it is contracting. See if any of the features of the lump you felt when the muscle was relaxed change when it contracts. A lump inside the muscle becomes fixed and more difficult to feel when the muscle contracts. A lump beneath the muscle may become more difficult to palpate when the muscle is contracted. A lump superficial to the muscle, or breaking through its fibrous sheath, becomes more prominent.

A gap or hollow that appears in the muscle when it contracts usually means that the fibres are ruptured (see below).

A lump that appears only when the muscle contracts is probably a bunch of ruptured fibres knotting up.

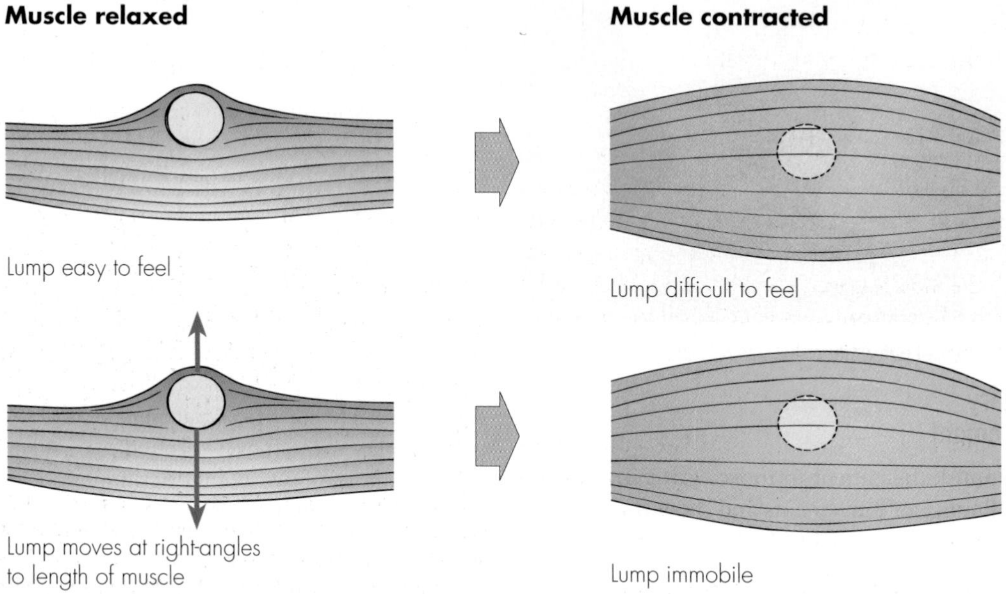

Muscle relaxed   **Muscle contracted**

Lump easy to feel   Lump difficult to feel

Lump moves at right-angles to length of muscle   Lump immobile

FIG 4.3 Principal features of an intramuscular lump.

Strength

Muscle power can be classified according to the MRC scale. However, it is often better not to use numbers but to describe the strength:

- **M0**: no active contraction at all,
- **M1**: barely perceptible flicker of contraction but insufficient to cause any movement,
- **M2**: weak contraction producing some movement but insufficient to lift the limb against the pull of gravity,
- **M3**: weak contraction but can move the limb against the pull of gravity only,
- **M4**: fairly strong contraction but not full strength; can produce movement against gravity and some added resistance,
- **M5**: full strength.

Remember that muscle strength can be impaired by pain, wasting, denervation or other disease processes.

Innervation and blood supply

You will know if a muscle is innervated after testing its motor function, but you must also examine the integrity of the whole nerve and the spinal segment supplying the muscle by testing all of its other motor, sensory and reflex functions. This means that you must know which nerves and which spinal segments innervate the main muscle blocks in the body (see Revision panel 1.9, page 27).

Examine the pulses in the limb.

Ruptured muscle fibres

Muscle fibres usually rupture during an excessively strong or unusually sudden contraction of the muscle. Pathological rupture can follow a normal contraction if the muscle is weakened by some degenerative process. The rupture usually occurs at the musculotendinous junction.

History

Age Muscle rupture can occur at all ages but is most common in athletic young men at play, and elderly men performing excessive or unaccustomed physical exercise.

Symptoms Sometimes there is pain, swelling and bruising at the time of the rupture, but in the elderly patient the original incident is often not noticed and the patient presents with weakness, a limp or a swelling of the muscle.

Site The muscles commonly affected are the biceps brachii and the quadriceps femoris – two muscles which often have to withstand sudden severe strains.

Examination

The diagnostic feature of a bundle of ruptured muscle fibres is the appearance of a lump in the muscle on one or both sides of a depression when the muscle contracts. The lumps are the bunched-up free ends of the contracted ruptured fibres.

The lumps cannot be felt when the muscle is relaxed because they have the same consistence as the adjacent muscle, but the hollow between the broken fibres may be palpable and visible.

The lump (or lumps) which appears when the muscle contracts is firm in consistence, has indistinct

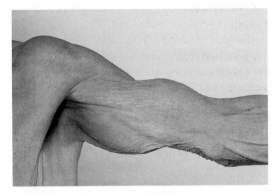

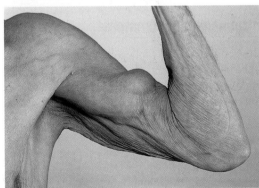

FIG 4.4 A rupture of the long head of the biceps. In the upper photograph the muscle is relaxed and its contours are normal. In the lower photograph the muscle is contracting and the ruptured fibres are bunched up into a firm mass in the middle of the arm.

Relaxed

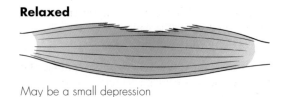

May be a small depression

Contracted

A lump appears on one or both
sides of a sharp depression

FIG 4.5 The clinical features of ruptured muscle fibres.

edges and cannot be moved independently of the muscle.

The local arteries, nerves, bones and joints are normal unless the rupture is caused by attrition or a chronic musculoskeletal disease such as rheumatoid arthritis.

Do not forget to examine the neighbouring bones and joints.

If a significant number of fibres are ruptured, the strength of the muscle will be reduced. If all the fibres are ruptured, the movement normally produced by the muscle will be absent.

Intramuscular haematoma

This condition usually follows a direct injury or tear of the muscle fibres and the intramuscular blood vessels. It can follow a severe cramp or a violent, sudden muscle contraction. Although some of the muscle fibres are ruptured, not enough are divided to produce the physical signs of a ruptured muscle.

History

Symptoms The two main symptoms are pain and swelling in the muscle. The pain is present at rest but is exacerbated by any movement of the muscle, passive or active. The patient may also have noticed a diffuse swelling of the limb or a tender lump in the muscle.

Cause The patient can often recall the initial injury. Trivial injuries only cause intramuscular bleeding if there is a haematological or vascular abnormality.

Ask the patient if he or she is taking anticoagulants and, if male, whether he has haemophilia.

Examination

Site The muscles of the lower limbs, especially the gastrocnemius, are most often affected.

Tenderness The lump is tender for a few days, and all movements of the muscle are very painful. Although the tenderness subsides quite quickly, the pain caused by contraction of the muscle may persist for weeks.

Shape and size Haematomata are usually ovoid, with their long axis parallel to the muscle fibres.

The size of the lump depends upon the amount of bleeding. This is not always easy to assess, because the edge of the lump is usually indistinct.

Composition The composition of a haematoma depends upon the state of the blood within it. The blood in most haematomata is coagulated, so the lump feels hard. Sometimes the central portion stays fluid, making the lump soft and fluctuant.

Local tissues The surrounding tissues, including the adjacent muscle, should feel normal, but contraction of the muscle causes pain and makes the lump more difficult to feel.

Lymph glands The lymph glands at the root of the limb should not be enlarged.

Muscle hernia

When a muscle contracts, it becomes shorter and thicker. If it is contained by a fibrous sheath, the tension within the sheath rises. If there is a defect in the fibrous sheath, the muscle will bulge through it, especially when it contracts. This is called a muscle hernia.

History

Symptoms The patient may notice the lump when looking at or feeling the muscle, or experience a slight ache in the muscle and find a lump when trying to pinpoint the source of the discomfort.

Examination

Site Although all muscles are surrounded by a fibrous sheath, only those with a thick covering are likely to cause symptomatic muscle herniae. The commonest muscle hernia is through the thick fascia which covers the anterior compartment of the lower leg.

Shape and size Muscle herniae can be of any size. Their characteristic feature is that they change in size according to the tension in the muscle. When the muscle contracts, it bulges through the fascial defect. When the muscle is relaxed, there is no lump – just a hole.

Occasionally these signs are reversed. The muscle may bulge through the defect when relaxed but be pulled back into its compartment when it retracts. Do not be confused by this variation. Provided the lump comes and goes as the muscle tension changes and there is a palpable defect in its covering fascia, it is a muscle hernia.

Intramuscular and intermuscular lipomata

There is not much fat inside a muscle, but there are often small collections of fat around the nutrient blood vessels and in the loose areolar tissue which separates the different sections of a group of muscles. Lipomata can develop in this fat. Histologically they are no different from any other lipomata, but the site gives them some distinctive physical signs.

History

Symptoms An intramuscular or intermuscular lipoma may interfere with the function of the muscle and cause pain when the muscle is being used, but it rarely makes the muscle weak.

The patient may have felt, or seen, a lump appear during exercise. If an intramuscular lipoma suddenly bursts out of a muscle during exercise, the patient experiences a sharp pain and notices the sudden appearance of the lump. They will then believe that the exercise caused the lump. The lump may change in size and shape as the muscle contracts.

Muscle lipomata are rarely multiple.

Examination

Site Any muscle can be affected. There is more fat between the flat muscles of the trunk than between the muscles of the limbs, so deep lipomata are more common on the back of the trunk.

Shape and size If there is only a thin layer of muscle or fascia covering the lipoma, its typical multilobular shape will be palpable.

These lipomata are often quite large (5–10 cm in diameter) because they grow unnoticed within or between the muscles for many years. They may become larger, smaller or disappear when the muscle contracts, according to their relation to the main bulk of the muscle.

Edge Their edge is difficult to feel. When a lipoma has herniated through the thick layer of fibrous tissue surrounding the muscle, you may feel a sharp edge, corresponding to the defect in the fascia, but there is usually a lot more of the lipoma deep to this edge that you cannot feel.

Composition The consistence varies with the tension in the muscle. When the muscle is relaxed, the lipoma has its typical soft consistence and may seem to fluctuate. When the muscle contracts, the lipoma, if it is still palpable, becomes hard and tense.

Relations Intermuscular and intramuscular lipomata are tethered to their site of origin and usually become fixed when the muscle contracts. An intermuscular lipoma may become impalpable when the muscle overlying it contracts.

Myositis ossificans

This is calcification, and sometimes ossification, in part of a muscle. It is an uncommon condition that may follow an injury that has caused extensive intramuscular haemorrhage, sometimes associated with a fracture of the adjacent bone. The muscles most often affected are the brachialis, after a supracondylar fracture of the humerus, and the quadriceps femoris, after a fracture of the femur or a direct blow such as a kick.

History

Previous injury The patient will know about their previous fracture or, when not associated with a fracture, remember a previous major soft tissue injury.

Symptoms The principal symptoms are caused by an inability of the muscle to relax. The nearby joint becomes stiff because there is a reduction of all the movements normally permitted by relaxation of the affected muscle (e.g. myositis of the quadriceps femoris restricts knee flexion but there is full extension). All forced movements are painful. If the intramuscular ossification is extensive, the joint may become completely fixed.

Examination

Site The common sites for myositis ossificans are the lower part of the brachialis muscle and the lower part of the quadriceps femoris muscle.

Tenderness The mass of ossified muscle is not normally tender, but forced passive movements may cause pain.

Temperature The mass has a normal temperature.

Shape The ossification takes the shape of the muscle in which it is occurring. It is usually an elongated mound filling the muscle and fixed to the underlying bone.

Surface The surface is smooth but irregular.

Composition The mass is bony hard and dull to percussion.

Relations In most cases the ossification in the muscle is continuous with the callus that developed around the fracture. Thus the mass is often mistaken for a bony swelling.

Normally the muscles over the callus of a healing fracture will work normally, whereas ossifying muscles cannot work properly and cannot be moved over the callus. The muscle fibres can be felt running into the mass.

Local tissues There may be other evidence of the previous trauma – bone and joint deformities, or nerve and artery damage – so it is important to examine the whole limb very carefully.

Myosarcoma

True tumours of muscle are rare. Those that arise from smooth muscle are called leiomyosarcomata. Those that arise from striated muscle are called rhabdomyosarcomata.

Almost all of the soft tissue sarcomata occurring in the limbs will actually be fibrosarcomata arising from the intermuscular and intramuscular fibrous septae or the fibrous tissue at the origin or inser-tion of the muscles. These tumours are described below. True

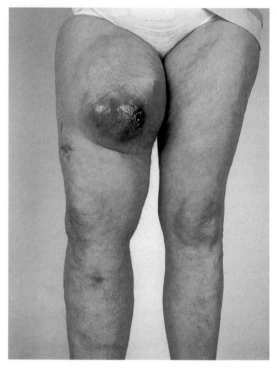

FIG 4.6 A large rhabdomyosarcoma of the thigh arising in the quadriceps muscles.

rhabdomyosarcomata are uncommon and clinically cannot often be differentiated from fibrosarcomata.

The diagnostic features of a tumour arising in or from a muscle are:

■ it moves freely when the muscle is relaxed, especially in a direction at right-angles to the length of the muscle;

■ it becomes immobile when the muscle contracts and its physical features may change; it may become more or less prominent, harder or softer, and change shape.

FIBROUS TISSUE

The fibrous tissue that covers muscles and links them to bone in the form of tendons, fibrous insertions, aponeuroses, tendon sheaths etc. is tough, durable and stable. It causes little trouble during life but is sometimes the site of malignant change.

Three tumours can arise from this tissue. The pure benign fibroma is very rare and can be forgotten, but the fibrosarcoma is one of the commonest mesodermal soft tissue malignant tumours. The third variety is a less common, locally invasive and recurrent tumour known by various names, but most often as Paget's recurrent desmoid tumour.

Fibrosarcoma

This is a malignant tumour of fibrous tissue. It is locally invasive and also spreads via the bloodstream to the lungs and liver. Spread to the lymph glands is an uncommon, but not unheard of, event. Distant spread is a late event and the primary will often grow locally for years before metastasizing.

History

Age Fibrosarcomata are more common in elderly patients but they can occur at any age.

Duration The patient has often known of the existence of a lump for months – sometimes years – before he comes to the doctor to complain of it.

Symptoms The reasons for complaint include:

- growth of the lump, causing disfigurement or interference with muscle movements,
- pain in the lump itself or from invasion of nearby structures,
- muscle weakness caused by infiltration of nearby muscles,
- general debility, from multiple metastases.

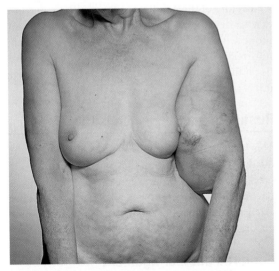

FIG 4.7 A slow-growing fibrosarcoma of the arm. The overlying skin is stretched and many distended subcutaneous veins are visible. There was no ischaemia or paralysis in the arm or forearm.

Examination

Site Fibrosarcomata can occur anywhere in the body but more occur in the limbs than elsewhere.

Colour If a large vascular tumour is near the skin, it may make the skin shiny and pink.

Temperature Sarcomata, even slow-growing ones such as fibrosarcomata, have an abnormal blood supply and usually feel warmer than the surrounding tissue.

Shape Their shape depends upon their site of origin. If a tumour grows in the middle of a soft tissue, it will be roughly spherical. If it arises close to a bone, it will be hemispherical, with its deep surface fixed to the bone.

Surface The surface is usually smooth but may be bosselated.

Edge The edge of slow-growing tumours is well defined. Fast-growing and invasive tumours have an indistinct edge.

Composition The consistence of fibrosarcomata is firm or hard. They are rarely stony hard because they do not ossify and their marked vascularity tends to keep them soft. They may be so vascular that they can pulsate, have an audible bruit and a palpable thrill.

Relations The relations of the tumour to the surrounding tissues depend entirely on its site of origin, size and invasiveness. Fibrosarcomata are usually firmly fixed to nearby structures and often invade neighbouring bones, nerves and arteries.

Lymph drainage On rare occasions the local lymph glands may be enlarged by secondary deposits.

State of local tissues Take particular care to test the integrity of any nerves running close to the mass of the tumour. A nerve deficit is more likely to indicate infiltration than stretching of the nerve, and is almost diagnostic of a locally malignant lesion.

Paget's recurrent desmoid tumour

This very rare condition is mentioned because it is an interesting variety of sarcoma. It occurs most often in middle-aged women, usually in the fascia covering the abdominal muscles, i.e. the rectus sheath and the external oblique aponeurosis. However, it can occur in other sites such as the plantar fascia of the foot or the palmar fascia of the hand. The malignant change affects a wide area because after an extensive

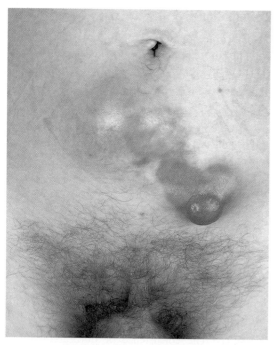

FIG 4.8 A large Paget's recurrent desmoid tumour arising from the anterior sheath of the rectus abdominis muscle.

and apparently adequate excision of the presenting lump, new lesions may appear years later, in fascia that was apparently healthy at the time of operation.

The lump has the same features as a fibrosarcoma, but is less vascular and very slow growing.

TENDONS AND TENDON SHEATHS

Ruptured tendons

When the tendon of a muscle is divided the muscle becomes ineffective. To assess the integrity of a tendon you must know its site of insertion and the movement that contraction of its parent muscle would normally produce.

Tendons can be ruptured by direct violence, especially if they have been weakened by rubbing over a fracture callus or the osteophytes and new bone produced by arthritis – a process called **attrition**. However, in most cases tendons rupture at a site that has been weakened by avascularity and degeneration (e.g. the Achilles tendon and long head of the biceps) or ischaemic pressure necrosis, such as that caused by a haematoma in the fibro-osseous sheath of the extensor pollicis longus. The tendon of the biceps

brachii, the Achilles tendon and various tendons in the hands are the tendons most often ruptured.

Ruptured biceps tendon

If the long, thin tendon of the long head of the biceps muscle ruptures, the muscle belly retracts into the middle of the arm, where it can be seen as a lump and be made more prominent by asking the patient to flex their elbow against a resistance. This condition is common in the elderly. It does not cause any significant weakness of the shoulder joint.

Ruptured Achilles tendon

Rupture of the Achilles tendon follows a sudden contraction of the gastrocnemius muscle during exercise. The patient feels a sudden severe pain, as if shot in the leg, and cannot walk properly. If the rupture happens during walking or running, the patient may fall down.

Examination reveals pain on attempting to plantar flex the foot and to stand on the toes of the affected leg, but some degree of plantar flexion is still possible using the long flexor and peroneal muscles. The gap in the tendon is easy to feel, even though there is often a considerable amount of oedema around the tendon and the ankle joint.

The rupture may be bilateral or the patient may have ruptured the other side in the past.

Rupture of the Achilles tendon is easy to miss but easy to detect with *Simmond's test*. Lie the patient prone with the feet beyond the edge of the couch, fully relaxed. Squeeze the calf. The foot will plantar flex if the Achilles tendon is intact but will not move if it is ruptured.

Ruptured quadriceps tendon

This is an avulsion of the tendinous insertion of the quadriceps femoris from the upper border of the patella. It usually occurs in elderly people and is uncommon. There is a loss or reduction of knee extension and a visible and palpable gap between the quadriceps muscle and the upper border of the patella.

Ruptured patellar ligament

This rare event is caused by an excessively strong contraction of the quadriceps femoris muscle in athletic young men. The obvious abnormality is an inability to extend the knee joint. The patella lies

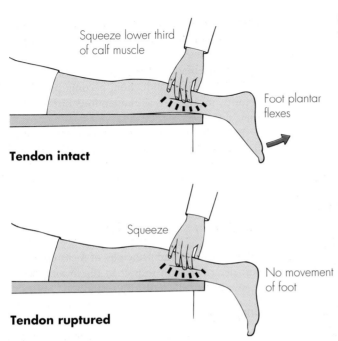

Squeeze lower third of calf muscle

Place the patient prone with the feet hanging freely over the end of the couch.

Foot plantar flexes

Tendon intact

Squeeze

Squeeze the calf muscles. If the Achilles tendon is intact, the foot will plantar flex.

No movement of foot

Tendon ruptured

FIG 4.9 Simmond's test for a ruptured achilles tendon.

high in the supracondylar groove of the femur, with a visible and palpable gap below it, in the area normally occupied by the hard, tense patellar ligament.

Ruptured extensor pollicis longus

Any of the finger tendons can be cut by penetrating injuries, but these present as an acute emergency with the appropriate history of trauma. In these cases it is important to check which finger movements are lost and confirm that this is due to the tendon injury and not to muscle paralysis caused by an associated nerve injury.

Some tendons, especially the tendon of the extensor pollicis longus, lie in a position which makes them liable to constant friction if arthritic changes (rheumatoid arthritis or osteoarthritis) occur in the underlying joint, or increasing pressure if their surrounding fibro-osseous sheath becomes tight or inflamed. When the tendon ruptures there is no pain, just a sudden loss of movement. In the case of the extensor pollicis longus, the patient cannot extend the distal phalanx of the thumb. Palpation will reveal the absence of tension in the tendon during extension of the thumb and the loss of the ulnar border of the anatomical 'snuff box' at the base of

the thumb. This is often seen complicating Colles' fracture and rupture of the extensor tendons of the fingers complicating rheumatoid arthritis.

Mallet finger

This is a rupture of the extensor tendon of a finger just proximal to its insertion. It is described on page 154.

Trigger finger

The movement of a tendon through its sheath can be impeded in two ways:

- by thickening of the tendon,
- by thickening of the tendon's sheath.

A trigger finger is a finger which gets fixed in flexion and can only be extended by excessive voluntary effort or sometimes physical assistance from the other hand. When extension actually occurs it does so with a jerk, just as the trigger of a gun moves when the resistance of its spring is overcome. The cause of this abnormality is a thickening of the tendon or the tendon sheath just where the tendon enters the sheath, which stops the tendon sliding freely into the sheath during extension.

Stenosing tenovaginitis
(of de Quervain)

This is an example of the restriction of tendon movement caused by thickening of the tendon sheath and/or the paratenon (i.e. a tenovaginitis or a tenosynovitis). The tendons involved are the extensor pollicis brevis and the abductor pollicis longus where they lie in their fibrous sheath on the lateral side of the wrist, just above the styloid process of the radius. The cause of the inflammation is usually repeated excessive movement of the tendons, e.g. typing.

All movements of the proximal phalanx of the thumb, especially abduction, become painful, and crepitus may be felt as the tendons move through their sheath.

Palpation reveals a tender, sausage-shaped swelling just above the styloid process of the radius.

BONES AND BONE IRREGULARITIES

EXAMINATION OF BONES

The basic plan follows a format similar to that described at the beginning of the chapter and includes inspection, palpation (including measurement), movement and percussion.

Inspection

The overlying skin may give an indication of the underlying pathology. An old tethered scar or a discharging sinus may indicate old or active osteomyelitis.

Redness and oedema of the skin may be caused by underlying infection or malignant growth.

If there is a bony deformity, record its site and angle.

Palpation

If there is a localized swelling, you must elicit all the physical signs pertaining to a swelling (described on pages 29–32).

Feel the whole length of the bone to assess its shape and compare it to the normal side.

Note the temperature of the skin. Conditions which increase bone blood flow, such as infection, tumours and Paget's disease, may raise the temperature of the surrounding tissues.

Measurement

Measure the length of the bone and the length of the limb. There are three measurements you can obtain:

1. the true length of individual bones,
2. the apparent length of the whole limb,
3. the real length of the whole limb.

The methods and principles of measurement are best described with respect to the lower limb, but they apply equally to the upper limb.

Bone length

This is a simple measurement because you are not measuring across any joints. Choose recognizable anatomical points at either end of the bone and measure between them. Do the same on the other side.

Bony points have to be felt through the overlying skin and muscle and it is difficult to get the end of the tape measure on identical points on both sides. The easiest method is to hold the measure between thumb and index finger and then press the back of the index finger firmly up against the bony point or edge that you are using as a landmark.

Apparent length of the limb

When a patient lies flat and 'straight' on a couch the limbs may appear to be of different length. This may be caused by a bone or joint abnormality. It is customary to record the apparent length, because when it is compared with the true length it gives some indication of the degree to which the skeleton has adapted its position to keep both legs parallel and both feet flat on the ground when the patient stands up, or alternatively an indication of the effect of a joint deformity on the length of the limb.

Method Ask the patient to lie straight on the bed. (Ask a child to lie like a soldier standing to attention.) Choose a point in the mid-line of the trunk – the umbilicus or xiphisternum – and measure from this central point to the tips of both medial malleoli. These lengths will be the apparent lengths of the limbs.

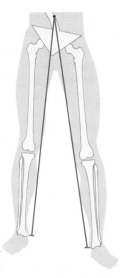

FIG 4.10 The apparent length of the limbs is measured from a central point with the patient lying comfortably straight. It is not possible with this measurement to tell whether any difference in limb length is caused by a bone or a joint abnormality.

Real length of the limb

To find out the real length of the limb (i.e. the combined length of the limb bones and joints, unaffected by the position of the spine, pelvis or hip joints) you must measure between bony points at each end of the limb with the joints in identical positions. The customary points to use in the leg are the anterior superior iliac spine and the tip of the medial malleolus.

The position of the joints profoundly affects this measurement. Figure 4.12a shows the measurements between the iliac spine and the medial malleolus in a patient, lying straight in bed, with disease of the left hip which has caused some fixed abduction. In order to lie straight in the bed the patient has tilted his pelvis and adducted the other hip. If you measure between the iliac spine and malleolus in this position, you are bound to get different measurements, because one hip is abducted and the other adducted.

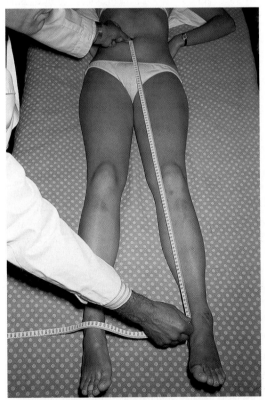

Measuring *apparent* limb length using the umbilicus as the measuring point.

FIG 4.11 MEASURING LIMB LENGTH.

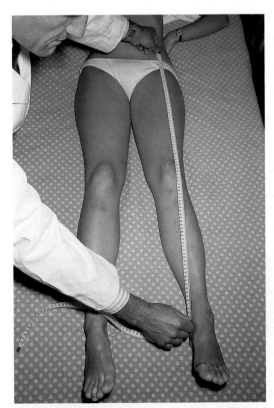

Measuring *real* limb length using the anterior superior iliac spine as the measuring point.

Before measuring real limb length, place the joints of both limbs in identical positions (see Figs 4.12b and c).

Begin by getting the pelvis square to the sagittal plane by checking that both iliac spines are in the same plane at a right-angle to the line of the spine. After doing this you may find the femur on the diseased side abducted or adducted. Place the good leg in the same position. Check that the positions of the knee joints are identical – if one has some fixed flexion, flex the good side to the same degree.

Now you can measure on both sides, from anterior superior iliac spine to medial malleolus, and get a true comparison of real leg lengths.

Joint deformities

Record the deformity of a joint in terms of the angle by which the distal bone is deviated from the

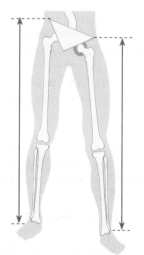
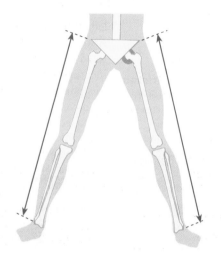
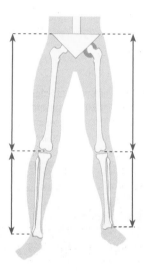

(a)

No
You cannot detect the real length of the limbs like this because the joints are in different positions

(b)

Yes
To measure the true lengths of the limbs you must put the joints in identical positions. This patient has a fixed abduction of the left hip so the right hip was abducted to the same degree before measuring

(c)

To detect the site of bone shortening you must measure the length of each bone

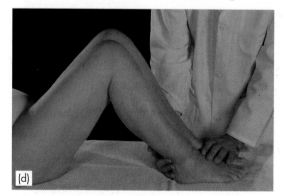

(d)

A quick method of detecting difference in bone length is to put the heels together, with the knees flexed, and look from the side and the end of the bed. This patient has shortening of the right tibia and femur.

FIG 4.12 MEASURING LIMB LENGTH.

sagittal plane (i.e. the angle of varus or valgus – see page 128). Bones may also be rotated on their long axis. Assess the angle of rotation from the displacement of the bony protuberances.

Movement

Examine the joints at both ends of the bone. Also make certain that each bone moves as one piece. A fracture of a long bone may be obvious by painful abnormal movement within the bone itself. Furthermore a false joint that has developed in the shaft of a long bone as a result of non-union of a fracture may also produce abnormal movements, which if longstanding may actually be pain free.

Percussion

The bone may not be tender when touched but painful if percussed. This indicates an abnormality deep inside the bone. Many of the long bones can be percussed using the heel of your hand. Other bones, such as the pelvis and vertebral column, have to be firmly struck with the side of a clenched fist to elicit deep tenderness. Percussion is seldom indicated and need not be part of a routine examination.

FRACTURES

The clinical signs of a fracture

Inspection

Look for the following signs.

- **Deformity** Measure and record any:
  angulation
  rotation
  displacement
  shortening.
  These may be better assessed on X-rays (see next column).
- **Swelling**
- **Any compound wounds** (i.e. any wounds that reach to the site of the fracture) These should be assessed accurately and measured and recorded using the Gustillo classification:
  – Grade 1: wounds less than 1 cm
  – Grade 2: wounds measuring 1–10 cm
  – Grade 3: wounds greater than 10 cm plus:
    A: no periosteal stripping
    B: periosteal stripping
    C: neurovascular damage.

Palpation

- **Bony tenderness**
- **Crepitus**
- **Soft tissue damage** This is often graded as follows:
  Grade 0: little or no soft tissue injury;
  Grade 1: superficial abrasion with moderate swelling and bruising;
  Grade 2: deep abrasion, tense swelling with bruising and blistering;
  Grade 3: extensive contusion, tense swelling, compartment syndrome and/or vascular damage.

Movement

- **Abnormal/painful movement** Do not cause the patient extra discomfort just to confirm abnormal movement. Furthermore, such abnormal movement may cause further soft tissue damage and further periosteal stripping.

X-rays

In the case of bone fractures, X-rays are almost a continuity of the clinical examination. When considering ordering the appropriate views, follow the 'Rule of twos'.

- **Two views**: usually an anterior/posterior view (AP) and a lateral view.
- **Two joints**: include the joint above and the joint below the bone under consideration.
- **Two sides**: useful for comparison, particularly in children, because it allows comparison of the epiphyseal lines in immature bones and distinguishes them from the fracture line.

All X-rays should be centred on the area of maximal tenderness.

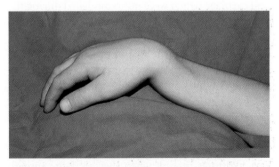

FIG 4.13 The classical dinner-fork deformity of a Colles' fracture, in this case in a child with a Colles' type fracture through the distal epiphysis of the radius and ulna.

BONE DISEASES AND DEFORMITIES

It is vital to make an accurate diagnosis of any bony lump, as bony swellings can be entirely benign or highly malignant lesions. The clinical presentation may provide some useful hints as to the underlying nature of the lesion, although radiological assistance is usually required. The actual site of a lesion in a long bone may give some clue as to the underlying pathology, as is demonstrated in Figure 4.14.

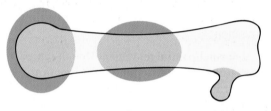

Expanding one end	Centre	On surface, at end
Osteoclastoma	Callus	Exostosis
Osteosarcoma	Secondary tumour	Ecchondroma
	Enchondroma	

FIG 4.14 Relationship between the site of a bony lump and its cause.

Exostosis

As the word implies, an exostosis is a lump which sticks out from the bone. The lump is mainly cancellous bone with a covering of cortical bone and a cartilaginous cap. Exostoses are usually single but may be congenital and multiple.

Solitary (diaphyseal) exostosis

Exostoses are derived from small pieces of metaphyseal cartilage which were not remodelled during the growth of the bone and have become separated from the main cartilaginous epiphyseal plate. Although isolated and left on the side of the shaft (diaphysis) of the bone, they continue to grow and ossify and so produce a bony knob just above the epiphyseal line. They sometimes have an adventitious bursa over their cap. They are not neoplasms.

History

Age Exostoses present when they are large enough to cause symptoms – usually in teenage and early adult life.

Symptoms The patient may have felt the lump or it may have become noticeable and cosmetically disfiguring. Because exostoses are near joints, they sometimes interfere with the movement of the joint and its tendons. Patients may find the movements of the joint limited or associated with 'clicks' or 'jumps' as the tendons slip over the lump.

The overlying bursa, if present, may become enlarged and inflamed.

Examination

Position Exostoses are usually found adjacent to the epiphyseal line of the bone, just on the diaphyseal side. The majority occur at the lower end of the femur and upper end of the tibia.

Shape and size Initial palpation gives the impression of a sessile, smooth, hemispherical protuberance, but with careful palpation it is often possible to feel that the base is quite narrow and that the exostosis leans away from the joint.

Exostoses are usually 1–2 cm in diameter when they are first noticed, but if they are not removed they may enlarge until all their cartilaginous cap is ossified, and become so large (4–5 cm across) that they interfere with joint movement.

Surface Their surface is smooth.

Composition Exostoses are bony hard but their consistence may be masked by a soft, fluctuant bursa overlying their cap.

Relations They are fixed to the underlying bone. It is important to palpate the lump while the adjacent

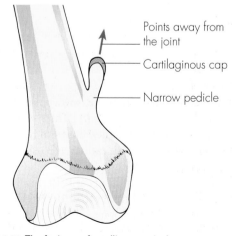

Points away from the joint

Cartilaginous cap

Narrow pedicle

FIG 4.15 The features of a solitary exostosis.

joint is moving to feel which muscles and tendons lie close to the lump and to measure the range of joint movement.

Local tissues The rest of the bone and the nearby joint should be normal.

Multiple exostoses
(diaphyseal aclasis)

This is a hereditary condition. It is carried in an autosomal dominant manner, so half the patient's children can be expected to have the abnormality. Boys are more susceptible than girls. All the bones that ossify in cartilage can be affected, with the exception of the spine and skull. Because this condition is caused by a widespread generalized abnormality of bone remodelling at the epiphyseal line, as opposed to the sporadic event that produces a solitary exostosis, the long bones may be a little shorter than normal.

The clinical features of each exostosis are similar to those described for the solitary variety. They are multiple and especially common on the limb bones. They can grow to a considerable size up to 5–10 cm in diameter.

Callus

Perhaps the commonest cause of thickening of a bone is callus. Callus is the buttress of new bone formed around a fracture site to unite and strengthen it while the cortical bone is being slowly repaired.

History

In the majority of cases the patient knows of the injury and the subsequent discomfort associated with the fracture that caused the callus, but this is not always the case. Some fractures are caused by minor stress, or stress that the patient does not connect with the breaking of bones, such as coughing causing a fracture of the ribs. Furthermore, not all fractures cause severe pain, so the absence of a history of trauma or pain does not necessarily exclude the possibility that the lump might be callus, but makes it unlikely.

Examination

Position The thickening of a bone by callus should be greatest at the site of the fracture, but it may be asymmetrical if the stresses on the bone do not run directly down the centre of the shaft.

Tenderness Mature callus is not tender. Once a fracture has united, there is no local tenderness, and if an area of thickening in a bone is tender, it is unlikely to be callus around a united fracture. It may be callus around non-union, but other signs of non-union will be present.

Shape Callus usually causes a fusiform enlargement of the whole bone – thickest at the site of the fracture.

Surface Newly formed callus has an irregular surface but it becomes smooth as time passes. In young people callus is eventually completely resorbed.

Local tissues Callus may surround a deformed bone – angulated or rotated – if the fracture was not set properly.

Paget's disease of bone
(Osteitis deformans)

This condition occurs in later life. Normally, bone is continually repaired and replaced throughout life. This process follows the same pattern as the original ossification. The ossified cartilage that is reorganized into mature bone is called osteoid bone. In Paget's disease the repair process stops at the osteoid bone stage so that the healthy, mature bone is gradually replaced by thick, bulky, very vascular osteoid bone. If the repair process stops a stage earlier, the old bone, which has been absorbed by the osteoclasts, is replaced by fibrous tissue. This makes the bone very weak.

Paget's disease of bone usually affects many bones but can affect just one bone in the whole skeleton (monostotic Paget's disease). Osteogenic sarcoma complicates 1 per cent of cases.

History

Age The patient is rarely under 50 years of age, often much older.

Symptoms Pain is the commonest symptom. As the bones enlarge and become more vascular, the patient feels a deep-seated aching, gnawing pain in the bone. They can usually tell that it is deep-seated but may have difficulty in appreciating its skeletal origin. The back is the commonest source of pain.

Make a careful note of any change in the nature and severity of the pain. This may indicate malignant change.

Deformity The bone grows bigger and bends. The typical complaints are:

- enlargement of the skull so that the patient's hat no longer fits and the frontal bones become prominent;
- curvature of the spine, causing a kyphosis and increasing difficulty with fitting clothes; patients occasionally complain that they are getting shorter;
- bowing of the legs.

Headache This pain is caused by the changes in the vascularity of the skull bones but is mentioned as a separate symptom because the patient rarely associates the headache with the skull changes.

Deafness Paget's disease in the temporal bones may affect the middle ear and cause otosclerosis and deafness. The patient may also develop vertigo.

Examination

General appearance The patient with generalized disease has a large head, a bent back, arms that seem too long (because of the kyphosis) and bow legs.

Cardiovascular system Examine the cardiovascular system with care. The increased bone blood flow causes an increased cardiac output. The heart may be enlarged, there may be an aortic ejection murmur and the blood pressure may be elevated. It is claimed that Paget's disease can cause a high-output heart failure, but this is a very uncommon occurrence. What is common is the exacerbation of any myocardial ischaemia, secondary to coronary vessel disease, by the extra demands placed upon the heart of an old person.

Respiratory system The patient may have râles and rhonchi at both lung bases if the kyphosis is severe

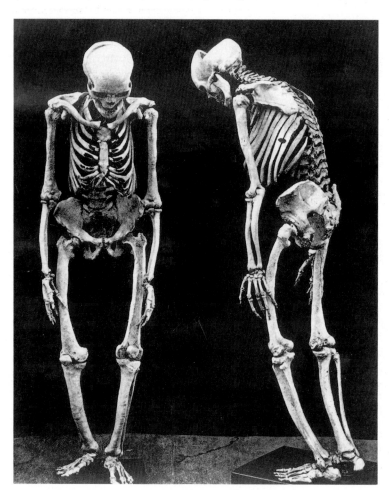

FIG 4.16 The skeleton of a man who had extensive Paget's disease. All the bones are thick. The kyphosis makes the arms seem long. The left femur is split in the coronal plane, revealing the thickening of the cortical bone. (Reproduced by kind permission of the Curator of the Pathology Museum of the Royal College of Surgeons, and the Medical Illustration Unit.)

enough to interfere with the movements of the chest wall.

Skeleton

- **Skull** the enlargement occurs in the vault. The dome looks swollen and the enlarged frontal bones make the forehead bulge forwards. Deafness is common.
- **Spine** The disease usually affects the whole skeleton, so producing an even kyphosis. The shoulders are rounded and the head and neck protrude anteriorly.
- **Legs** The femur and the tibia may bow in both anterior/posterior and lateral directions. The sharp anterior edge of the tibia becomes so prominent that the description 'sabre tibia' is apt, although this expression is usually reserved for bowing caused by syphilis and yaws.

When examining the skeleton, look for any localized bony enlargement, especially in the areas where the pain is severe or has changed. A swelling of

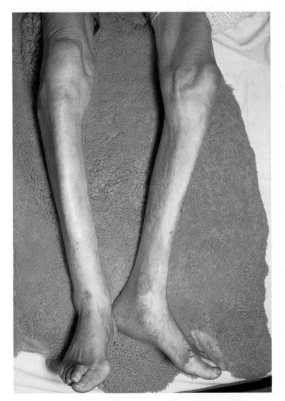

FIG 4.17 'Sabre tibiae'. The anterior edge of the tibia is normally straight and sharp. In this patient, Paget's disease has made these edges thick and curved.

the bone that is painful, a little tender and warm to the touch suggests the presence of sarcomatous change.

Central nervous system The patient may have a conduction deafness and difficulty when standing, caused by middle ear and vestibular apparatus damage. The function of other cranial nerves can be affected if the thickening of the bones reduces the size of the foramina in the base of the skull. Blindness can occur if the optic nerves are compressed.

Spinal nerves may also be damaged by collapse of the vertebrae.

Acute osteomyelitis

Bone can become infected by organisms which reach it through the bloodstream or directly through a wound. Blood-borne organisms are probably trapped in thrombi or haematomata caused by minor trauma, usually in the capillary loops in the part of the shaft adjacent to the epiphyseal line known as the metaphysis.

The common infecting organisms are streptococci and staphylococci.

History

Age Patients with acute osteomyelitis are usually between 1 and 12 years old.

Symptoms The site of infection is painful, though in the early stages this is only a deep-seated ache. When pus forms and the intramedullary tension increases, the pain becomes intense and throbbing.

There is usually some swelling around the painful area, but this is not marked as it is caused by diffuse oedema of the overlying tissues, not swelling of the bone.

The patient may notice that the adjacent joint is swollen and stiff.

The infection causes a loss of appetite and general debility. Most patients feel hot and sweaty and may suffer from rigors.

Examination

Site The bones commonly infected are the tibia, femur, humerus, radius and ulna.

Colour The skin over the painful area may be red or reddish-brown.

Temperature The skin does not become palpably hot until the infection has spread through the bone into the subperiosteal layer.

Tenderness The swollen area is tender and the whole bone is sensitive. Percussion on the end of the bone is painful.

Consistence Any swelling is soft and indistinct because it is caused by oedema of the overlying structures. If there is pus near the surface, there may be an area which fluctuates.

Lymph glands The local lymph glands will only be enlarged if the infection has spread outside the bone.

Surrounding structures The overlying skin may be oedematous. The neighbouring joint may be swollen by an effusion and its movements limited and slightly painful. If the joint movements are very restricted and painful, the infection has probably spread into the joint and caused a septic arthritis.

The subcutaneous veins of the limb are often dilated.

General examination The patient looks ill and feverish. Their face may be flushed and their temperature raised. If the patient has a septicaemia, they may be hypotensive, sweating, possibly shaking and have a dry tongue and oliguria.

BENIGN TUMOURS OF BONE

Benign tumours of bone fall into two categories: those arising from cortical bone (the so-called 'ivory' osteoma) and those which are primarily cartilage tumours but arise within or on the surface of long bones (enchondroma and ecchondroma). An exostosis (described earlier in this chapter) is not a benign neoplasm.

Osteoma

History

The patient complains of a lump which they have either felt or had drawn to their attention. These lumps are not painful and rarely occur in a site that interferes with joint or tendon movements.

Examination

Site Osteomata are common on the surface of the vault of the skull, frequently the forehead.

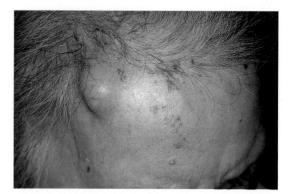

FIG 4.18 An osteoma of cortical bone – an 'ivory' osteoma – on the forehead, which has been present for 40 years.

Shape and size They are sessile, flattened mounds with a smooth surface.

Consistence Osteomata are bony hard – hence the name 'ivory' osteoma.

Relations Nearby muscles and fascia move freely over the lump, which is obviously fixed to and an integral part of the underlying bone.

Chondroma

A chondroma can grow inside a long bone only if a piece of the cartilage from which the bone developed fails to become converted to bone.

An **en**chondroma is a chondroma growing in the centre of the bone; an **ec**chondroma is a chondroma growing on the surface of the bone. There is no pathological difference between these two varieties of chondromata.

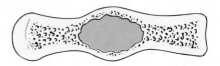

ENchondroma

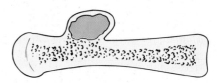

ECchondroma

FIG 4.19 The two varieties of chondromata that are found in long bones.

When the chondromata are multiple and congenital (but not familial), the condition is called **dyschondroplasia** or **Ollier's disease**.

History

Age Chondromata usually present in teenage or early adult life.

Symptoms The patient notices either that a bone is gradually expanding or that a lump is appearing on the side of a bone.

Neither type of chondroma is painful, but an ecchondroma may interfere with joint and tendon movement.

Examination

Site Chondromata are common in the bones of the hands and feet but may occur anywhere. Large, long bones are rarely affected, except when the patient

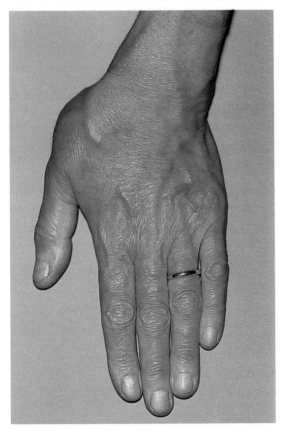

FIG 4.20 A large ecchondroma of the metacarpal bone of the thumb.

has congenital and multiple chondromata (Ollier's disease).

Temperature The overlying skin has a normal temperature.

Shape Enchondromata cause a fusiform enlargement of the shaft of the bone. Ecchondromata form a sessile lump on the surface of the bone.

Surface The surface of both varieties is smooth.

Consistence As chondromata are usually covered by a thin layer of cortical bone, they feel hard.

MALIGNANT TUMOURS OF BONE

Malignant tumours in bone are either primary or secondary. The secondary deposit is by far the most common and is usually a metastasis from one of the carcinomata listed below.

There are four primary tumours of bone:

- osteosarcoma
- reticulum cell sarcoma (Ewing's tumour)
- giant cell tumour (osteoclastoma)
- multiple myeloma.

These are all relatively rare tumours.

Secondary (metastatic) tumour

The primary cancers that commonly metastasize to bone are to be found in the lung, breast, kidney, thyroid and prostate. The first four tend to produce lytic-type lesions as seen on radiographs, while prostatic secondaries tend to appear sclerotic.

These are the five to keep uppermost in your mind, but also remember that any tumour can metastasize to bone.

The bones most often afflicted by secondary deposits are the vertebral bodies, pelvic bones, ribs and the upper ends of the femur and the humerus, because these bones contain red bone marrow and so have a good blood supply.

History

General features Patients often give a history of a previous disease and its treatment (e.g. a mastectomy for a lump in the breast). If not, they are likely to be complaining of symptoms related to the primary growth, such as a cough with haemoptysis, or difficulty with micturition.

Some patients develop bony secondary deposits with no signs or symptoms to indicate the site of the primary lesion.

Symptoms The commonest symptom is pain. Low back pain or pain in the pelvis and hip is often the first indication of the existence of secondary deposits.

Acute pain will occur if there is a pathological fracture, such as the collapse of a vertebral body or a fracture of the femur. The patient rarely notices any swelling at the site of a metastasis unless it is in a superficial bone such as the vault of the skull, the clavicle or a rib.

Examination

If the metastases are deep-seated, they may present no physical signs except pain on movement and tenderness on percussion.

When superficial, they may cause a swelling of the bone which appears rapidly and grows steadily.

The consistence of a secondary deposit in a bone may vary from hard and bone-like to soft, compressible and even pulsatile.

Carcinoma of the kidney is a source of very vascular secondary deposits, so vascular that in certain more advanced cases they may pulsate dramatically and even be misdiagnosed as aneurysms.

Osteosarcoma

This is a malignant sarcoma of bone. It is seen in two groups of patients:

- the young
- the elderly with Paget's disease.

Sarcoma complicating Paget's disease has already been described (see page 119).

Osteosarcoma spreads early and rapidly by the bloodstream.

History

Age Primary osteosarcoma occurs in childhood and the teenage years.

Symptoms Pain is the predominant symptom. It usually begins before the patient notices a lump and is a persistent ache or throb.

Swelling of the bone may be noticed and in some instances this increases rapidly.

The development of general malaise, cachexia and loss of weight may precede or coincide with the appearance of local symptoms.

Pulmonary metastases may cause a cough and haemoptysis.

Abdominal discomfort and jaundice may follow the enlargement and destruction of the liver by metastases.

Patients will often relate the onset of their symptoms to an injury, but there is no evidence that

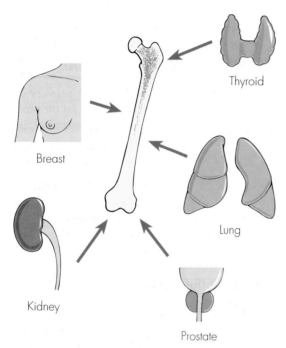

Breast

Thyroid

Kidney

Lung

Prostate

FIG 4.21 Common sources of bone metastases.

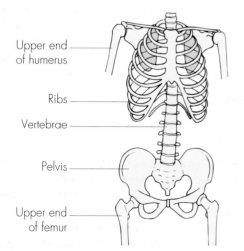

Upper end of humerus

Ribs

Vertebrae

Pelvis

Upper end of femur

FIG 4.22 Common sites for skeletal metastases.

trauma causes sarcoma. The injury simply focuses patients' attention on symptoms which they had previously dismissed as trivial and insignificant.

Examination

Site The commonest place to find an osteosarcoma is the lower end of the femur. The upper end of the tibia is the second most common site, followed by the upper end of the humerus.

Colour The overlying skin may be reddened and the subcutaneous veins visibly distended.

Tenderness The swelling may be slightly tender ·but not exquisitely so like osteomyelitis. Any red, warm, non-tender bony swelling should, in the first instance, be considered to be a tumour and not an infection.

Temperature The skin over the swelling is usually warm, sometimes quite hot.

Shape The swelling tends to appear on one side of the lower end of the bone, making it asymmetrical.

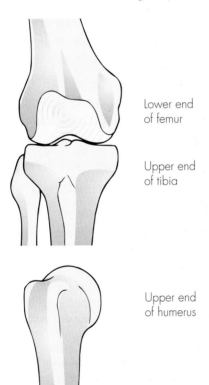

Lower end of femur

Upper end of tibia

Upper end of humerus

FIG 4.23 The common sites to find osteosarcomata.

Surface Its surface is smooth unless it has spread into the surrounding tissues, when it becomes irregular.

Consistence Bony sarcomata feel firm but not bony hard. It is a clinical aphorism that benign tumours of bone feel hard whereas malignant tumours of bone feel soft. A very vascular tumour may pulsate.

Relations The structures overlying a small osteosarcoma are mobile but become fixed to it if the tumour spreads locally beyond the bone.

Lymph drainage The draining lymph glands will not be enlarged in the early stages of the disease, which may be another indication that the red, warm swelling is not an infection. However, when the tumour invades the surrounding soft tissues, it may then spread to local lymph glands.

Local tissues The nearby joint often becomes stiff and develops an effusion. The adjacent artery and nerves are only involved in advanced local disease.

General examination Take particular care to examine the chest and the abdomen because the lungs and the liver are common sites for metastases. There may be generalized wasting, and wasting of the muscles of the affected limb.

Reticulum cell sarcoma
(Ewing's tumour)

This is a tumour which appears most often, but not exclusively, in the centre of long bones – a feature that helps distinguish it from osteosarcoma and osteomyelitis. The cells of this tumour have a distinct reticulate staining. In many instances the tumour represents a secondary deposit from an adrenal neuroblastoma, but there is a primary variety whose cell of origin is not known.

History

Age Ewing's tumour occurs in childhood and the teenage years.

Symptoms The commonest symptom is a persistent ache or pain made worse by movement.

As the femur is the bone most often affected, many children present with a limp.

These tumours can sometimes present as a pyrexia of unknown origin (PUO) and cause rigors and night sweats.

There may be weight loss and malaise, especially if the lesion is a metastasis from a neuroblastoma.

Examination

Site The mid-shaft of the femur is the commonest site to find these tumours, but the tibia and the humerus can be affected.

Colour The overlying skin may be reddened.

Tenderness The swelling is usually a little tender.

Temperature The increased vascularity makes the whole area feel warm.

Shape The tumour causes a symmetrical fusiform enlargement of the shaft of the bone, the upper and lower limits of which are indistinct.

Surface The surface of the swelling is smooth.

Consistence When the bone is so expanded that the tumour mass is palpable, it feels firm and rubbery, not bony hard.

Relations The overlying structures can be moved over the mass because, although they are displaced, they are not usually infiltrated.

Lymph drainage The lymph glands should not be palpable.

Local tissues The arteries and nerves of the limb are rarely involved.

General examination There may be pyrexia and generalized wasting. The lungs and liver may reveal evidence of secondary deposits and, very rarely, a primary neuroblastoma may be palpable in the abdomen as a lobulated mass in the upper part of the abdomen, which may cross the mid-line.

Giant cell tumour
(Osteoclastoma)

These tumours are sometimes classified as having a variable malignant potential because approximately one-third are entirely benign, one-third invade nearby tissues and only one-third metastasize.

History

Age The patient is usually between 20 and 40 years old.

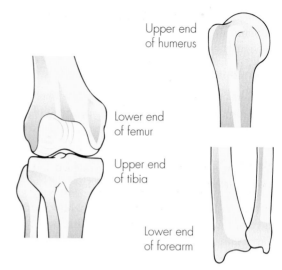

Upper end of humerus

Lower end of femur

Upper end of tibia

Lower end of forearm

FIG 4.24 The common sites for giant cell tumours of bone.

Symptoms The usual presenting symptom is pain. The pain is a dull ache, but may become acute if there is a pathological fracture.

The patient may also notice swelling of the lower end of the femur or the upper end of the tibia.

The nearby joint may get stiff if the swelling disturbs the tendons around it, or if the tumour invades the bone just beneath the articular cartilage.

Examination

Site The common sites to find giant cell tumours are the lower end of the femur and the upper end of the tibia (i.e. either side of the knee), and the upper end of the humerus and the lower end of the radius (i.e. away from the elbow).

Colour The colour of the skin is normal.

Tenderness The swelling may be tender.

Temperature These tumours are not usually vascular and the temperature of the overlying skin should be normal.

Shape Giant cell tumours usually cause a diffuse expansion of the end of a bone but it may be asymmetrical and noticeable on one side only.

Surface Their surface is smooth.

Consistence If the outer layer of bone is reasonably thick, the lump feels bony hard. If it is thin, it may feel firm and slightly pliable. When it is very thin it crackles and bends when touched, and feels like a broken egg shell.

It does not pulsate unless very thin walled and malignant.

Relations The surrounding structures are usually freely mobile over the swelling.

Lymph drainage The local lymph glands should not be enlarged.

Multiple myeloma
(Plasmacytoma)

This is a disease of the blood and bone marrow in which multiple deposits of myeloma cells (plasmacytes) are found throughout the bones containing red bone marrow – the vertebral bodies, ribs, pelvis, skull and proximal ends of the femur and the humerus.

The patient presents complaining of general malaise, loss of weight and intractable pain in the skeleton – mostly the back and chest wall.

There may be signs of involvement of other parts of the blood-forming tissues – enlarged lymph glands, hepatomegaly and splenomegaly.

Occasionally a deposit in a subcutaneous bone causes a palpable lump and is the presenting symptom.

The urine may contain Bence–Jones protein.

JOINTS

EXAMINATION OF A JOINT

Use the same basic approach to examine a joint as for other aspects of the musculoskeletal system – inspection, palpation and movement: look at it, feel it and move it.

Inspection

Overlying skin What is the colour of the overlying skin and are there any associated sinuses or scars?

Shape What is the shape of the joint? Is there any general or localized swelling? Are there any deformities?

Malalignment of a joint in the coronal plane, the plane of abduction and adduction, is known as a **valgus** or a **varus** deformity. Figure 4.25 illustrates these terms. When the part of the limb below the joint is angled away from the mid-line (abducted), there is a valgus deformity; when the part of the limb below the joint is angled towards the mid-line (adducted), there is a varus deformity. Students often get these deformities confused. The easiest way to remember them is to remember one deformity and work out the rules. For example: knock-knees = genu valgum (the tibia is angled away from the mid-line).

Do the muscles that move the joint look normal or wasted? What do the other joints in the limb look like? In what position does the patient hold the joint?

Palpation

Skin Feel the temperature and texture of the skin over the joint.

Subcutaneous tissues Are the subcutaneous tissues normal or thickened?

Muscles Feel the texture of the local muscles for wasting and tone. The muscles may be in spasm if joint movement is painful.

Joint capsule Is the capsule thickened? Is the thickening diffuse or localized?

Synovium Is the synovial membrane thickened and palpable? Is there excess synovial fluid (i.e. an effusion)?

Bones Define the contours of the bones that form the joint. Check that they are in their correct anatomical positions.

Movement

Active movement Ask the patient to move the joint through its full range of movements. Record the degree of any limitation of movement and any associated discomfort.

Strength of movements Make the patient move the joint against resistance so that you can assess the strength of the muscles producing each movement.

Record the power of such movements as described on page 107.

Passive movements Move the joint through its full range of movement with the patient's muscles relaxed. Note any crepitus (grating sensations) felt during this passive movement and any pain or discomfort.

Ligaments Check the integrity of each ligament associated with the joint by stretching it. This will also reveal any abnormal movements.

General examination of the limb

Examine the arteries, nerves, lymph glands and the other joints of the limb.

The majority of joints have simple movements (e.g. extension and flexion) and their examination presents no problem. The examination of the two complex joints of the lower limb, the hip and the knee, which are frequently diseased or deranged, deserves a detailed description.

Examination of the hip joint

Position

First examine the patient standing up if possible. This gives you the opportunity of inspecting the patient from the front, the side and then from the back. You may either assess their gait at this stage or after the rest of the examination has been completed (see below). Then ask the patient to lie flat and straight on the couch, and check that the pelvis is square to the mid-line by feeling the positions of the anterior superior iliac spines.

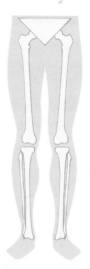

Normal

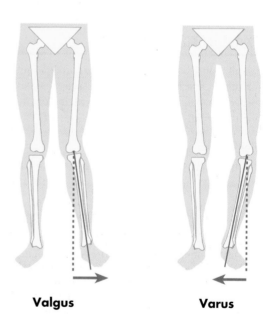

Valgus   **Varus**

FIG 4.25 The definition of a varus and a valgus deformity. In valgus deformity the distal bone forming the joint is abnormally abducted. In a varus deformity it is abnormally adducted. Remember, knock-knees = genu valgum.

Revision panel 4.1	
The causes of joint deformities	
Skin	Contractures
Fascia	Contractures
Muscle	Paralysis, fibrosis, spasm
Tendon	Division, adhesion
Ligament	Rupture, stretching
Capsule	Rupture, fibrosis
Synovium	Inflammation
Bone	Changes in shape, trauma, pressure atrophy

Inspection

Skin Remember that sinuses and scars from the hip joint are often on the buttock and posterior aspect of the upper thigh, so look at the skin over the back of the joint as well as the front.

Shape Check the contours of the thigh and buttock. Asymmetrical skin creases indicate joint displacement. Note any muscle wasting or rotational deformity. Also note any increased lumbar lordosis or scoliosis.

Position When the hip joint is painful or distended by an effusion it is held slightly flexed and abducted. This flexion deformity may also be fixed. In cases of true shortening, once the anterior superior iliac spines are level, the degree of shortening may be apparent by noting that the heels are not level. This should stimulate an accurate assessment of shortening and limb length measurement (see pages 114–16).

Palpation

The capsule and synovium of the hip joint cannot be felt but the muscles and the bony contours can be examined. Place the fingers of one hand over the head of the femur, i.e. just below the inguinal ligament and lateral to the femoral pulsation. Note any tenderness and then rotate the leg to allow the detection of any crepitations arising in the joint.

Relationship between pelvis and femur

In cases of shortening, the position of the greater trochanter with respect to the pelvis (i.e. acetabulum) can be checked in three ways.

1. **Bilateral palpation**. To compare the two sides, put your thumbs on the anterior superior iliac spines and your fingers on the tops of the greater trochanters. You will appreciate any difference in the distance between these points through the position of your fingers.
2. **Nélaton's line**. Turn the patient on their side. Imagine a line drawn from the anterior superior iliac spine to the ischial tuberosity. The top of the greater trochanter should just touch this line. If it lies above the line, there is shortening of the neck of the femur or a dislocation of the hip.
3. **Bryant's triangle**. This gives a measurement of the distance between the top of the greater trochanter and the coronal plane of the iliac spine. Lie the patient supine. Imagine a horizontal line passing through the anterior superior iliac spine. Measure the vertical distance between this line and the top of the greater trochanter.

Nélaton's line and *Bryant's triangle* are now very rarely used clinically (radiographs are much more

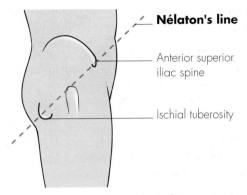

Nélaton's line

Anterior superior iliac spine

Ischial tuberosity

FIG 4.26 Nélaton's line is a line drawn through the anterior superior iliac spine and the ischial tuberosity. It should just touch the top of the greater trochanter.

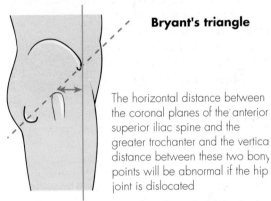

Bryant's triangle

The horizontal distance between the coronal planes of the anterior superior iliac spine and the greater trochanter and the vertical distance between these two bony points will be abnormal if the hip joint is dislocated

FIG 4.27 Bryant's triangle measures the vertical distance from the anterior superior iliac spine to the greater trochanter, and the horizontal distance between the coronal planes of the iliac spine and trochanter.

accurate), but they are useful ways of remembering the normal relationships of the bony landmarks.

Movement

Test for fixed flexion Other fixed deformities (e.g. abduction or adduction) will be clearly visible from the position of the thigh when you set the pelvis square with the spine, but fixed flexion can be masked by a lumbar lordosis.

Place your left hand underneath the hollow of the lumbar spine. Grasp one leg and flex the hip and knee until the lumbar spine straightens and presses against your left hand. If the other hip joint is normal, the thigh on that side will remain flat on the couch. If the other hip lifts off the couch, this will indicate a loss of extension in that hip, which is

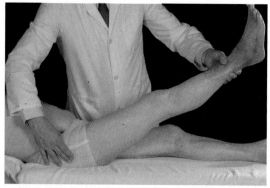

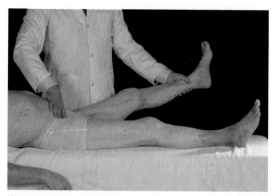

When testing movements such as flexion, place your fingers on the great trochanter and your thumb on the iliac spine so that you detect any tilting of the pelvis.

Keep your fingers and thumb stretched across the iliac spines when testing abduction and adduction to detect any movement of the pelvis.

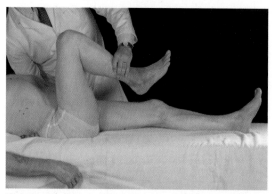

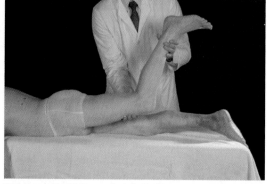

Measure the degree of fixed flexion by flexing the good hip until the lumbar spine straightens and presses on your other hand placed beneath the lumbar spine. No fixed flexion in the left hip. 25° fixed flexion in the right hip. This is *Thomas' test*.

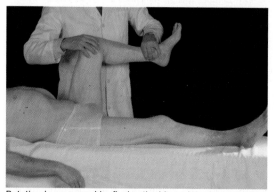

Rotation is measured by flexing the hip and the knee to 90° and rotating the femur by moving the foot back and forth across the line of the limb.

With the patient lying on their front, lift each thigh and assess hip extension.

FIG 4.28 SOME IMPORTANT ASPECTS OF THE EXAMINATION OF THE HIP JOINT.

referred to as a fixed flexion deformity, and the angle of elevation, or fixed flexion, should be recorded. This is called *Thomas' test* for fixed flexion. Now flex the other leg to check the opposite joint.

Passive movements You can only test the movements of a joint by keeping one of the bones that forms the joint still, and moving the other bone. A false impression of hip movement may be obtained if the pelvis

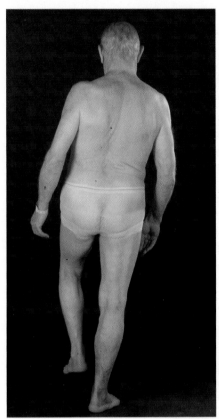

Ask the patient to stand on one leg. They should raise the pelvis on the opposite side. This is *Trendelenburg's test*.

FIG 4.28 continued

moves during the examination. Therefore during all passive movements of the hip you must continually check that the pelvis is not moving by keeping the thumb and little finger of one hand resting upon the two anterior superior iliac spines.

Flexion Flex the good hip and knee until the thigh presses against the abdomen and get the patient to hold the leg in this position. Then flex the hip under consideration, using your other hand to check that no further pelvic movement takes place. Record the degree of flexion and any fixed flexion deformity.

Abduction and adduction Keeping the left hand firmly on the pelvis, abduct or adduct each leg until the pelvis begins to move, and record the range of movement.

Rotation Both internal and external rotation can be assessed by rolling the whole limb, but the best way is to flex the hip and knee to 90°. The foot can then be moved laterally to assess internal rotation and medially to assess external rotation. The range of movement can then be measured by comparing the position of the leg to the mid-line.

Abnormal movements The only abnormal movement you are likely to meet, except those caused by acute trauma, is 'telescoping' of the joint, caused by a dislocated head of the femur sliding up and down the outer aspect of the ilium. This abnormal movement is detected by pushing and pulling the femur along its long axis while steadying the pelvis and feeling the top of the greater trochanter. It is sometimes easier to do this by flexing the hip to 90° and pulling the thigh upwards.

Extension Do this last, as you need to turn the patient on their face. Put your hand under the knee and lift up the thigh, again steadying the pelvis with your other hand. A normal hip extends only 5–2°.

With the patient standing Look for deformities and abnormal skin creases if this has not already been done.

Trendelenburg test Ask the patient to stand on one leg. The opposite side of the pelvis should rise to help balance the trunk on the leg by bringing the centre of gravity over the weight-bearing foot. This involves the use of the hip abductors – gluteus medius and minimus. If the opposite side of the pelvis falls and the patient has difficulty standing, the test is positive. A positive test means one of the following:

- paralysis of the abductor muscles,
- an unstable joint (e.g. congenital dislocation of the hip or a fracture of the neck of the femur),
- approximation of the insertion and origin of the abductor muscles preventing their proper function by a severe coxa vara or a dislocation of the hip.

Assessing the gait Make the patient walk. Observe their gait from the front, the rear and the side.

Any instability of a joint becomes more noticeable during the stresses of walking.

Examine the nerves and arteries of the limb Joint disease is often secondary to neurological abnormalities.

Examination of the knee joint

Inspection

Skin Look at the skin all round the joint – front and back – for discolouration, scars and sinuses. Erythema may suggest inflammation, whereas bruising may indicate trauma. Note any skin conditions that are often associated with joint problems, such as psoriasis and arthritis.

Shape The contours of the knee joint are easy to see and any bony or joint swelling distorts them at an early stage. The size of the whole joint should be compared with the other side, but the areas in which minor degrees of swelling caused by a small effusion are first apparent are the hollows either side of, and above, the patella. Assess any swelling in terms of whether it is confined to the limits of the synovial cavity or extends beyond the joint boundaries, which would suggest infection, tumour or injury. Note any localized swellings that may represent bursitis, meniscal cyst or lesions such as exostoses. Look for any evidence of muscle wasting, particularly of the quadriceps muscle.

Position A knee joint that is swollen and painful is most comfortable when slightly flexed. Also look for any degree of genu valgus or varus.

Palpation

Skin Note any increase in temperature that may indicate active arthritis or infection.

Synovium The synovium of the knee joint can be felt on either side of the patella, and in the suprapatellar pouch. In some diseases it becomes thickened and rubbery, or 'boggy'. A thickened synovium is usually hyperaemic and makes the overlying skin warm.

Bony contour Check the position of the patella. It should be in the patellar groove of the femur, but it may be displaced laterally or superiorly if there is lengthening or rupture of the patellar ligament.

Check the position of the knee joint. When students are asked to put their index finger on the line of the knee joint, they invariably point to a spot 2.5 to 5 cm above it. Remember that the main bulge of the knee is formed by the lower end of the femur. The easiest way to find the joint line is to flex the knee until you can feel the anterior curved edge of the femoral condyles and can slide your finger downwards over this edge until you reach the tibial plateau.

It is important to relate areas of tenderness to the joint line and the points of attachment of the collateral ligaments.

Effusions Effusions of the knee joint are common and easy to detect because the excess synovial fluid collects in the front of the joint where it can be seen and felt. There are three tests for detecting an effusion in the knee joint.

1. **Visible fluctuation**. A small quantity of fluid present does not make the whole joint look swollen, but if you press gently on one side of the joint, the other side may bulge outwards. Get the leg in a good oblique light so the hollows on either side of the patella are visible. Stroke the joint just to one side of the patella and watch the hollow on the other side of the patella to see if it gradually fills out as the effusion is pushed into it. This is the most sensitive way of detecting a small effusion. It cannot be used if the joint is full and tense.

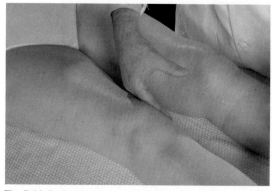

The fluid displacement test: compress one side of the knee and note the joint distending on the opposite side.

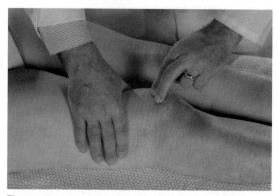

The patellar tap test: squeeze any fluid out of the suprapatellar pouch using the right hand and then press down on the patella. A tap or click will indicate an effusion.

FIG 4.29 TESTING FOR A KNEE EFFUSION.

2. **Palpable fluctuation**. When the knee joint is full of fluid it is possible to press on one side and feel the increase in pressure transmitted over to the other side. Place the palm of the left hand above the patella, and the thumb and index finger either side of it. Press posteriorly and distally to squeeze any fluid in the suprapatellar pouch down into the joint behind and either side of the patella. Place the thumb and index finger of the right hand either side of the patella and see if you can feel fluctuation or fluid displacement between your thumb and finger.

3. **Patellar tap**. When the joint is full of fluid the patella is lifted off the femur. If it is pressed or tapped, it can be felt to move backwards and hit the femur. This test is also helped by emptying the suprapatellar pouch into the space behind the patella with the left hand.

Surrounding tissues Pay particular attention to the bulk and strength of the quadriceps muscle, but remember the quadriceps of the patient's dominant leg will always be slightly bulkier. Any substantial wasting can be measured by comparing the circumference of the thighs at the same distance above the joint line.

Movements

Ask the patient to move the joint themself before checking passive movement. Record the extent of the active knee movements in degrees. Remember that when the leg is straight the angle between the femur and tibia is 0°. At full flexion the angle is usually 135–150° and full extension 0° to minus 10°.

Flexion Bend the knee as much as possible. When there is hip joint disease you may have to turn the patient on to their side to see the full extent of knee flexion. Record the degrees of flexion from the zero position of normal extension.

Extension Lift the leg off the bed by the heel and ask the patient to relax. Record any limitation to extension as well as any excess extension. In women the knee joint often extends 5° or 10° past the 0° mark.

Rotation There are small degrees of rotation of the tibia on the femur, but these are not easy to detect unless the knee is slightly flexed.

Abnormal movements The knee joint is a hinge joint which depends entirely on muscles and ligaments for its stability. If the ligaments are ruptured or stretched, abnormal movement can occur. Thus by testing for abnormal movements such as abduction and adduction, and antero-posterior glide or sliding of the tibia on the femur, you are really checking the stability of the knee and the integrity of its ligaments.

1. **Lateral ligaments**. Let the leg rest extended on the couch. If standing on the patient's left side, place the fingers of your right hand under the right knee joint and the butt of your hand firmly against the medial aspect of the joint. Keep this hand firm and use it as a fulcrum to try to adduct the knee joint by pulling the ankle towards you with your left hand. There should be only the slightest movement in the joint. If it moves easily, the lateral collateral ligament is

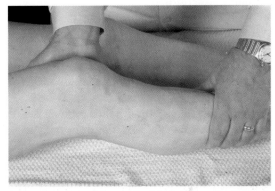

Assess the collateral ligaments of the knee by using the heel of your hand as a fulcrum and then stressing the collateral ligaments by pulling laterally and medially.

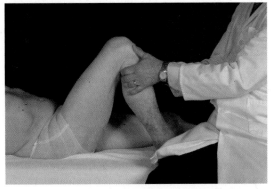

Assess the cruciate ligaments by flexing the knee to about 70°, fixing the foot, and then pulling the tibia towards you or pushing it away. Any significant movement or glide will indicate cruciate damage.

FIG 4.30 TESTING THE LIGAMENTS OF THE KNEE JOINT.

ruptured. If you stay on the same side of the patient, the same action on the other leg will abduct the joint and test the medial collateral ligament.

To test the ligaments on the other side of the joint, change your hands around so that your right hand lies on top of the joint with the fingers resting on the side of the joint. Pull this hand towards you and push the ankle away from you with the other hand.

An alternative method is to tuck the patient's leg under your arm and then, with your hands on each side of the knee joint to detect movement, move the tibia from side to side with your body.

2. **Cruciate ligaments**. Remember the anterior cruciate ligament stops the tibia sliding anteriorly. The posterior ligament stops the tibia sliding posteriorly.

Flex the knee to about 70°. Grasp the upper end of the tibia with both hands and pull it towards you. This is the **anterior draw test**, and any significant movement suggests a torn anterior cruciate ligament, possibly associated with damage to the lateral ligaments as well. Now repeat the test but this time pushing the tibia backwards – the **posterior draw** *test*. Any significant displacement indicates rupture of the posterior cruciate ligament. Always compare the degree of movement between both sides.

In normal knees there should be little or no movement.

Note. It is not necessary to sit on the patient's foot and crush their toes to death to perform this procedure, but it does help if the foot is fixed by the pressure of your buttock as you sit beside the leg, facing the patient's head, so that both of your arms are in front of you and in line with the leg.

Clicks There are some special tests which make the joint click if there is a torn cartilage. Do not try these tests. They are difficult to perform and to interpret.

Normal joints sometimes click. If the patient is complaining of clicking, find out exactly when it occurs, if it is painful, and ask the patient to reproduce it for you, but do not indulge in excessive manipulation just to hear it.

Gait Ask the patient to stand up and walk about. Observe the gait carefully.

EXAMINATION OF THE SPINE

Many pains that are felt in the front of the trunk and down the limbs are caused by disease of the spine. The general surgeon must always bear this in mind

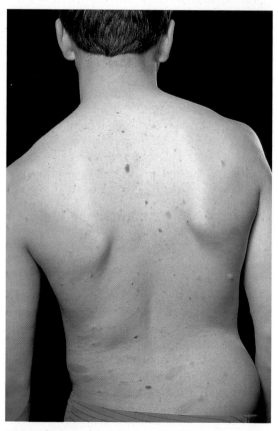

FIG 4.31 Scoliosis of the spine secondary to neurofibromatosis.

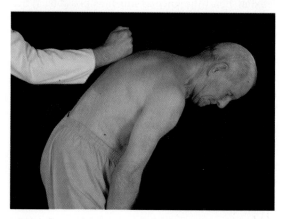

FIG 4.32 Percussion over the spine will reveal tenderness that may indicate infection or metastatic disease.

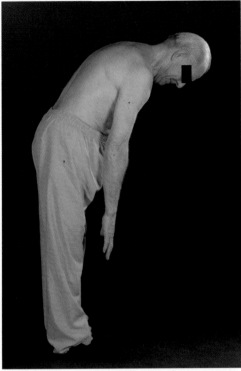

Flexion: ask the patient to attempt to touch their toes and record the degree of flexion.

FIG 4.33 EXAMINING THE SPINE.

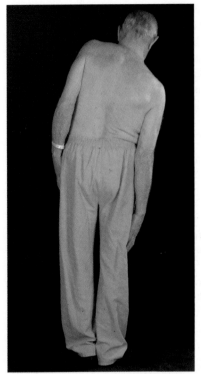

Assess lateral flexion by asking the patient to slide their hand down their side as far as possible.

and make the examination of the spine part of their routine examination. The routine is the same as that for examining any other joint.

Inspection

Skin colour This is usually normal, but note any erythema.

Scars and sinuses Note any scars from previous surgery or trauma, any sinuses that might indicate previous sepsis or tuberculosis, and any fat pad or hairy patch that might suggest spina bifida.

Shape of the back Assess the patient's posture and note any kyphosis, scoliosis or lumbar lordosis. Record any bony deformity or abnormality relating to the muscles of the back.

Palpation

Temperature Note any change in skin temperature.

Revision panel 4.2
Some causes of scoliosis and kyphosis

Scoliosis
  Congenital
  Idiopathic
  Neuromuscular
    Cerebral palsy
    Spina bifida
    Muscle dystrophies
    Poliomyelitis
  Trauma
  Postural
Kyphosis
  Congenital
  Tuberculosis
  Ankylosing spondylitis
  Osteoporosis
  Secondary carcinoma

The bony landmarks Check the bony landmarks, such as the lumbar vertebral spines, for any tenderness. In a similar way, check the sacroiliac joints and also look for any step at the lumbo-sacral junction that may indicate spondylolisthesis. Percuss over the spine lightly, as marked pain may indicate tuberculosis or other infections, or metastatic disease.

Movement

These movements should be performed by the patient while standing upright, apart from rotation. It is not practicable to perform passive movements of the spine.

Flexion Ask the patient to bend forwards and seek to touch their toes. Flexion may be recorded in terms of how far towards the toes the patient can actually reach.

Extension Ask the patient to arch their back. This movement is very limited and is seldom more than about 30°.

Lateral flexion Ask the patient to slide their hand down their side as far as possible. Record the distance reached on both sides.

Rotation This part of the examination should be performed with the patient sitting to fix the pelvis. Ask the patient to twist from side to side and assess the angle between the plane of the shoulder blades and pelvis.

Nerves

A full neurological examination is essential in all patients with any spinal abnormality.

Test for irritation of the roots of the sciatic nerve with the straight-leg raising test.

It is advisable to palpate the abdomen and do a rectal examination to exclude intra-abdominal and pelvic lesions which might be affecting the spine or the spinal nerves.

DISEASES OF JOINTS

The main object of this chapter is to ensure that you can examine the muscles and the skeleton properly. The two commonest joint abnormalities that you will find are swelling and deformity.

Swelling of a joint must be caused by one or more of:

- bony enlargement
- synovial thickening
- an effusion.

Deformity of a joint is invariably be caused by one or more of:

- skin contractures (e.g. scar following burns)
- fascial contracture (e.g. Dupuytren's contracture)
- muscle spasm or weakness
- tendon division or fixation
- capsule fibrosis
- bone deformity.

Detailed descriptions of the diseases affecting joints are to be found in orthopaedic textbooks. The following section describes the signs and symptoms of the four common diseases of joints.

Osteoarthritis

This condition can affect any joint. It is believed to be caused by prolonged wear and tear, and exacerbated by injury and any disturbance of the normal stresses and strains associated with the transference of weight across the joint. The common causative factors are therefore:

- age
- previous fractures involving the articular surface and cartilage
- previous joint diseases
- malalignment of the skeleton following trauma or bone disease.

The articular cartilage becomes thin and ultimately wears through. The bone at the edges of the cartilage hypertrophies, but the bone beneath the cartilage degenerates.

History

Age Most patients with osteoarthritis are over 50 years old, but secondary osteoarthritis following trauma or disease may begin in early adult life.

Symptoms The principal symptom is pain, which comes on gradually, but steadily increases until all movements of the joint are very painful. This is a very slow process. Associated with the pain is an increasing stiffness. If the arthritis is secondary to an old injury, the stiffness may precede the onset of the pain.

Weakness The stiffness and pain lead to disuse atrophy, so the muscles controlling the joint become weak.

Deformity As the stiffness increases, the joint often develops a degree of fixed flexion and the limb may lie with a degree of abnormal abduction or adduction.

Limping Pain, stiffness, weakness and deformity of the joints in the lower limb interfere with walking.

Swelling The whole joint is often swollen by bony osteophytes and an effusion. The synovium is not usually thickened.

Examination
Inspection

Colour The skin should not be reddened or discoloured.

Contour The joint is usually swollen.

Deformity The joint may be fixed in an abnormal position.

Relations Other joints in the same limb, and the same joint in the other limb, may be similarly diseased. Nearby muscles are wasted.

Palpation

Skin The skin temperature is normal, not hot.

Tenderness Pressure on the joint, especially if it is swollen, may cause pain, but local tenderness is uncommon except during an acute exacerbation when there is an effusion.

Synovium The synovium is not usually palpable.

Muscle bulk The bulk of the muscles that control the joint is reduced.

Bony contours The bone at the edge of the articular cartilage may feel irregular and protuberant.

Movement

All movements of the joint are painful at their extremes and some movements are reduced.

(Make sure that you assess the limitation of movement accurately by asking the patient to do active movements before you perform passive movements.)

Not all movements of the joint will be equally affected. For example, early osteoarthritis of the hip may cause limitation of abduction and medial rotation long before it affects flexion, extension, adduction and lateral rotation.

Crepitus

The joint often crackles and clicks during movement. Although the patient can feel a grating sensation associated with the crepitus, it is not usually painful.

Abnormal movements

There should be no abnormal movements because all the ligaments should be intact.

Arteries and nerves in the limb

These structures should all be normal.

Other joints

Osteoarthritis is sometimes bilateral and symmetrical. The joints most often affected are the hip, knee, spine and fingers.

General examination

Osteoarthritis is not associated with any other generalized disease, so the rest of the examination should be normal. As many of the patients with osteoarthritis are old and overweight, they frequently have unrelated diseases such as coronary, cerebral and peripheral artery disease.

The detection of these diseases is important because their existence may alter the management of the patient.

Rheumatoid arthritis

Rheumatoid arthritis is a generalized inflammatory joint disease. Its cause is unknown. The synovial membrane becomes thickened by hyperaemia and lymphocyte infiltration. There may be an effusion. As the disease progresses, the cartilage becomes damaged and eroded and eventually the joint is destroyed.

Near the joints there may be nodules consisting of necrotic collagen surrounded by fibroblasts.

History

Age Rheumatoid arthritis may appear in patients of all ages, but the common time of onset is between the ages of 30 and 40 years.

Sex Women are affected three times more often than men.

Symptoms The main symptoms are pain and swelling, which usually begin together. The commonest first complaint is of swollen, stiff fingers.

Wasting As the disease progresses, the joint movements are restricted and the muscles which control the joint waste away and become weak. As the joints of the upper limbs are often the first to become affected, the patient complains that she keeps dropping things, and cannot carry a shopping basket.

General malaise The patient may feel ill, listless and lose weight. The muscles ache, especially after exercise, and tender, painful nodules appear around the joints.

Skin rashes The patient may complain of skin irritation and rashes, especially if the joint changes are part of another generalized disease such as Reiter's syndrome or systemic lupus erythematosus.

Examination

Inspection

The disease usually starts in the small joints at the end of the limbs – fingers, wrists, toes and ankles – before it moves to the larger joints of the limb and ultimately to the joints of the trunk. The manifestations of the disease in the hands are described on page 158.

Contour The joints are evenly enlarged. The finger joints become fusiform.

Colour The skin overlying the joint may be red and, if there is much swelling, shiny and taut.

Deformity As the disease advances, it affects the ligaments and tendons around the joint as well as the articular surfaces, so causing a variety of joint deformities. For example there is usually ulnar deviation at the wrist joint and hyperextension of the proximal interphalangeal joints.

Wasting The muscles which control the affected joints will be wasted.

Other joints Many joints are affected and the condition is frequently symmetrical.

Palpation

Temperature The skin over the joint is warm.

Tenderness In the acute stage of the disease the joint is tender to light palpation. As the disease becomes chronic, the tenderness subsides but the pain during movement persists.

Synovium Soft tissue thickening can often be felt around the joint. It is only possible to be certain that this is thickened synovium in those joints where it has a clearly palpable edge beyond the joint line. There may also be an effusion in the joint.

Muscle bulk The muscles which control the joint feel thin and atrophic.

Bony contours Until the joint surfaces are destroyed and pathological dislocations occur, the general bony contour of the joint remains normal, but it is often obscured by the synovial thickening.

Arteries and nerves in the limb The other structures in the limb should be normal. Patients with long-standing rheumatoid arthritis sometimes get a peripheral arteritis, which causes gangrene of the tips of the toes and fingers, and ulceration of the skin of the lower third of the leg. Swelling of the joints around the wrist may cause a carpal tunnel syndrome.

Movement

Active movements are limited by pain and reduced in power. Passive movements are limited by pain and fibrous contractures. Abnormal movements appear when the disease has weakened the ligaments, or tendons have ruptured.

General examination

Apart from other joint involvement, there may be generalized wasting and anaemia. There are three systemic diseases associated with rheumatoid joint disease:

1. *Still's disease*: a disease in which children get arthritis, splenomegaly and lymphadenopathy;
2. *Reiter's syndrome*: urethritis, conjunctivitis, skin rashes and arthritis;
3. *Systemic lupus erythematosus*: a collagen disease in which there is a scaly, red rash on the face, debility and manifestations in all tissues of a small vessel arteritis.

Psoriasis and rheumatoid arthritis often coexist. The connection between these two apparently very different diseases is not understood.

Tuberculous arthritis

Any joint can become infected with the human or bovine tubercle bacillus. The joints of the vertebral column are most often affected. The infection reaches the joint via the bloodstream and produces typical pathological changes in the synovium – giant cells, lymphocytes, infiltration and caseation. As the disease progresses, the effusion in the joint becomes purulent and the articular cartilage and the bone are destroyed.

History

Age Tuberculous arthritis tends to occur in young adults and children. Mild symptoms may be present for many years before the patient complains or seeks advice.

Symptoms The common joint symptoms of pain and swelling usually begin simultaneously, but in the hip or the spine where the swelling is not so apparent, pain is the presenting feature.

The pain limits movement of the joint and this usually interferes with walking, bending and stooping. If an abscess forms in the joint, it may point onto the skin and then discharge. The resulting chronic sinus, with a seropurulent discharge, persists until the disease is cured or dies out.

General malaise and loss of weight are common symptoms.

Social history It is important to enquire about social conditions, such as diet, housing and international travel, as well as the existence of any family history of tuberculosis.

Local examination

Inspection

Contour The joint (especially the knee) is diffusely swollen.

Colour The colour of the skin over the joint is normal.

Sinuses There may be a discharging sinus near the joint, or the scars of healed sinuses.

Muscle wasting There is usually marked muscle wasting, especially of the quadriceps femoris muscles when the knee joint is diseased.

Palpation

Skin The skin over the joint is not hot but the inflammatory hyperaemia in the underlying synovium may make it slightly warmer than normal.

Tenderness The joint is tender for a short period in the early acute phase of the disease, but once the infection is established, the joint is not usually painful.

Synovium The swelling around the joint feels soft and pliable – something like unbaked dough. There is always an effusion in the joint.

Bony contour The bones are only deformed or destroyed in long-standing severe disease.

Movement

Movements are only limited if they are painful. In these circumstances there is usually a pronounced protective muscle spasm. There should be no abnormal movements.

When the disease is advanced and has destroyed the joint, it becomes fixed by a fibrous ankylosis.

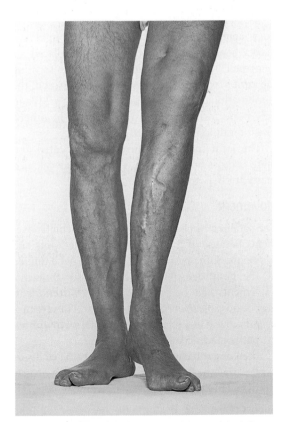

FIG 4.34 The end-result of severe tuberculosis of the left knee joint: a fibrous ankylosis, shortening and wasting of the limb and healed sinuses.

General examination

There may be evidence of tuberculosis elsewhere, such as in the lungs or the kidneys, so the general examination should be complete and thorough.

Neuropathic joints
(Charcot's joint)

The brain is unable to protect a joint which has lost its pain and position sense from harmful stresses and strains. The resulting frequent minor injuries ultimately destroy the bones and the ligaments of the joint. A neuropathic joint is therefore a painless, disorganized joint. The possible causes of loss of joint sensation are:

- diabetic neuropathy
- tabes dorsalis
- syringomyelia
- leprosy
- cauda equina lesions such as myelomeningocele.

Tabes dorsalis used to be the commonest cause of a Charcot's joint in Great Britain, but now that untreated tertiary syphilis is rare, the commonest cause is diabetes.

History

Age Neuropathic joints occur in middle and old age. However, in cases of syringomyelia, the condition often dates from an earlier age and there is often dissociation of sensory loss, with loss of pain and temperature sense but not of touch.

Symptoms The patient notices that the joint is becoming swollen and deformed and gives way frequently but is not painful, except in the early stages of the disease when there may be a few pain fibres but no proprioceptive fibres functioning.

Revision panel 4.3
The causes of a disorganized, painless (Charcot) joint

Diabetic neuropathy
Tabes dorsalis
Syringomyelia
Leprosy
Cauda equina lesions (e.g. myelomeningocele)

The mechanical weakness of the joint together with the sensory defects of the neuropathy make the patient's gait unstable.

Previous illness The patient will probably know if they have had diabetes for many years, but may not know if they have had syphilis. Other neurological conditions are usually obvious.

Local examination
Inspection

Colour The colour of the skin over the joint is normal.

Contour The joint is usually swollen and obviously deformed. There is no common pattern of deformity for any particular joint.

Palpation

Tenderness The joint is not tender and movements in any direction do not usually cause pain.

Synovium The synovium is not thickened, but there is always an effusion.

Bony contours Displacement of the bony landmarks reveals that the bones are displaced or deformed. The normal shape of the bones forming the joint may completely disappear as a result of the combination of bone destruction in some areas and new bone formation and hypertrophy in others. The joint fluid is often greatly increased.

The joint may be subluxed or dislocated and there is gross bone erosion with irregular calcified masses in the capsule.

Movement

The patient may be unable to perform normal movements because of the destruction of the joints and ligaments. Some passive movements may be limited by the bony deformities, while grossly abnormal movements may be possible in other directions. It may be possible to dislocate the joint and then reduce it, and move it in a variety of abnormal ways without the patient feeling any pain or discomfort.

The knee and elbow joints may become so disorganized that the limb becomes flail-like, with grossly abnormal but painless movements.

Nerves of the limb Examine the nerves of the limb with great care. Vibration sense, position sense and deep pain sensitivity are usually all reduced or absent. The motor innervation should be normal.

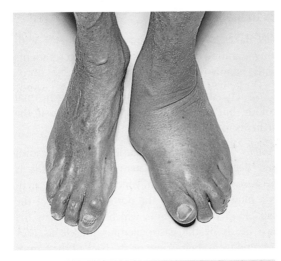

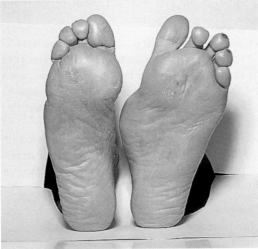

A totally disorganized, but painless, left ankle and foot. This *Charcot* ankle and foot was caused by diabetic peripheral neuropathy.

FIG 4.35 TWO VIEWS OF A CHARCOT JOINT.

General examination

Look for the signs of diabetes and syphilis. Take particular care to examine the whole of the nervous system for evidence of any other neurological disease process, such as syringomyelia, and test the urine for sugar.

Ankylosis

An ankylosed joint is a fixed joint. If the bones that form the joint are fixed together by bone, this

is referred to as a bony ankylosis. If the bones are fixed by dense fibrous tissue, this is a fibrous ankylosis.

A **bony ankylosis** is absolutely fixed and painless, even when stressed.

A **fibrous ankylosis** moves a little, and forced movement causes pain.

Semimembranosus bursa and Baker's cyst

The common forms of subcutaneous bursae are described in Chapter 3.

The normal anatomically constant bursae around joints, usually between the joint and those tendons which cross it, do not enlarge very often. The one which gives most trouble is the bursa between the semimembranosus tendon and the posteromedial aspect of the femoral condyle.

This presents as a swelling behind the knee and is often confused with the other common swelling in this site, a Baker's cyst.

Semimembranosus bursa

History

The common complaint is of a swelling behind the knee joint that interferes with knee movements, particularly flexion.

The swelling tends to grow slowly and does not usually cause pain.

Examination

Age The patient is usually a young or middle-aged adult.

Colour The skin over the swelling is of normal colour and temperature.

Position The swelling lies in the popliteal fossa and is covered only by skin. It lies above the level of the joint line, slightly to the medial side of the fossa.

Consistence It is firm in consistence but clearly cystic because it fluctuates and often transilluminates. It may have a fluid thrill.

Variability Semimembranosus bursae often appear to empty into the knee joint with firm pressure, or during flexion of the knee joint, but this does not actually occur because the bursa does not connect

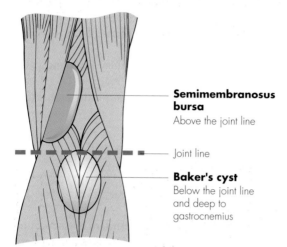

Semimembranosus bursa
Above the joint line

Joint line

Baker's cyst
Below the joint line and deep to gastrocnemius

FIG 4.36 A semimembranosus bursa appears above the joint line. A Baker's cyst appears below the joint line, deep to the gastrocnemius muscle.

with the joint. The fluid is just moving into the deeper recesses of the bursa between the tendons.

Lymph glands The local lymph glands should not be enlarged.

Adjacent tissues The knee joint and other nearby tissues are normal.

Baker's cyst

A Baker's cyst is a pulsion diverticulum of the knee joint, caused by chronic disease in the joint.

History

Previous illness The patient will usually give a history of chronic aches, pains and swelling of the knee joint, often known to be caused by osteoarthritis or rheumatoid arthritis.

The use of the knee is already limited when the patient notices a swelling behind it which further interferes with knee flexion. The swelling itself is not painful. It often fluctuates in size. The patient may have arthritis in other joints.

Examination

Age Baker's cyst appears in elderly patients with long-standing osteoarthritis or in younger patients with rheumatoid arthritis.

Colour The skin over the cyst is usually a normal colour, but may be a little red and warm if the arthritis in the knee joint is active.

Position The lump is below the level of the knee joint and deep to the gastrocnemius muscle. This is because the diverticulum, which becomes the cyst, is a blow-out through the posterior aspect of the capsule of the knee joint, which is covered by the two heads of the gastrocnemius muscle as they descend from their origin on the back of the femur.

Some of the cyst may bulge out between the heads of the gastrocnemius.

Consistence The swelling is soft and fluctuant but will not usually transilluminate because of the density of the muscles which cover it. It is dull to percussion and the fluid content can often be reduced into the joint. Cyst fluid that has moved into the joint can sometimes be seen as a swelling, which appears at each side of the patella as the cyst is compressed.

The knee joint usually shows evidence of arthritis, with limited movements, crepitus and often an effusion.

Adjacent tissues Sometimes these cysts rupture and cause pain and swelling in the calf; this is usually misdiagnosed as a deep vein thrombosis.

Differential diagnosis It is usually easy to differentiate between a Baker's cyst and a semimembranosus bursa (see Fig. 4.36).

Remember the other common cause of a swelling behind the knee joint – a popliteal aneurysm. This is easy to diagnose if it has an expansile pulsation, but easy to confuse with one of the above swellings if it is thrombosed. Remember to feel the pulses at the ankle and to palpate the other leg – popliteal aneurysms are often bilateral.

5

Conditions peculiar to the hands

The hand is mankind's greatest physical asset and, anatomically, one of his most distinctive features. It has enabled humans to use the tools that their brains have invented, and is indispensable to their well-being. Everything that the doctor does to the hand should be aimed at restoring or maintaining its function.

When you examine the hand there are four systems to assess: the muscles, bones and joints; the circulation; the nerves; and the skin and connective tissues. The general examination of these systems is described in other chapters, but the important points relating to the hand are repeated here and assembled into a system of examination designed to ensure that you do not miss any important abnormalities.

A PLAN FOR THE EXAMINATION OF THE HAND

Examine each system in turn.

The musculoskeletal system (bones, joints, muscles and tendons)

Inspection

Look for any abnormality of the shape, size and contour of the hand. Look for local discolouration, scars and sinuses. Look for muscle wasting by assessing the size of the thenar and hypothenar eminences and the bulk of the muscles between the metacarpal bones (the interossei). Look at the wrist joint.

Palpation

Feel the bony contours, the tender areas, and any localized swellings. Feel the finger joints to assess the cause of any swelling of these joints.

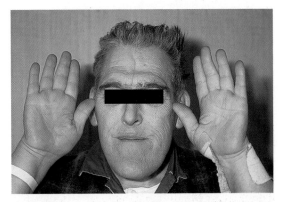

FIG 5.1 The large spade-like fingers and hands of acromegaly.

Movement

Check the range and ease of movement of all the joints:

- the carpometacarpal joint of the thumb (flexion, extension, abduction, adduction and opposition),
- the metacarpophalangeal joints of the fingers (flexion, extension, abduction and adduction),
- the interphalangeal joints (flexion and extension).

Inability to move these joints may be caused by joint disease, soft-tissue thickening, divided tendons or paralysed muscles.

The circulation

Inspection

Pallor of the fingers indicates arterial insufficiency or anaemia. During an episode of vasospasm the fingers may be white or blue. Observe the degree of filling of the veins on the back of the hands. Ischaemic atrophy of the pulps of the fingers makes the fingers thin and pointed. Ischaemic **ulcers**, small **abscesses** and even frank **gangrene** may be visible.

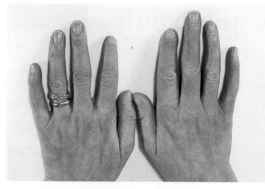

FIG 5.2 Acrocyanosis. A persistent blue discolouration of the skin of the hands caused by mild vasospasm, usually induced by a drop in ambient temperature.

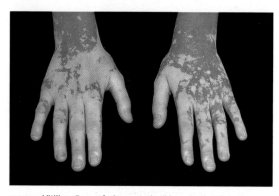

FIG 5.3 Vitiligo (loss of pigmentation) in a dark-skinned patient.

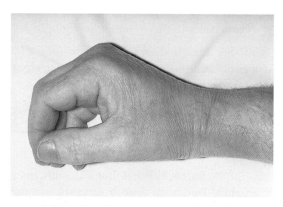

FIG 5.4 Inflammatory changes at the wrist. Such findings often occur from superficial thrombophlebitis when an intravenous infusion site becomes inflamed. In this patient this was flitting thrombophlebitis migrans secondary to carcinoma of the pancreas.

Palpation

Feel the temperature of the skin of each finger.

Feel both pulses (radial and ulnar) at the wrist. Sometimes the digital arteries can be felt on either side of the base of the fingers.

Capillary return A crude indication of the arterial inflow to the fingers can be obtained from watching the rate of filling of the vessels beneath the nail after emptying them by pressing down on the tip of the nail.

Allen's test Ask the patient to clench one fist tightly and then compress the ulnar and radial arteries at the wrist with your thumbs. After 10 seconds, ask the patient to open the hand. The palm will be white. Release the compression on the radial artery and watch the blood flow into the hand.

Slow flow into one finger caused by a digital artery occlusion will be apparent from the rate at which that finger turns pink.

Repeat the procedure, but release the pressure on the ulnar artery first.

Auscultation

Listen with the bell of your stethoscope over any abnormal areas. Vascular tumours and arteriovenous fistulae may produce a bruit, sometimes a palpable thrill.

Measure the blood pressure in both arms.

The nerves

Sensory nerves

When there is loss of sensation you must find out which type of sensation is lost (e.g. light touch, pain, position sense, vibration sense), as described in Chapter 1, and the distribution of the sensory loss. Does it correspond to the innervation of one nerve or to a dermatome? The following gives details of the areas of skin innervated by the three nerves of the hand.

Median nerve The median nerve innervates the palmar aspect of the thumb, index and middle fingers, the dorsal aspect of the distal phalanx and half of the middle phalanx of the same fingers, and a variable amount of the radial side of the palm of the hand.

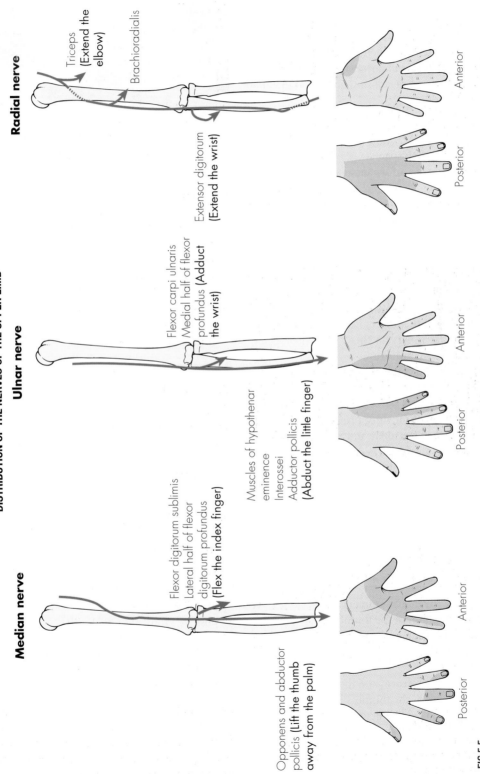

DISTRIBUTION OF THE NERVES OF THE UPPER LIMB

Median nerve

Flexor digitorum sublimis
Lateral half of flexor
digitorum profundus
(Flex the index finger)

Opponens and abductor
pollicis (Lift the thumb
away from the palm)

Posterior

Anterior

Ulnar nerve

Flexor carpi ulnaris
Medial half of flexor
profundus (Adduct
the wrist)

Muscles of hypothenar
eminence
Interossei
Adductor pollicis
(Abduct the little finger)

Posterior

Anterior

Radial nerve

Triceps
(Extend the
elbow)

Brachioradialis

Extensor digitorum
(Extend the wrist)

Posterior

Anterior

FIG 5.5

Ulnar nerve The ulnar nerve innervates the skin on the anterior and posterior surfaces of the little finger and the ulnar side of the ring finger, the skin over the hypothenar eminence, and a similar strip of skin posteriorly. The ulnar nerve sometimes innervates all of the skin of the ring finger and the ulnar side of the middle finger.

Radial nerve This innervates a small area of skin over the lateral aspect of the first metacarpal and the back of the first web space.

The dermatomes of the hand are:

- C6 – thumb
- C7 – middle finger
- C8 – little finger.

Motor nerves

The muscles that control the movements of the hand lie within the hand and in the forearm (i.e. they are intrinsic and extrinsic). All the long flexors and extensors of the fingers lie in the forearm, and the nerves that innervate them leave their parent nerves at or above the elbow.

The nerves that innervate the intrinsic muscles have a long course in the forearm before they reach the hand. Thus it is necessary to examine all the motor functions of the three principal nerves in the upper limb (median, ulnar and radial) if you wish to find the level at which a nerve is damaged. A rapid assessment of the motor function of these three nerves in the hand can be obtained by looking for the following physical signs.

A **median nerve palsy**, which may follow penetrating injuries, lacerations at the wrist, dislocation of the carpal tunnel and carpal tunnel compression, may present as follows.

If the injury is at wrist level:

- wasting of the thenar eminence
- absent abduction of the thumb
- absent opposition of the thumb.

If the injury is at or above the cubital fossa:

- wasting of the forearm and thenar eminence
- loss of flexion of the thumb and index finger
- hand held in the benediction position, with ulnar fingers flexed and index finger straight.

An **ulnar nerve palsy**, which may follow damage or compression at the elbow, penetrating injuries,

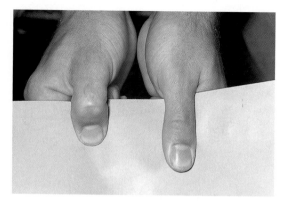

FIG 5.6 A positive Froment's test on the right hand (i.e. on the left of the picture) indicating an ulnar nerve palsy and inability to adduct the thumb due to paralysis of adductor pollicis. This means that the thumb flexes to grip paper due to contraction of the flexor pollicis longus.

fractures of the medial epicondyle, lacerations at the wrist and long-standing marked cubitus valgus, may present as follows.

If the injury is at wrist level:

- wasting of the hypothenar eminence and hollows between the metacarpals
- absence of flexion of the little and ring fingers
- claw hand, with ring and little finger hyperextended at the metacarpophalangeal joint and flexed at the interphalangeal joints
- absence of adduction and abduction of the fingers with a positive *Froment's test*.

If the injury is at the level of the elbow:

- wasting of intrinsic muscles
- claw hand, but with terminal interphalangeal joints not flexed as half of flexor digitorum profundus now paralysed
- positive Froment's test.

If the injury is high above the elbow:

- all the above
- the flexor carpi ulnaris also paralysed.

A **radial nerve palsy**, which may follow fractures of the shaft of the humerus, penetrating injuries and pressure in the axilla from prolonged resting with the arm suspended over a chair or over a crutch, may present in the following ways.

FOUR QUICK TESTS OF THE MOTOR AND SENSORY INNERVATION OF THE HAND

Motor innervation

Median nerve

Abduct the thumb

Radial nerve

Extend the wrist

Ulnar nerve

Abduct the fingers

Sensory innervation
Test sensation in these three areas

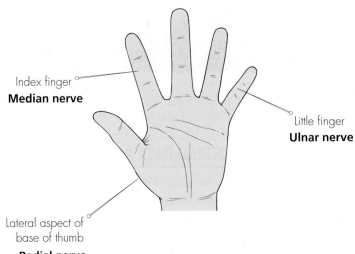

Index finger
Median nerve

Little finger
Ulnar nerve

Lateral aspect of
base of thumb
Radial nerve

FIG 5.7

If there is an injury in the axilla:

- absence of extension of the wrist (wrist drop)
- loss of triceps action.

If the injury is at the level of the middle third of humerus:

- wrist drop
- sparing of the brachioradialis (when paralysed, this weakens elbow flexion).

If the injury is to the posterior interosseous:

- hand held in radial deviation when attempting extension
- no wrist drop
- an inability to maintain finger extension against forcible flexion.

If the injury is to a superfical branch of the nerve:

- no motor loss.

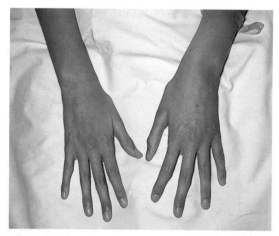

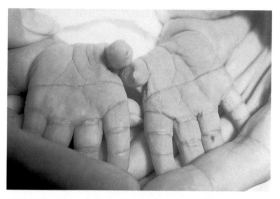

FIG 5.9 The abnormal palmar creases associated with Down's syndrome.

FIG 5.8 Arachnodactyly – long spindly fingers associated with Marfan's syndrome (see page 220).

The examination of the motor function of these three nerves can be simplified by using three screening tests:

1. **median nerve**: abduction of the thumb;
2. **ulnar nerve**: abduction of the little finger;
3. **radial nerve**: extension of the wrist.

As you perform each of these tests, feel the muscle you are testing to check whether or not it is contracting.

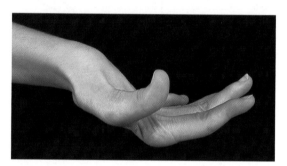

FIG 5.10 The hyperextensibility of the thumb and metacarpophalangeal joints of Ehlers–Danlos syndrome.

The skin and connective tissues

Much will have been learnt about the skin after studying its circulation and innervation. Be careful to note any colour changes and any inflammatory processes. It is also important to palpate the palmar fascia, as thickening and contraction of this structure are a common cause of contraction deformities (Dupuytren's contracture). Also note any change in the shape or configuration of the hand and digits and any abnormal skin creases. Hyperextensibility of the joints may indicate a connective tissue disorder such as Ehlers–Danlos syndrome.

The wrist, elbow, shoulder, thoracic outlet, neck

Examine the wrist, elbow, shoulder, thoracic outlet and neck because abnormalities at these sites can cause symptoms in the hand.

RECORDING DATA ABOUT THE HAND

Almost every issue of the Medical Insurance Societies' publications contains references to errors that have arisen because of inadequate or misleading records of lesions in the hand.

Never forget to state which hand you are describing. Write the words in full: RIGHT or LEFT. A bad R can easily be confused with an L.

Name the digits

Some people prefer to number rather than name the digits, the first digit being the thumb, the second digit the index finger and so on. But unless you remember to write the word 'digit' every time, you will eventually make a mistake because the first finger, which is the index finger, is the second digit. **Do not use this system; always use names: thumb, index, middle, ring and little finger.**

Left hand

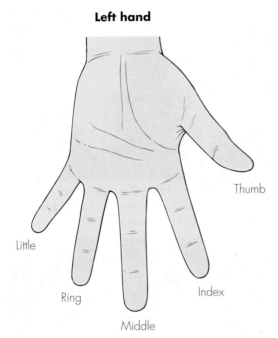

FIG 5.11 The names of the digits of the hand.

It is acceptable to number the toes, as the first toe is the great toe.

ABNORMALITIES AND LESIONS OF THE HAND

Congenital abnormalities

There are three common skeletal abnormalities in the hand:

1. part of the hand (usually a digit) may be absent
2. there may be an extra digit
3. the digits may be fused (syndactyly).

All these abnormalities are rare, but immediately recognizable.

Dupuytren's contracture

This is a thickening and shortening of the palmar fascia and the adjacent connective tissues that lie deep to the subcutaneous tissue of the hand and superficial to the flexor tendons. The cause of this change in the fascia is not known. As the thickening increases, it becomes attached to the skin of the palm.

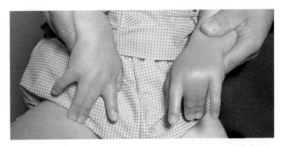

FIG 5.12 Syndactyly. Fusion of the middle and ring fingers of each hand.

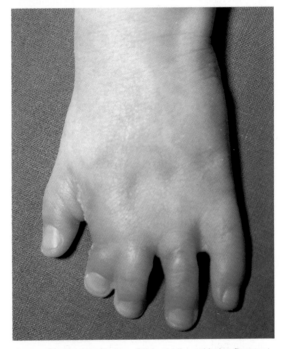

FIG 5.13 Syndactyly. Fusion of the middle and index fingers, in this case associated with a marked failure of finger growth and other bony abnormalities.

It is known to occur in response to repeated local trauma and in association with cirrhosis of the liver, but in most cases there is no obvious predisposing cause.

History

Age Dupuytren's contracture usually begins in middle age but progresses so slowly that many patients do not present until old age.

Sex Men are affected ten times more often than women.

Symptoms A **nodule in the palm**. The patient may notice a thickening in the tissues in the palm of the hand, near the base of the ring finger, many years before the contractures develop.

Contraction deformities. The patient notices an inability fully to extend the metacarpophalangeal joint of the ring finger, and later the little finger. If the contraction of the palmar fascia becomes severe, the finger can be pulled so far down into the palm of the hand that it becomes useless.

There is no pain associated with this condition. Very rarely, the nodule in the palm may be slightly tender.

Development The nodule gradually enlarges and the strands of contracting fascia become prominent. Deep creases form where the skin becomes tethered to the fascial thickening, and the skin in these creases may get soggy and excoriated. The deformity of the fingers slowly worsens.

Multiplicity Dupuytren's contracture is commonly bilateral and can also occur in the feet.

Cause Dupuytren's contracture may follow repeated trauma to the palm of the hand, which is probably why it used to be found in shoe repairers and other manual workers, but nowadays it is uncommon to find a convincing cause.

Systemic disease There may be symptoms of epilepsy or cirrhosis of the liver. There is a higher incidence of the condition in patients suffering from these diseases. The reasons for these associations are unexplained.

Family history Dupuytren's contracture can be familial. If so, it is inherited in an autosomal dominant manner.

Revision panel 5.1
Factors associated with Dupuytren's contracture

Alcoholism
Epilepsy
Diabetes
Repeated trauma
Family history

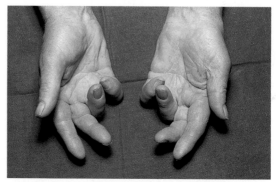

The anterior view shows the typical deformity: flexion of the metacarpophalangeal and proximal interphalangeal joints and extension of the distal interphalangeal joints.

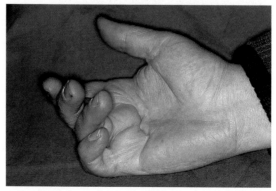

This view shows the puckering of the skin of the palm and the taut strands of palmar aponeurosis.

FIG 5.14 DUPUYTREN'S CONTRACTURE.

Examination

The palm of the hand Palpation of the palm of the hand reveals a firm, irregular-shaped nodule with indistinct edges, 1–2 cm proximal to the base of the ring finger. Taut strands can be felt running from the nodule to the sides of the base of the ring and little fingers, and proximally towards the centre of the flexor retinaculum. These bands get tighter if you try to extend the fingers.

The skin is puckered and creased, and tethered to the underlying nodule.

The deformity The metacarpophalangeal joint and the proximal interphalangeal joint are flexed because the palmar fascia is attached to both sides of the proximal and middle phalanges. The distal interphalangeal joint tends to extend. The ring finger is most affected and may be pulled down so far that its nail digs into the palm of the hand.

The flexion deformity is not lessened by flexing the wrist joint.

Local tissues The rest of the hand is normal. There may be some thickening of the subcutaneous tissue on the back of the proximal phalanges of the affected fingers, sometimes called *Garrod's pads*.

General examination Dupuytren's contracture is sometimes associated with epilepsy and cirrhosis of the liver. There may be systemic evidence of these diseases. These are rare associations.

The condition may be present in the feet.

Congenital contracture of the little finger

This is a congenital deformity of the little finger. The patient is rarely aware of the fact that they have a deformity, accepting it as the normal shape of their little finger.

It is mentioned here because, although it is the opposite deformity to a Dupuytren's contracture, the student who is unaware of its existence may misdiagnose it.

Pick up a tea cup with your thumb and index finger and hook your little finger in the manner of the affected snob at a tea party. You will find that you have extended your metacarpophalangeal joint and flexed both of the interphalangeal joints. Someone with a congenital contracture of the little finger has this deformity all the time and cannot straighten the finger.

Volkmann's ischaemic contracture

Volkmann's ischaemic contracture is a shortening of the long flexor muscles of the forearm, caused by fibrosis of the muscles, secondary to ischaemia. The common causes of the ischaemia are direct arterial damage at the time of a fracture near the elbow (most often a supracondylar fracture), a tight plaster which restricts blood flow, and arterial embolism.

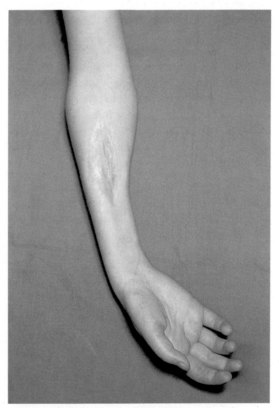

FIG 5.16 Volkmann's ischaemic contracture. Wasting, fibrosis and contraction of the muscles of the forearm following ischaemic damage, causing flexion and ulnar deviation of the wrist joint and flexion of all the finger joints. Further contraction will turn this into a permanently clawed hand.

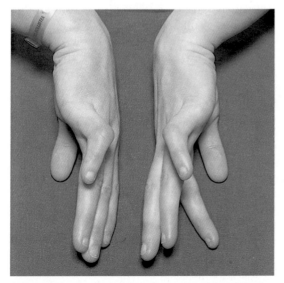

FIG 5.15 Congenital contracture of the little finger. Extension of the metacarpophalangeal joint and flexion of the proximal interphalangeal joint.

History

Age Supracondylar fractures are common in children and young adults, so Volkmann's contracture most often begins between the ages of 5 and 25.

Cause The patient usually knows the cause of the deformity because they can clearly relate the loss of finger extension to their injury. Indeed, the loss of finger movements frequently begins while the arm is immobilized for the treatment of the fracture.

Symptoms When muscles become ischaemic, they are usually **painful**. If a patient complains of pain under their plaster at a point distant from the site of the fracture, remove the plaster and examine the muscles carefully.

Movements of the fingers, especially extension, become **painful and then limited**. This is more noticeable if there is no restriction of movement caused by a coexisting fracture. If the forearm is not in a plaster cast, the patient soon discovers that they can extend their fingers if they flex their wrist.

If the blood supply of the hand is also diminished, the skin of the hand will be **cold and pale**.

Ischaemia of the nerves in the anterior compartment (the median and anterior interosseous nerves) often causes 'pins and needles' (**paraesthesia**) in the distribution of the median nerve, and sometimes the severe burning pain of ischaemic neuritis.

Development As the acute phase passes, the pain slowly fades away, but the restriction of finger extension increases and the hand becomes claw-like. The patient may present with a fully developed deformity.

Examination

Inspection The skin of the hand is usually pale and the hand looks wasted. All the finger joints are flexed and the anterior aspect of the forearm is thin and wasted. The deformity is called a 'claw hand'.

Palpation In the acute phase the forearm is swollen and tense, but once this has passed the forearm feels thin, the hand is cool and the pulses at the wrist may be absent. In the later stages the fibrosis and shortening make the forearm muscles hard and taut.

Movement **Extension of the fingers is limited but improves as the wrist is flexed.** This is an important sign, as it differentiates Volkmann's ischaemic contracture from Dupuytren's contracture. Further flexion of the fingers (beyond the deformity) is present but the grip is weak. All other hand movements are present but may be difficult to perform with the fingers fixed in an acutely flexed position.

Passive forced extension of the fingers is painful in the acute stage and uncomfortable in the established condition. An important diagnostic feature of ischaemic contracture is that all the muscles, even the damaged ones, have some function, whereas when a claw hand is caused by a nerve lesion, some of the muscles will be completely paralysed.

State of local tissues The abnormalities in the arteries and nerves of the forearm and hand have already been described. If the contracture follows a fracture, the vessels and nerves above the level of the fracture should be normal.

The heart, great vessels, subclavian and axillary arteries must be examined carefully in case they are the source of an arterial embolus.

Palpate the supraclavicular fossa for a cervical rib or subclavian artery aneurysm.

Carpal tunnel syndrome

This is a condition in which the median nerve is compressed as it passes through the carpal tunnel – the space between the carpal bones and the flexor retinaculum. The compression can be caused by skeletal abnormalities, swelling of other tissues within the tunnel, or thickening of the retinaculum. It is often associated with pregnancy, rheumatoid arthritis, diabetes, myxoedema, previous trauma and osteoarthritis.

History

Age and sex Carpal tunnel syndrome is common in middle-aged women – especially at the menopause.

Local symptoms **Pins and needles in the fingers**, principally the index and middle fingers, is the common presenting symptom. Sometimes the thumb is involved.

Theoretically the little finger should never be affected, as it is innervated by the ulnar nerve, but occasionally patients complain that the whole of their hand tingles.

Pain in the forearm. For some (so far unexplained) reason, patients often complain of a pain which radiates from the wrist, up along the medial side of the forearm. This is usually an aching pain, not pins and needles.

Loss of function. As the compression increases, the axons in the nerve are killed and objective signs of **nerve damage** appear. Because the sensitivity of the skin supplied by the median nerve is reduced, the patient notices that she drops small articles and cannot do delicate movements. Note that this is not caused by a loss of muscle power, but by the loss of fine discriminatory sensation. Ultimately, if the nerve damage is severe, there may be a **loss of motor function**, which presents as weakness and paralysis of the muscles of the thenar eminence and the first two lumbricals (see median nerve palsy on page 146).

Exacerbations at night. Patients are often woken in the middle of the night by their symptoms. This feature is difficult to explain but is so characteristic that it is considered to be pathognomonic of the condition.

General symptoms An increase of weight commonly exacerbates carpal tunnel syndrome symptoms. A change in weight may be secondary to another disease such as myxoedema, diabetes or steroid therapy, or to physiological water retention, as in pregnancy.

If the condition is secondary to rheumatoid arthritis or osteoarthritis, the patient may have symptoms of arthritis in the wrist and other joints.

Examination

Inspection The hand usually looks quite normal, except in the advanced case where there may be visible wasting of the muscles forming the thenar eminence.

Palpation Pressure on the flexor retinaculum does not produce the symptoms in the hand, but holding the wrist fully flexed for 1 or 2 minutes may induce symptoms. Light-touch sensitivity and two-point discrimination may be reduced in the skin innervated by the median nerve (palm, thumb, index and middle finger). The loss of muscle bulk in the thenar eminence may be easier to feel when these muscles are contracting.

The wrist pulses and the colour and temperature of the skin should be normal.

Movement All movements of the joints of the hand, active and passive, should be present.

Abduction, adduction and opposition of the thumb may be weak, but the muscles that cause these movements are rarely completely paralysed.

General examination There are two important aspects of the general examination.

First, you must **exclude other causes of paraesthesia in the hand**, such as cervical spondylosis, cervical rib, peripheral neuritis, and rare neurological disease. This requires a detailed examination of the head, neck and arm.

Second, you must **look for evidence of the cause of the carpal tunnel syndrome**, such as pregnancy, rheumatoid arthritis, osteoarthritis and myxoedema.

Claw hand

Claw hand is a deformity in which all the fingers are permanently flexed. Although an ulnar nerve paralysis makes the hand claw-like, because it causes flexion of the ring and little fingers, it does not cause a true claw hand, because only part of the hand is involved.

The causes of claw hand are neurological and musculoskeletal.

Neurological causes

Remember these causes by thinking of the course of the nerve fibres from the spinal cord through the brachial plexus into the peripheral nerves. Although the deformity is caused by a loss of motor function, there is often an associated sensory loss.

Spinal cord Poliomyelitis, syringomyelia, amyotrophic lateral sclerosis.

Brachial plexus Trauma to medial roots and cord – especially birth injuries to the lower cord as in Klumpke's paralysis; infiltration of the brachial plexus by malignant disease.

Peripheral nerves Traumatic division of the median and ulnar nerves; peripheral neuritis.

Musculoskeletal causes

Volkmann's ischaemic contracture This only causes a claw hand at rest, as the deformity can be reduced or abolished by flexion of the wrist.

Joint disease Asymmetrical muscle tension, bone and joint deformities and subluxation of the finger joints caused by rheumatoid arthritis may produce a claw-like hand.

Trigger finger

This is a condition in which a finger gets locked in full flexion and will only extend after excessive voluntary effort, or with help from the other hand. When extension begins, it does so suddenly and with a click – hence the name trigger finger. The condition is caused by a thickening of the flexor tendon, paratenon, or a narrowing of the flexor sheath, preventing movement of the tendon within the flexor sheath.

History

Age and sex There are two groups of patients affected by this condition – middle-aged women and very young children. The thumb can be affected in neonates and infants, but this is a rare condition.

Symptoms The patient complains that the finger clicks and jumps as it moves, or gets stuck in a flexed position.

A trigger finger is not usually a painful condition, even when force is required to extend it.

The disability gradually gets more severe, but a fixed, immovable flexed finger is uncommon.

Cause Occasionally the patient can recall an injury to the palm of the hand which may have caused the tendon or tendon sheath to thicken, but in most cases there is no indication of the cause.

Examination

Inspection The patient will show you how the finger gets stuck and how it snaps out into extension. The finger looks quite normal.

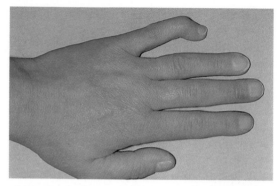

FIG 5.17 A mallet finger. The patient's inability to extend the terminal phalanx of the little finger is only noticeable when he holds his fingers out straight.

Palpation and movement The thickening of the tendon or tendon sheath can be felt at the level of the head of the metacarpal bone. During movement, the thickening can be felt snapping in and out of the tendon sheath.

General examination Trigger finger is not associated with any systemic musculoskeletal disease.

Mallet finger

This is a fixed flexion deformity of the distal interphalangeal joint of a finger, caused by an interruption of the extensor mechanism: either a rupture of the extensor tendon or an avulsion fracture of its insertion. It is also known as 'baseball' finger because the commonest cause of the injury is a blow on the tip of the finger by a ball or hard object which forcibly flexes it against the pull of the extensor tendon, which then ruptures or pulls off the bone.

History

The patient usually remembers the original injury but, if it is not painful, may not complain about it until the deformity is established and a nuisance.

Symptoms The inability to extend the tip of a finger is not a great disability, but to a person with an occupation that requires fine finger movements, including full extension of the distal interphalangeal joints, the deformity can be a serious handicap. Some patients complain that the deformity is disfiguring.

Revision panel 5.2
The causes of claw hand (main en griffe)

Combined ulnar and median nerve palsy
Volkmann's ischaemic contracture
Advanced rheumatoid arthritis
Brachial plexus lesion (medial cord)
Spinal cord lesions
    Syringomyelia
    Poliomyelitis
    Amyotrophic lateral sclerosis

Examination

When the patient holds out their hand, with the fingers extended, the distal phalanx of the affected finger remains 15–20° flexed. If you flex the distal interphalangeal joint to 90°, the patient can extend it back to the 20° position but cannot get it straight.

An X-ray is required to decide whether the tendon is ruptured or avulsed.

Chilblains
(Erythema pernio)

A chilblain is an area of oedema in the skin and subcutaneous tissues that follows a local change in capillary permeability induced by cold. Chilblains are by far the most common of the group of conditions known as **cold sensitivity states**. In addition to the oedema, there is vasospasm and interstitial infiltration with lymphocytes.

History

Age Chilblains first appear in childhood or early adult life.

Sex Woman are affected more often than men.

Occupation An outdoor occupation increases the chances of a susceptible subject getting chilblains.

Symptoms The patient complains of a **swelling** on the side or back of a finger (or toe) that has developed within a few minutes or hours of exposure to cold. The swelling is **painful**, especially in a warm environment, and often **itches**. The overlying skin may ulcerate and weep serous fluid. As chilblains usually follow exposure to the cold, they are more common in **winter**.

Chilblains are often **multiple** and occur on the toes, heels and lower leg, as well as the hands.

Development Chilblains first appear in childhood and adolescence and then appear regularly every winter until the patient reaches middle age. After the susceptibility to chilblains subsides, most patients continue to have some cold sensitivity problems in the hands, such as Raynaud's phenomenon (see next page).

Family history The tendency to get chilblains is often familial.

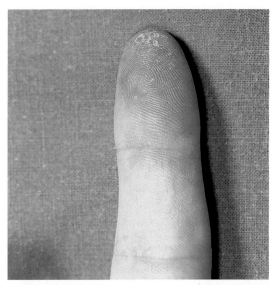

FIG 5.18 Patchy areas of discolouration and coldness, which are sometimes painful, sometimes hypoaesthetic, caused by digital artery embolism.

Examination

Position Chilblains usually occur on the backs and sides of the fingers.

Colour At first the skin over the swelling is pale, but it quickly turns a reddish-blue colour.

Temperature The temperature of the skin over the swelling is normal or slightly cooler than normal.

Shape and size The lumps on the fingers are flattened, elongated mounds, with indistinct edges that fade away into the normal finger. They vary in size. On the fingers they are usually 0.5–2 cm wide, but on the legs they can be 4–5 cm across.

Surface The oedema involves the skin and subcutaneous tissues and often collects in an intradermal blister, which can burst and leave a superficial ulcer. If the acute superficial ulcer fails to heal, it may become deeper, destroying the full thickness of the skin and leaving a permanent scar.

Composition Although the lump is mainly oedema fluid, there is often sufficient cellular infiltration to make it feel firm and sometimes hard.

Lymph glands The axillary or inguinal lymph glands will not be enlarged unless the chilblain is infected – a rare event.

Local tissues There may be evidence of long-standing arterial insufficiency – absent wrist pulses, loss of the finger pulps, recurrent paronychia and scars from previous chilblains. The changes should be distinguished from the painful hypoaesthetic patchy areas of discolouration and coldness that can result from arterial emboli. The nerves of the hands should be normal.

General examination The other extremities may be cold and show Raynaud's phenomenon or acrocyanosis.

Raynaud's phenomenon

The symptoms and signs which are commonly called *Raynaud's phenomenon* are a series of colour changes in the hands following exposure to cold.

To remember the order of the colour changes, remember the initials WBC (the same as 'white blood count'): white, blue and crimson (red).

White. The skin of one, or a number, of the fingers turns white.

Blue. After a variable time, the skin turns a purple-bluish colour but is still cold and numb.

Red. When the vasospasm relaxes, the skin turns red and hot and feels flushed, tingling and often painful.

One or two of these phases may be absent. The fingers may go white and then turn red, or return to normal after the blue phase, or just turn blue.

The orthodox explanation of these changes is as follows.

The **white** phase is caused by severe arteriolar spasm, making the tissues bloodless.

The **blue** phase is produced by a very slow trickle of deoxygenated blood through dilated capillaries. Venous congestion may also be caused by persistent venous spasm.

The **red** phase is the period of high blood flow (reactive hyperaemia) that follows relaxation of the arteriolar spasm. The increased blood flow through the dilated vessels makes the skin red, hot and painful.

There are many causes of Raynaud's phenomenon. These are described in Chapter 7 because Raynaud's phenomenon is not a condition peculiar to the hands alone, although they are invariably affected. It can also occur in the feet, ears, nose and lips.

In between attacks the tissues look quite normal. Ultimately the arteries suffer permanent structural damage, which causes permanent tissue damage.

Scleroderma

Scleroderma is an uncommon disease in which the skin and subcutaneous tissues become thickened and stiff. Although it is a systemic disease affecting the bowel, especially the oesophagus and colon, as well as the skin, it often appears in the hands many years before it develops in other sites. Structural changes in the hands may be preceded for many years by Raynaud's phenomenon. The aetiology of the disease is unknown. The principal abnormality is found in the collagen fibrils, which are thick and stiff.

History

Age Scleroderma commonly begins in the late 30s, but may not become severe for many years.

Sex Females are more often affected than males.

Symptoms There is **thickening of the fingers**. The patient notices that the skin of her fingers is slowly becoming **pale and thick**, and the movements of the interphalangeal joints are reduced.

Many patients present with the colour changes of **Raynaud's phenomenon** years before the skin changes begin.

Painful splits and **ulcers** appear in the skin of the fingertips.

Some patients get **multiple, recurrent small abscesses** around the nails; these abscesses throb and ache and finally discharge a small bead of pus.

Development Although the symptoms may begin in one hand or even one finger, they gradually spread to involve all the digits of both hands.

Systemic effects If the disease affects the oesophagus, the patient will complain of dysphagia. Involvement of the colon causes constipation and colicky abdominal pain.

Local examination

Colour The skin of the hands has a white, waxy appearance caused by the combination of ischaemia and skin thickening.

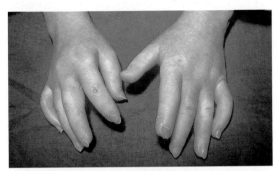

Thick, stiff fingers with pale, waxy, thick skin.

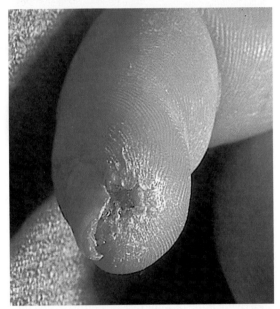

An ischaemic ulcer on the fingertip. These slowly destroy the pulp of the finger and make it pointed.

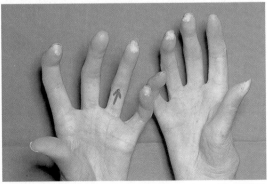

Calcinosis in the pulps of the fingers of a patient with CREST syndrome.

FIG 5.19 THE EFFECT ON THE HANDS OF SCLERODERMA.

Temperature The hands are cool, especially at the fingertips.

Shape and size The hands and fingers look swollen and the **skin thickened** but the pulps of the fingertips may be **wasted**. There are often small scars on either side of the finger nails, and on the pulps, where previous abscesses have pointed and discharged.

Nodules There may be small, hard subcutaneous nodules in the finger pulps and on the dorsal aspect of the hands and fingers. These are patches of calcified fat. This abnormality is called **calcinosis**.

Pulses The pulses at the wrist are usually palpable, but Allen's test often reveals occlusions of the digital arteries.

Nerves The nerve supply of the hand is normal.

Joints The thick skin reduces the range of all movements of the finger joints. The interphalangeal joints are particularly affected, and the most noticeable abnormality is an inability to straighten the fingers.

General examination

Other signs of scleroderma may be visible.

Face. The skin of the face looks tight and shiny and the mouth is small – **microstomia**. There are often multiple telangiectases all over the face (and sometimes on the hands).

Wasting. There may be generalized wasting if the dysphagia is causing malnutrition.

Abdominal distension. Scleroderma in the large bowel inhibits peristalsis and causes chronic constipation and abdominal distension.

The combination of **C**alcinosis, **R**aynaud's phenomenon, **E**sophageal problems (dysphagia), **S**cleroderma and **T**elangiectases is known as the **CREST** syndrome.

Flexor sheath ganglion

A ganglion is an encapsulated myxomatous degeneration of fibrous tissue. When a ganglion occurs on the anterior aspect of a flexor sheath it can interfere with the grip and cause pain and disability out of proportion to its size.

History

Age and sex Flexor sheath ganglia are most common in middle-aged men.

Symptoms The patient complains of a sharp pain at the base of one finger whenever they grip something tightly.

They may also complain of a lump at the site of the pain.

Examination

Colour and temperature These are normal.

Site A small tender nodule can be felt on the palmar surface of the base of a finger, superficial to the flexor sheath.

Tenderness Direct pressure on the lump is usually **very painful**.

Shape The nodule is spherical or hemispherical.

Size Flexor sheath ganglia are usually quite small; some cause symptoms when they are only 2–3 mm in diameter.

Surface and edge The surface of the nodule is smooth and the edge sharply defined.

Composition The nodule feels solid and hard. It is usually too small to permit the assessment of any other features such as fluctuation or translucence.

Lymph glands The local lymph glands should not be enlarged.

Local tissues The rest of the hand is normal.

Comment

Benign giant cell tumours of the flexor sheath present in an identical manner and are indistinguishable from flexor sheath ganglia.

Heberden's nodes

Heberden's nodes are bony swellings close to the distal finger joints. They are non-specific and do not indicate any particular disease.

History

The patient complains of swelling and deformity of their knuckles. There may be a history of an old injury to the finger or aching pains in both the lumps and the joints.

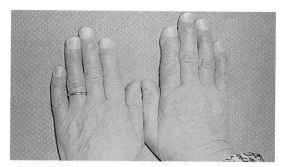

FIG 5.20 Heberden's nodes. This patient had full, painless movements of all her finger joints but large Herberden's nodes on the base of the distal phalanges of both index and middle fingers.

Examination

Heberden's nodes are commonly found on the dorsal surface of the fingers just distal to the distal interphalangeal joint. They are not mobile and can be easily recognized as part of the underlying bone.

The joint movements may be slightly restricted by osteoarthritis, and there may be radial deviation of the distal phalanx. The index finger is the finger most often affected. Small adventitious bursae may develop between the skin and the nodes. Similar nodes may appear near the proximal interphalangeal joint.

Comment

Heberden's nodes do not indicate any specific underlying bone or joint disease and have no clinical significance. They should not be confused with rheumatoid nodules, which are areas of necrosis surrounded by fibroblasts and chronic inflammatory cells and are found in all types of connective tissue. Patients with rheumatoid nodules invariably have other evidence of rheumatoid arthritis.

Rheumatoid arthritis in the hand

The symptoms and signs of rheumatoid arthritis are described in Chapter 4, but, as this disease affects the hand so often, its manifestations in the hand are described here. All the deformities of rheumatoid arthritis result from the combination of uneven pull by the tendons and destruction of the joint surfaces.

Thickening of the joints

The joints most affected are the metacarpophalangeal and the proximal interphalangeal joints. Swelling of these joints gives the finger a fusiform, spindle shape.

Ulnar deviation of the fingers

The fingers are pulled towards the ulnar side of the hand, causing a varus deformity at the metacarpophalangeal joints. In advanced disease the varus deformity can be as much as 45–60°.

Flexion of the wrist

The wrist joint develops a fixed flexion deformity and usually some ulnar deviation.

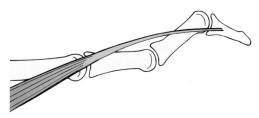

The *swan neck* deformity is caused by fibrotic contracture of the interosseus and lumbrical muscles.

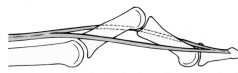

The *boutonnière* deformity develops when the proximal interphalangeal joint pokes through the centre of the extensor expansion following rupture of its central portion.

FIG 5.21 The finger deformities of rheumatoid arthritis.

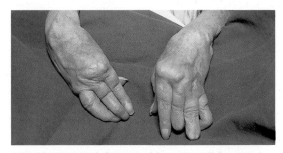

FIG 5.22 Rheumatoid arthritis in the hands. These hands are grossly deformed. The joints are swollen, the wrists flexed and the fingers deviated. In the right hand the index finger has a 'swan neck' deformity, whereas the ring finger has a *boutonnière* deformity.

'Swan neck' deformity of the fingers

This deformity is hyperextension of the proximal interphalangeal joint and flexion of the distal interphalangeal joint. It is caused by fibrotic contraction of the interosseous and lumbrical muscles.

Boutonnière deformity

The joint deformities of this abnormality are the opposite of those of the 'swan neck' deformity: flexion of the proximal interphalangeal joint and hyperextension of the distal interphalangeal joint.

It is caused by the projection and trapping of the flexed proximal interphalangeal joint through a rupture of the central portion of the extensor tendon expansion.

Tendon ruptures

In severe rheumatoid arthritis, any tendon may undergo attrition (damage from friction) and rupture. This causes a variety of deformities. The commonest tendons to rupture are the long extensor tendons of the fingers and thumb.

Compound palmar 'ganglion'

This is a term that is applied to an effusion in the synovial sheath that surrounds the flexor tendons. **It is not a ganglion.** In the UK it is now invariably secondary to rheumatoid arthritis, but in many other parts of the world it is almost always caused by a tuberculous synovitis.

History

The commonest presenting symptom is **swelling** on the anterior aspect of the wrist and sometimes in the palm of the hand. Pain is uncommon.

The patient may notice **crepitus** during movements of the fingers.

Paraesthesia may occur in the distribution of the median nerve.

Examination

Distension of the flexor tendon synovial sheath produces a soft, fluctuant swelling which can be felt on the anterior aspect of the wrist and lower forearm, and in the palm of the hand. Because the swelling passes beneath the flexor retinaculum, compression of the lump on one side of the retinaculum makes it distend on the other side.

Crepitus may be felt during palpation and when the patient moves their fingers. This is caused by the presence of fibrin bodies within the synovial sheath – commonly called 'melon seed bodies'.

There are no local signs of inflammation.

General examination All the joints should be examined to exclude rheumatoid arthritis, and the chest should be examined (and X-rayed) to exclude tuberculosis.

THE NAILS

Inspection of the nails often yields useful information about the patient's general health.

The nails are usually pale pink. The commonest cause of loss of this colour is anaemia.

Another sign of anaemia in the hands of white-skinned races is loss of skin crease colour. When the hand is relaxed, the palmar skin creases are slightly darker than the rest of the skin, but if the skin of the palm is stretched, the creases turn a deep red. This deep red colour is not visible if the patient is anaemic.

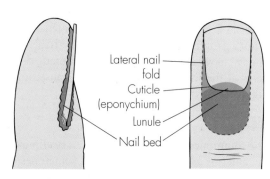

Lateral nail fold
Cuticle (eponychium)
Lunule
Nail bed

FIG 5.23 The anatomy of the nail.

Splinter haemorrhages

Splinter haemorrhages are small extravasations of blood from the vessels of the nail bed caused by minute arterial emboli. They are long, thin, red-brown streaks, their long axis running towards the end of the finger. Their colour and shape make them look like splinters of wood beneath the nail.

The presence of splinter haemorrhages is an important physical sign because they are usually caused by emboli from a bacterial endocarditis or a fulminating septicaemia. They may also occur in rheumatoid arthritis, mitral stenosis and severe hypertension.

Clubbing

Clubbing of the nails is a term used to describe the loss of the normal angle between the surface of the nail and the skin covering the nail bed.

If you look at your finger from the side, you will see that the plane of the nail and the plane of the skin covering the base of the nail bed form an angle of 130–170°.

In clubbed nails there is hypertrophy of the tissue beneath the nail bed, which makes the base of the nail bulge upwards and distorts nail growth so that the nail becomes curved. The planes of the nail and the skin covering the nail bed then meet at an angle greater than 180°.

It is possible to have a very curved nail but still have a normal nail/nail-fold angle, so do not look only at the shape of the nail when assessing clubbing: look at the whole finger.

The terminal phalanx may enlarge to make the end of the finger bulbous.

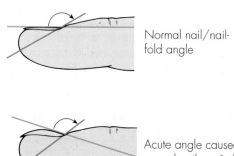

Normal nail/nail-fold angle

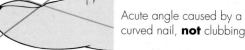

Acute angle caused by a curved nail, **not** clubbing

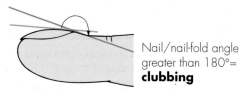

Nail/nail-fold angle greater than 180°= **clubbing**

Normal and abnormal nail/nail-fold angles.

FIG 5.24 CLUBBING.

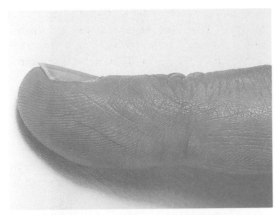

A normal finger.

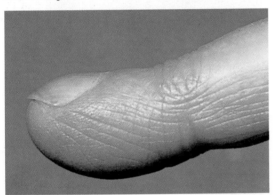

A nail/nail-fold angle greater than 180° = clubbing.

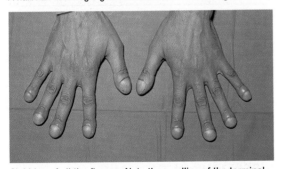

Clubbing of all the fingers. Note the swelling of the terminal phalanges.

FIG 5.24 continued

Spoon-shaped nails
(koilonychia)

A normal nail is convex transversely and longitudinally, the degree of curvature varying considerably from person to person. Loss of both these curves produces a hollowed-out spoon-shaped nail (koilonychia).

When a patient complains that their nails have changed from a normal to a spoon shape, it is very likely that they have developed anaemia following chronic loss of blood, usually from menorrhagia or haemorrhoids.

Subungual haematoma and melanoma

A blow on a nail can cause bleeding beneath it. A collection of blood beneath the nail is called a subungual haematoma. If it appears at the time of the injury, the patient usually makes their own diagnosis and only comes for treatment if it is painful.

Sometimes the patient does not notice the injury and comes complaining of a brown spot beneath the nail. The clinical problem in this case is to decide whether the brown spot is haemosiderin or melanin – a haematoma or a mole.

The features of the spot sometimes help. A haematoma is usually reddish-brown, with sharp edges. A melanoma is brown with a greyish tinge, and has indistinct edges.

Inspection with a small hand-lens may solve the problem by revealing small blood vessels in the lesion, which means it is cellular.

Revision panel 5.3
The signs of clubbing

Increased nail/nail-fold angle
Increased longitudinal and transverse nail curvature
Bulbous terminal phalanges
Spongy nail bed

Revision panel 5.4
Some causes of clubbing

Congenital
Carcinoma of the bronchus
Chronic lung disease
    Alveolitis
    Bronchiectasis
    Cystic fibrosis
Congenital cyanotic heart disease
Ulcerative colitis/Crohn's disease

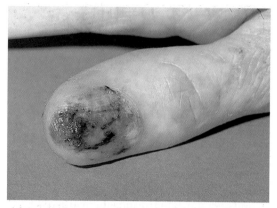

FIG 5.25 A subungual malignant melanoma of the thumb.

If the patient has watched the lesion for a few weeks, they will be able to tell you if it has moved down the nail with nail growth, or stayed still. Haematomata move down the nail; melanomata do not move.

If it is not possible to make a definite clinical diagnosis, the patient should be managed as if they had a melanoma until you prove otherwise.

Glomus tumour

This is a very rare tumour but is mentioned because it can cause a great deal of pain, and often occurs beneath the nail. It is an **angioneuromyoma**.

The patient complains of severe pain every time they touch the nail. Examination usually reveals a

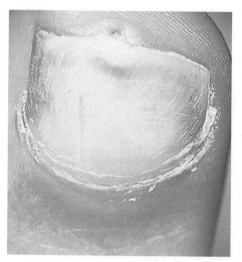

FIG 5.26 A subungual glomus tumour.

small, purple-red spot beneath the nail. The colour is due to the angiomatous nature of the tumour; the pain comes from its abnormally rich nerve supply. Glomus tumours can occur in any part of the skin but are most often found in the hands.

Changes in the nails associated with generalized diseases

- **Psoriasis**: pitting, ridges, poor growth.
- **Myxoedema**: brittle nails.
- **Cirrhosis of the liver**: white nails.
- **General debilitating illnesses**: transverse furrows (*Bean's lines*).
- **Anaemia**: koilonychia.
- **Telangiectasia**: Rendu–Osler–Weber syndrome.
- **Gout** (and **pseudogout**).

INFECTIONS IN THE HAND

Infections in the hand cause severe pain and swelling. They are more likely to present in an emergency department than in a routine surgical outpatient clinic, but two varieties are so common that they deserve a description in this chapter.

Paronychia

This is an infection beneath the skin at the side or base of the nail, and which develops into a small abscess.

Revision panel 5.5 **Common nail abnormalities**	
Loosening	Psoriasis Fungal infections
Pitting	Psoriasis
Transverse ridges	Systemic illness Local damage (paronychia)
Longitudinal ridges	Myxoedema
Thickening and twisting (onychogryphosis)	Trauma Age
Clubbing	See Revision panel 5.4

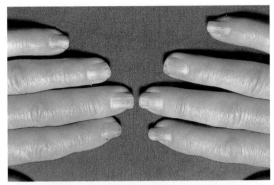

Pits and furrows in the nails in a patient with psoriasis.

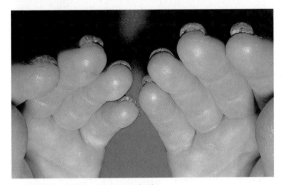

Thickening of the nails in psoriasis.

FIG 5.27 NAIL CHANGES IN PSORIASIS.

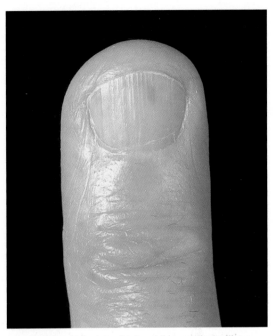

FIG 5.29 Telangiectasia under the nail in a patient with Rendu–Osler–Weber syndrome.

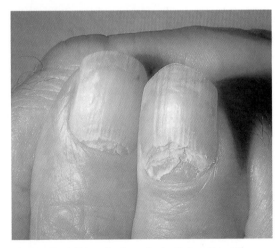

FIG 5.28 The brittle nails of a patient with hypothyroidism (myxoedema).

The patient complains of a painful, tender spot close to the nail that may have throbbed all night and kept them awake. They may remember picking or cutting a piece of cuticle or split skin (hang nail) a few days before the pain began.

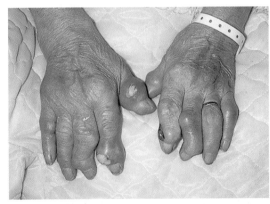

FIG 5.30 The gouty tophi of a patient with long-standing gout.

The skin at the base and side of the nail is red, shiny and bulging and the whole area is exquisitely tender.

In the early stages the pus collects between the nail and the overlying skin, but later it spreads deep to the nail so that movement of the nail is painful and pus is visible through it.

Paronychia are more common in fingers with a poor circulation.

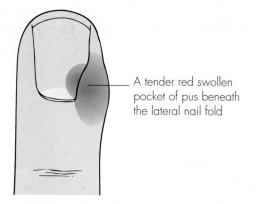

A tender red swollen pocket of pus beneath the lateral nail fold

FIG 5.31 A paronychia.

Chronic paronychia

Normally a paronychia subsides after the pus has drained out, but if there is a foreign body present or the infecting organism is an unusual bacterium or a fungus, the wound may fail to heal and continue to discharge. The patient may then present with a discharging sinus in a discoloured area close to the nail, with unhealthy bluish granulation tissue protruding from it. Biopsy is an essential part of the management of such a case to exclude other conditions such as malignant melanoma and squamous cell carcinoma.

Pulp space infections

These are infections, usually followed by abscess formation, in the subcutaneous tissue which forms the pulp of the fingertip.

They present with throbbing pain, swelling and redness. Sometimes there is a history of a penetrating injury such as a prick with a needle. On examination, there is swelling and tenderness and sometimes a pus-filled blister. If the blister is opened, you will see a hole in the skin leading to the subcutaneous abscess.

If neglected or poorly treated, the skin of the pulp, and the distal phalanx, may necrose.

The only lesion likely to be mistaken for a pulp space infection is a rapidly growing, vascular, secondary tumour deposit in the distal phalanx. Although this will be red, hot and tender, it will progress much more slowly than an infection and not suppurate. There may also be clinical evidence of the primary lesion.

6

Conditions peculiar to the feet

CONGENITAL AND ACQUIRED DEFORMITIES OF THE FOOT AND ANKLE

There are many congenital abnormalities of the foot, such as polydactyly, but the most important ones clinically and functionally are those related to club foot.

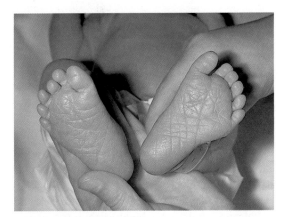

FIG 6.1 An infant demonstrating polydactyly on both feet.

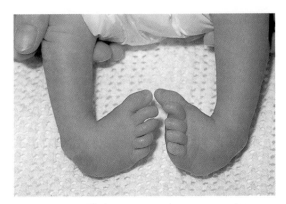

FIG 6.2 Severe bilateral clubbed feet. The varus deformity is so gross that the feet are pulled upwards as well as inwards, making this a talipes calcaneovarus.

Club foot
(Talipes)

These deformities of the ankle and foot develop in utero and are usually present at birth. They are classified according to the skeletal deformity but are collectively known as talipes or club foot. However, these are inappropriate terms when used in such a broad, non-specific manner. Similar deformities can also develop in adult life after injury, paralysis and other musculoskeletal disorders.

There are two main types of deformity.

1. The ankle may be abnormally extended so that weight bearing is on the toes – an equinus deformity; or abnormally dorsiflexed so that weight bearing is on the heel – a calcaneous deformity.

Lateral view

　　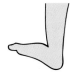

Normal　　　　Equinus　　　Calcaneous

Superior view

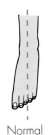　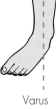　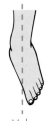

Normal　　　　Varus　　　　Valgus

FIG 6.3 The deformities of the foot.

2. The foot may be deviated into a varus or valgus position, which usually means that there is also some associated inversion and eversion, respectively. These terms are defined below.

There are, therefore, eight types of deformity – four simple and four mixed. Each is prefixed with the term 'talipes' to indicate that the site of the abnormality is the ankle–foot (talipes):

simple:

- talipes varus
- talipes valgus
- talipes equinus
- talipes calcaneous

mixed:

- talipes equinovarus
- talipes equinovalgus
- talipes calcaneovarus
- talipes calcaneovalgus.

Of these eight variations, only two are common: talipes equinus caused by a short Achilles tendon, and talipes equinovarus – the true 'club foot'.

The clinical examination of the foot should follow the pattern described for bones and joints in Chapter 4: look, feel and move. The obvious deformities of the true club foot will be the equinus at the ankle, the varus of the heel with supination of the subtalar joint, and the adduction of the forefoot. The joint movements may be limited and the muscles that effect the joint movements wasted.

The nerves and arteries are usually normal when the abnormality is a congenital skeletal deformity, but there may be neurological abnormalities if the deformity has been acquired since birth.

Flat feet
(Pes planus)

The foot has a longitudinal and a transverse arch. If the longitudinal arch flattens to the extent that the medial border of the foot rests on the ground, the patient has pes planus.

Pes planus is usually associated with a mild valgus deformity of the hind foot which results in pronation of the forefoot and subsequent loss of the medial arch.

All children are flat-footed when they start walking, but the arch develops as they grow more active.

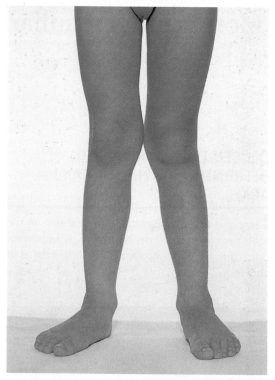

FIG 6.4 Flat feet (pes planus). The medial border of the foot rests on the ground. There is also mild genu valgum (knock-knees).

However, the infantile pattern may persist into adult life and the deformity may become fixed by secondary changes in the bones.

Contrary to popular opinion, flat feet rarely cause trouble in adult life as the body weight is spread over a large flat area.

Hollow or high-arch foot
(Pes cavus)

This is the opposite to flat foot; the longitudinal arch is accentuated. Pes cavus is secondary to muscle imbalance with relative weakness of the intrinsic (small muscles) of the foot. Usually no specific cause is found, but it is important to examine the peripheral nerves thoroughly. Peripheral neuropathies, especially Charcot–Marie–Tooth disease, spina bifida and poliomyelitis, can all present with pes cavus.

The high arch is clearly visible and easy to diagnose. The toes are always 'clawed' (hyperextension of the metatarsophalangeal joints and flexion of the interphalangeal joints) and the patient cannot

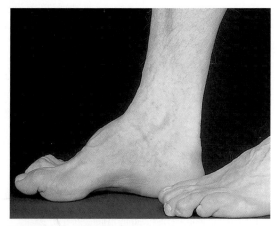

FIG 6.5 A high-arched foot (pes cavus).

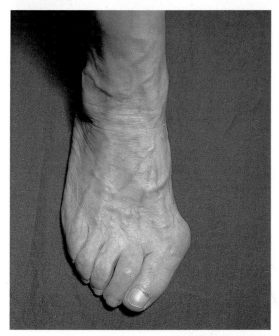

FIG 6.6 Significant hallux valgus. There is a tendency for the second toe to rise up over the great toe, while the remaining toes are deviated towards the lateral side of the foot.

straighten their toes. Extension of the metatarsophalangeal joints and the high arch make the ball of the foot more prominent and lift the tips of the toes off the ground so that they do not participate in weight bearing. Consequently callosities develop on the ball of the foot beneath the heads of the metatarsal bones, and on the dorsal aspect of the toes where they rub against shoes.

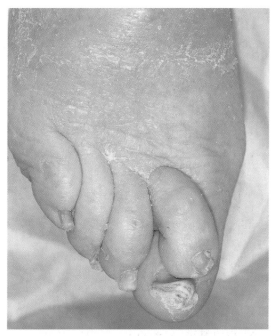

FIG 6.7 Marked over-riding of the second toe over the great toe.

Unlike the flat foot, the high-arched foot frequently causes pain and discomfort.

Hallux valgus

A valgus deformity at the metatarsophalangeal joint of the great toe is a common abnormality. It can be congenital or acquired. The acquired variety is more common in women than men and is often attributed to poorly fitting footwear.

The valgus deformity is obvious to the patient and the doctor. In itself it causes little trouble, but two secondary effects are the source of much discomfort.

Bunion

This is the name given to the bursa which forms over the medial aspect of the prominent head of the first metatarsal. It often swells up and sometimes becomes infected. The patient has difficulty in finding a comfortable pair of shoes because the bunion is painful when rubbed or touched. The fluctuant subcutaneous swelling is easy to feel and distinguish from the underlying bony prominence.

As a result of prolonged abnormal stresses across the deformed metatarsophalangeal joint, the joint

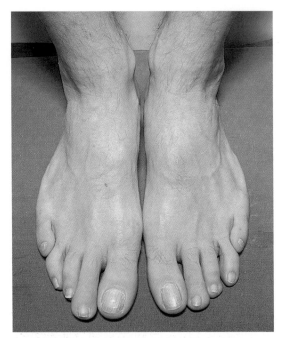

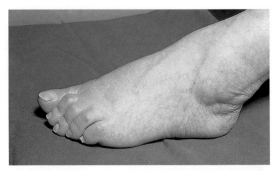

FIG 6.9 A row of hammer toes. The tips of some of the toes are off the ground and there are callosities over the flexed proximal interphalangeal joints. The distal interphalangeal joints of the fourth and fifth toes are only slightly hyperextended.

FIG 6.8 Digiti quinti varus. This is the opposite deformity to hallux valgus and affects the fifth toe. It is a common congenital abnormality and rarely causes symptoms.

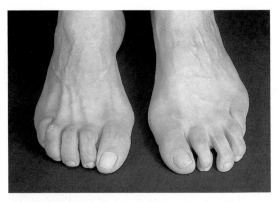

FIG 6.10 Bilateral claw toes. Claw toes are caused by hyperextension of the metatarsophalangeal joint and the flexion of both interphalangeal joints. The tip of the toe points directly downwards and may not reach the ground.

surfaces degenerate and **osteoarthritis** develops. This causes pain in the joint during movement and weight bearing, and hypertrophy of the bone, which makes the deformity more obvious.

Clinical examination reveals the deformity, the adventitious bursa (the bunion), pain on moving the joint, limited movements and, sometimes, crepitus.

Hallux rigidus

The first metatarsophalangeal joint is often afflicted by osteoarthritis even when it is in normal alignment. This causes pain and a progressive reduction of joint movement.

A stiff, painful metatarsophalangeal joint secondary to osteoarthritis is known as hallux rigidus.

The pain may become less severe when the joint becomes fixed by a fibrous ankylosis.

Hammer toe and claw toe

A hammer toe is caused by a fixed flexion of the proximal interphalangeal joint. The middle phalanx points downwards so much that the distal interphalangeal joint has to hyperextend to enable the pulp

of the toe to rest on the ground. There is also hyperextension of the metatarsophalangeal joint.

The cause of hammer toe is not understood, except that it must ultimately result from an imbalance of muscle tone.

A hammer toe causes pain and discomfort when the skin over the proximal interphalangeal joint rubs on the sole or top of the shoe, respectively.

A claw toe is caused by a contracture of its long flexor tendon. This causes flexion of both interphalangeal joints and a secondary extension of the metatarsophalangeal joint. The tip of the toe rests upon the ground and may develop a painful callosity. As the metatarsophalangeal joint extension develops, the tip of the toe may be lifted off the ground and a callosity may develop over the proximal interphalangeal joint.

Callosities and corns

Continual pressure and friction on small areas of the skin of the foot caused by poor-fitting shoes or skeletal deformities stimulate thickening of the skin. A patch of thickened hyperkeratotic skin is called a callosity. If it is pushed into the skin so that it appears to have a deep central core, it is often called a corn, but there is no real difference between a corn and a callosity.

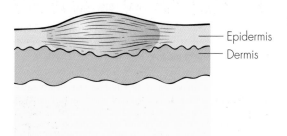

Callosity

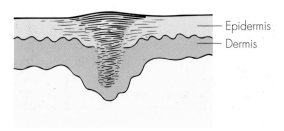

Corn

FIG 6.11 Callosities and corns are patches of thickened, hard epidermis. A callosity protrudes above the surface of the skin; a corn is pushed into the skin.

Plantar wart
(Verruca plantaris)

This is a wart on the sole of the foot. It is caused by a virus similar to that which causes warts on the hands but, because it gets pushed into the sole of the foot, it has different physical characteristics.

History

The patient is usually a child or young adult and the main complaint is of pain in the sole of the foot during walking.

Examination

Site Plantar warts are usually found on the ball and the heel of the foot.

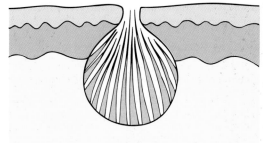

A diagrammatic representation of a plantar wart (verruca). The fine fronds get pushed down into the sole of the foot.

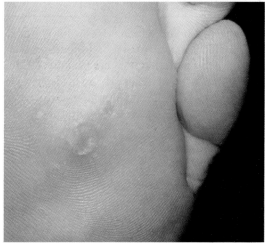

The tips of the embedded fronds of the wart and the surrounding skin become thick and hard. The patient has the sensation of standing on hard stone.

FIG 6.12 THE PLANTAR WART. (By kind permission of Professor David Gawkrodger.)

Colour The painful spot is pearly white in colour, with occasional brown flecks caused by haemorrhage.

Tenderness Pressure on the wart is very painful, in contrast to corns and callosities, which are not very tender when pressed.

Size The area of tenderness may be a few millimetres, or 1 cm, in diameter.

Surface When the wart is small, it is covered by apparently normal skin, but as it enlarges the skin breaks down to reveal a circular pit and the ends of the grey-white filiform strands which are the substance of the wart.

Edge A plantar wart has clearly demarcated edges, as it is really a pit containing a wart. This gives it a 'punched-out' appearance, in contrast to the indistinct edge of a corn or callosity.

Consistence Because the wart is pushed into the hard, thick skin of the foot it is rarely possible to feel a well-defined lump. The fine strands in the centre of the wart are soft.

Multiplicity There may be more than one plantar wart.

Local structures The local lymph glands, arteries and nerves should be normal.

Trophic and ischaemic ulcers

The presentation of ischaemia in the lower limb is described in Chapter 7, but as ischaemic ulcers are very common in the feet, they are mentioned here.

Ischaemic ulcers are caused by an inadequate circulation of blood in the skin. Trophic ulcers are ulcers secondary to an inadequate sensory nervous system.

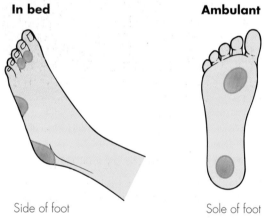

In bed   **Ambulant**

Side of foot   Sole of foot

FIG 6.13 The sites of ischaemic and trophic ulcers.

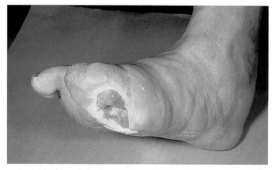

FIG 6.14 A trophic ulcer on the sole of the foot. This patient had undergone previous toe amputations for ischaemia.

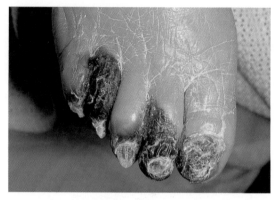

FIG 6.15 Gangrene of the toes.

Both occur in those parts of the feet which are subjected to repeated pressure and trauma, the prime cause of both types of ulcer.

Prolonged pressure on one part of the foot causes ischaemic damage of the tissues, and pain. If the circulation is inadequate, the tissues cannot repair themselves and an ischaemic ulcer develops. If the nerves are inadequate, the patient does not feel the pain and continues to damage the area until it is beyond repair.

These ulcers occur on the heel, the ball of the foot, over the head of the fifth metatarsal and over the tips and knuckles of the toes.

When a patient is ambulant, the main pressure areas are on the sole of the foot (i.e. the heel and ball of the foot and the tips of the toes). When a patient is lying in bed, the main pressure areas are on the back of the heel and lateral side of the foot.

Whenever you examine a patient with an ulcer on their foot:

1. examine the circulation (pulses, etc.),
2. examine the sensory nerves (light and deep touch and pain sensation),
3. test the urine for sugar.

Ischaemic ulcers are usually secondary to atherosclerosis of the iliac and femoral arteries and can be accompanied by gangrene of the toes. Trophic ulcers are usually secondary to conditions such as diabetic peripheral neuropathy, leprosy and primary neurological abnormalities.

THE TOE NAILS

The toe nails may show the same changes in response to local or generalized disease that have been described

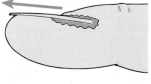

The normal nail is slid forwards as a thin plate

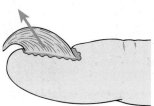

In onychogryphosis the nail heaps up and curls over the end of the toe

FIG 6.16 Onychogryphosis.

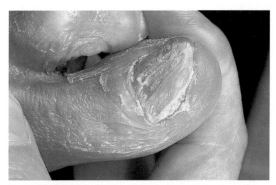

The nail is thick, growing upwards and beginning to curl around the end of the toe like a claw.

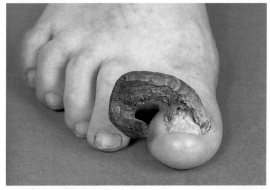

A severe degree of onychogryphosis with the nail heaped up and curling over the side of the toe.

FIG 6.17 ONYCHOGRYPHOSIS.

for the finger nails (pages 162–4). Paronychia and other forms of infection are far less common, but fungal infection (athlete's foot) between the toes and near the nails is very common.

Onychogryphosis

The normal nail is a thin plate which slides along the nail bed. When the sliding mechanism goes wrong, the nail begins to thicken and heap up until it appears to be growing vertically out of the nail bed. It then curves over the end of the toe and looks like an animal's claw. This deformity of the nail is called onychogryphosis. It can occur in young people after an injury to the nail bed, but is most common in elderly people, in whom it is presumed to be a failure of the sliding mechanism caused by old age.

Ingrowing toe nail

This is a common condition in which the side of the nail, usually the lateral side of the great toe nail, appears to be growing or digging into the substance of the toe.

It is a misnomer because, although the nail may be excessively curved in its transverse plane, it is growing normally as a thin plate sliding forwards on the nail bed.

If you remove an ingrowing toe nail, you invariably find that it has an irregular edge, which is damaging the skin. The damage is exacerbated when the skin at the side of the toe is forced upwards during walking.

The usual cause of the irregularity of the nail is an attempt by the patient to cut off the corner, which has ended with the nail being torn off, leaving a jagged spike at the edge.

History

Age and sex Ingrowing toe nails are commonly found in adolescent and young adult males. The excessive use of the feet in games such as football, and less stringent hygiene in young boys and men, may contribute to the sex incidence.

Symptoms The principal symptom is pain. The toe is sore and painful when walking. If it gets badly infected, it throbs at night. There may be a purulent or serous discharge from beneath the lateral nail fold. The toe becomes swollen and wide because the skin at the lateral nail fold becomes prominent, oedematous and soggy.

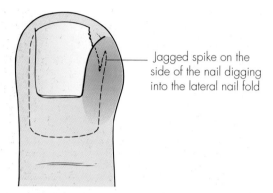

FIG 6.18 The jagged, irregular edge of the nail beneath the lateral nail fold is the real cause of the pain and infection known as 'ingrowing toe nail'. The nail is damaged by misguided efforts to cut off the corner of the nail.

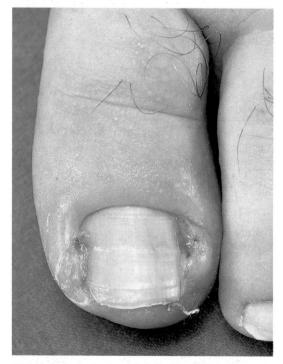

FIG 6.19 An ingrowing toe nail. Both sides of the nail are pushing into the soft tissues, which are infected and producing exuberant granulation tissue.

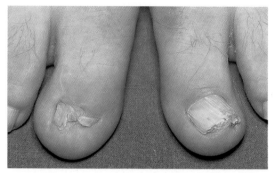

FIG 6.20 This patient had the right nail bed excised 4 years before this photograph was taken. It shows two spikes of nail growing up the corners of the nail bed that were not excised. The nail of the left foot (on the right in the photograph) shows the thickening that precedes the appearance of an onychogryphosis. A fungus infection can cause a similar thickening.

Examination

Site The symptoms of ingrowing toe nail invariably occur in the great toe. The lateral side of the nail (between the great and second toe) is affected more than the medial side, but both sides and both great toes are commonly abnormal.

Colour The skin of the lateral nail fold is reddish-blue. Red granulation tissue may be visible between the skin fold and the nail.

Tenderness The swollen skin and the nail are tender. When there is extensive infection, the whole toe is tender and movement of the interphalangeal joint is painful.

Shape The increase in the bulk of the lateral nail fold makes the great toe wide and spatulate.

The nail itself does not look abnormal. If the nail fold can be pulled away from the nail without causing too much pain, it may be possible to see the extent to which the nail is digging into the tissues and the jagged spikes on the edge of the nail.

Local lymph glands The inguinal lymph glands may be enlarged if there has been long-standing infection, but this is uncommon.

Complications Inadequate excision of the nail bed may result in the re-growth of spikes of nail from the residual corners of the nail bed.

Subungual exostosis

When an exostosis grows on the dorsal surface of the distal phalanx it soon impinges upon the nail bed, causing pain and distortion of the nail.

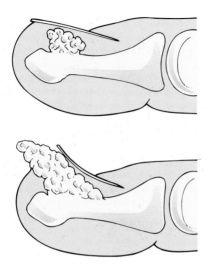

FIG 6.21 A diagrammatic representation of a small and a large subungual exostosis.

History

Age Subungual exostoses present in all age groups, but young and middle-aged adults are most often affected.

Symptoms The patient complains of pain in the toe, especially when it is pressed. The toe may swell slightly and the nail become pushed up and deformed.

Examination

In the early stages the toe looks normal, but pressure on the nail causes severe pain. At this stage, when there are no visible changes in the nail, the diagnosis can only be made from a radiograph. As the exostosis grows, the nail bulges upwards and then a swelling appears between the toe and the end of the nail. The skin overlying this swelling (which is the exostosis) is hard, rough and fissured.

If the exostosis is not removed, it will continue to grow and form a prominent mass on the dorsal surface of the toe, with the nail tipped up and displaced posteriorly.

The cracks and fissures on the skin covering the exostosis may become infected.

Subungual melanoma

The features of malignant melanoma are described in Chapter 2.

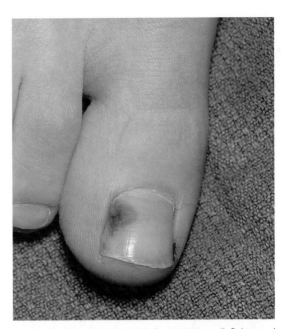

FIG 6.22 A brown patch beneath the great toe nail. Subungual melanoma or haematoma? The latter will migrate down the toe with nail growth, but do not wait too long to detect this sign – remove the nail and biopsy the lesion.

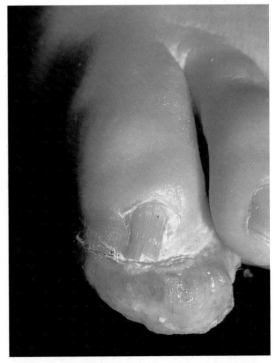

FIG 6.23 An advanced amelanotic malignant melanoma that initially started subungually.

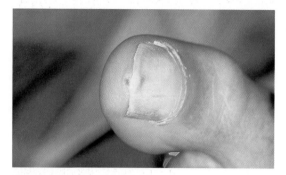

FIG 6.24 A subungual glomus tumour.

Beware of the brown spot beneath the nail. It may be a subungual haematoma or a melanoma. Assume it is the latter unless there is a definite history of injury and clear evidence that the brown area is moving down the nail with nail growth. Also beware of the amelanotic malignant melanoma – any fungating lesion like this should be treated with great suspicion. Other more benign conditions can also occur subungually, such as a glomus tumour.

Dupuytren's and ischaemic contractures

Do not forget that both these conditions may occur in the feet. Their presentation and signs are

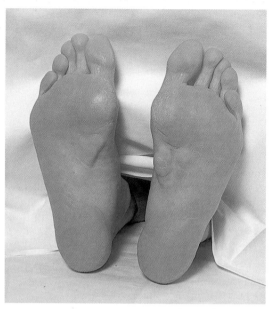

FIG 6.25 Dupuytren's contracture of the feet. There are bilateral thick nodules in the plantar fascia but no flexion deformities of the toes.

similar to those in the hands (see pages 149–52), except that Dupuytren's contracture in the foot usually involves the whole of the plantar fascia and all of the toes.

7

The arteries, veins and lymphatics

The examination of the arteries, veins and lymphatics requires special techniques, which are described before the detailed descriptions of the history and clinical features of individual conditions.

THE ARTERIES

CLINICAL ASSESSMENT OF THE ARTERIAL CIRCULATION OF THE LOWER LIMB

Always examine the patient in a warm room.

Inspection

COLOUR

The first, most notable, feature of an ischaemic limb is its colour. The skin may be as white as marble or show varying degrees of redness or blueness, which become more obvious in the lower parts of the leg and the toes. Sometimes excessive deoxygenation of the blood in the skin capillaries gives the foot a purple-blue cyanosed appearance, but the blue fades to white within a few seconds when the patient lies down. A black skin of ethnic origin masks these subtle colour changes, making the diagnosis of mild and moderate arterial insufficiency in black and coloured races more difficult.

In acutely ischaemic legs, blue streaks around white patches produce a mottled discolouration. When the cyanotic areas become fixed, the ischaemia is irreversible.

Gangrene turns the skin a permanent blue/black colour which is usually first seen in the toes (see pages 170 and 183).

THE VASCULAR ANGLE

The vascular angle, which is also called *Buerger's angle*, is the angle to which the leg has to be raised before it becomes white. In a limb with a normal circulation the toes stay pink, even when the limb is raised by 90°. In an ischaemic leg, elevation to 15° or 30° for 30–60 seconds may cause pallor. A vascular angle of less than 20° indicates severe ischaemia. This test is useful as a comparator. When both limbs are raised together, the ischaemic foot goes white while the normal foot remains pink.

CAPILLARY FILLING TIME

After elevating the legs, patients should be asked to sit up and dangle their feet over the side of the couch. A normal leg and foot will remain a healthy pink colour, whereas an ischaemic leg slowly turns from white (after elevation) to pink and then takes on a suffused purple-red colour. The latter is caused by de-oxygenated blood filling the dilated capillaries. The time taken for the colour of the foot to change from white to pink is the capillary filling time, and depends upon the degree of arterial obstruction. In severe ischaemia it may be as long as 15–30 seconds. A red-purple foot is indicative of severe ischaemia.

VENOUS FILLING

In a warm room the veins of a normal foot are dilated and full of blood, even when the patient is lying horizontally. In an ischaemic foot the veins collapse and sink below the skin surface to look like pale-blue gutters. This appearance is called **guttering of the veins**.

PRESSURE AREAS

Inspect all areas subjected to pressure or trauma during walking or bed rest very carefully, because these are the first sites to show evidence of trophic changes, ulceration and gangrene. It is important to look at the bottom, back and lateral surfaces of the heel, and the ball of the foot. It is also important to look at the skin over the malleoli. The skin over the head of the fifth metatarsal must be carefully inspected, as must the tips of the toes, and between the toes where pressure of one toe nail against the side of the adjacent toe can cause ulceration.

Pressure necrosis is manifest by thickening of the skin, a purple or blue discolouration, blistering, ulceration or patches of black, dead, gangrenous skin.

Many textbooks state that loss of hair on the skin of the lower leg, foot and toes is a sign of ischaemia. **This is a very unreliable sign and does not need to be recorded.**

Palpation

TEMPERATURE

The skin temperature can only be assessed reliably if both lower limbs have been exposed to the same ambient temperature for a full 5 minutes. Uncover the limbs and perform some other part of the physical examination to allow the skin temperature to adjust to the temperature of the surrounding air. Most clinicians prefer to use the backs of their fingers to assess temperature. The cool, dry backs of the fingers are ideal temperature sensors.

The whole limb should be assessed to discover which parts are warm or cold, and the level at which these changes occur. A blue or even red foot can be very cold.

CAPILLARY REFILLING

Press on the tip of a nail, or the pulp of a toe or finger, for 2 seconds and then observe the time taken for the blanched area to turn pink after you have stopped pressing. This gives a crude indication of the rate of blood flow in the capillaries and the pressure within them.

FEEL ALL THE PULSES

Pulses are most easily felt where an artery is superficial and crosses a bone. In the neck, shoulder and upper limbs the **carotid, subclavian, brachial** and **both wrist arteries** are close to the skin and easy to palpate.

The **femoral pulse** in the groin lies halfway between the symphysis pubis (in the mid-line) and the anterior superior iliac spine (the mid-inguinal point). The artery is so superficial it can usually be felt, even when it is pulseless.

The **dorsalis pedis artery** runs from a point on the anterior surface of the ankle joint, mid-way between the malleoli, towards the cleft between the first and second metatarsal bones. In 10 per cent of subjects, the anterior tibial artery is absent and replaced by a branch of the peroneal artery.

The **posterior tibial artery** lies one-third of the way along a line between the tip of the medial malleolus and the point of the heel, but is easier to feel 2.5 cm higher up, where it lies just behind the medial malleolus.

It is often helpful to feel the dorsalis pedis and posterior tibial pulses in both limbs simultaneously. Stand at the end of the bed or couch and feel the dorsalis pedis artery of each foot, simultaneously, by placing the pulps of all the fingers of each hand along the line of the artery, with your thumbs beneath the arch of the foot. From this position, the hands can be rotated over the foot, until the pulps of your fingers lie in the groove between the Achilles tendon and the medial malleolus. The pulps of the fingers

---

Revision panel 7.1
Routine for assessing the arterial circulation

Inspection
    Colour when:
        horizontal
        elevated (vascular angle)
        dependent
    Venous filling
    Look at the pressure areas and
    between the digits
Palpation
    Skin temperature
    Capillary refilling time
    Palpate the pulses
Auscultation
    Listen for bruits
    Measure the blood pressure
    Reactive hyperaemia time

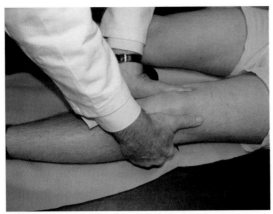

Palpating the popliteal pulse with the knee extended.

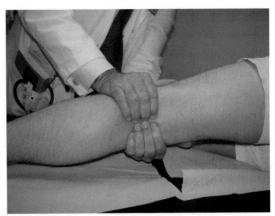

The position of the fingers when feeling the popliteal pulse with the knee fully extended and the patient supine – method 1 in the text. (The patient has rolled over to one side to reveal the back of the knee.)

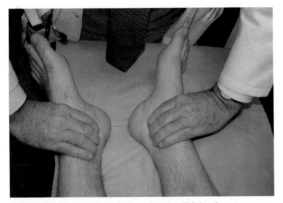

Simultaneous palpation of the posterior tibial pulses.

FIG 7.1 PALPATION OF THE PERIPHERAL PULSES.

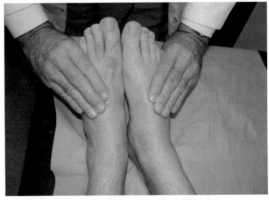

Simultaneous palpation of the dorsalis pedis pulses.

can then be pulled up against the back of the tibia, trapping the posterior tibial pulse against the bone.

The **popliteal pulse** is difficult to feel because it does not cross a prominent bone and is not superficial. There are three ways to feel it and all three may have to be tried before deciding that the pulse is present or absent.

1. The **most convenient** technique for feeling the popliteal pulse is to extend the patient's knee fully and place both hands around the top of the calf with the thumbs placed on the tibial tuberosity and the tips of the fingers of each hand touching behind the knee, over the lower part of the popliteal fossa. The pulps of all the fingers are then pulled forwards against the posterior part of the tibial condyle, trapping the popliteal artery between them and the posterior surface of the tibia. The pulsating artery can be felt in the mid-line (provided the fingers are held still). If in doubt, count any pulse you feel against the rate detected by a second examiner feeling the radial or superficial temporal pulse to check for synchronization.

2. **Flexing the knee to 135°** loosens the deep fascia and may make the lower half of the artery easier to feel, but moves the vessel further from the surface and may make palpation of the upper half of the artery more difficult as it sinks into the large fat pad between the femoral condyles.

3. It is sometimes worth turning the patient into the **prone position** and feeling along the course of the artery with the fingertips of both hands.

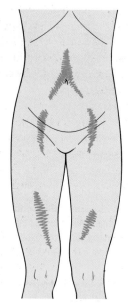

FIG 7.2 The common sites to hear bruits over the arteries of the lower limbs.

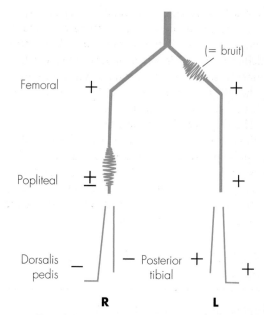

FIG 7.3 Record the pulses and bruits on a simple diagram.

Remember:

■ when a popliteal pulse is very easy to feel, the artery may be aneurysmal

■ the popliteal pulse should be palpable if the foot pulses are easy to feel and there are no adductor canal or femoral artery bruits.

TEST THE MUSCLES AND NERVES

Severe ischaemia causes loss of muscle and nerve function, ultimately producing an immobile, numb limb.

Auscultation

Use your stethoscope to listen along the course of all the major arteries, especially if the pulses are weak. It is an important part of the routine examination to listen to the arteries in the neck, the abdomen, the groin and the thigh. **Always remember to listen over the adductor canal.** Bruits are caused by turbulent flow beyond a stenosis or an irregularity in the artery wall. Do not press too hard over a superficial artery with the bell of your stethoscope, as pressure can distort flow and cause a bruit. Bruits may change in volume and character if there are changes in blood flow.

Before finishing the physical examination of the lower limb you should always measure the blood pressure in **both arms** to exclude significant subclavian or innominate artery disease.

Pressure measurement with the Doppler flow detector

Ultrasound can be used to detect blood flow and produce images of deep structures. The ultrasound is generated by exciting a piezo-electric crystal to vibrate at its resonant frequency in response to a small electric current. In the small hand-held Doppler ultrasound instruments used in the clinic, the sound waves are focused into a beam and directed towards the vessel to be examined by placing the probe over the surface of the vessel after abolishing any air between the probe and the skin with a coupling jelly. Moving red cells alter the frequency of the reflected ultrasound according to the Doppler principle. The chosen vessels, usually the dorsalis pedis, posterior tibial or peroneal arteries at the ankle, are located by insonating over their known anatomical course and listening for regular changes in sound generated by the pulsatile flow. A sphygmomanometer cuff, previously placed around the ankle, is then inflated until the noise created by the flow ceases. The pressure at which this occurs is the systolic blood pressure. This can be measured in all three ankle vessels.

The **pressure index** is the ratio between the pressure measured by this technique and the pressure in the brachial artery. It is normally unity or 1.1, i.e. both foot and brachial artery pressures should be almost identical. Ratios above 1.0 indicate stiff, calcified limb vessels (often diabetic arteries), which cannot be squashed by the external pressure applied by the sphygmomanometer cuff. Ratios below 1 indicate occlusive disease upstream to the foot vessels.

The Doppler ultrasound flow detector is a very useful tool because it can detect pulsatile flow when the pulse pressure is impalpable to the fingers. The pressure index provides a rough indicator of disease severity. A more accurate assessment of the severity of the disease can be obtained by measuring the pressure before and after exercise.

SYMPTOMS PRODUCED BY ARTERIAL INSUFFICIENCY

Severe limb pain of sudden onset

This occurs when the arterial blood supply of a limb is suddenly interrupted, with no time for collaterals to form. The pain comes from ischaemic muscles and nerves, which develop irreversible changes within a few hours.

The *symptoms* are easy to remember, as each begins with **P**:

- **P**ain, usually very severe and of sudden onset
- **P**araesthesiae ('pins and needles') and numbness, which develop over a few hours and eventually progress to
- **P**aralysis.

The *three principal physical signs* also begin with **P**:

- **P**allor
- **P**ulselessness, and the limb feels
- **P**erishingly cold to the touch.

The limb looks white and feels cold. These findings can be compared with the appearance of the other side if the symptoms are unilateral. The capillary circulation is poor, with a prolonged refilling time after digital compression. The veins are empty and the limb may become blue and develop a blotchy, blue-white appearance. The femoral pulse may be present if the arterial occlusion is at the division of the common femoral artery into the superficial and profunda femoris arteries or is situated more distally. Similarly in the upper limb, the subclavian and

axillary pulses may be palpable, whereas the distal pulses, e.g. brachial, wrist and ankle pulses, are not.

Muscle tenderness, a bad prognostic sign, especially in the muscles of the anterior and posterior calf compartments, should be sought by gently pressing the bellies of these muscles.

A full neurological examination should concentrate on power, sensation and reflexes.

The Doppler ultrasound probe should be used to confirm the absence of pulsatile blood flow in the peripheral arteries. If any pulsatile flow is detected, it is likely to be severely diminished in height and intensity.

If the ischaemia persists, the leg becomes mottled and marbled, the muscles become hard, and the skin begins to blister and develop gangrene, which usually starts in the toes before spreading proximally. The causes of acute limb ischaemia are shown in the Revision panel 7.3.

General examination

Examine the heart and general circulation with care to ascertain the cause of the sudden arterial occlusion, such as the following.

An **arterial embolus** is suspected if the patient is fibrillating, has had a recent heart attack, or is known

---

Revision panel 7.2
The symptoms and signs of acute ischaemia

Pain, becoming
Painless (numb)
Pallor
Paralysis
Pulseless

Revision panel 7.3
Causes of acute arterial ischaemia

An arterial embolus
Thrombosis on an atheromatous plaque
Thrombosis of an aneurysm (usually popliteal)
Arterial dissection (usually aortic)
Traumatic disruption
External compression, e.g. cervical rib, popliteal entrapment

to have heart valve disease. Patients may never have had any symptoms of arterial ischaemia, e.g. intermittent claudication, before the embolus occurs.

An **acute arterial thrombosis** is suspected if the patient has already experienced symptoms of chronic arterial ischaemia, such as intermittent claudication or even rest pain (see below).

A **thrombosed aneurysm** is suspected if other arteries, such as the popliteal artery of the opposite limb, are found to be dilated.

An **aortic dissection** is suspected if the patient presents with severe chest and/or back pain. Other pulses such as the left subclavian artery may be absent.

A **traumatic arterial disruption** is suspected if there is a clear history of injury or vascular intervention.

Cervical rib is suspected if there is a palpable supraclavicular swelling. Patients with cevical ribs may have experienced neurological symptoms in the arm and hand for many years. (Special investigations are required to diagnose the other causes of subclavian artery compression.)

Also exclude two of the major **non-arterial causes** of an acute limb pain of sudden onset – **acute venous thrombosis** (see page 206) and **spinal cord compression** or **infarction**.

Intermittent claudication

Strictly speaking, *intermittent claudication* means intermittent limping (Latin *claudicatio* = to limp, a word derived from the disability of the Emperor Claudius). This term is used to describe a cramp-like pain in a muscle which appears during exercise. It is caused by an inadequate blood flow to the muscles. The pain stops the patient using the muscle and, if the affected muscle is in the leg, causes them to limp and then stop walking.

History

Age The majority of patients presenting with intermittent claudication are males, over the age of 50, with smoking-related atherosclerotic disease of the lower limb vessels. But claudication can develop in young adults with Buerger's disease or after an arterial embolism or a traumatic occlusion of a major artery.

Sex Claudication is more common in men than in women. There may be impotence if the occlusive disease is at the aortic bifurcation.

Pain The pain of intermittent claudication is quite specific and must fulfill three criteria.

1. The patient must experience the pain in a muscle, usually the calf.
2. The pain should only develop when the muscle is exercised.
3. The pain must disappear when the exercise stops.

Walking distance **Limitation of walking** is the principal complaint. The patient finds they can only walk a limited distance before an ache begins in the muscles of the leg, which then becomes a cramp and then stops them walking any further. The distance walked by the time walking has to stop is called the **claudication distance**. This should be recorded. If necessary, the patient should be observed walking to see when the pain develops. They should also be asked how long they have to wait until the pain goes away and whether they can then walk the same distance again. Some patients complain of an ache or cramp which does not stop them walking and which fades away if they force themselves to continue walking. Others find they can prevent the pain developing by walking slowly.

The severity of the pain and the time taken for it to begin and cease vary from patient to patient. Any muscle can be affected. The calf muscles are most often affected, but a claudication pain can arise in the thigh, buttock or foot muscles and in the muscles of the upper limb and forearm.

Patients may also describe **numbness** and **paraesthesiae** in the skin of the foot at the time that the muscle pain begins. This is the result of blood being shunted from the skin to the muscle.

Pains that begin when at rest or immediately the patient stands up, and pains that occur in tissues other than muscles and that do not abate with rest are not claudication pains.

Onset and progression The pain of claudication usually begins insidiously. The walking distance gradually shortens over a few months before becoming static. In a third or more of affected patients, the walking distance then increases, with spontaneous remission of the symptoms as the collateral circulation develops.

It is always important to ask about rest pain in a patient with claudication, as its presence signifies the onset of critical limb ischaemia. Patients with rest pain may have had intermittent claudication in the affected limb for many years before the onset of rest pain.

Examination of the legs in patients with claudication

Inspection The appearance of the limb on inspection is often remarkably normal, although if the condition is severe, there may be some blanching on elevation of the legs.

Palpation The foot and leg may be cold. The pulse immediately above the affected group of muscles is likely to be weak or absent. Thus, if claudication is experienced in the calf, the popliteal pulse is usually impalpable but the femoral pulse is likely to be present. The femoral pulse is likely to be absent if the pain is felt in the thigh muscles. Thus the level of the symptoms and signs often indicates the level of disease. It is possible to have claudication in the calf with palpable ankle pulses, but careful examination often reveals a bruit in the thigh, and if the pulses are re-examined after exercise, they may no longer be palpable.

The Doppler pressures are invariably reduced and fall still further with exercise.

Auscultation The common sites to find bruits in association with intermittent claudication are over the aortic bifurcation, the iliac and common femoral arteries and the superficial femoral artery at the adductor hiatus.

Examination of the motor and skeletal systems

This should be normal.

Differential diagnosis

Other causes of a claudication-like pain include osteoarthritis of the hip and knee, spinal stenosis, prolapsed intervertebral disc and venous claudication.

The hip and knee should always be carefully examined, as should the spine, especially if all the pulses are palpable (see Chapter 4).

Venous claudication should be considered if the limb is swollen or if there is lipodermatosclerosis of the gaiter skin.

Rest pain

Rest pain is a term used to describe the continuous, unremitting pain caused by severe ischaemia. In contrast to the pain of intermittent claudication, which only appears during exercise, this pain is present at rest throughout the day and the night.

History

Age Most patients with arterial disease severe enough to cause rest pain are 60 or more years old, but Buerger's disease and trauma can cause rest pain in young men.

Symptoms Patients complain of a continuous, severe aching pain which stops them sleeping. Rest pain is usually experienced in the most distal part of the limb, namely the toes and forefoot. If any gangrene is present, the patient feels the pain at the junction of living and dead tissues.

Rest pain is often relieved by putting the leg below the level of the heart, so patients hang their legs over the side of the bed or prefer to sleep sitting in a chair. The painful part is very sensitive. Movement or pressure exacerbates the pain. The patient often sits in bed with the knee bent, holding the foot still to try and relieve the pain. Strong analgesic drugs are the only means of providing relief. Rest pain is unremitting and gets steadily worse.

Systematic questions It is important to enquire about symptoms suggestive of pre-existing arterial disease in the affected limb, such as claudication, and any symptoms which indicate the presence of atherosclerosis elsewhere. Chest pains, a previous myocardial infarction, fainting, weakness, paraesthesiae in the upper limbs, episodes of blurred vision or stroke are all important indications of serious vascular disease elsewhere.

Family history Arterial disease is often familial, so it is important to ascertain the cause of death of parents and siblings and whether they had any symptoms of vascular disease.

Risk factors These include cigarette smoking, hypertension, diabetes and hypercholesterolaemia.

Examination

General appearance Patients with rest pain usually look drawn and haggard because of continuous pain and sleepless nights. They are often unwilling to lie flat on a couch with the leg horizontal for more than a short period because elevation of the leg exacerbates the pain.

An arcus senilis (see Fig. 8.14, page 227) is not diagnostic of vascular disease but is worth noting.

Xanthelesmata and xanthomata (see Fig. 3.47, page 103), which are cholesterol deposits around the eye and in the subcutaneous tissues, are indicative of hypercholesterolaemia. Pallor suggesting anaemia or a rubicund appearance suggesting polycythaemia (rubra vera) is worthwhile noting, as both these conditions can predispose to claudication and rest pain.

General examination The whole cardiovascular system must be examined with care. The blood pressure must be measured in both arms and recorded, the heart examined, the major arteries auscultated and the abdominal aorta felt in case it is dilated and aneurysmal (see below).

Inspection **When dependent**, a painful ischaemic foot is a deep reddish-purple colour. The tips of the toes may be grey or white if they are completely bloodless. There may be black patches of gangrene on the toes or the heel.

When horizontal, the foot rapidly becomes pale or marble white and the veins empty, becoming guttered. Further elevation of the leg increases the pallor. If the foot is not white when horizontal, it will certainly become so when elevated to 20°.

It is possible to have severely ischaemic toes and a good circulation in the rest of the foot. In these circumstances, the description above applies to the toes only. The pain is unlikely to be an ischaemic pain if the whole foot is painful but stays pink above an angle of 20°. The foot may be swollen and blue if the patient has been sitting with the leg dependent to ease the pain.

The pressure areas on the heel and the skin between the toes may be gangrenous, ulcerated or infected. Ischaemic changes often develop at the site of the nail beds.

Palpation The skin temperature from mid-calf downwards is usually reduced, even when the foot is dependent and congested. Capillary re-filling is retarded.

In general, rest pain is caused by a combination of large and small vessel disease, so it is common to find that the popliteal and femoral pulses are absent. Small vessel disease should be suspected if these pulses are palpable. The likely cause is then diabetes or Buerger's disease.

AUSCULTATION
Bruits may be heard over the iliac and femoral arteries.

OTHER SIGNS
There may be muscle wasting caused by disuse, and if the patient has been sitting holding the ischaemic foot for many weeks, there may be a fixed flexion deformity of the knee and hip joint.

Examination of the nervous system is important because a severe, constant pain in the lower limb may be caused by a neurological abnormality. The nervous system may be abnormal in diabetics, but these patients rarely have very severe rest pain, as the diabetes destroys the limb's pain sensation.

Gout may cause severe pain in the foot, with redness and tenderness.

Very occasionally, an **abscess** or **foreign body** needs to be excluded.

Pre-gangrene and gangrene

Pre-gangrene

This term is used by clinicians to describe the changes which indicate that a tissue's blood supply is so precarious that it will soon be insufficient to keep the tissue alive.

The principal symptom of pre-gangrene is rest pain, which is described in detail above.

The principal signs are pallor of the tissues when elevated, congestion when dependent, guttering of the veins, thick and scaling skin, and wasting of the pulps of the toes or fingers. The limb is cold and has poor capillary refilling. Ischaemic tissue is tender. Any further reduction in the blood supply will result in tissue death, or **gangrene** (see below). These symptoms must therefore be treated with the utmost urgency.

Gangrene

Gangrene is the term used to describe dead tissue. Dead tissue is brown, dark blue or black, and gradually contracts into a crinkled, withered, hard mass. These changes can happen if a patch of skin, a toe or the whole of the lower limb becomes ischaemic. The nerves in the dead part die and therefore gangrenous tissues are not painful. The junction between the living and dead tissue gradually becomes distinct, provided there is adequate venous drainage and the

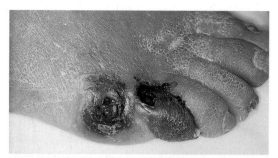

Gangrene of the fifth toe caused by atherosclerotic obstruction of the iliac and femoral arteries.

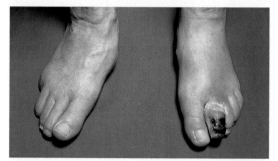

Infected (wet) gangrene caused by a mixture of infection and mild ischaemia in a diabetic.

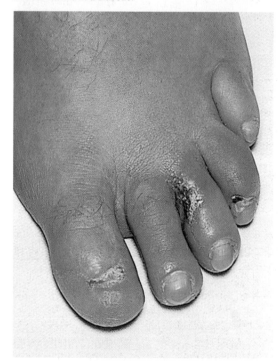

Infected gangrene between the second and third left toes in a diabetic.

FIG 7.4 THE COMMON SITES AND CAUSES OF GANGRENE.

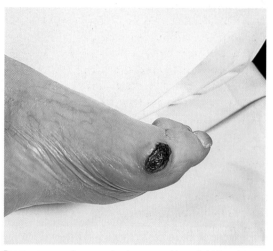

Pressure necrosis over a bunion caused by a tight bandage and mild occlusive vascular disease.

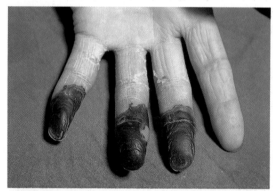

Gangrene of the fingertips caused by emboli from a subclavian aneurysm.

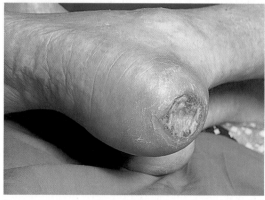

Pressure necrosis on the heel following a prolonged period of unconsciousness (normal circulation).

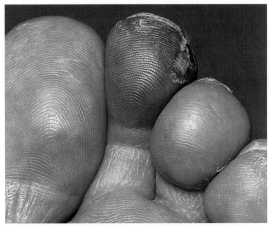

A blue ischaemic toe caused by emboli from a femoral artery stenosis.

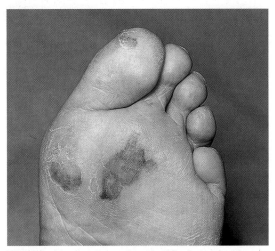

Multiple ischaemic areas on the sole of the foot caused by emboli from the left side of the heart.

FIG 7.4 continued

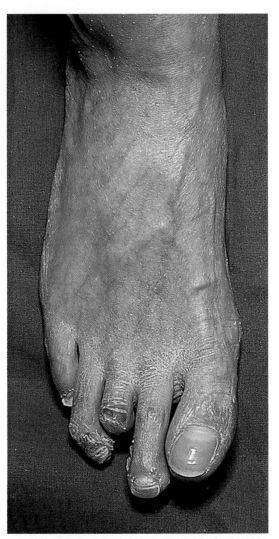

Long-standing ischaemia of the toes with gangrene of the third toe that has proceeded to auto-amputation.

proximal blood supply remains intact. This junction is known as the **line of demarcation**. The dead tissue may eventually separate and fall off. The living tissue on the proximal side of the line of demarcation is usually ischaemic and so is often constantly painful (rest pain) and tender. If the gangrene is the result of local trauma and the surrounding tissues are normal, they are not usually painful.

Gangrene usually develops in the extremities of the limbs – the tips of toes and fingers, and in areas of skin subjected to pressure. The dead tissue does not become shrivelled if its venous drainage is impaired or if it becomes infected. In these circumstances the gangrene becomes soft and boggy and the line of demarcation often becomes purulent.

A hard, shrunken, non-infected patch of gangrene with a clear line of demarcation is called **dry gangrene**. A soft, swollen, infected patch of gangrene without a clear margin is called **wet gangrene**. However, it is better to use the terms **infected** and **non-infected** rather than **wet** and **dry**. This difference is important because sometimes, as in diabetics, the gangrene is actually secondary to the infection not the ischaemia.

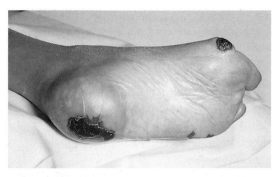

FIG 7.5 An ischaemic foot with patches of gangrene on all the pressure areas: the heel, the head of the first metatarsal and the base of the fifth metatarsal.

Diabetic gangrene is often associated with gas in the tissues (tissue-crepitus) and a foul smell.

Venous gangrene, which may complicate a massive deep vein thrombosis and phlegmasia caerulia dolens, usually affects all of the toes.

Ischaemic ulceration

An ischaemic ulcer is the aftermath of gangrene. By definition, it is caused by an inadequate blood supply.

History

Ischaemic ulcers are common in the elderly, who often also have symptoms of coronary or cerebral vascular disease. Patients sometimes remember a minor precipitating injury.

Symptoms Ischaemic ulcers, except those associated with a neurological abnormality, are very painful. They cause rest pain.

They do not bleed, but discharge a thin serous exudates, which can become purulent. They are usually indolent and often get slowly deeper and larger. Ischaemic ulcers may occasionally penetrate into joints, making movements very painful. The causes of ischaemic ulcers are:

- large artery obliteration: atherosclerosis, embolism,
- small artery obliteration: Buerger's disease, athero-embolism, diabetes, scleroderma and physical agents such as prolonged local pressure, radiation, trauma and electrical burns.

Systematic questions and past history The patient may give a history of prior claudication or symptoms of generalized vascular disease such as chest pain.

Examination

Site Ischaemic ulcers are found at the tips of the toes or fingers and over the pressure points.

Size Ischaemic ulcers vary in size from small, deep lesions, a few millimetres across, to large, flat ulcers 10 cm or more wide on the lower leg.

Shape The ulcers are most often elliptical.

Tenderness The ulcer and the surrounding tissues are often very tender. Removing a dressing can cause exacerbation of the pain that lasts for several hours.

Temperature The surrounding tissues are usually cold because they are ischaemic. Warm, healthy tissue suggests another cause for the ulceration.

Edge The edge of an ischaemic ulcer is either punched out, if there is no attempt at healing by the surrounding tissues, or sloping, if the ulcer is beginning to heal (see Chapter 1, page 33). The skin at the edge of the ulcer is usually a blue-grey colour. There is no lipodermatosclerosis in the surrounding skin unless venous disease coexists (see page 204).

Base The base of the ulcer usually contains grey-yellow slough covering flat, pale, granulation tissue.

Depth Ischaemic ulcers are often very deep. They may penetrate down to and through deep fascia, tendon, bone and even an underlying joint.

Discharge This may be clear fluid, serum or pus.

Relations The base may be stuck to, or be part of, any underlying structure. It is quite common to see bare

---

Revision panel 7.4
The causes of ischaemic ulceration

Large-artery obliteration
    Atherosclerosis
    Embolism
Small-artery obliteration
    Scleroderma
    Buerger's disease
    Embolism
    Diabetes
    Physical agents
        Pressure necrosis
        Radiation
        Trauma
        Electric burns

bone, ligaments and tendons exposed in the base of an ischaemic ulcer (see above).

Lymph drainage Infection in an ischaemic ulcer usually remains confined to the ulcer, so that the local lymph glands are not normally enlarged.

State of the local tissues Surrounding tissues may show signs of ischaemia – pallor, coldness and atrophy.

Distal pulses These are invariably absent.

Doppler pressures The Doppler pressure index is invariably reduced.

Neurological examination If the ulcer is caused by a neuropathy (see below), there may be a loss of superficial and deep sensation, weakness of movement and a loss of reflexes.

General examination There may be evidence of vascular disease elsewhere. The urine should be tested for sugar.

Neuropathic ulceration

Tissue ischaemia is usually painful. Pain is the mechanism by which the body appreciates that any part of the skin is becoming deprived of blood. The feet and buttocks become painful after prolonged standing or sitting, encouraging movement to remove the pressure from the painful part. When pain sensation is lost this warning is lost, and any compressed tissue may become permanently damaged.

Neuropathic ulcers are therefore only indirectly caused by local ischaemia. The main cause is lack of sensation in the tissues, allowing unrecognized trauma to occur.

Neuropathic ulcers are deep, penetrating ulcers which occur over pressure points, but the surrounding tissues are healthy and may have a good circulation. The diagnostic features are:

- the ulcers are painless,
- the surrounding tissues are unable to appreciate pain,

> **Revision panel 7.5**
> **The causes of chronic ulceration**
>
> Infection
> Repeated trauma
> Ischaemia
> Oedema
> Denervation
> Localized destructive disease (tuberculosis, carcinoma)

> **Revision panel 7.6**
> **The causes of neuropathic ulceration (ulcers secondary to a loss of sensation)**
>
> **Peripheral nerve lesions**
>   Diabetes
>   Nerve injuries
>   Leprosy
> **Spinal cord lesions**
>   Spina bifida
>   Tabes dorsalis
>   Syringomyelia

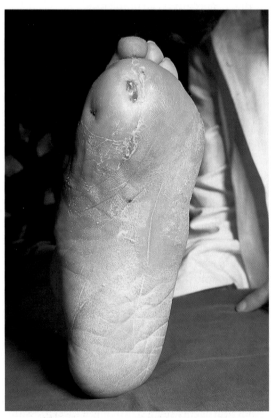

FIG 7.6 Trophic ulcers on the sole of the foot in a patient with diabetic peripheral neuritis. The circulation was good and all the pulses were present, but there was a total loss of pain sensation. The great toe had been amputated 2 years earlier for similar ulceration.

- the surrounding tissues may have a normal blood supply.

These ulcers can easily be mistaken for ischaemic ulcers, which is why a neurological examination is always important. The causes of neuropathic ulceration are:

- peripheral nerve lesions: diabetes, nerve injuries, leprosy,
- spinal cord lesions: spina bifida, tabes dorsalis and syringomyelia.

However, all these conditions may occur in patients with vascular disease and so true ischaemic and neuropathic ulcers may occur together and the combined effect of both diseases may be synergistic.

Careful examination of the arterial and neurological systems is required to identify the major cause.

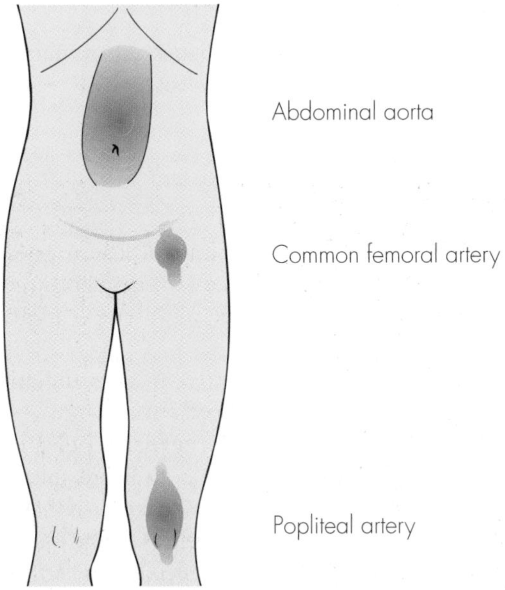

The common sites to find aneurysms.

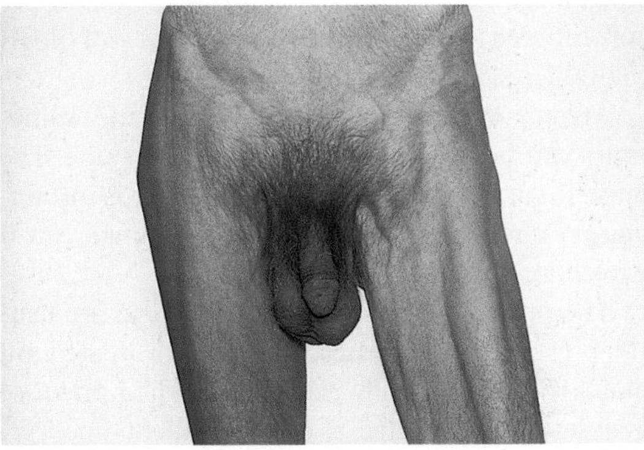

An aneurysm of the left common femoral artery compressing the femoral vein and causing distension of the long saphenous vein.

FIG 7.7 ANEURYSMS.

Pulsatile swellings (aneurysms)

An aneurysm is a localized dilatation of an artery. The majority of aneurysms are associated with atherosclerosis, but some are caused by a primary weakness in the connective tissues of the arterial wall.

The causes of aneurysms are shown in the Revision panel 7.7.

In a **true aneurysm** all the layers of the arterial wall are involved (intima, media and adventitia). In a **false aneurysm** the arterial wall is breached and the wall of the aneurysm consists of blood clot and compressed surrounding normal tissues.

Although an aneurysm can develop in any artery, most occur in the abdominal aorta and the femoral and popliteal arteries.

Berry aneurysms are believed to arise in a congenitally weak area of the circle of Willis. They are associated with hypertension and are responsible for many subarachnoid haemorrhages in middle

Revision panel 7.7
The causes of aneurysms

Congenital
- A localized weakness
  - Berry aneurysm
  - Marfan's syndrome
  - Ehlers–Danlos syndrome
  - Arterial dilatation associated with a congenital arterio-venous fistula

Acquired aneurysm
- Trauma
  - Direct injury
- Infection
  - Bacterial arteritis (mycotic)
  - Syphilis
  - Acquired immunodeficiency syndrome
- Degeneration
  - Atherosclerosis

False aneurysms
- Trauma
- Post-arterial surgery

age. It is debatable if these are truly congenital, but the weakness responsible for their development may indeed be inherited.

Syphilitic aneurysms of the thoracic aorta were once common but are now extremely rare.

History

Age Atherosclerotic aneurysms are rare before the age of 50. Thereafter, their frequency increases with age.

Sex Men are affected 10 to 20 times more often than women.

Other causative factors A family history, cigarette smoking and hypertension are well-recognized risk factors.

Symptoms Many aneurysms cause no symptoms during life and are discovered by chance during a routine physical examination or screening programme.

The commonest presenting symptom is dull, aching pain. With abdominal aneurysms, this is usually experienced over the swelling in the centre of the abdomen, but the pain often radiates to the back and may be experienced only in this site. The abdominal pain is caused by stretching of the artery, and the back pain by erosion of the lumbar vertebrae.

Some patients with abdominal aneurysms present with sciatica or loin pain as a consequence of local pressure on the nerves.

Acute pain occurs if the vessel suddenly stretches or begins to tear. This becomes a very severe pain if the aneurysm ruptures and a large haematoma forms (see Chapter 15). The patient may collapse from the accompanying hypotensive shock or suddenly die.

A few thin patients notice a pusatile mass. This is a common presentation for femoral aneurysms but is rare for abdominal aneurysms.

Occasionally patients notice their abdomen pulsating when they lie in the bath or in bed.

Severe ischaemia of the lower limb follows thrombosis of an aneurysm. This is a rare event in aortic and femoral aneurysms but is a common presentation of popliteal aneurysms.

Less severe ischaemia may be caused by emboli originating in the aneurysm. One of the best examples of this complication is the multiple small emboli which may block the digital arteries of a patient with a subclavian aneurysm.

Peripheral emboli in the lower limb may cause intermittent claudication or rest pain.

The aorta, femoral and popliteal arteries are closely related to the inferior vena cava, femoral and popliteal veins, respectively. Dilatation of an artery may block its adjacent vein by direct pressure, or cause it to thrombose. Patients may then present with a swollen, blue, painful limb.

Very occasionally aneurysms rupture into an adjacent vein. The resulting acute arterio-venous fistula may cause severe cardiac embarrassment. The tissues distal to the fistula become cyanosed, the neck veins are elevated and there is usually a loud machinery murmur over the aneurysm.

Systematic questions and past history Coronary or cerebral vascular disease can coexist.

Examination
Abdominal aneurysms

The abdominal aorta divides into the iliac arteries at about the level of the umbilicus. Consequently most abdominal aneurysms are felt in the upper umbilical and epigastric regions.

Iliac artery aneurysms present as a pulsating mass in the iliac fossa or hypogastrium.

Aneurysms produce an expansile pulsation. In order to feel the expansion, both hands must be placed on either side of the mass to confirm that the hands are pushed apart as well as being pushed upwards. Many lumps in the upper abdomen transmit aortic pulsation and may be misdiagnosed as aneurysms. Real difficulty may occasionally be encountered if the aorta is encased by pathologically enlarged lymph glands.

Aneurysms feel firm and smooth, and sometimes can be moved a little from side to side. The presence of tenderness implies that there is inflammatory change or that the wall of the aneurysm is stretching and likely to rupture.

The pulses at the groins and in the legs are usually present and the vessels often slightly dilated. All pulses must be carefully palpated and their presence or absence documented, as in some patients aneurysmal and occlusive disease may coexist.

The signs and symptoms of a ruptured aneurysm are described on page 416. When an aneurysm ruptures it becomes very painful and tender. The patient

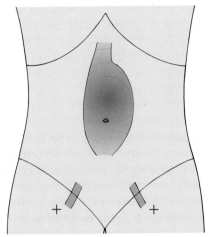

The position of an aneurysm of the abdominal aorta. If there is a gap between the top of the aneurysm and the costal margin, the aneurysm probably begins below the origin of the renal arteries. The femoral pulses are usually palpable.

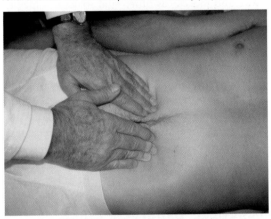

Assess the width of the abdominal aorta by placing your hands on either side of the pulse in the epigastrium.

FIG 7.8 ASSESSMENT OF AN ABDOMINAL AORTIC ANEURYSM.

may collapse with signs of hypovolaemia – pallor, tachycardia and hypotension.

An expanding retroperitonal haematoma may be felt as a large mass in the abdomen spreading down into the iliac fossa or posteriorly into the loins.

Femoral aneurysms

These usually arise in the common femoral artery and produce a bulge just below the inguinal ligament. They have an expansile pulsation. A mass of enlarged lymph glands may transmit pulsation and can be misdiagnosed as an aneurysm (see the differential diagnosis of groin lump, page 430). The other

pulses in the leg must be documented, as there is often an associated popliteal aneurysm. Femoral and popliteal aneurysms are often bilateral, but do not necessarily develop or present at the same time (see below).

Popliteal aneurysms

Aneurysms of the popliteal artery are occasionally noticed by patients if they bulge out of the popliteal fossa. They may be found by chance in patients presenting with claudication. Popliteal aneurysms should always be excluded in patients presenting with an **idiopathic calf vein** thrombosis.

Unfortunately, popliteal aneurysms often thrombose before they are noticed and present with **acute ischaemia** of the lower limb (see above).

The diagnosis is confirmed by finding an **expansile pulsation** in the popliteal fossa. The pulse is easy to feel. The examiner's fingers are pushed apart and away by the pulse, which can often be felt on both sides of the popliteal fossa. **A popliteal aneurysm should always be suspected when a popliteal pulse is easy to feel.** A bruit may be present above or over an enlarged segment of the vessel.

A **thrombosed popliteal aneurysm** is smooth and solid and does not pulsate or flucuate. It can be moved slightly from side to side, but never moves up and down. It may be confused with a **Baker's cyst** or **semimembranosus bursa** (see Chapter 4), but its size does not change when the knee is flexed and it occupies the whole length of the mid-line of the popliteal fossa.

The ankle pulses will not be palpable.

The legs should be examined for signs of venous obstruction, as this is a common complication of popliteal aneurysms.

False aneurysms

A false aneurysm is a large haematoma whose centre contains fluid blood which connects with the lumen of the blood vessel. The commonest cause is a therapeutic or diagnostic vascular puncture or a stab wound. Following the arterial puncture, a haematoma forms outside the artery. At first, thrombus plugs the defect, but pulsatile blood pressure gradually pushes out the haemostatic plug from the defect in the artery wall and excavates the haematoma to form a cavity connected to the vessel.

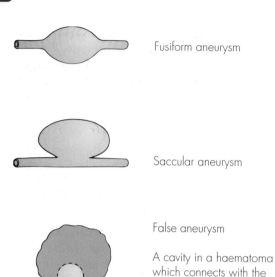

Fusiform aneurysm

Saccular aneurysm

False aneurysm

A cavity in a haematoma which connects with the lumen of the artery

FIG 7.9 The types of aneurysm.

The symptoms, signs and complications of false aneurysms are exactly the same as those of a true aneurysm except:

- there is a history of trauma or iatrogenic intervention, followed by
- the sudden appearance of a swelling;
- false aneurysms tend to occur at unusual sites, e.g. wrist or ankle, though iatrogenic false aneurysms are now most common in the groin.

False aneurysms also occur when a surgical graft separates from the native vessel. A pulsatile mass beneath an incision in the groin at the site of a previous vascular anastomosis is most likely to be a false aneurysm.

HAEMORRHAGE

A major vascular disruption, which may be the result of a **penetrating, blunt** or **hyperextension injury** is likely to result in severe hemorrhage. The bleeding may be **concealed**, as when, for example, a serrated or spiculated end of a fractured long bone pierces an artery or a ruptured aneurysm bleeds into the tissues or a body cavity, or may be revealed, as when an aneurysm erupts through the skin or a congenital vascular malformation bleeds onto the skin surface.

Concealed haemorrhage from an arterial injury is suspected if a large swelling rapidly develops in association with signs of hypovolaemia, i.e. pallor, sweating, venoconstriction, tachycardia and eventually hypotension. The pulses distal to the injury will not be palpable if the artery has been transected, when the limb may show signs of acute ischaemia (the six Ps, see page 179).

In patients presenting with visible (**revealed**) haemorrhage, the diagnosis is straightforward. There is usually a jet of bright-red, high-pressure, pulsatile blood coming out of an obvious cutaneous defect or wound. (Venous bleeding, in contrast, is dark red and wells up out of the wound.) The pulses distal to the injury may be absent if the artery has been transected. Direct pressure or proximal arterial compression over a bony point should arrest the bleeding until definitive treatment can be administered.

When the bleeding is coming from the site of a penetrating wound it is important to assess local nerve and muscle, as other vital structures may be damaged. This may be difficult because the arrest of the haemorrhage must take precedence.

Artery, vein, nerve and muscle injuries commonly coexist.

When the haemorrhage occurs into a body cavity or is deeply seated, there may be no signs of swelling and the **symptoms of hypovolaemia** predominate. Haemorrhage into the peritoneum or retroperitoneum often causes pain as well as collapse (see page 416).

TRANSIENT AND PERMANENT WEAKNESS, PARALYSIS AND BLINDNESS

Transient cerebral ischaemia

A **transient ischaemic attack** (**TIA**) is an episode of sudden paralysis, paraesthesiae or speech loss caused by a sudden reduction in the blood flow to a part of the brain. To be classified as transient, the symptoms must recover completely within 24 hours. (TIA is a poor term, as it does not indicate which tissue in the brain is ischaemic.)

Persistant cerebral ischaemia

Persistant cerebral ischaemia causes a **stroke**. This is a sudden episode of prolonged cerebral malfunction caused by cerebral infarction or haemorrhage, both caused by vascular disease, which usually takes the form of a prolonged weakness or paralysis of half the body (a **hemiplegia**) and sometimes an associated **sensory** or **speech defect**, which may predominate. The malfunction does not begin to recover for several days and may never recover completely.

Ischaemia of the mid-brain that damages the vital centres in this area may cause coma and cardiovascular and respiratory instability.

It is important to remember that the right side of the brain controls the left side of the body, and vice versa.

The speech area (*Broca's area*) is invariably in the left temporo-parietal area in right-handed people, although it can be in the right hemisphere in left-handed patients.

Strokes are more commonly caused by **infarction** than by cerebral haemorrhage and are usually **embolic** or **thrombotic**, though an **arterial wall dissection** can occlude an artery's lumen.

Stroke caused by **cerebral haemorrhage** produces identical cerebral symptoms but is more common in women and is associated with hypertension.

Both types of stroke usually cause upper motor neurone signs, with reduced power, spastic tone and brisk reflexes in the limbs, associated with an up-going plantar reflex (*Babinksi's sign*). A cerebral haemorrhage can only be differentiated from an infarct with certainty by computerized tomography (CT) scanning, not by the history or physical signs.

Transient ischaemic attacks

Transient ischaemic attacks are caused by **emboli** or **hypoperfusion**.

The emboli that cause TIAs come from the carotid arteries, heart valves and the great vessels. Platelet clumps and cholesterol crystals originally attached to ulcerated plaques break off and are swept up into the retinal or cerebral vessels. Retinal emboli cause transient loss of vision, known as **amaurosis fugax** (fleeting blindness), which seems to the patient like a curtain coming across the visual field or a grey veil blocking out all or part of the vision in one eye.

Anyone presenting with a brief episode of weakness, paraesthesiae or loss of sensation in one half of the body which lasts a few minutes or several hours and then recovers completely must be suspected of having a TIA.

There are usually no physical signs by the time the patient presents, but evidence of previous ischaemic episodes – facial weakness, expressive dysphagia, upper motor neurone lesions and cholesterol emboli in the retinal vessels or areas of retinal infarction – should be sought.

The detection of a **carotid bruit** over the carotid artery just below the angle of the jaw indicates the presence of at least some stenosis in the region of the carotid bifurcation. However, a severe internal carotid artery stenosis can be present without any bruit, and a loud bruit can be caused by a stenosis of the external carotid artery.

Arrhythmias and cardiac murmurs suggest a cardiac source for the emboli. A low pulse pressure and an ejection systolic murmur suggest the presence of **aortic valve disease**, while an irregularly irregular or very slow pulse suggests a possible cause of Stokes–Adams attacks.

Transient hypoperfusion

Whereas emboli are common, hypoperfusion is rare because auto-regulation usually ensures adequate cerebral perfusion unless there is a very severe reduction in carotid blood pressure and flow. Episodes of hypoperfusion usually occur with much greater frequency than embolic attacks – often several times a day or week – and can be brought on by exercise or vasodilatation. They may cause 'global' brain ischaemia and present with dizziness and collapse rather than motor cortical symptoms.

Differential diagnosis

The differential diagnosis of a TIA is shown in Revision panel 7.8.

A history from a bystander or relative may be very helpful in making the diagnosis. Any history of aura, twitching, tongue biting or incontinence is indicative of **grand mal epilepsy**, whereas **petit mal** causes patients to lose touch temporarily with their surroundings.

Hypoglycaemic attacks These occur during periods of food abstinence, especially at night. Patients often describe hunger, malaise and vague abdominal pain, which is accompanied by trembling, dizziness and blurred vision. They may also notice incoordination, slurred speech, diplopia and drowsiness. The blood and urinary sugar is low during an attack, the symptoms of which can be instantly relieved by glucose.

Migraine Migrainous attacks are usually associated with severe unilateral headache, often situated over one eye and associated with photophobia and vomiting and occasionally transient blindness. There are no physical signs and the diagnosis relies entirely on the history.

Vertebrobasilar insufficiency Sometimes it can be quite difficult to separate TIAs from vertebrobasilar insufficiency, but the symptoms of the latter are often precipitated by neck movements or looking up. Neurological signs may indicate pathology in the hind-brain or cerebellum. Bruits may be heard over the origin of the vertebral artery.

Subclavian steal syndrome Occasionally patients present with transient motor or sensory symptoms, even loss of consciousness, after arm exercise. The presence of a weak brachial and radial pulse, reduced blood pressure in the affected arm, and a bruit over the subclavian artery should suggest the diagnosis of subclavian steal syndrome.

This syndrome occurs when the first part of the subclavian artery is blocked and blood flows down the vertebral artery because, during arm exercise, it acts as a collateral vessel to supply the arm. This steals blood away from the hind-brain and gives rise to hind-brain and cerebellar symptoms.

Multiple sclerosis, acute glaucoma, retinal tears and temporal arteritis can cause **transient blindness**. Multiple sclerosis can cause considerable diagnostic

confusion, but multiple lesions occurring in time and space eventually indicate the likely diagnosis.

Other intracranial disease Patients with a **subdural haematoma** may experience fluctuations in their level of consciousness and will almost always develop some localizing neurological signs before eventually developing signs of **raised intracranial pressure**. This is also true of **cerebral tumours** and **metastases**, which can initially cause diagnostic confusion until the patient eventually develops signs of fixed and expanding defects.

Completed strokes

A full neurological examination is essential in all patients who present with a completed stroke, in order to exclude a vascular cause as well as a neurological dysfunction caused by space-occupying lesions, abscesses, haematomata and multiple sclerosis. The blood pressure and heart must be carefully assessed. The superficial temporal arteries should be palpated. The carotid bifurcation and lower neck should be auscultated for bruits. A stethoscope placed over the closed eye can occasionally detect intracerebral bruits in patients with a stenosis of the carotid siphon.

COLD, BLUE DIGITS, HANDS AND FEET

Intermittent colour changes in the skin of the periphery of the limbs suggest the presence of vasospasm or recurrent minor episodes of arterial occlusion, the many causes of which are listed in Revision panel 7.9 and must be excluded before the diagnosis of vasospastic disease is accepted. To do this, the supraclavicular fossa must be inspected and palpated for a fullness or occasionally a bony lump caused by a cervical rib or a dilated subclavian artery. The subclavian, axillary, brachial, radial and ulnar pulses must all be palpated and auscultated. The blood pressure should be measured in both arms, and Doppler pressures must be measured in the radial, ulnar and brachial pulses. Abnormalities in any of these examinations may require special tests such as plain radiographs, Duplex scanning and arteriography.

Patients not found to have a physical obstruction of their blood vessels are likely to be suffering from excessive vasospasm of the small vessels in their hands in response to cold and emotional stimuli.

Revision panel 7.8
The differential diagnosis of a transient ischaemic attack

Grand or petit mal epilepsy
Stokes–Adam's attacks from a tight aortic stenosis
Arrhythmias
Vasovagal attacks
Hypoglycaemia
Migraine
Vertebrobasilar disease
Subdural haematoma
A space-occupying lesion in the brain

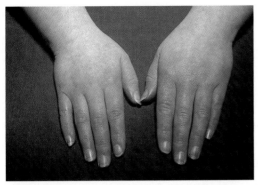

Hands showing the transition from the blue to the red phase. Ten minutes earlier the fingers of both hands had been white and numb.

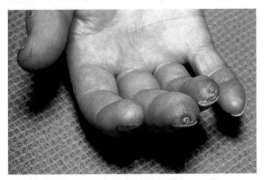

Ischaemic ulceration of the fingertips. This usually indicates permanent, rather than spastic, occlusion of the digital vessels.

FIG 7.10 RAYNAUD'S PHENOMENON.

Some conditions can be diagnosed by the physical appearances they produce, but their aetiology is still largely conjectural and there is a considerable overlap between each condition.

Raynaud's phenomenon

This is the best known vasospastic disorder. The term is used to describe a series of colour changes in the skin of the hands or feet following exposure to cold. The condition can be most distressing in cold climates, especially in winter.

- The skin first turns **white** and becomes cold and numb.
- It next turns **blue** but remains cold and numb.
- Finally, it turns **red**, hot and painful.

Many attacks are brought on by cold or emotion and many do not pass through all the classic colour changes.

History

Sex Ninety per cent of those affected are women, and many are cigarette smokers. It affects 5–20 per cent of the population.

Past history It is worthwhile asking patients if they have a history of **frostbite**, have ever worked in a **cold storage** environment or have regularly used **vibrating tools**.

Joint problems, rashes and swallowing difficulty indicate the likelihood of **scleroderma** or another **collagen vascular disease**.

Examination

Those conditions that, in addition to the colour changes, cause permanent damage to the digital

---

Revision panel 7.9
The causes of Raynaud's phenomenon

Atherosclerosis and Buerger's disease
Platelet emboli from:
    subclavian aneurysm (secondary to cervical rib)
    atherosclerotic stenosis of subclavian artery
Collagen disease
    Scleroderma
    Systemic lupus erythematosus
    Rheumatoid arthritis
Vibrating tools
Irritation of nerves
    Cervical spondylosis
    Cervical rib
    Spinal cord disease
    Old poliomyelitis
Repeated immersion in cold water
Working in a cold environment
Previous frostbite
Blood abnormalities
    Cold agglutinins
    Cryoglobulins
    Polycythaemia
Drugs
    Ergot
General diseases
    Hypothyroidism
    Diabetes
    Malnutrition

arteries, such as scleroderma, vibration injury and blood abnormalities, gradually cause atrophy of the pulps of the fingers, poor nail growth and ulceration of the fingertips.

If the digital arteries become occluded, the fingers waste, especially the pulps, and become thin, stiff and pointed. The hand is cold and the joints may be stiff. Sometimes there are small, painful, ischaemic ulcers on the fingertips which are slow to heal, or small scars at the site of the resolution of previous patches of ischaemia. Both are very painful and tender. The patient may eventually get rest pain and gangrene of the fingertips.

Repeated infections around the nails (**paronychia**) are common.

Many patients eventually develop the signs of scleroderma, evidence that the phenomenon is a secondary abnormality, not a primary disease.

If the cause of the colour changes is solely vasospasm, the hands will look normal between attacks, making the diagnosis of the underlying cause far more difficult. As has been shown, the symptoms are often secondary to many other conditions and the diagnosis of idiopathic Raynaud's disease is only made when these have been excluded. The common causes are the collagen vascular diseases, especially scleroderma, the excessive use of vibrating tools, and cold exposure. Patients with scleroderma, systemic lupus erythematosus and rheumatoid arthritis may show the characteristic changes in their skin and face.

Primary Raynaud's disease

When all the other causes of Raynaud's phenomenon have been excluded, one is left with the diagnosis of primary Raynaud's disease.

This is quite common in teenage girls. It is mild, familial and often associated with chilblains. It often disappears in the late twenties, but a few women have symptoms all their life and occasionally the disease becomes very severe.

If the phenomena start in adult women, often around the menopause, they are likely to be the first sign of scleroderma.

It is always worthwhile measuring the Doppler pressures at the wrist, especially if the pulses are impalpable. The digital vessels may also be insonated with the Doppler flow detector, and in patients with collagen diseases, pulses in these may well be absent near the tips of the fingers.

Some doctors use a cold exposure test – dipping the hands in cold water and re-mapping and re-measuring the Doppler digital pressures in the fingers – to reproduce the symptoms and confirm the existence of a cold sensitivity. This can also be carried out at the bedside using **thermographic equipment**.

Acrocyanosis

This is a condition, usually affecting women, in which the hands and feet are persistently blue and cold. The colour of the skin does not vary with the environmental temperature as it does in Raynaud's phenomenon, but the blueness may come and go. The hands may be pink and normal between attacks, or cold with sweaty palms. As the attack subsides, the hands may become warm, sweaty and painful. The fingers are susceptible to chilblains. The diagnosis is based solely on the colour, temperature and appearance of the hands.

Erythrocyanosis crurum puellarum frigidum

This condition affects the posterior and medial aspects of the lower legs of young (15–25 years old) girls in response to cold. The legs are often fat and hairless. The affected areas become red/blue (**erythrocyanotic**) and swollen. Dusky reddish purple blotches appear and may feel cold to the touch. The swollen area is tender and may progress to chilblains and superficial ulceration. The swelling is often more noticeable than the discolouration, and if it spreads around the ankle, can be mistaken for lymphoedema. When the chilblains break down and ulcerate, they must be differentiated from other forms of leg ulcer.

Erythromelalgia

This is a condition in which the patient complains of **burning red extremities**. These symptoms may be exacerbated by the pressure of bedclothes against the skin. The condition is much commoner in women. It appears to result from the release of vasodilator neurochemicals, with 5-hydroxytryptamine accumulating in the tissues. It must be differentiated from gout, Buerger's disease, systemic lupus erythematosus, rheumatoid arthritis and peripheral neuritis.

Examination of the extremities confirms that they are red and the patients complain that dependency causes an increase in the pain.

Hyperhidrosis (excessive sweating)

This condition (see Chapter 3, page 99) is closely associated with vasospastic disorders. The excessive sweating is unrelated to heat and affects especially the palms of the hands, the soles of the feet and the axillae. Excessive sweating from the groins and face may also be troublesome. It is more common in women and is socially embarrassing, particularly during the patient's first clinic consultation.

Hyperhidrosis can be caused by **thyrotoxicosis**, which must be excluded by careful examination and special tests.

Large limbs

Local gigantism, multiple arterio-venous fistulae and the Klippel–Trenauney syndrome all cause a limb to grow larger and thicker than its fellow.

Multiple arterio-venous fistulae throughout a single limb is known as the **Parkes Weber syndrome**. This is a congenital abnormality. The limb, as well as being enlarged, feels hot. The subcutaneous veins are often dilated. There may be palpable thrills and audible machinery murmurs over the major sites of fistulation.

A tourniquet inflated around the root of the limb should cause slowing of the pulse (the *Branham–Nicoladoni sign*). This is a consequence of reducing the venous return by abolishing the shunt. The differential diagnoses are the other causes of limb hypertrophy mentioned above. Rarely, patients with a swollen, lymphoedematous limb are misdiagnosed as having a hypertrophic limb.

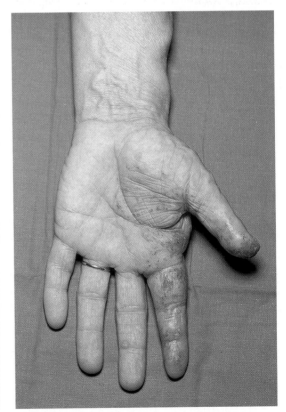

FIG 7.11 A congenital arterio-venous fistula of the hand, anterior and posterior views. The index finger and thenar eminence are enlarged, the veins are distended and the thenar eminence is pulsatile. There is ischaemic ulceration on the tip of the thumb. A bruit could be heard, on auscultation, all over the hand.

HYPERTENSION

Patients with *high blood pressure* rarely present to a surgical outpatients, but renal artery stenosis, adrenal tumours and coarctation of the aorta are important, surgically correctable causes of hypertension. The renal function must be assessed and the abdomen should be auscultated for bruits in all atherosclerotic patients who are found to be hypertensive.

A 'moon' face, abdominal striae and a 'buffalo' hump (see Chapter 8) are indicative of **Cushing's syndrome**, while the presence of neurofibromata suggests the possibility of a **phaeochromocytoma**.

Coarctation of the aorta is a rare but important condition. Knowledge of the physical signs enables early detection before symptoms develop. This can lead to a surgical correction, which prolongs life. Coarctation is a congenital narrowing of the aorta just beyond the left subclavian artery close to the site of the ligamentum arteriosum, which is the remnant of the ductus arteriosus. Provided the ductus closes normally, a coarctation usually remains symptomless until adult life, but if the ductus remains patent, patients rapidly develop symptoms and often have other cardiac abnormalities.

The symptoms and signs include:

- **dyspnoea** on exertion,
- **cerebrovascular accidents** associated with hypertension in the upper half of the body,
- **collateral arteries** visible and palpable over the scapulae, and
- **weak** or **delayed femoral pulses**.

There will be a strong cardiac impulse as the left ventricle hypertrophies in an attempt to overcome the resistance to aortic blood flow caused by the coarctation. A **systolic murmur** is usually present to the left of the vertebral column at the T4/5 level, just over or beyond the stenosis.

Ophthalmoscopic examination may reveal retinal haemorrhages, exudates and papilloedema.

INTESTINAL ISCHAEMIA

Ischaemia of the bowel may have an acute or chronic onset.

Acute obstruction of the superior mesenteric artery by an embolus or by thrombosis causes acute abdominal pain, peritonitis and shock (see Chapter 15, page 414).

Chronic atherosclerotic occlusion or stenosis of the coeliac or mesenteric vessels can cause **intestinal angina** – abdominal pain that develops 30–60 minutes after eating – causing fear of eating and weight loss.

A reduced blood flow in the arteries of the colon, particularly the splenic flexure, can cause **ischaemic colitis** with diarrhoea and sometimes rectal bleeding.

The only physical sign in the chronic syndromes may be the presence of an **abdominal bruit**.

THE VEINS

CLINICAL ASSESSMENT OF THE VENOUS CIRCULATION OF THE LOWER LIMB

Anatomy and physiology

The veins of the lower limb are divided into **superficial** and **deep systems**, separated by the deep fascia of the leg. At certain points there are veins that pass through the deep fascia to provide a communication between the two systems. Normally the valves in these **communicating veins** only allow blood to pass from the superficial into the deep system. The deep veins have many valves to ensure that blood only flows upwards against the force of gravity towards the heart.

Blood flow in the erect position is mostly produced by the **calf muscle pump**. Within the soleal muscles of the calves are large venous sinusoids – the **soleal sinusoids** – which are compressed during contraction of the calf muscles, e.g. during walking, so that blood is forced out of the calf veins into the popliteal veins and on towards the heart. During calf muscle relaxation, the intramuscular veins open but blood is prevented from refluxing back into them from the proximal deep veins by the valves in the popliteal veins. The negative pressure in the deep veins then sucks blood in from the superficial system through the communicating veins to reduce the superficial venous pressure, incrementally, with each calf muscle contraction.

The superficial veins all eventually join either the **great** (long) or **lesser** (short) **saphenous system**. These two major subcutaneous veins end where they communicate with the femoral and popliteal veins, respectively.

Both superficial systems are also joined to the deep veins by a number of other **communicating (perforating) veins**, the most important of which are in the calf.

The main tributaries of the saphenous veins are the veins that become varicose because they, unlike the saphenous veins, do not contain a strong coat of smooth muscle in their wall. They lie in a more superficial position and are not bound down to the deep fascia.

The deep veins accompany the arteries of the lower leg join to form the popliteal vein, which also receives blood from the calf muscle sinusoids.

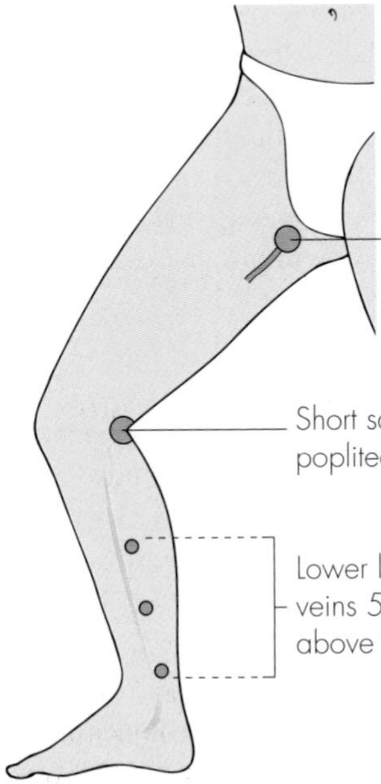

Deep vein thrombosis usually starts in the sinusoids and venae commitantes. The thrombus may then extend up into the popliteal vein, the femoral vein, the iliac veins and even into the vena cava.

Symptoms of lower limb venous disease

Most patients with venous disorders complain of **unsightly veins** in their lower limbs, **pain** or **discomfort** when standing and **minor ankle swelling**. They also may complain of **skin changes** (lipodermatosclerosis, eczema, pigmentation and ulceration) in the skin of the gaiter region. Superficial veins may occasionally **bleed**.

Superficial vein thrombosis causes painful lumps or cords.

Deep vein thrombosis presents with **calf pain** and **leg swelling** or **pleuritic chest pain**, **haemoptysis** and **dyspnoea** if it is complicated by a pulmonary embolism.

Examination of the veins of the lower limb
Inspection

The lower limbs need to be properly exposed with the patient standing erect on a low stool in a warm,

Long saphenous – femoral vein junction

Short saphenous – popliteal vein junction

Lower leg communicating veins 5, 10 and 15 cm above the medial malleolus

FIG 7.12 The common sites where the superficial veins connect with the deep veins.

Revision panel 7.10
Routine for assessing the venous circulation

Ask the patient to stand up
Inspection
    Site and size of visible veins
    Effect of elevation and dependency
    Ankle oedema
    Skin colour
Palpation
    Palpate the trunks of long and short saphenous veins
    Palpate the sapheno-popliteal junction
    Feel for fascial defects
    Feel the texture of the skin and subcutaneous tissues
Percussion
    Percussion wave conduction
Auscultation
    Listen for bruits over prominent varices
Tourniquet tests
Doppler ultrasound

well-lit examination room. Many patients with venous disorders have visible, dilated and tortuous subcutaneous veins, which are described as **varicose veins**.

Both limbs must be examined from **in front** and **behind** to ensure that all aspects of the legs are examined. The site and course of all the varicosities should be recorded on anterior and posterior outline drawings of the lower limb.

A blue-tinged bulge in the groin, which disappears on lying down, is likely to be a saphena varix.

Some varicose veins are large and prominent, whereas others are minute and intradermal. The latter may cause a blue patch, which can arise from a single feeding vein. Intradermal veins are called **spider veins** or **venous stars**. Slightly larger intermediate veins are often called **reticular veins**. Large, prominent, distended veins on the medial side of the lower calf are often called **blow outs** if they lie in close proximity to the site of **incompetent calf communicating veins**.

The network of small dilated venules that develops beneath the lateral and/or the medial malleolus of limbs with severe venous hypertension is called an **ankle flare** or a **corona phlebectactica**.

Distended veins crossing the groins and extending up over the abdominal wall are collateral veins and indicate the presence of a deep venous obstruction. Cross-pubic collateral veins may be visible if one iliac system is obstructed.

The skin of the lower medial third of the leg, the gaiter region, must be carefully inspected. Venous hypertension caused by venous outflow obstruction or severe reflux may cause an area of skin pigmentation, tenderness and subcutaneous induration, called **lipodermatosclerosis**, and eventually **eczema** and **ulceration**.

Palpation

The examiner's dominant hand should be gently run over the course of the main veins and their tributaries because dilated veins can sometimes be more easily felt than seen, especially in fat legs. Veins in the lower leg often lie in a gutter of indurated subcutaneous fat. Dilated long and short saphenous veins are usually easy to feel. The termination of a distended short saphenous vein is easier to feel if the patient is asked to bend the knees slightly to relax the deep fascia covering the popliteal fossa.

Carefully palpate the **sapheno-femoral junction** (2.5 cm below and lateral to the pubic tubercle) and the **sapheno-popliteal junction**, which has a variable termination in the popliteal fossa (high or low). The patient should be asked to cough while the dilated veins are palpated to see if there is any impulse or thrill (a cough impulse) indicating that the valves at their junctions with the deep veins are incompetent and the back flow is turbulent.

Palpate the skin of the calf to define any areas of induration and tenderness (lipodermatosclerosis). Palpate the medial side of the calf for deficits in the deep fascia which may be the sites of incompetent calf communicating (perforating) veins. (This is an unreliable technique, as large surface varicosities produce lacunae in the subcutaneous fat of the calf similar to the perforating vein deficits.)

Percussion The distended, dilated trunks of the long and short saphenous systems will always transmit a **percussion wave** in an orthograde direction whether the valves are competent or not. The more distended the vein, the better the wave is transmitted. If a percussion wave is transmitted retrogradely, i.e. downwards while the patient is standing, the valves must be incompetent.

Percussion can also be used to help define the terminations of the long and short saphenous veins by placing the fingers of one hand gently over the upper end of the dilated saphenous trunk and percussing the vein below it using the middle finger of the other hand to 'flick' the distended varicosities. The process can then be repeated in reverse, with the upper end of the vein being 'flicked' and the lower hand detecting a downward percussion wave, to check the competence of the valves.

Auscultation

Listen with your stethoscope over any large clusters of veins, especially if they remain distended when the patient lies down and the limb is elevated. A **machinery murmur** over such veins indicates that they are secondary to an arterio-venous fistula.

Tourniquet tests

Many clinicians have abandoned tourniquet tests as a means of assessing varicose veins in favour of more sophisticated investigations, but these tests are simple to perform and, if correctly carried out,

Leg horizontal, superficial veins empty

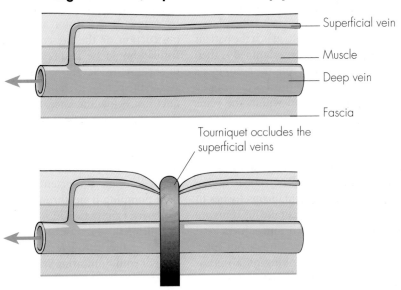

Superficial vein

Muscle

Deep vein

Fascia

Tourniquet occludes the
superficial veins

The patient stands up

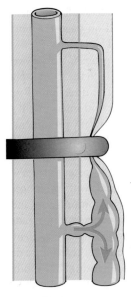

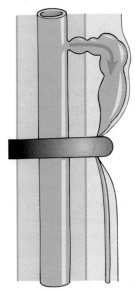

An incompetent communicating
vein below the tourniquet fills
the superficial veins below the
tourniquet

An incompetent communicating
vein above the tourniquet fills
the superficial veins above the
tourniquet

By moving the tourniquet up and down the leg it is possible to determine
the level of the incompetent communicating veins

FIG 7.13 The principles of the tourniquet test.

can provide useful information on the major sites of communicating vein incompetence.

The patient should lie on a couch which has a small foot stool attached to it, onto which the patient can rapidly stand. The limb to be examined is then elevated – often by placing it on the examiner's shoulder – to empty the veins, a process that can be expedited by stroking the blood within the veins towards the heart.

A tourniquet made from a long length of 1 cm diameter soft rubber tubing is then pulled tight around the upper thigh and held in place by strong artery forceps (Spencer Wells). The rubber tubing must press firmly into the subcutaneous tissues of the thigh to ensure that the subcutaneous veins are completely occluded. The Velcro tourniquets used by many house officers for venesection do not apply enough pressure, but the soft tubing on a stethoscope is an effective alternative if rubber tubing is not available, provided it is long enough. The patient is then asked to stand up quickly and the legs are observed for 10–15 seconds. If the saphenofemoral junction is the only site of superficial to deep valvular incompetence, the veins above the tourniquet will rapidly fill but those below it will remain collapsed. This can be confirmed by suddenly releasing the tourniquet and watching the veins below the site of the tourniquet rapidly distend from above, as blood regurgitates down the long saphenous vein. If the veins below the tourniquet fill immediately the patient stands up, there must be other sites of superficial to deep incompetence below the level of the tourniquet.

This test can be repeated with the tourniquet moved progressively down the whole length of the leg to try to define all the sites of superficial to deep vein incompetence, but it is easier and simpler to apply it once below the knee to exclude short saphenous incompetence.

Tourniquet tests are often difficult to interpret in patients with recurrent varicose veins, and the value of applying multiple tourniquets in an effort to locate the precise level of calf communicating veins has never been scientifically verified.

A modification of the tourniquet test is to empty the limb as described above and apply direct digital pressure over the upper end of the long saphenous vein while the patient stands up to see if this prevents retrograde filling. This is called the *Trendelenburg test*.

Venous hypertension caused by proximal vein obstruction or the presence of an arterio-venous fistula should be suspected if varicose veins fail to collapse on elevation. This can be confirmed by asking the patient to stand up after placing a tourniquet just below the knee, to cut off both long and short saphenous reflux, and then to stand repeatedly on tiptoe and relax. In a normal limb this exercise will empty the superficial veins by sucking the blood in the surface varicosities into the deep veins, through competent perforating veins, and then pumping it up through the popliteal vein to the heart. Failure to achieve superficial vein emptying during this exercise indicates deep vein obstruction or reflux through incompetent valves in the deep or communicating veins. This is called *Perthés' walking test*.

Doppler flow detector studies

The simple directional Doppler ultrasound flow probe described on page 178 can be used to assess venous reflux. The patient is asked to stand up and the ultrasound probe is placed over the termination of the long and then the short saphenous veins using coupling jelly. The direction of venous blood flow, augmented by rapid intermittent manual compression of the calf and any prominent varicosities in the lower limb, is then assessed. A **uniphasic signal** on squeezing, with no sound on releasing the compression, indicates competent valves with forward flow. A **biphasic signal**, with prolonged retrograde flow on releasing the compression, indicates reflux and valvular incompetence. Retrograde flow can also be confirmed by asking the patient to perform the Valsalva manouevre, i.e. taking a deep breath, pinching off the nose, closing the mouth and attempting a forced expiration. This causes venous flow to reverse if the valves are incompetent.

The Doppler ultrasound flow detector can also be used in association with the tourniquet test to demonstrate retrograde flow in the saphenous trunks when the tourniquet is released.

The simple hand-held Doppler flow detector cannot detect retrograde flow in either the deep or calf perforating veins with any accuracy. The detection of

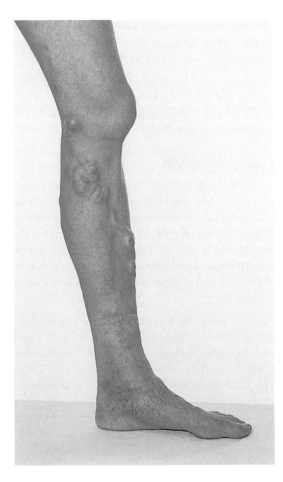

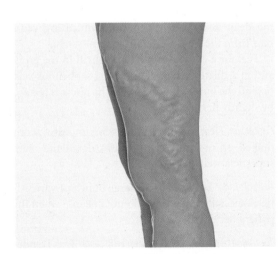

FIG 7.14 Varicose veins are, by definition, dilated and tortuous, and usually have incompetent valves. They occur on both the medial and lateral sides of the leg.

deep vein flow abnormalities requires more sophisticated Duplex scans.

Varicose veins

A varicose vein is a dilated, tortuous vein. The cause of 'primary' varicose veins is unknown, but the erect stance and abnormalities in the components and structure of the vein wall may be important factors.

'Secondary' varicose veins may be secondary to a proximal venous obstruction, destruction of the valves by thrombosis or an increase in flow and pressure caused by an arterio-venous fistula.

Varicosities do not cause symptoms, apart from unsightliness. Symptoms are caused the physiological malfunction that follows the valvular incompetence and retrograde flow.

Consequently, many patients have massive varicose veins but no symptoms, whilst others have severe symptoms with very few visible varicose veins. To add to the confusion, many patients with normal veins have symptoms similar to those caused by venous disease.

History

Age Varicose veins affect all age groups but are more common in older people. In children they are usually caused by a congenital vascular abnormality.

Sex Ten times more women than men attend hospital with venous complaints, but surveys in the community have shown there is little difference in the incidence of varicose veins between the sexes.

Ethnic groups Varicose veins are said to be less common in Africa and the Far East than in Europe and North America.

Occupation Many patients with symptomatic varicose veins have occupations that involve standing for prolonged periods. It is doubtful if standing, by itself, causes varicose veins, but it certainly exacerbates leg symptoms.

Symptoms Many patients with varicose veins have no symptoms. The **disfiguring effect** of the veins is often the principal complaint.

The next commonest complaint is **pain**. This is usually a dull ache felt in the calf and lower leg that gets worse throughout the day, especially when the patient is standing up for prolonged periods. It is relieved by lying down for 15 or 30 minutes or by wearing compression hosiery. The pain is often experienced in the dilated varicosities.

Night cramps and **itching** are common complaints.

Mild swelling of the ankle by the end of the day is common, but marked ankle oedema is not, and other causes of oedema should be eliminated before accepting that it is caused by the varicose veins. Some patients present with red, painful, tender lumps caused by **acute superficial thrombophlebitis** (see below).

Lipodermatosclerosis, **eczema** and **ulceration** are important complications which indicate the need for treatment. Always exclude conditions which may obstruct the iliac veins and cause secondary varicose veins, such as pregnancy and abdominal tumours.

Previous history Most patients with varicose veins have had them for years and many have had various forms of treatment such as operations and injections. It is important to exclude a previous deep vein thrombosis that may have accompanied previous illnesses, operations, accidents or pregnancies. All women should be asked if they had swelling of their legs or a deep vein thrombosis during pregnancy.

Family history It is common to find the patient's mother and sisters also have varicose veins. A definite family history is obtained in one-third to one-half of the patients who present with varicose veins.

Local examination

Inspection Look for large visible veins. Record their site, extent and size on large drawings of the front and back of the limbs. The skin of the leg should be inspected, especially the skin of the lower third of the medial side of the calf, for signs of chronic venous hypertension, lipodermatosclerosis, pigmentation, induration and inflammation as well as eczema and ulceration.

Palpation Assess the texture of the skin and subcutaneous tissue of the lower leg by palpation. There may be pitting oedema or thickening, redness and tenderness. These changes are caused by chronic venous hypertension and are known as **lipodermatosclerosis**, a term which indicates that there is a progressive replacement of the skin and subcutaneous fat by fibrous tissue, induration and an associated inflammation caused by the fibrin deposition which proceeds the fibrosis.

Palpation along the course of the veins just behind the medial border of the tibia may reveal defects in the deep fascia where the **communicating veins** pass from the superficial to the deep system.

Feel for a **cough impulse** and **thrill** in the groin and in a dilated trunk of the short saphenous vein behind the knee. This is easier if the fascia is relaxed by slightly flexing the knee.

Percussion Test whether a percussion impulse is conducted up or, more significantly, down the main superficial veins.

Auscultation Listen over any large bunch of varicosities, especially if the veins do not collapse when the patient lies down.

Tourniquet and Doppler flow detector tests The Trendelenburg and tourniquet tests must be carried out to detect the site of any incompetent superficial to deep communicating veins. Confirm the presence of reflux with the Doppler flow detector.

Revision panel 7.11
The causes of varicose veins in the lower limbs

Secondary
Obstruction to venous outflow by:
    pregnancy
    fibroids/ovarian cyst
    abdominal lymphadenopathy
    pelvic cancer (cervix, uterus, ovary, rectum)
    ascites
    iliac vein thrombosis
    retroperitoneal fibrosis
Valve destruction
    Deep vein thrombosis
High flow and pressure
    Arterio-venous fistula (especially the
    acquired traumatic variety)
Primary
Cause not known; often familial
Probably a weakness of the vein wall that permits valve ring dilatation
Very rarely, congenital absence of valves

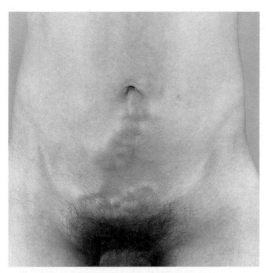

FIG 7.15 Dilated, tortuous collateral veins crossing the abdomen in a patient with an inferior vena cava thrombosis. The common cause of inferior vena cava obstruction is intra-abdominal malignant disease.

General examination

Because varicose veins are so common, it is tempting to omit a full general examination. Never do this. Always examine the abdomen and make sure the patient is not pregnant.

Inspection of the abdomen may reveal dilated **collateral veins** crossing to the other groin or up over the abdomen and chest to join the tributaries of the superior vena cava. The direction of flow in these veins is detected by placing two fingers on the veins, sliding one finger along the vein to empty it and then releasing the other finger and watching which way the empty segment fills (*Harvey's test*). This test may have to be repeated moving the fingers in either direction before the direction of blood flow can be confirmed.

A rectal or vaginal examination may be required to exclude a pelvic or abdominal cause for the varicose veins. In men it is important to feel the testes. Massive enlargement of the abdominal lymph glands by metastases from small testicular tumours can cause inferior vena cava obstruction.

Venous ulceration

Many patients with venous ulcers do not have visible varicose veins. Approximately 50 per cent of all venous ulcers are associated with primary varicose veins. The remainder are the result of post-thrombotic deep vein damage (see below).

History

Age Venous ulcers usually follow many years of venous disease, so the majority are seen in patients over the age of 40, many of whom have had recurrent ulceration for some years before seeking medical help. Post-thrombotic disease can cause ulceration in young adults, and ulcers can occur in children and teenagers with congenital venous malformations.

Sex Venous ulcers are more common in women than in men.

Symptoms Patients have often had aching pain, discomfort and tenderness of the skin (lipodermatosclerosis and pigmentation) for many months or years before an ulcer appears. Some ulcers are painful, but many are not. The discharge may be very smelly, leading to depression and social isolation. There is often an episode of trauma that initiates the breakdown of the skin, but sometimes itching and scratching may start an ulcer.

Previous history A majority of venous ulcers are caused by deep and communicating vein damage, so there is often a history of venous thrombosis during an illness or pregnancy. The patient may have had previous episodes of ulceration.

Cause The ulcer invariably begins after the skin of the leg has been knocked and damaged. Sometimes the initial incident is remembered, but often not.

Examination

Site Venous ulcers are commonly found around the gaiter area of the lower leg and usually begin on the medial aspect. Ulcers situated lower down on the foot or higher up on the fleshy part of the calf are rarely caused by venous disease.

Shape and size Venous ulcers can be of any shape and any size.

Edge The edge is gently sloping and, when healing begins, pale pink as new epithelium migrates across its surface.

Base This may be covered with yellow slough but becomes covered with pink granulation tissue when

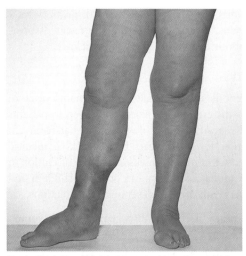

The 'gaiter' area. This photograph shows the medial aspect of the lower third of the leg narrowed and hardened by **venous lipodermatosclerosis**. This is the area in which most venous ulcers develop.

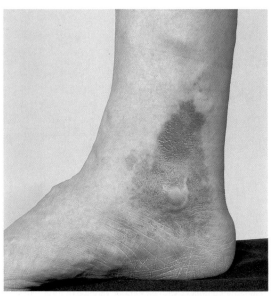

Chronic venous insufficiency causes *pigmentation* of the skin and dilated **intradermal venules**. The venules first appear in a triangular area over and below the medial malleolus, with the apex of the triangle over the first or second lower leg communicating vein. This is known as the **ankle-flare** or **corona phlebectatica**.

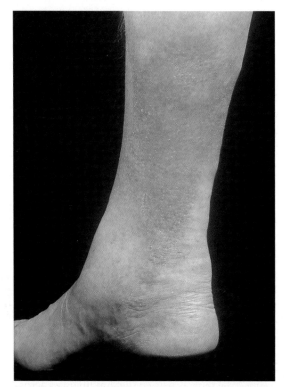

Acute lipodermatosclerosis usually begins on the medial side of the gaiter area and is painful, hot, red and tender. It is often misdiagnosed as cellulitis or acute thrombophlebitis.

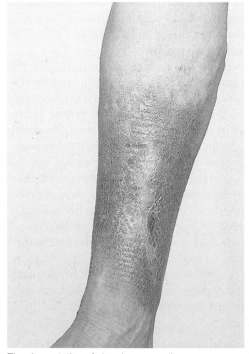

The pigmentation of chronic venous disease may cover the whole of the lower limb.

FIG 7.16 THE CUTANEOUS MANIFESTATIONS OF CHRONIC VENOUS INSUFFICIENCY.

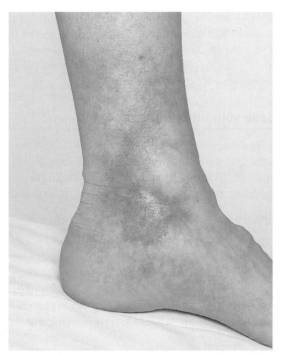

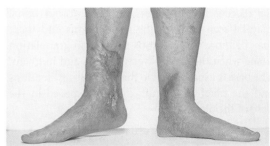

Subcutaneous fibrosis, following chronic lipodermatosclerosis, and/or painful ulceration may cause a **fixed flexion** of the ankle joint.

Atrophie blanche is the name given to white scars in the skin that appear without the skin ever having broken down or ulcerated.

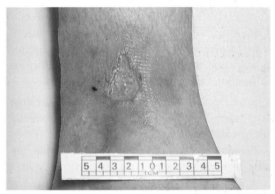

A chronic, recurrent, infected, enlarging venous ulcer. The base contains little healthy granulation tissue and many areas of avascular fibrous tissue.

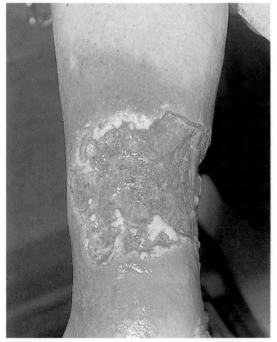

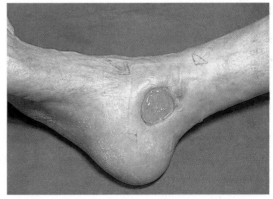

An acute venous ulcer. The surrounding lipodermatosclerosis is clearly visible. In the acute stages, when tissues are dying and sloughing, venous ulcers can be very painful.

A healing venous ulcer. The surrounding skin looks healthy, the granulation tissue in the base of the ulcer is clean and pink, and the edges of the ulcer are sloping and made of new epithelium.

FIG 7.16 continued

the ulcer is healing. Areas of white fibrous tissue may be seen between the granulations and there may be more white fibrous tissue than granulation tissue when the ulcer is very chronic and indolent. The base is usually fixed to the deep tissues. Tendons and the tibial periosteum may be exposed in the base of the ulcer.

Depth Venous ulcers are usually shallow and flat.

Discharge The discharge is usually seropurulent but can occasionally be blood stained.

Surrounding tissues The surrounding tissues usually show the signs of chronic venous hypertension – induration, inflammation, pigmentation and tenderness, i.e. lipodermatosclerosis. There may be old white scars (atrophie blanche) from previous ulceration and many dilated intradermal and subcutaneous veins. Movements of the ankle joint may be limited by scar tissue, which may cause an equinus deformity of the joint. Occasionally true cellulitis occurs.

Local lymph glands Ulcers are usually colonized rather than infected, so the inguinal lymph glands should not be enlarged or tender.

Remember that squamous cell carcinoma can arise in a chronic venous ulcer, particularly in a patient known to have a long-standing venous ulcer which has enlarged, become painful and malodorous, and especially if the edge of the ulcer is found to be raised or thickened. Malignant change is also suggested by finding enlarged inguinal lymph glands. Biopsy is indicated should any of these changes appear.

Malignant change in a chronic venous ulcer is known as a **Marjolin's ulcer** (see Chapter 3, page 94).

The lower limbs The whole of both lower limbs must be examined for the presence of varicose veins, competent and incompetent communicating veins and skin changes, as described above. Most patients have bilateral disease and the majority of patients with venous ulcers have incompetent communicating veins.

It is also important to assess the arterial circulation and the nerves, to exclude an ischaemic or neuropathic cause of the ulcer.

General examination

The abdomen should be examined to exclude an abdominal cause of venous insufficiency, and the other leg should be examined for signs of venous disease.

Look for any general features of the many other causes of skin ulceration such as ischaemia, rheumatoid arthritis, skin tumours, pyoderma gangrenosum, collagen diseases, anaemia, polycythaemia, neuropathic ulcers and sickle cell disease.

Deep vein thrombosis

Only a quarter of deep vein thromboses cause symptoms and signs. Many occur spontaneously, but in more than half there is a predisposing cause such as an operation, bed rest, thrombophilia, or recent air travel.

History

Patients complain of **pain** and **swelling** in the calf or the whole leg. The onset of symptoms is sudden and they are usually severe enough to make walking difficult. The first indication may be a pulmonary embolism, which causes symptoms such as **pleuritic pain**, **breathlessness**, **haemoptysis** and **collapse**.

Examination

Swelling of a leg, particularly if it is unilateral, is the most significant physical sign. The ankle may be the only site of swelling if the thrombosis is confined to the calf. Swelling of both ankles needs to be differentiated from other causes of oedema.

The swelling may extend up to the groin if the iliac vein is thrombosed.

The muscles that contain the thrombosed veins may become hard and tender. A change in texture of the muscle is more significant than tenderness because, although there are many conditions that make a muscle tender, there are few that make it stiff and hard.

Stretching the calf muscles by forced dorsiflexion is known as *Homan's sign*. This sign is a poor discriminator and should be abandoned.

The superficial veins may be dilated and the leg may feel hot. A large, swollen limb that is made pale by severe oedema is called **phlegmasia alba dolens**. When the venous thrombosis blocks almost all the main outflow veins, the skin of the leg becomes congested and blue. This is called **phlegmasia caerulea dolens**.

Venous gangrene can develop when there is very severe venous outflow obstruction. Venous gangrene usually affects the peripheral tissues (toe or fingers).

Chest signs If the patient has had a pulmonary embolus, the neck veins may be dilated and there may be central cyanosis and signs of right ventricular hypertrophy. A fixed-split second heart sound may be heard and there may be a pleural rub.

The post-thrombotic limb

The symptoms and signs that follow the damage caused by a deep vein thrombosis – obstruction and valvular incompetence – may appear months or years after the thrombosis. The initiating thrombosis may have passed unrecognized, but more often it produced clinical signs and required treatment. The earliest symptoms are usually a slowly progressive **swelling of the leg** that becomes **painful** as the day wears on. Initially the skin of the gaiter area becomes pigmented, but eventually it becomes a hard inflamed, indurated, pigmented plaque (lipodermatosclerosis). These changes may spread around the whole circumference of the gaiter area.

Varicose veins become more prominent and, if the thrombosis obstructs the venous outflow at the base of the limb, collateral veins may develop across the groins and the pubis, and the superficial veins will not empty when the patient is asked to carry out heel-raising on the spot with a mid-thigh tourniquet in place (*Perthes' test*).

A small group of patients develop true **venous claudication**. This is a severe calf and sometimes thigh pain caused by walking. It must be differentiated from intermittent claudication caused by arterial insufficiency. These patients usually have a swollen, tender limb, multiple varicose veins, collateral veins and lipodermatosclerosis, all indicating the likelihood of a previous deep vein thrombosis. The pain of venous claudication is usually accompanied by an increase of the swelling, and the pain fades very slowly.

Superficial thrombophlebitis

Deep vein thrombosis begins in normal veins, the vein wall becoming secondarily inflamed. In superficial thrombophlebitis, the inflammation of the vein wall is invariably the cause of the thrombosis.

The causes of superficial thrombophlebitis are given in Revision panel 7.12.

An occult carcinoma should be suspected when the episodes occur in the arms of patients over the age of 45 years, especially if they are transient and migrate. Thrombophlebitis migrans is, however, a rare condition.

History

Patients complain of the sudden appearance of a painful lump on their arm or leg. The pain usually subsides in 3–7 days, leaving a tender lump or subcutaneous cord which takes several weeks to disperse. There may be a preceding injury such as a venepuncture or, if the vein is varicose, a direct injury.

Examination

The swelling is in the subcutaneous tissues. It has an elongated, **cord-like shape** and may be several centimetres long, running along the long axis of the limb. The lump is tender. The overlying skin is at first red and inflamed before becoming pigmented and brown. Enlargement of the local lymph glands is rare and other tissues in the limb are normal, unless the condition is secondary to varicose veins.

The whole patient must be examined for an occult carcinoma, even if they have varicose veins.

Axillary vein thrombosis

Thrombosis of the axillary/subclavian vein may follow excessive use of the limb, especially above the head, or compression of the vein by musculoskeletal abnormalities such as a **cervical rib**.

Revision panel 7.12
The causes of superficial thrombophlebitis

Varicose veins
Occult carcinoma
  Bronchus
  Pancreas
  Stomach
  Lymphoma
Thromboangiitis obliterans (Buerger's disease)
Polycythaemia
Polyarteritis
Idiopathic
Iatrogenic
  Intravenous injection and injuries

History

The patient complains of a **sudden discomfort** and **swelling** of the arm. The arm, forearm and hand swell up, and there is discomfort on the medial side of the upper arm and in the axilla. The arm may feel hot and if it becomes very swollen, movements may become restricted. The patient may give a history of unusual activity in the preceding 24 hours, such as painting a ceiling.

Examination

The whole arm is swollen, congested and blue, and the surface veins usually distended. When the hand is raised above the level of the heart, the veins at the back of the hand do not collapse. The axillary vein may be palpable and tender. Distended cutaneous veins develop across the anterior chest wall and over the scapula to provide collateral drainage. The supra-clavicular fossa must be carefully palpated to exclude a causative mass such as a cervical rib, a subclavian aneurysm, or lymph glands enlarged by secondary malignant disease.

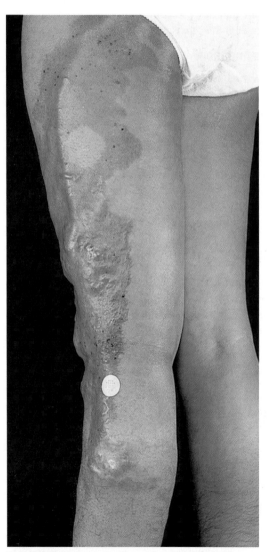

The dilated, anatomically abnormal varicose veins of a congenital venous deformity. There are also patches of port-wine staining.

FIG 7.17 CONGENITAL VARICOSE VEINS.

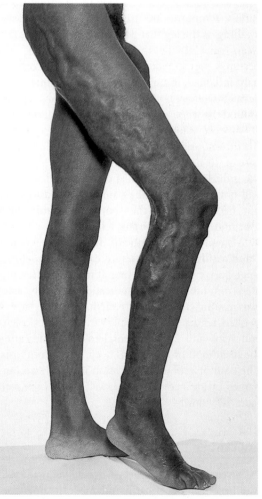

This patient had the abnormal dilated veins on the lateral side of the leg typical of the Klippel–Trenaunay syndrome, with marked overgrowth of the length and circumference of the leg.

Congenital vein abnormalities

Klippel–Trenaunay syndrome

This is a rare syndrome in which dilated veins develop early in life, often on the outer side of the leg, which is longer than the normal leg and covered in cutaneous angiomata (port-wine stains).

Venous angiomata

These are localized hamartomatous overgrowths of small to middle-sized veins. They mostly occur in the subcutaneous tissues and skin. They have a blue discolouration and become distended when dependent, collapse on elevation and are compressible.

THE LYMPHATICS

Primary abnormalities of the lymphatic vessels are rare. Disease in the lymph glands that interrupts the flow of lymph is common.

Lymphangitis

When bacterial infection spreads through the tissues, the bacteria get into the lymphatics and pass along in the lymph to the draining lymph glands. Inflamed lymphatics close to the skin are visible as thin, tender, red streaks on the skin. Lymphangitis is most often seen as a complication of infection starting in the hands or feet.

History

The patient complains of a throbbing pain at the site of the primary infection, tenderness along the red streaks and tenderness in the groin or axilla.

Examination

Inspection of the limb reveals the red, tender lymphatics. The overlying skin may be slightly oedematous. The axillary or inguinal lymph glands are usually swollen and tender.

The site of the primary infection is often not obvious. It may be a small crack between the toes or alongside a finger nail.

If a lymph gland in an oedematous limb with poor lymphatic drainage becomes infected, the infection quickly spreads throughout the oedematous tissues – **cellulitis**.

Lymphoedema

Lymphoedema is the accumulation of lymph in the interstitial spaces as a consequence of defective lymphatic drainage. The oedema fluid is rich in protein, in contrast to the oedema of heart and kidney failure, which has a low protein content.

The causes of lymphoedema are given in Revision panel 7.13.

The commonest cause of lymphoedema is secondary disease in the lymph glands. Primary lymphoedema is only diagnosed when all the causes of secondary lymphoedema have been eliminated, or there is a clear family history of the condition.

History

Age Primary lymphoedema may present at birth, in young adults or, much less often, in middle age. Secondary lymphoedema presents in middle and old age and is common after treatment for cancers.

Revision panel 7.13
The causes of lymphoedema

Primary
    Congenital genetic disorders causing dilatation, incompetence, aplasia or obliteration of the lymphatics

Secondary
    Neoplastic infiltration of lymph glands by:
        secondary carcinoma
        lymphomas (Hodgkin's/non-Hodgkin's)

Infection
    Filariasis
    Lymphogranuloma inguinale
    Tuberculosis
    Recurrent non-specific infection

Iatrogenic
    Surgical excision of lymph glands
    Irradiation of lymph glands

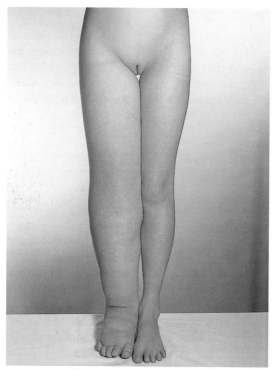

Lymphoedema of the right leg.

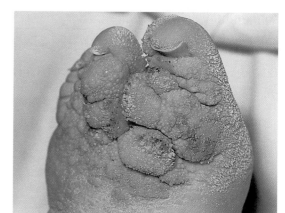

Severe long-standing lymphoedema. The skin is thickened and hyperkeratotic.

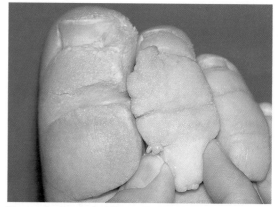

Stemmer's sign. An inability to pinch the skin together on the dorsum of the toes.

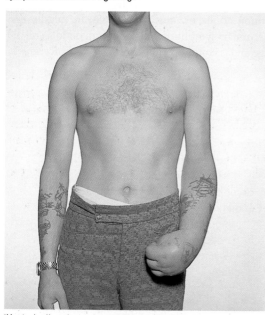

'Hysterical' oedema. Immobility and dependency, in this case caused by a 'hysterical' paralysis, can cause severe oedema. This is not a true lymphoedema, but a gravitational oedema. The limb is often bluish in colour because of the concomitant venous congestion – hence the name **hysterical oedeme blue**.

FIG 7.18 LYMPHOEDEMA.

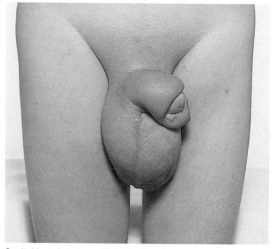

Genital lymphoedema. This usually affects the penis and scrotum but may be confined to the scrotum. In about 50 per cent of patients there is also mild lymphoedema of the legs.

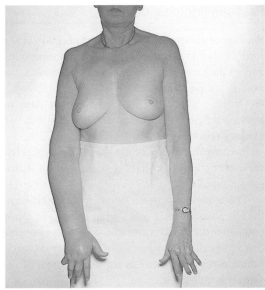

Secondary lymphoedema. This patient's right arm lymphoedema was caused by infiltration of the axillary lymph glands by metastases from a carcinoma in the right breast. Some carcinomata of the breast present in this way.

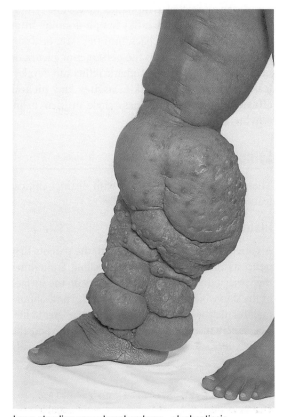

Long-standing gross lymphoedema– elephantiasis.

FIG 7.18 continued

Family history Many forms of primary lymphoedema are familial, and abnormal genes have now been discovered in several of them.

Sex Females are affected three times more often than males. Even secondary lymphoedema is more common in women, because tumours of the uterus and ovary metastasize to the iliac lymph glands, and carcinoma of the breast spreads to the axillary lymph glands.

Geography Filariasis – infestation with the parasite *Wuchereria bancrofti*, which is found in tropical and sub-tropical countries – is a common cause of lymphoedema (**elephantiasis**).

Symptoms The patient notices a slowly progressive swelling of the limb or genitalia. Primary lymphoedema most often affects the lower limb, often beginning after a sprained ankle or another form of trivial injury. The swelling takes many years to develop and is often bilateral.

In contrast, the swelling of secondary lymphoedema may appear in a few weeks and may progress rapidly.

The swelling is not painful There is no discomfort in the swollen limb apart from that caused by the increased weight, which may produce a mechanical disability.

Patients with lymphoedema often develop severe episodes of **acute cellulites**, which may be accompanied by septicaemia. Acute cellulitis is often preceded by a prodromal period of sweating, rigors and malaise, which is then followed by the development of pain, tenderness, redness and swelling in the limb. The infection often gets in through cracks between the toes caused by athlete's foot (Tinea pedis). Vesicles may appear on the skin and leak a clear, colourless fluid.

Examination

The swollen limb

Lymphoedema has no special characteristics. It is often said that lymphoedema does not pit – this is incorrect. All oedema pits. The longer the lymphoedema has been present, the denser the accompanying fibrosis and the firmer and more 'doughy' the oedema; nevertheless, lymphoedema always pits if you press hard enough and long enough.

Lymphoedema of the lower limb affects the toes much more often than other forms of oedema. If it has been present for years, the toes are squashed together and become **square** in cross-section. This hardly ever occurs with other types of oedema. *Stemmer's sign* is an inability to pinch the skin together on the dorsal surface of the second toe. This indicates the presence of lymphoedema and is a consequence of secondary thickening and hyperkeratosis of the skin. Sometimes thick scales grow outwards, looking like warts.

Lymphoedema is usually diagnosed when other general causes of oedema (cardiac, renal, hypoproteinaemia) and other local causes (venous obstruction, multiple arterio-venous fistulae, local gigantism and excessive fat deposition – lipodystrophy) have been excluded. It is therefore essential to examine the whole patient once the presence of oedema has been confirmed, especially the heart, the abdomen and the veins of the limb.

The lymph glands

The lymph glands are often slightly thickened and enlarged in patients with primary lymphoedema. They will almost certainly be enlarged and hard if they are infiltrated with primary or secondary tumour.

All the areas that drain to any palpable glands must be carefully examined.

General examination

A full examination of the patient must be carried out to look for any possible causes for secondary lymphoedema.

Revision panel 7.14
The causes of lymphadenopathy

Infection
 Non-specific
 Glandular fever
 Tuberculosis
 Toxoplasmosis
 Syphilis
 Cat-scratch fever (*Rochalimaea henselae*)
 Filariasis
 Lymphogranuloma (inguinale)
Metastatic tumour
Primary reticuloses
Sarcoidosis

Post-mastectomy oedema

Swelling of the arm is a common complication of any form of mastectomy or combination of lumpectomy and radiotherapy which damages or removes the axillary lymph glands.

Oedema which develops in the first days or weeks after the initial treatment is likely to be an **axillary vein thrombosis**.

Swelling after this time may be caused by scar tissue constricting the axillary vein, especially if it progresses rapidly.

Though lymphoedema caused by obliteration of the lymphatics can appear within months or many years after the initial treatment, it is always possible that late swelling may be caused by **recurrent carcinoma**, especially if there is any enlargement of the axillary lymph glands.

Lymphatic reflux

A relatively small number of patients have dilated ecstatic incompetent lymphatics that allow lymph and chyle (which is the milky lymph draining from the intestine) to reflux back into the skin, or drain into large cavities such as the peritoneum, pleura or intestine. Patients with lymphatic reflux can develop **leaky vesicles** on their skin, **ascites** and **pleural effusions** and may even pass chyle in their urine (**chyluria**).

Lymphangiomata

These are rare malformations with distinct clinical features that are easy to recognize.

History

A patient or, in the case of a child, the parents first notice a small soft subcutaneous swelling. Sometimes there may be associated **small vesicles** on the surface of the skin which may weep clear fluid. These abnormalities may be present at birth or appear later in life. The subcutaneous swellings slowly enlarge and the vesicles increase in number, but neither are usually painful.

Examination

The skin over the subcutaneous cysts usually contain many small vesicles. Lymphangiomata tend to occur at the junction of the leg, arm or neck with the trunk.

The subcutaneous swellings cannot be compressed or emptied. They are often indistinct and multiple. They fluctuate and transilluminate if they are of a reasonable size, and have the same signs as a cystic hygroma (see Chapter 11, page 281).

Lymphadenopathy is described in the chapter on the neck (Chapter 11), but as lymphoedema is so often secondary to lymph gland disease, you should refresh your knowledge of the causes of lymph gland enlargement (see Revision panel 7.14).

8

General and facial appearance

(Scalp, head, eyes, nose, ears and chest wall)

COLOUR

One of the first things that one notices about a patient is the colour of their skin: not their racial colour, though it is important to record their racial origin, but changes from what you would expect to be their normal colour. Although minor colour variations are easier to appreciate in white-skinned people, they are also visible in dark-skinned races.

The skin may be pale or tinged blue, yellow or brown.

Pallor

Normal skin colour varies according to the thickness of the skin, the state of the skin circulation and the degree and type of pigmentation. If the skin thickness and circulation appear to be normal, pallor of the skin usually indicates anaemia. Anaemia is best detected by looking at the colour of the mucous membranes.

- Look at the colour of the conjunctiva on the inner side of the lower eyelid.
- Look at the colour of the buccal mucous membrane.
- Stretch the skin of the palm and look at the colour of the palmar creases.

Cyanosis

Cyanosis is the purple-blue colour given to the skin by de-oxygenated blood. It is most apparent in areas with thin skin but a rich blood supply, such as the lips, tongue, finger nails and ear lobes. Cyanosis is difficult to see in black skin and when the patient is anaemic.

The causes of cyanosis can be divided into two categories: central, when the defect lies in the cardiopulmonary circulation, and peripheral, when there is excessive de-oxygenation in the tissues, usually because of inadequate tissue perfusion.

If the cyanosis is caused by a central abnormality, it will be generalized and the patient's extremities are likely to be warm.

If the cyanosis is caused by a peripheral abnormality, the extremities will be blue and cold, but central organs such as the tongue will be pink.

Polycythaemia

An excess of circulating red blood cells gives the patient a purple-red, florid appearance. This may be mistaken for cyanosis. It differs from cyanosis in that it heightens the colour of all the skin, especially the cheeks, neck and backs of hands and feet. The discolouration of cyanosis is usually limited to the tips of the hands, feet and nose.

Jaundice

Jaundice is a yellow discolouration of the skin, caused by an excess of bile pigments in the plasma.

The yellow colour is first visible against the white background of the sclera, but as the jaundice increases, the whole skin turns yellow.

The colour changes with the depth of the jaundice. White skin first turns a pale lemon yellow. As it deepens, it becomes yellow-orange, sometimes almost brown, and in those rare conditions in which severe jaundice may exist for many years, such as biliary cirrhosis, the skin eventually turns a yellow-grey-green colour.

It is not possible to diagnose the cause of jaundice from its presence. The most useful diagnostic features are the sequence of events preceding its onset and the presence or absence of pain.

Jaundice can be caused by excessive haemolysis – pre-hepatic jaundice; by liver malfunction – hepatic jaundice; or by obstruction of the bile ducts – post-hepatic jaundice.

The common causes of these three types of jaundice are:

- **pre-hepatic** jaundice – haemolytic anaemia,
- **hepatic** jaundice – infectious hepatitis,
- **post-hepatic** jaundice – gallstones and carcinoma of the pancreas.

Figure 8.1 describes the principal premonitory symptoms, pain and fluctuations of jaundice that accompany the common diseases that cause jaundice.

Brown pigmentation

An increase in the natural brown pigmentation of the skin can be generalized or localized.

Causes of generalized pigmentation

- Addison's disease is the important cause of increased pigmentation to remember, because if it is not diagnosed and treated, it can cause sudden death. The brown pigmentation of Addison's disease is visible in the buccal mucous membrane.
- Arsenic and silver poisoning.
- Haemochromatosis.
- Gaucher's disease.

Causes of localized pigmentation

- Pregnancy: round the areolae and along the mid-line of the abdomen.
- Chronic venous hypertension: lower medial third of the lower leg.
- Erythema ab igne: frequently seen on parts of the legs exposed to heat.
- Ultraviolet and high-voltage irradiation.
- Café au lait patch: associated with neurofibromatosis.
- Various forms of melanoma.
- Pellagra: nicotinic acid deficiency.
- Rheumatoid arthritis.
- Acanthosis nigricans.

Vitiligo

Vitiligo is the name given to white, de-pigmented areas of skin. It commonly occurs without a generalized cause, but it can be secondary to leprosy, scleroderma, syphilis, and some organ-specific autoimmune diseases such as Hashimoto's thyroiditis, Addison's disease, pernicious anaemia and diabetes.

Excoriation/pruritus

This is itching of the skin caused by a local or general abnormality. The presence of multiple scratches on the skin is usually very obvious and noticed during your initial inspection. Itching of the skin is caused by:

- **skin diseases:**
  urticaria
  eczema
  (psoriasis does not usually cause itching)
- **local irritation:**
  clothing/washing powder
  parasites – fleas, scabies
  discharges – vaginal and rectal
- **occult disease:**
  subclinical jaundice with bile salt retention
  Hodgkin's disease
  leukaemia
  uraemia
  food sensitivity
  polycythaemia
  thyrotoxicosis.

If a skin disease or local irritation is the initiating stimulus, the cause of the pruritis and excoriation is usually obvious on inspection, so the causes to remember are the occult diseases. Any patient presenting with an itching, but otherwise normal, skin should be suspected of having subclinical jaundice, Hodgkin's disease or uraemia until you prove otherwise.

Revision panel 8.1
Causes of a generalized increased skin pigmentation

Sunlight
Pregnancy
Addison's disease
Renal failure
Haemochromatosis
Drugs (e.g. busulphan)

THE DISTINGUISHING FEATURES OF THE FOUR COMMON DISEASES THAT CAUSE JAUNDICE

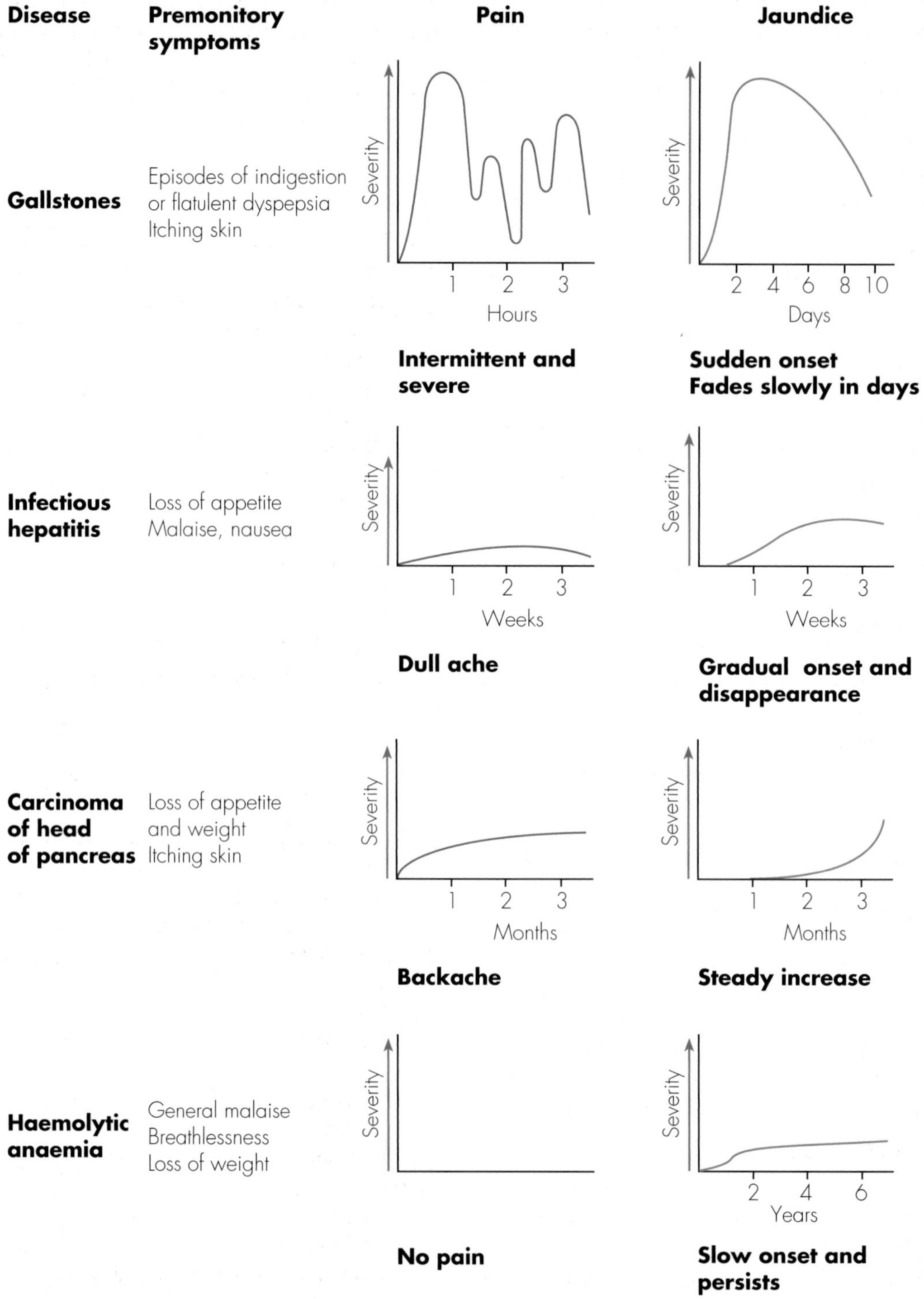
Disease
Premonitory symptoms
Pain
Jaundice
Gallstones
Episodes of indigestion or flatulent dyspepsia
Itching skin
Severity
1 2 3
Hours
Intermittent and severe
Severity
2 4 6 8 10
Days
Sudden onset
Fades slowly in days
Infectious hepatitis
Loss of appetite
Malaise, nausea
Severity
1 2 3
Weeks
Dull ache
Severity
1 2 3
Weeks
Gradual onset and disappearance
Carcinoma of head of pancreas
Loss of appetite and weight
Itching skin
Severity
1 2 3
Months
Backache
Severity
1 2 3
Months
Steady increase
Haemolytic anaemia
General malaise
Breathlessness
Loss of weight
Severity
No pain
Severity
2 4 6
Years
Slow onset and persists

FIG 8.1

GENERAL APPEARANCE

When you look at a patient's size, shape and physical characteristics you will subconsciously put them into one of four categories: their body will look normal, wasted, overweight, or have some skeletal or sexual characteristics that look out of proportion.

The following sections describe the principal conditions that cause these three changes in body build.

Wasting

There are many causes of wasting. Almost all serious diseases cause some loss of appetite and weight, so only the common conditions are listed in Revision panel 8.3.

Severe wasting of the upper half of the body with oedema of the lower half is a common physical appearance in the elderly and is usually caused by advanced carcinoma which has either destroyed the liver and so caused hypoproteinaemia or formed large intra-abdominal masses which have obstructed the vena cava or iliac veins.

The degree of wasting is apparent from the way in which the skeleton, particularly the shoulder girdle, and the folds of loose skin on the arms, trunk and buttocks become visible.

This clinical picture can also be caused by the combination of two diseases: a disease which causes wasting, such as carcinoma, and congestive heart failure. Although you should always try to make one diagnosis, many elderly people have more than one disease.

Overweight

Patients with normal skeletal and sexual proportions but whose bodies are bigger than they should be are most likely to be obese from overeating, but three serious pathological conditions cause an increase in weight that can easily be mistaken for obesity: water retention, myxoedema and Cushing's syndrome.

Water retention

Nephrosis and other causes of water retention (renal, cardiac or hepatic) cause an increase in weight. The whole body swells but the swelling is most noticeable in the dependent parts. These patients have oedema of the legs, or the sacral region if they have been confined to bed, but also in the loose tissues of the face, especially in the skin below the eyes. The swelling around the eyes is often the first symptom and is present when the patient wakes up. Cardiac oedema is also most apparent in the dependent parts and similarly tends to disperse to other areas (not resolve) at night in response to the change of body position.

Revision panel 8.2
The common causes of itching

General
  Cholestasis (subclinical jaundice)
  Hodgkin's disease
  Lymphoma
  Renal failure (uraemia)
  Food sensitivities
  Iron deficiency
  Polycythaemia
Skin disease
  Infestations (e.g. scabies)
  Insect bites
  Eczema
  Urticaria
  Prickly heat
  Clothing/washing powder sensitivities

Revision panel 8.3
The common causes of wasting

In children
  Severe gastroenteritis
  Malabsorption syndromes
In young adults
  Tuberculosis
  Reticuloses
  Anorexia nervosa
In middle age
  Diabetes
  Thyrotoxicosis
  Carcinoma
In old age
  Carcinoma
  Senility
  Gross cardiorespiratory disease
All age groups
  Starvation

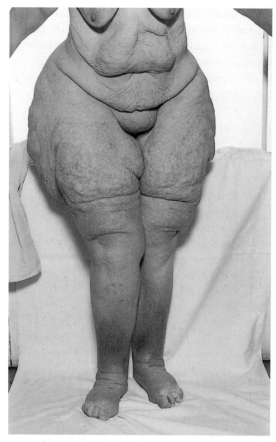

FIG 8.2 Gross obesity usually affects the whole body, but may, as in this patient, be predominantly confined to the buttocks and thighs.

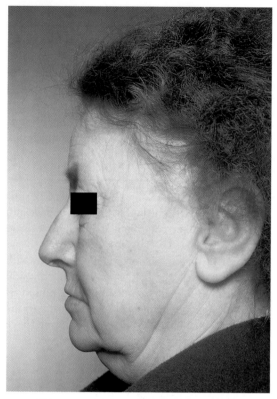

FIG 8.3 This woman has myxoedema. There is some loss of hair, especially the outer third of the eyebrows, heaviness of the face and creamy skin, but none of these features is diagnostic. This photograph is included to emphasize that early myxoedema is extremely difficult to recognize (see also Fig. 11.39, page 302).

Myxoedema

Myxoedema, which is caused by a deficiency of thyroid hormone, causes a puffy face, a generalized, non-pitting increase in the subcutaneous tissues of the trunk and limbs, a 'peaches and cream' complexion and a dulling of thought, speech and action (see pages 301–3).

Cushing's syndrome

Cushing's syndrome is caused by an excess of adrenal glucocorticoids. One in four patients with Cushing's syndrome has an adrenal adenoma; the remainder have a pituitary abnormality, either an adenoma or excess hypothalamic stimulation.

The patient puts on weight, particularly on the face, neck and trunk. The arms and legs stay thin. The face becomes 'moon-shaped' and the rounded, thickened shoulders are often described as a 'buffalo hump'.

There is excess of lanugo hair, an increase in skin pigmentation and red (fresh) striae in the skin that has been stretched, particularly the skin of the abdomen. Hypertension is common.

Revision panel 8.4
The common causes of an increase in weight

Obesity
Pregnancy
Interstitial fluid retention (renal, cardiac or hepatic failure)
Localized fluid retention (massive ovarian cysts, ascites)
Myxoedema
Cushing's syndrome

Skeletal or sexual disproportion

There are a variety of skeletal abnormalities and a few rare disorders of general body development usually associated with chromosomal abnormalities that will be apparent from your initial general inspection.

Paget's disease of bone
(Osteitis deformans, see page 119)

This is a disease in which normal bone is absorbed and replaced by primitive vascular (osteoid) bone. This makes the bones thick but soft.

The skull enlarges. The bones of the vault bulge outwards above the eyes and ears so much that the patient may complain that they have had to buy a larger hat.

The spine bends into a marked kyphosis which reduces the patient's height and may make respiration difficult. The bending of the spine makes the arms look longer.

The long bones of the limbs become thicker and curve forwards and outwards.

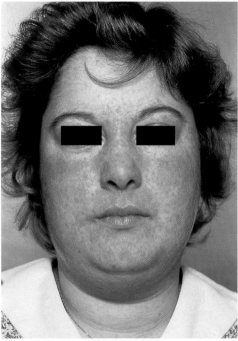

A round 'moon' face, some early hypertrichosis and an unusually florid acneiform rash.

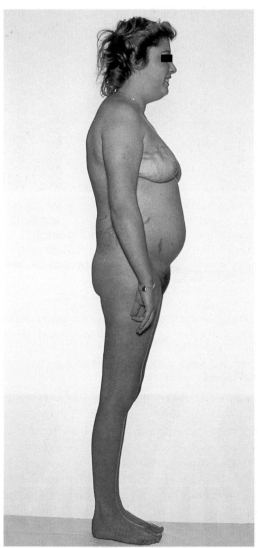

An increase of fat on the trunk and shoulders but thin arms and legs. Red striae on the abdomen and breasts.

FIG 8.4 CUSHING'S SYNDROME.

Revision panel 8.5
The common causes of hair loss

Local
    Male balding
    Alopecia areata
    Skin infections
General
    Hypothyroidism
    Cytotoxic drugs
    Hypopituitarism
    Iron deficiency
    Severe illness

Acromegaly

The deformities of acromegaly are caused by the stimulation of growth after normal growth has ceased. The primary abnormality is a pituitary acidophil adenoma secreting too much growth hormone.

The patient has a large face and large hands. There is overgrowth of the soft tissues of the face, nose, lips and tongue and of the facial air sinuses and jaw. The enlargement of the hands is caused by overgrowth of the small bones of the fingers, particularly the distal phalanges.

Giant (tall) acromegalics usually have a kyphosis which makes the arms look longer than they really are, but many acromegalics are not tall or kyphotic. Their joints are often enlarged by exuberant osteoarthritis.

The big nose, protuberant jaw and large hands have been compared to the facies of Punch of 'Punch and Judy'.

The skin is greasy, not dry, and there is no loss of mental faculties. These two features help distinguish early acromegaly from myxoedema.

Marfan's syndrome

Although this is a rare syndrome, you must know of its existence because of the blindness, caused by lens dislocation, and the vascular catastrophes, such as dissecting aneurysm and aortic incompetence, that often accompany it. It is caused by an abnormality of the mucopolysaccharides that form the ground substance of intercellular cement.

Patients with Marfan's syndrome are tall and thin, with very long fingers and toes (arachnodactyly) and a high arched palate.

When this syndrome causes only minor skeletal changes it is difficult to recognize.

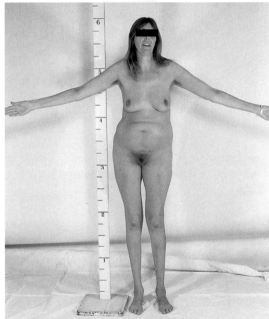

Tall, slim, with a high-arched palate, long arms, and long spindly fingers.

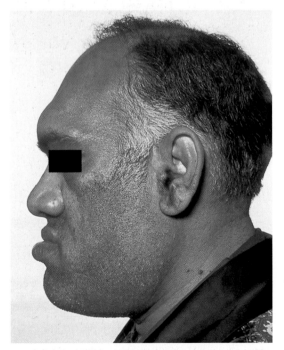

FIG 8.5 Acromegaly. A heavy head with a prominent nose, chin and lips. These patients also have long arms and large hands and feet.

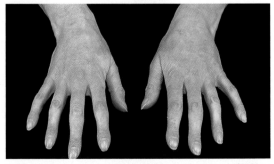

The long, spindly fingers of a patient with Marfan's syndrome.

FIG 8.6 MARFAN'S SYNDROME.

Klinefelter's syndrome

Klinefelter's syndrome is a congenital abnormality in which a male has an extra female (X) chromosome. Thus, instead of being a normal XY male, he is XXY, and testosterone production is subnormal.

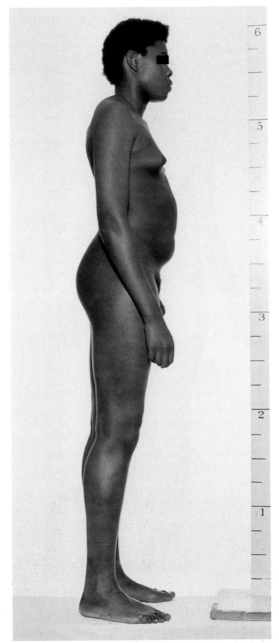

A tall male with a female body shape, a female distribution of body fat and hair, and atrophic testes.

FIG 8.7 KLINEFELTER'S SYNDROME.

The patients are tall, with a female distribution of fat around the breast and pelvis, but normal male hair growth on the face and pubis.

The testes are very small and soft and do not produce spermatozoa, so the patients are sterile.

Turner's syndrome

Turner's syndrome is a congenital abnormality in which a female has only one female (X) chromosome. Thus, instead of being a normal XX female, she is XO.

There are no skeletal abnormalities, but the patient has a masculine shape – wide shoulders and narrow pelvis – and is invariably shorter than average for a woman.

The most distinctive feature, when present, is 'webbing' of the shoulders. This is a thickening of the neck and a prominence of the skin folds that run from the neck to the shoulders.

The breasts and pubic hair are usually underdeveloped.

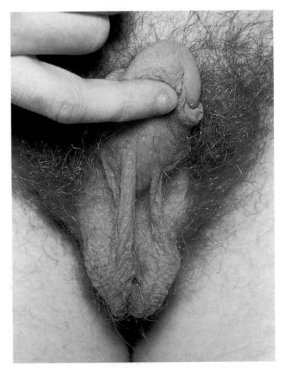

The small, underdeveloped scrotum, containing atrophic testes, of a patient with Klinefelter's syndrome.

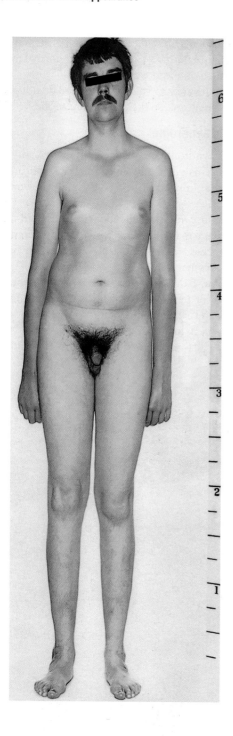

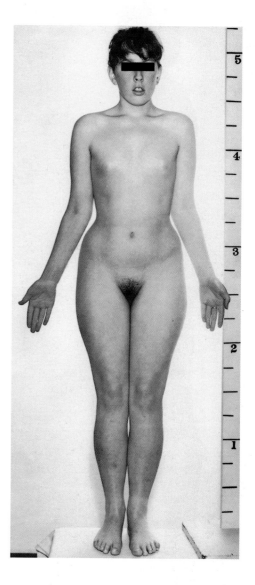

FIG 8.8 A comparison between the body build of a young man with Klinefelter's syndrome – a tall male with a female distribution of body fat – and a young woman with Turner's syndrome – a short female with a masculine shape and amenorrhoea. The 'webbing' of the shoulders is not very pronounced in the female patient.

Dwarfism

There is a multitude of causes of dwarfism, many of which are obscure endocrine abnormalities. The common causes are as follows.

- **Rickets**. Bowed long bones. Scoliosis. Prominent costochondral junctions ('rickety rosary'). Transverse groove across rib cage at attachment of diaphragm (Harrison's sulcus).
- **Achondroplasia** (the circus dwarf). Large head. Flattened bridge of nose. Stunted trunk, hands and fingers. Waddling gait. Umbilicus below the mid-point of vertical height.
- **Renal dwarfism**.

- **Cretinism**.
- **Pituitary deficiency**.

Signs and stigmata of congenital syphilis

This is now a rare condition.

In infants

Signs of congenital syphilis rarely appear before 7 years of age. Any symptoms that do occur are usually similar to the symptoms of the secondary stage of acquired syphilis: snuffles, condylomata around the mouth and anus, and a ham-coloured, symmetrical, transient rash.

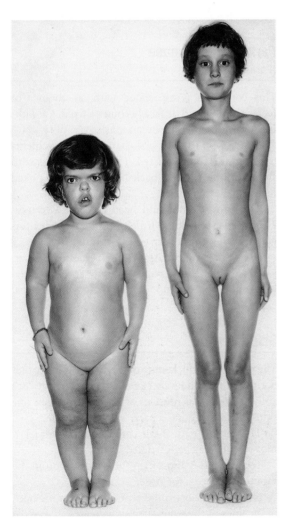 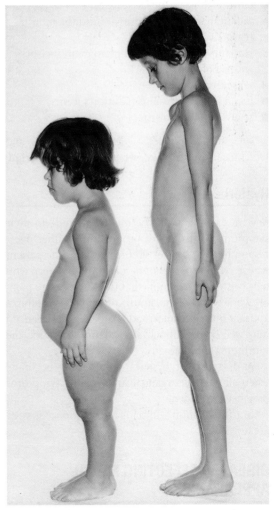

FIG 8.9 An achondroplastic child standing beside a normal child of the same age. The facial and skeletal abnormalities are all obvious. Note that the umbilicus of the achondroplastic child is below the mid-point of the vertical height.

In children and young adults

Congenital syphilis causes:

- interstitial keratitis
- deafness
- periostitis (sabre tibia)
- synovitis (Clutton's joints).

These conditions leave permanent defects, aptly described as making the patient blind, deaf and lame.

The stigmata of the infection remain with the patient for the rest of their life. They are:

- remnants of interstitial keratitis (loss of vision)
- nerve deafness
- depressed bridge of nose (saddle nose)
- perforated palate or nasal septum
- radiating scars and creases around the mouth (rhagades)
- Hutchinson's teeth (small permanent incisors with a notched border)
- sabre tibiae
- painless joint effusions (Clutton's joints)
- retardation of growth.

Interstitial keratitis, nerve deafness and Hutchinson's teeth are known as **Hutchinson's triad**.

Hysteria

Beware of patients whose mental attitude to their symptoms seems out of proportion – either over-responding to them or ignoring them. The patient whose symptoms do not fit any known pattern who tells you with a big smile that they have severe pain, or who, while complaining of severe symptoms, appears quite unconcerned ('la belle indifference') may well be neurotic, hysterical, or fabricating the symptoms and the signs.

A diagnosis of hysteria should only be made when all possible organic causes for the symptoms have been excluded.

In this situation your clinical experience is your greatest help.

DISEASES AFFECTING FACIAL APPEARANCE

The appearance of the face has a major effect on the patient's general appearance. Those general conditions that affect the face have already been described. This section deals with diseases that particularly affect facial expression and appearance.

Bell's palsy

Bell's palsy is a paralysis of the facial nerve affecting the muscles of facial expression.

The absence of tone in the facial muscles makes the affected side of the face look smooth and sloppy. The corner of the mouth droops, the nasolabial creases become asymmetrical and less noticeable, and the lower eyelid droops. The asymmetry of the mouth can be increased by asking the patient to bare their teeth. If they are asked to shut their eyes, you will see that the lids fail to close on the affected side.

Parkinson's disease
(Paralysis agitans)

This condition is associated with an absence of facial expression. The face becomes a fixed, unblinking mask – the Parkinsonian mask.

In addition to the facial changes, all movements become stiff and restricted. The patient walks with short, shuffling steps, back bent, and head poked forwards.

The hands, limbs and head develop a tremor. The repetitive shaking of the thumb and index finger gives the appearance of 'pill-rolling'.

In its florid state, Parkinson's disease presents an unmistakable clinical picture, but it can be detected long before this if you look out for the loss of facial expression.

Scleroderma

The progressive thickening of the skin of the face that occurs with scleroderma can also reduce the patient's ability to use their muscles of facial expression. The skin thickens and has a pale, waxy appearance.

The mouth gets small (**microstomia**) and jaw movements may be restricted.

Telangiectases appear on the cheeks, around the mouth and across the nose.

Fine, white, horizontal scars appear on the neck in the lines of the transverse skin creases.

When the patient smiles and laughs the face does not respond fully. This is different from Parkinson's

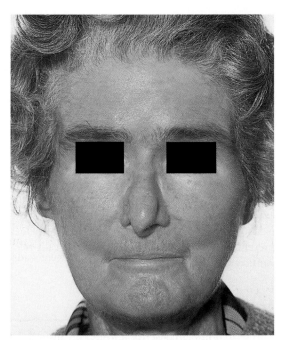

Note the tight skin, small mouth, fine wrinkles around the mouth and small telangiectases.

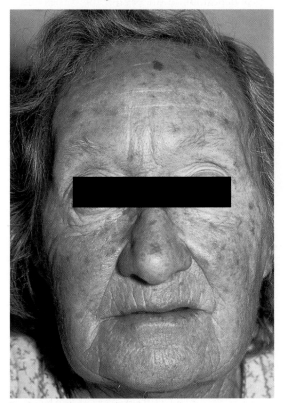

The telangiectases of scleroderma.

FIG 8.10 SCLERODERMA.

disease, in which there is not a flicker of facial expression even though the tissues of the face are obviously normal.

Myasthenia gravis

Remember that myasthenia gravis causes weakness of all muscles but particularly the muscles of the eyelids. Suspect it in any patient who complains of tired, drooping eyelids or weakness of the face and jaw.

The weakness is transitory; power and movement return if the muscles are allowed to rest.

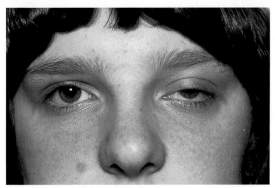

FIG 8.11 Myasthenia gravis: heavy, drooping eyelids, much worse on the patient's left side. The eye signs of generalized diseases are often asymmetrical, even unilateral.

Cretinism

A cretin is a child deficient in thyroid hormone. It is a condition that should only be seen in neonates because it should be recognized soon after birth and cured by giving the child thyroid hormone.

In an advanced case, the face is broad and flat, the eyes are wide apart and the tongue protrudes from the mouth.

If the condition is not treated, growth is slowed, so that the child is short, fat and mentally retarded.

Down's syndrome

Down's syndrome is a congenital abnormality usually associated with an extra chromosome 21.

Males and females and all races are equally affected. The prime abnormalities are mental retardation, floppiness and a short stature. The old name (mongolism) describes the dominant facial features: the outer ends of the palpebral fissures slant upwards and there are prominent epicanthic folds. The face is flattened, and the tongue protrudes.

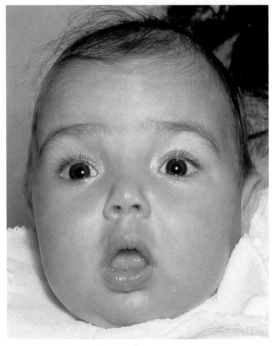

FIG 8.12 Congenital hypothyroidism (cretinism). The head is broad, the eyes wide apart, the tongue protrudes from the mouth and all movements and responses are slow and sluggish.

Affected children often have a squint and one-third have congenital heart disease.

The Down's baby is distinguishable from the cretin because their skin and hair are smooth and fine, not coarse and thick, and though they are more floppy than a normal baby, they are not slow and sluggish like a cretin.

THE EYES

This book cannot discuss the many diseases of the eye that affect facial appearance, some of which are part of generalized medical conditions, but does present a few easily recognizable and surgically relevant conditions.

Arcus senilis

This term is used to describe a white rim around the outer edge of the iris. It is a rim of sclerosis and cholesterol deposition in the edge of the cornea and is common in the elderly.

It has no great clinical significance, except in patients below the age of 40, when it may be associated with hyperlipoproteinaemia. It is not associated with generalized degenerative arterial disease, although both conditions often coexist.

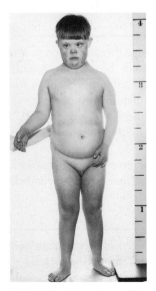
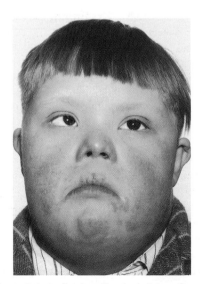
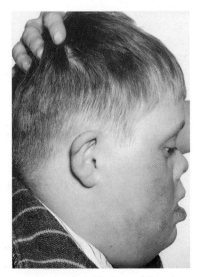

FIG 8.13 Down's syndrome. These three photographs show the short stature, floppiness and typical facial features of Down's syndrome.

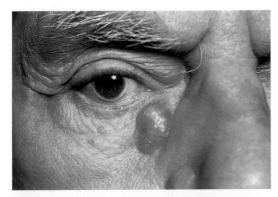

FIG 8.14 Arcus senilis: a thin white rim around the iris. It is a common abnormality and does not indicate advanced arterial disease. Note that the patient also has a basal cell carcinoma.

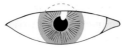

Normal

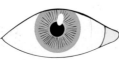

Mild exophthalmos
Sclera visible below the inferior limbus

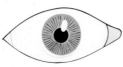

Severe exophthalmos
Sclera visible all round the iris

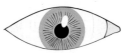

Lid retraction
Elevation of the upper eyelid

FIG 8.15 The relations of the eyelids to the iris.

Xanthelasma
(Xanthoma)

Xanthelasmata are fatty plaques in the skin of the eyelids. They look like masses of yellow, opaque fat. They are confined to the skin and are not painful or tender.

Xanthelasmata are very common. One or two on the eyelids do not indicate any underlying disease, but if the patient has extensive, multiple, growing lesions, you should exclude any underlying abnormality of cholesterol metabolism, diabetes or arterial disease.

Exophthalmos
(Proptosis)

Exophthalmos is the forward protrusion of the eye from its normal position in the orbit.

In the normal eye (Fig. 8.15), the lower eyelid just touches the lower edge of the iris (the inferior limbus), provided the lower lid is normal, while the upper lid crosses the eye mid-way between the pupil and the superior limbus.

The first sign of exophthalmos is the appearance of sclera below the inferior limbus. The proptosis has to be considerable before sclera is visible above the superior limbus.

The position of the upper eyelid is also altered by the tone of the levator palpebrae superioris muscle. Retraction of the upper eyelid will reveal sclera above the superior limbus, but you will not mistake this for exophthalmos if you remember to check the position of the lower eyelid.

When the eye is pushed forwards, four secondary physical signs appear.

1. The patient can look up without wrinkling the forehead.
2. Convergence for very close vision is restricted.
3. The patient blinks less often than normal.
4. The patient may not be able to close their eyes and **corneal ulceration** may develop.

If the protrusion of the eye interferes with the venous and lymphatic drainage of the conjunctiva, it becomes oedematous and wrinkled. This is called **chemosis**.

The causes of exophthalmos are listed in Revision panel 8.7.

The commonest cause of both bilateral and unilateral exophthalmos is thyrotoxicosis.

Revision panel 8.6
The causes of ptosis

Inflammation
Tumours
Excess eyelid skin
Muscle weakness (myopathies, myasthenia)
Third nerve palsy

Revision panel 8.8 lists the causes of a pulsating exophthalmos. This is a rare condition but easy to recognize. It is usually associated with severe chemosis.

Ectropion

Deformities of the lower eyelid often cause the lid to evert. This reveals sclera below the inferior limbus and so mimics exophthalmos, but should not lead to a misdiagnosis because the eyelid looks deformed. When the eyelid becomes everted, its inner surface of shiny conjunctiva may become scarred, dull and immobile.

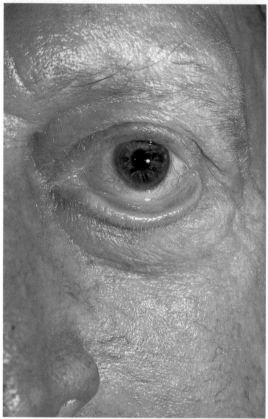

Ectropion: eversion of the lower eyelid.

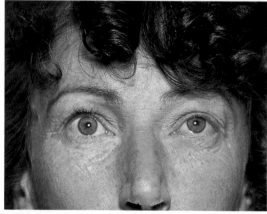

Proptosis: the sclera is visible between the inferior limbus and the left lower eyelid, but the lower eyelid is normal. Thus this is not ectropion but proptosis, caused, in this patient, by a retro-orbital tumour.

FIG 8.16

Revision panel 8.7
The causes of exophthalmos

Endocrine[a]
    Thyrotoxicosis (before, during and after its onset)
    Cushing's syndrome (rare)
Non-endocrine
    Congenital deformities of the skull[a] (craniostenosis, oxycephaly, hypertelorism)
Orbital or peri-orbital tumours
    Peri-orbital meningioma
    Optic nerve glioma
    Orbital haemangioma
    Lymphoma
    Osteoma
    Pseudotumour (granuloma)
    Carcinoma of antrum
    Neuroblastoma
Inflammation
    Orbital cellulitis
    Ethmoid or frontal sinusitis
Vascular causes
    Cavernous sinus arterio-venous fistula
    Cavernous artery aneurysm
Eye disease
    Severe myopia[a]
    Severe glaucoma (buphthalmos)[a]

[a]Likely to be bilateral.

Revision panel 8.8
The causes of pulsating exophthalmos

Carotid artery–cavernous sinus arterio-venous fistula
Aneurysm of the ophthalmic artery
Vascular neoplasm in the orbit
Cavernous sinus thrombosis

Subconjunctival haemorrhage

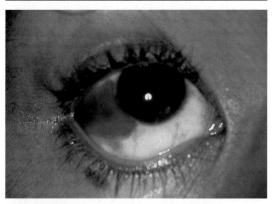

A subconjunctival haemorrhage may arise from a subconjunctival vessel or be blood which has tracked forwards from behind the eye – usually from a fracture of the base of the skull. When this patient looked to the left, white sclera could be seen to the right of the haemorrhage, confirming that the bleeding was solely from subconjunctival blood vessels.

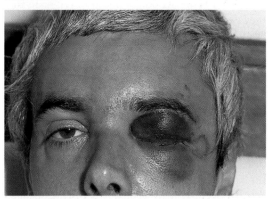

Extensive bleeding from a fracture of the base of the skull may cause a large peri-orbital haematoma as well as a subconjunctival haemorrhage.

FIG 8.17

Horner's syndrome

Horner's syndrome comprises the physical signs that follow interruption of the sympathetic nerve supply to the head and neck.

The pre-ganglionic sympathetic fibres of the head and neck arise in the first and sometimes second thoracic segments of the spinal cord. They synapse with the cells in the three cervical sympathetic ganglia whose fibres (post-ganglionic) are distributed to the structures of the head and neck along the nerves and blood vessels.

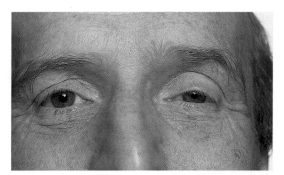

FIG 8.18 Horner's syndrome of the left eye. (See Revision panel 8.9.)

The sympathetic pathway to the face and eye can, therefore, be interrupted by trauma or disease anywhere between the appearance of the pre-ganglionic fibres from the spinal cord and their termination.

Absence of sympathetic tone causes myosis, ptosis, vasodilatation and anhidrosis.

The causes of Horner's syndrome are as follows (the common causes are in bold type).

- Brain lesions – **posterior inferior cerebellar artery thrombosis**.
- Spinal cord lesions – syringomyelia, tumours.
- Injuries to the lower roots of the brachial plexus.
- Surgical excision of the inferior cervical ganglion (**cervical sympathectomy**).
- Tumours in the apex of the lung (**Pancoast's tumour**).
- Tumours in the neck.
- Aneurysm and dissection of the carotid artery.

When these nerve fibres are interrupted by disease there may be a period before the paralysis when the sympathetic activity is increased. Stimulation of the sympathetic nerves makes the pupil dilate, the upper eyelid retract and the skin of the face pale,

---

Revision panel 8.9
Horner's syndrome

A small pupil (*myosis*)
Drooping of the upper eyelid (*ptosis*)
A warm, pink cheek (*vasodilatation*)
Absence of sweating (*anhidrosis*)
Nasal congestion (*nasal vasodilatation*)
Apparent enophthalmos

cold and sweaty. The causes of sympathetic nerve irritation are the same as the causes of paralysis.

THE NOSE

The appearance of the face is affected by the shape of the nose. In addition to the infinite variability of the shape of the normal nose, there are two pathological conditions which alter its shape.

Saddle nose

A nose whose bridge is depressed and widened is called a saddle nose. This deformity is caused by congenital abnormalities such as achondroplasia and hypertelorism, or destruction of the nasal cartilages, commonly caused by leprosy, cutaneous leishmaniasis and congenital syphilis.

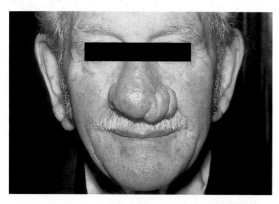

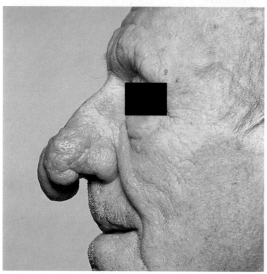

FIG 8.19 Two examples of rhinophyma.

Rhinophyma

Rhinophyma is a thickening of the skin over the tip of the nose caused by hypertrophy and adenomatous changes in its sebaceous glands. It is not caused by an excessive intake of alcohol.

SHAPE OF THE SKULL

There are a number of congenital deformities of the skull, all with long names that describe the skull's shape, but they are all very rare.

The abnormality of shape that you should look out for in neonates and young children is the progressive and disproportionate enlargement of the skull caused by hydrocephalus.

The normal scalp consists of hairy skin, subcutaneous fat and a fascial aponeurosis. All these structures can give rise to the common lesions of the skin and subcutaneous tissues described in Chapters 2 and 3, but some are so common on the scalp that they deserve special mention.

Hydrocephalus

Hydrocephalus is a pathological accumulation of cerebrospinal fluid within or around the brain – internal or external hydrocephalus.

Congenital hydrocephalus is caused by a failure of cerebrospinal fluid absorption, so that there is distension of the ventricles within the brain and of the subarachnoid space with which they communicate. Congenital hydrocephalus is often associated with a meningo-myelocele and spina bifida.

Acquired hydrocephalus is caused by a block of the aqueduct of Sylvius or the foramina over the fourth ventricle, by tumour or infection. In this type of hydrocephalus the distended ventricles do not communicate with the subarachnoid space.

Multiple sebaceous cysts

The scalp may be covered with sebaceous cysts of all sizes. They are diagnosed by their spherical shape and hard, tense composition (see also page 73). They are by far the commonest cause of a lump on the scalp. They rarely have a visible punctum.

A suppurating sebaceous cyst with granulation tissue bulging out of it is sometimes called **Cock's**

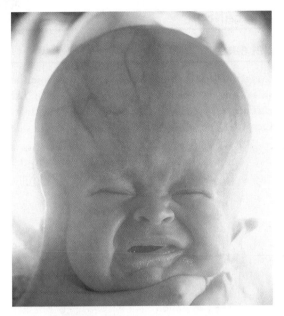

FIG 8.20 Congenital hydrocephalus. The bright light behind the baby's head reveals the thinness of the bones of the skull.

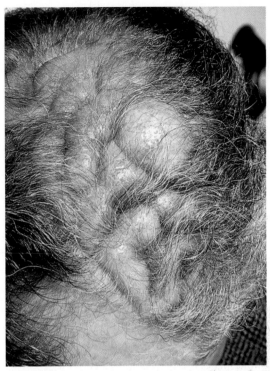

FIG 8.21 A 'turban tumour'. This one was a cylindroma.

peculiar tumour (see page 73). It is easily mistaken for a squamous cell carcinoma.

Turban tumour

There are four pathological conditions that can cause multiple lumps on the scalp which grow steadily, coalesce and eventually produce an irregular mass that covers the whole scalp and looks like a turban. All are rare.

As the term 'turban tumour' is purely descriptive, it can be applied to all four conditions. However, it is most often used to describe **multiple cylindromata**, which present as firm, pink nodules in the skin.

Multiple nodular basal cell carcinomata may also cover the scalp, but they are firm, retain their pearly-white appearance and covering of fine blood vessels, do not really look like a turban and can usually be diagnosed by examining one of the smaller lesions.

Multiple sweat gland tumours (**hidradenomata**) form soft, boggy swellings in the scalp. Although very soft (they feel like lumps of oedematous skin), they are not fluctuant and cannot be compressed or indented.

Finally, and rarest of all, is subcutaneous **plexiform neurofibromatosis** of the scalp. This is usually associated with neurofibromata in other sites and café au lait patches.

Pott's puffy tumour

Pott's puffy tumour is a diffuse oedematous swelling of the scalp over a patch of osteomyelitis in the skull. It is most often seen in the frontal region overlying frontal bone osteomyelitis caused by frontal sinusitis.

Cephalhaematoma

This is a subperiosteal haematoma. It occurs in neonates following a traumatic delivery, and in infants following direct trauma. The haematoma spreads beneath the pericranium (periosteum) to the fissures between the skull bones.

For a few days it forms a soft, fluctuant swelling covering one of the bones of the vault of the skull, but when the blood begins to resorb, the residual blood clot forms a ridge around the edge of the swelling. Ultimately all that is left of the swelling is

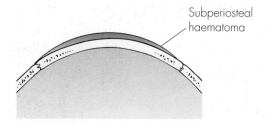

Subperiosteal haematoma

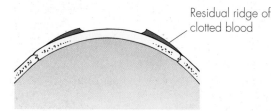

Residual ridge of clotted blood

FIG 8.22 A cephalhaematoma is a subperiosteal haematoma limited by the fissures between the bones. When the blood is absorbed, a ridge of clotted blood forms a rim around the edge of the haematoma.

a **hard, raised edge**, which is often compared to a dinner plate, and is easily mistaken for a depressed fracture if you do not observe that its lip is above the level of the rest of the skull.

Ivory osteoma

This is an osteoma of the cortical bone that forms the outer table of the skull. Ivory osteomata appear during adolescence and young adult life but cause no symptoms and need no treatment.

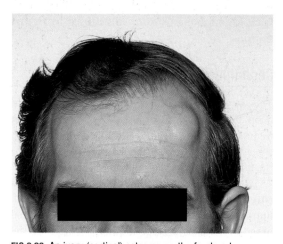

FIG 8.23 An ivory (cortical) osteoma on the forehead.

THE EARS

Bat ears

Congenital bat ears are ears which jut out from the side of the head rather than lying flat against it. Bat ears are not associated with any mental abnormalities. Cup-shaped ears that protrude from the side

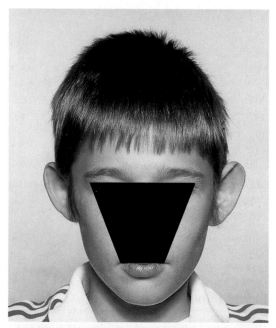

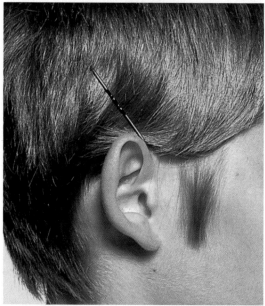

FIG 8.24 Bat ears: antero-posterior and lateral views.

of the skull are a feature of Down's syndrome, but these are not true bat ears.

If a patient complains that one ear has become prominent, look behind it for swellings in the sub-cutaneous tissue or bone that may be pushing it outwards. For example a mastoid abscess makes the ear more prominent.

Cauliflower ears

Cauliflower ears are ears distorted by multiple sub-perichondral haematomata. Unlike most other haematomata, those beneath the perichondrium of the ear are slow to resorb. Some actually absorb fluid and swell. The patient complains of a flattened, sometimes fluctuant, sometimes firm, swelling fixed to the cartilage of the ear, which fills the hollows of the ear and distorts its shape.

Cauliflower ears are common in boxers and wrestlers.

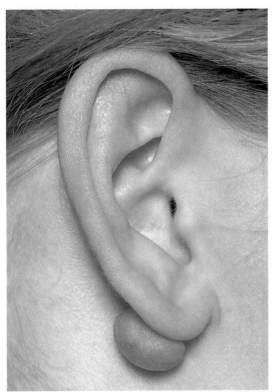

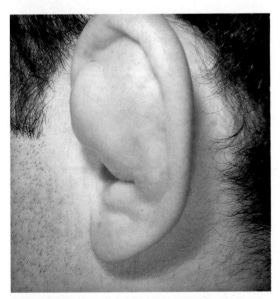

FIG 8.25 A 'cauliflower ear'. The swelling is a subperichondral haematoma and is almost blocking the external auditory meatus.

Keloid nodules

Many women have their ears pierced. If the hole becomes infected, or if the patient has an inherent tendency towards keloid scarring, the scar tissue may overgrow and produce a large nodule behind the lobe of the ear. The nodule is soft, spherical

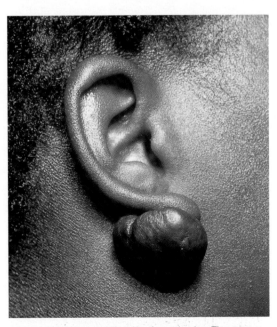

FIG 8.26 Keloid scars at the site of ear piercing. The mass of scar tissue usually protrudes from the posterior aspect of the ear lobe. Keloid scars are more common in black-skinned races.

and sometimes pedunculated. It is often misdiagnosed as an inclusion dermoid cyst but is usually a solid mass of keloid scar.

Accessory auricle

Accessory auricles are small pieces of cartilage separate from the pinna. They are found on the side of the face just in front of the tragus. They cause no symptoms and can be differentiated from the other two lumps that develop in front of the ear – an enlarged pre-auricular lymph gland or a parotid gland tumour – by the fact that they have been present from birth.

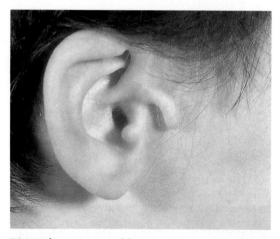

FIG 8.27 An accessory auricle.

MENINGOCELE

A meningocele is a protrusion of the meninges through a defect in the spinal canal or skull. It contains cerebrospinal fluid and is covered by skin.

A **meningo-myelocele** is a protrusion of the meninges plus part of the spinal cord or cauda equina through a defect in the spinal canal. It is not completely covered by skin, and the thin meninges rupture a few days after birth.

There are two other, uncommon, congenital abnormalities of spinal cord and canal development. A **myelocele** is an open, exposed spinal cord. The infant is stillborn or dies within a few days of birth. A **syringo-myelocele** is the bulge of a dilated spinal cord (**hydromyelia**) through the spinal canal.

The diagnosis of a meningocele, or meningo-myelocele, is made on the basis of its composition – soft, fluctuant and translucent; its site – in the midline of the lower back, or the back of the skull; and

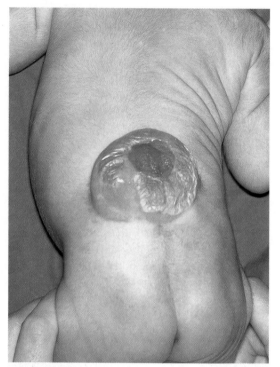

FIG 8.28 A meningo-myelocele of the spine.

the presence of neurological abnormalities below the level of the lesion.

THE CHEST WALL

There are a number of deformities and diseases which alter the shape of the chest wall and which, therefore, affect the general appearance of the patient – hence their inclusion in this chapter.

Funnel chest
(Pectus excavatum)

Funnel chest is a congenital depression of the body of the sternum. If it is deep, it may embarrass respiration and cause recurrent respiratory tract infection.

Pigeon chest
(Pectus carinatum)

Pigeon chest is the opposite deformity to funnel chest. The sternum sticks forwards like the keel of a boat. It may be a congenital deformity or be caused by chest disease in childhood, such as asthma.

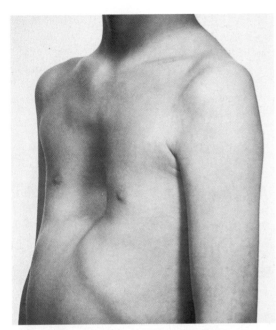

Funnel chest.

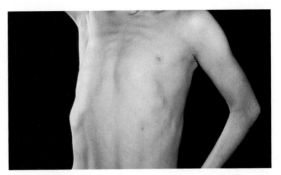

A rickety rosary.

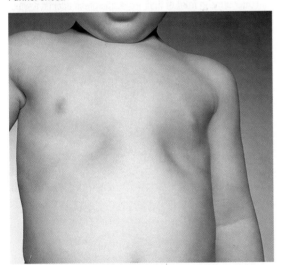

Pigeon chest.

FIG 8.29 DEFORMITIES OF THE CHEST WALL.

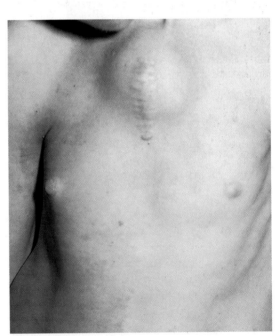

An aortic aneurysm eroding through the sternum.

Harrison's sulcus

This is a hollow in the thoracic cage, caused by the depression of the costo-chondral junctions of the fourth, fifth, sixth and seventh ribs.

This abnormality is a late effect of rickets. Rickets first causes an enlargement of the costo-chondral junctions – the rickety rosary – but later both these and the ends of the ribs soften and sink inwards. The resulting hollow is particularly noticeable over the lower group of ribs attached to the sternum.

Sprengel's shoulder

Sprengel's shoulder is caused by a congenital elevation of the scapula which distorts the whole shape of the chest and shoulder.

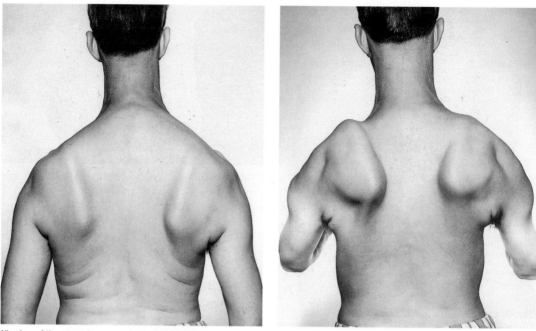

Winging of the scapulae, accentuated by asking the patient to hold out their arms in front of their trunk and press against a wall.

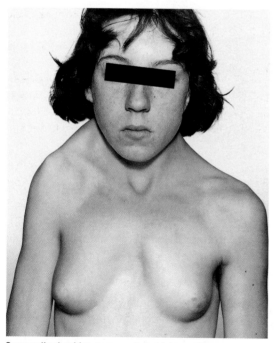

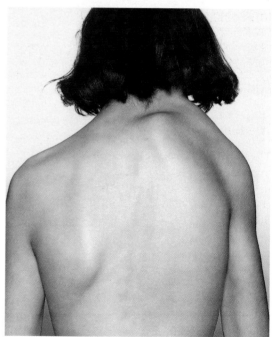

Sprengel's shoulder: a congenitally high scapula.

FIG 8.30 SOME ABNORMALITIES AFFECTING THE APPEARANCE OF THE CHEST WALL.

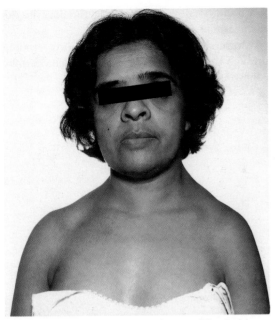
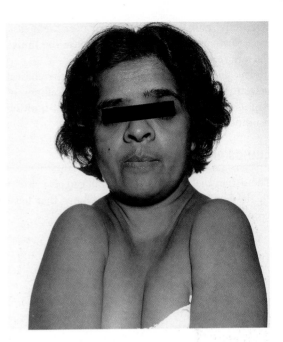

Craniocleidodysostosis: congenital absence of the clavicles.

FIG 8.30 continued

Craniocleidodysostosis

Craniocleidodysostosis is a rare inherited absence of the clavicles. The patient is able to pull the shoulders to the mid-line and distort the whole shape of the chest.

Winging of the scapulae

The scapula is normally held against the chest wall by the serratus anterior muscle. This muscle also rotates and moves the scapula forwards around the chest during those movements that involve holding the arm out forwards.

The nerve to the serratus anterior (the long thoracic nerve of Bell) may be divided or stretched by direct trauma, carrying heavy weights or wearing a knapsack, or affected by a viral neuritis. When the serratus anterior muscle is paralysed, the scapula pokes out from the chest wall – a deformity called 'winging'. If a patient complains of weakness of the arms or deformity of their back, remember to ask them to put their hands and arms out forwards and press against a wall. If the serratus anterior muscle is paralysed, the scapula will protrude backwards.

Myopathy affecting the serratus anterior muscle will also cause 'winging'.

Tietze's syndrome

This is a condition which occurs in young women. It is a painful swelling of the second, third and fourth costal cartilages. The cause is unknown, but the

> **Revision panel 8.10**
> **The causes of swellings of the chest wall**
>
> **Bony hard**
> Secondary carcinoma
> Chondroma
> Osteoma
> Exostosis (diaphyseal aclasis)
> Myeloma
> **Fluctuant**
> Tuberculous abscess of rib or lymph gland
> Empyema necessitas
> Infected haematoma
> **Pulsatile**
> An eroding aortic aneurysm

symptoms, pain and swelling in or near the breast, cause the patient great concern because she thinks she has a carcinoma of the breast.

The diagnosis is based solely upon the clinical detection of hard, immobile, tender swellings of the costo-chondral junctions. It is a self-limiting condition.

Lumps on the chest wall

The tissues that form the chest wall can give rise to all the benign and malignant swellings that have been described in Chapters 2, 3 and 4.

Chondromata and secondary tumours in the ribs are quite common.

Aneurysms of the arch of the aorta eroding through the sternum and causing sudden death by rupturing are now extremely rare.

9

The salivary glands

Saliva is produced by the paired parotid, submandibular and sublingual glands and many other small, unnamed glands scattered beneath the buccal mucous membrane.

The commonest surgical conditions affecting the salivary glands are:

- infection and calculus formation in the submandibular gland,
- tumours of the parotid gland.

Mumps is the commonest medical disease; all other diseases of the salivary glands are uncommon.

THE SUBMANDIBULAR SALIVARY GLAND

Submandibular calculi

Submandibular calculi are common because the submandibular gland lies below the opening of its duct on the floor of the mouth, and because the secretion of the submandibular gland contains a considerable quantity of mucus, two factors which encourage stasis in the duct. Calculi in the parotid gland are less common.

A salivary gland calculus is composed of cellular debris, bacteria, mucus, and calcium and magnesium phosphates – a mixture similar to the 'scale' (tartar) that the dentist scrapes off our teeth.

History

Age Most submandibular salivary calculi occur in young to middle-aged adults. They are rare in children.

Sex Males and females are equally afflicted.

Symptoms The main symptoms are **pain** and **swelling** beneath the jaw, caused by obstruction of Wharton's duct.

These two symptoms vary in predominance. Swelling is usually the principal complaint, because it appears before, and persists after, the pain. The pain is a dull ache, which occasionally radiates to the ear or into the tongue.

Both symptoms appear, or worsen, before and during eating. The swelling begins just before eating and the pain develops as the gland enlarges. Both symptoms last through the meal, but afterwards the pain goes away before the swelling. If the gland becomes irreparably damaged, the swelling persists between meals and the dull aching pain may also become constant.

Very rarely, the patient may notice **discomfort** and a **swelling in the floor of the mouth**.

Patients may be able to relieve their symptoms by pressing on the gland, and they may notice that this action produces a foul-tasting fluid in their mouth (purulent saliva).

Development The symptoms may recur and remit for periods of a few days or weeks if the stone moves about in the duct, sometimes obstructing it, sometimes not.

If the stone passes through the orifice of the duct, the symptoms disappear.

Persistent obstruction damages the gland, making it harder and more tender.

Previous history The patient may have had similar symptoms on the other side of the face. Simultaneous bilateral calculi are uncommon.

Examination
The lump

Position The submandibular gland lies beneath the horizontal ramus of the mandible on the mylohyoid muscle. It is 2–3 cm in front of the anterior border of the sternomastoid muscle and should not be

Superficial part

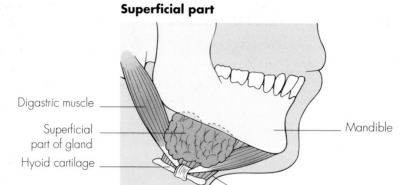

Digastric muscle

Superficial part of gland

Hyoid cartilage

Mandible

Mylohyoid muscle

Deep part

Lingual nerve

Deep part of gland

Hyoglossus muscle

Tongue

Genioglossus muscle

Jaw

Duct

Geniohyoid muscle

Hyoid cartilage

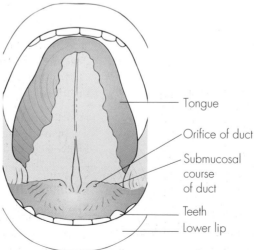

Tongue

Orifice of duct

Submucosal course of duct

Teeth

Lower lip

FIG 9.1 The anatomy of the submandibular gland.

confused with enlarged upper deep cervical lymph glands, which are deep to the sternomastoid muscle.

Colour and temperature If the gland is not infected, the overlying skin will have a normal colour and temperature. If the gland is infected, the skin becomes red, oedematous and hot.

Tenderness The gland is tender when it is tense (before and during eating) but is not usually tender between meals, unless it is infected.

Shape The shape of the superficial part of the submandibular gland, and hence of the swelling, is a flattened ovoid (almond shaped).

Size If the gland is enlarged solely by obstruction of its duct, it rarely becomes more than 3–5 cm across. If it becomes infected, it may get much bigger.

Surface Its surface is smooth but the lobules of the gland may make it bosselated.

Edge The anterior, posterior and inferior edges of the gland are distinct and easy to define, but the upper edge is wedged between the mandible and the mylohyoid muscle and is impalpable.

Composition A distended submandibular gland has a **rubbery**, hard consistence and will not fluctuate, transilluminate or reduce. It is dull to percussion and has no bruit.

Occasionally, prolonged pressure on the gland may make it a little smaller and produce a jet of saliva from the orifice of the submandibular duct.

Relations The skin is freely mobile over the swollen gland. The gland itself can be moved a little from side to side, but most movements are restricted by the tethering of the gland to the underlying muscles.

When the muscles of the floor of the mouth are tensed by asking the patient to push their tongue against the roof of the mouth, the gland becomes less mobile.

It is important to ascertain the relations of the lump to the floor of the mouth and the tongue by **bimanual palpation**. Feel the lump between the index finger of one hand inside the mouth (suitably gloved), and the fingers of the other hand on the outer surface of the lump.

It should be possible to appreciate that the lump is outside the structures that form the floor of the mouth. It should not be fixed to the mucosa of the floor of the mouth or to the tongue.

Lymph drainage The submandibular gland lymph drains to the middle deep cervical lymph glands, but there is also some lymphoid tissue within the gland which can contribute to its enlargement.

The local lymph glands are usually not enlarged unless the gland is infected.

Local tissues The nearby tissues, except the submandibular duct in the floor of the mouth, should be normal.

The floor of the mouth

Inspection Ask the patient to open their mouth and lift their tongue up to the roof of the mouth. This displays the orifices of the submandibular ducts on their small papillae on either side of the frenulum of the tongue.

If a stone is impacted at the end of the duct, its grey-yellow colour may be visible in the open orifice of the duct.

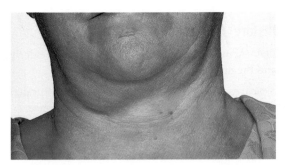

FIG 9.2 A swollen right submandibular gland. Although some of the swelling seems to spread over the jaw, the upper part of the lump is actually deep to the mandible.

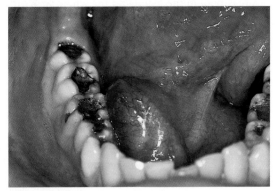

FIG 9.3 When a stone impacts at the end of the submandibular duct, the floor of the mouth looks asymmetrical. In this photograph there is a bulge over the patient's right duct. Palpation revealed a firm lump.

The presence of a stone in the duct makes that side of the floor of the mouth bulge upwards and look pink.

Press the gland gently and watch for any discharge from the orifice of the duct.

Palpation Feel along the course of the duct in the floor of the mouth for lumps and tenderness.

A stone in the duct will not feel stony hard if it is small and surrounded by inflammatory oedema. The lump caused by such a stone will feel soft with a hard centre.

General examination Examine all the salivary glands in case the symptoms are due to a systemic disease such as Sjögren's syndrome (see page 249), not just a stone.

Submandibular sialadenitis

Infection of a submandibular gland is invariably secondary to the presence of a stone in its duct or the damage done by a stone which has passed through the duct. The infecting organism is usually a staphylococcus.

The symptoms are identical to those caused by a stone except that when the gland is infected the **pain is severe, throbbing, continuous** and exacerbated by eating.

The physical signs of the lump in the neck are similar to those of the obstructed gland described above, with the addition of **heat** and **tenderness**. An infected gland may become quite big (5×10 cm). If the duct system becomes dilated (**sialectasis**), the pus may pool in the gland and the whole structure turn into a multilocular abscess, which may then point externally onto the skin.

Submandibular salivary gland tumours

The tumours that often occur in the parotid gland – **pleomorphic adenoma**, **cylindroma** and **carcinoma** – may occur in the submandibular gland, but they are rare.

The physical features of pleomorphic adenoma and carcinoma in the submandibular gland are identical to those of these tumours when they occur in the parotid gland, apart from the site.

The pleomorphic adenoma forms a painless, slow-growing, non-tender, hard, well-defined, spherical mass within the gland. Carcinoma causes an indistinct, hot, slightly tender, rapidly growing, painful mass. Numbness of the anterior two-thirds of the tongue indicates infiltration of the lingual nerve, and is diagnostic of carcinoma.

It may be difficult to distinguish a pleomorphic adenoma from enlargement of the lymph tissue within the gland. A long history of slow, gradual growth is the most useful distinguishing feature.

THE PAROTID GLAND

Acute bacterial parotitis

The commonest infection of the parotid gland is mumps. This is an **epidemic viral parotitis**; when it occurs in an epidemic with bilateral painful, swollen glands and excessive oedema, which spreads down into the neck, giving the child a double chin, it is easy to diagnose.

When it causes unilateral gland enlargement, little pain, no oedema, and there are no obvious contacts with the infection, it can be much more difficult to diagnose.

Remember, mumps is the commonest cause of parotitis.

Non-specific parotitis, usually a staphylococcal infection, is caused by:

- poor oral hygiene
- dehydration
- obstruction of Stensen's duct by stone or scar tissue.

In the days before the fluid balance of sick patients was properly controlled, fulminating parotitis with a subsequent septicaemia was a common cause of death.

History

Age   Acute parotitis is more common in the elderly and the debilitated.

Symptoms The patient complains of the sudden onset of pain and swelling in the side of the face.

The pain is continuous and throbbing, and radiates to the ear and over the side of the head.

Speaking and eating cause pain because any movement of the temporo-mandibular joint is painful.

The patient feels hot, sweaty and ill and may complain of shivering attacks (rigors).

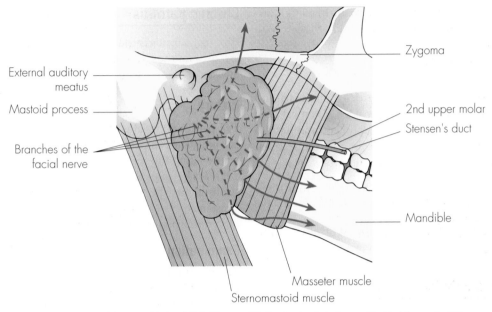

External auditory meatus

Mastoid process

Branches of the facial nerve

Zygoma

2nd upper molar
Stensen's duct

Mandible

Masseter muscle
Sternomastoid muscle

FIG 9.4 The anatomy of the parotid gland. **N.B.** The parotid gland extends below and behind the angle of the mandible. Lumps in this part of the gland are easily mistaken for enlarged upper deep cervical lymph glands.

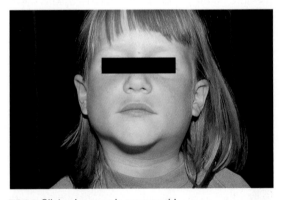

FIG 9.5 Bilateral mumps in a young girl.

Systematic questions The answers to these questions may reveal symptoms of another illness, such as a bronchial carcinoma, which has caused the debility and dehydration.

Previous history The patient may have recently undergone a major operation or suffered a severe medical illness.

Examination

The lump

Position The parotid gland lies in front of and below the lower half of the ear. It is wrapped around the

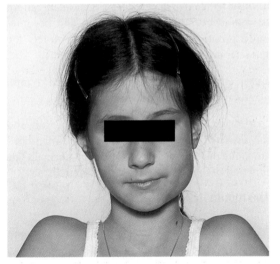

FIG 9.6 Unilateral mumps. A young girl with diffuse swelling of the left parotid gland caused by mumps. Much of the swelling is caused by oedema.

vertical ramus of the mandible, with its deep portion in between this bone and the mastoid process.

In acute parotitis the whole gland is swollen, so the whole of the face in front of the lower half of the ear bulges outwards.

Colour and temperature The skin over the swelling is dis-coloured a reddish-brown, feels hot, and is smooth and shiny.

Tenderness The swelling is very tender.

Shape The mass has the shape of the normal parotid gland: a semicircular anterior edge, a vertical edge just in front of the ear, and a bulge running into the gap between the mandible and the mastoid process.

Size The swollen gland may be three or four times larger than a normal gland.

Surface Its surface is smooth but difficult to define because of the oedema, inflammation and tenderness.

Composition The texture of the swelling is often described as **brawny**. This means that it has a firm consistence but is indentable. It is dull to percussion, not fluctuant and not compressible.

Relations If the overlying skin is red and oedematous, it will be tethered to the swelling. The swelling cannot be moved over the deep structures and becomes more prominent when the patient contracts the masseter muscles by clenching their teeth.

Lymph drainage The upper deep cervical lymph glands are usually enlarged and tender.

Local tissues Apart from the changes in the skin, and the restricted movements of the temporo-mandibular joint, the surrounding tissues are normal. The function of the facial nerve is *not* impaired.

The mouth

Inspection Remember that the orifice of Stensen's duct is opposite the second upper molar tooth. The mouth of the duct may be patulous and the buccal mucosa over the course of the duct slightly oedematous.

Palpation Feel the mouth of the duct for any thickening or lumps.

The parotid gland cannot be palpated bimanually because it lies behind the anterior edge of the masseter muscle and the vertical ramus of the mandible.

Gentle pressure on the gland may produce a purulent discharge from the orifice of the duct.

Chronic parotitis

Chronic parotitis is usually caused by a small calculus or a fibrous stenosis blocking the mouth of Stensen's duct.

History

The patient complains of recurrent swelling of the parotid gland. The swelling is particularly noticeable before eating and is associated with an aching pain.

In severe cases the gland becomes permanently swollen, but the pain does not usually become constant.

Chronic parotitis is sometimes bilateral.

Examination

The whole gland is easy to feel because it is slightly bigger and firmer than a normal gland and its edges are distinct. It is also tender and feels rubbery hard.

If there is partial obstruction to the flow of saliva, pressure on the gland may produce a copious squirt of fluid through the orifice of the duct.

Examine all the other salivary glands to exclude a general abnormality.

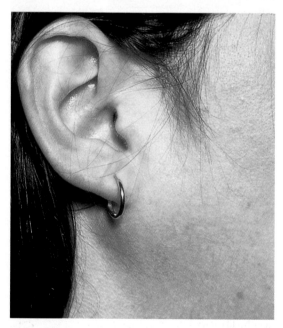

FIG 9.7 Chronic parotitis. A firm, slightly tender enlargement of the whole of the parotid gland caused by recurrent infection secondary to a stone in Stensen's duct.

Pleomorphic adenoma
(Mixed parotid tumour, sialoma)

This is a **true adenoma** of the parotid gland. Its mixed histological appearance gave rise to its old name, mixed parotid tumour, and its currently favoured name, pleomorphic adenoma. It has also been called a sialoma.

It is a slow-growing adenoma with an incomplete capsule. The small pieces of tumour that protrude through the defects in its capsule limit its treatment by enucleation and allow its rapid extension if it turns malignant. After many years of slow, benign growth, a small proportion of adenomata become locally invasive.

History

Age These tumours appear in early and middle adult life.

Sex They occur more often in males than in females.

Symptoms The patient complains of a **painless swelling** on the side of their face which has been present for months or years and which is **slowly growing**.

The lump may be more prominent when the mouth is open, or when eating. The latter symptom can cause confusion, so it is important to find out whether the lump just becomes more prominent because of contraction of the masseter muscle or actually increases in size.

Examination

Position The majority of parotid adenomata begin in the portion of the gland that lies over the junction of the vertical and horizontal rami of the mandible, just anterior and superior to the angle of the jaw.

Why the majority begin here is not known, for they can occur in any part of the gland.

Colour and temperature The temperature and colour of the overlying skin are normal.

Tenderness The lump is not tender.

Shape Most pleomorphic adenomata are spherical when they are small, but as they grow they become flat on their deep surface and slightly pointed superficially. They may become lobulated when very large.

Size These tumours can vary from pea-sized nodules to large, almost pendulous, masses, 20 cm across.

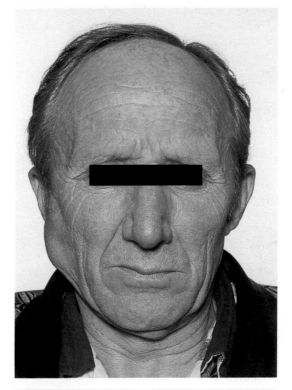

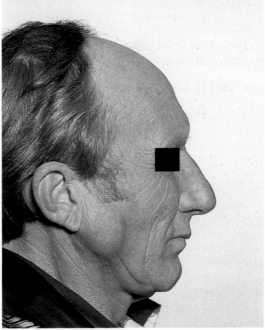

FIG 9.8 A pleomorphic adenoma. These photographs show the typical site, the healthy overlying skin, the absence of facial nerve involvement and the lobulation that develops as the tumour grows.

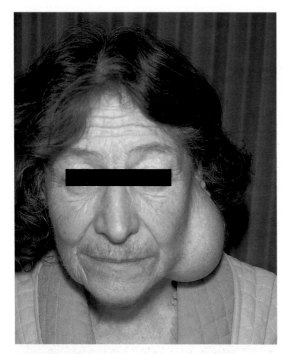

FIG 9.9 A very large, almost pendulous, pleomorphic adenoma of the parotid gland.

Surface Their surface is smooth, sometimes bosselated, and occasionally crossed by deep furrows.

The surface of any deep extension between the mandible and the mastoid process is impalpable.

Edge The edge is quite distinct and easy to feel.

Composition The tumour mass has a rubbery, hard consistence, is dull to percussion, not fluctuant or translucent, and not compressible.

Relations The overlying skin and the ear are freely movable, not attached to the lump.

Small tumours can be moved about over the deep structures, but large tumours are less mobile.

Lymph drainage The cervical lymph glands should not be enlarged.

Local tissues Apart from any distortion caused by the mass, the local tissues should be normal. In particular, the **facial nerve should function normally**. Paralysis of any facial muscles indicates infiltration of the nerve, which means that the lump is a carcinoma, not a benign adenoma.

Examine the inside of the mouth

A pleomorphic adenoma in the deep part of the parotid gland will push the tonsil and the pillar of the fauces towards the mid-line.

Differential diagnosis

Remember that the pre-auricular lymph gland may be enlarged by secondary infection or metastases from a tumour in the forehead, scalp, eyelids, cheek or external auditory meatus. The resulting firm, smooth swelling just in front of the tragus can be indistinguishable from a pleomorphic adenoma if it is not tender and there are no obvious abnormalities in its drainage area.

The most distinctive physical sign of an enlarged pre-auricular lymph gland is its mobility. Most tumours in the parotid gland can only be moved a short distance because they are tethered to the gland; the pre-auricular lymph gland lies outside the capsule of the parotid gland and is usually very mobile.

Adenolymphoma
(Warthin's tumour)

This is a cystic tumour which contains epithelial and lymphoid tissues. The epithelial element is believed to originate from embryonic parotid ducts that have become separated from the main duct system of the gland. The lymphoid element comes from normal lymph tissue that happened to be close to the developing gland.

The tumour arises on the surface of, or just beneath, the capsule of the parotid gland.

History

Age Adenolymphomata appear in middle and old age.

Sex They are more common in men than in women.

Ethnic group It does not occur in Negroes.

Symptoms The patient complains of a **slow-growing, painless swelling** over the angle of the jaw. The swelling may be bilateral.

Examination

Position The adenolymphoma usually develops in the lower part of the parotid gland, level with the lower

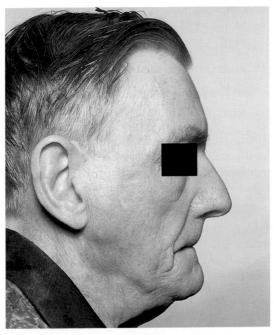

FIG 9.10 Warthin's tumour. An adenolymphoma of the parotid gland. This photograph shows the typical site of an adenolymphoma – just over the angle of the jaw. Although it looks similar to the pleomorphic adenoma shown in Fig. 9.8, it had a soft consistence.

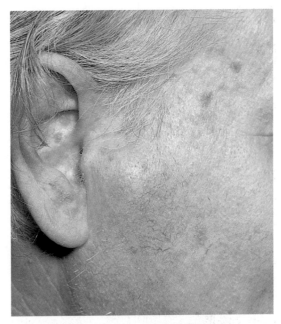

FIG 9.11 Carcinoma of the parotid gland. This patient complained of a painful swelling in front of his ear. The swelling was hot and the overlying skin reddened. Although the swelling was not very large, there was some weakness of the muscles of facial expression.

border of the mandible. This is slightly lower than the common site of origin of the pleomorphic adenoma.

Temperature and colour The overlying skin looks and feels normal.

Tenderness The lump is not tender.

Shape Adenolymphomata are spherical or hemispherical.

Size They are usually 1–3 cm in diameter.

Surface The surface is smooth and well defined.

Edge Its edge is distinct and sometimes makes the lump seem separate from the parotid gland.

Composition Adenolymphomata have a soft consistence, are dull to percussion and not translucent, but they often fluctuate. The fluctuation is sometimes a true sign of the fluid content of the cysts, but more often is a reflection of the soft, solid consistence and strong capsule.

Relations The lump can usually be moved a little in all directions and is not attached to the skin.

Lymph drainage The cervical lymph glands should not be enlarged.

Local tissues The adjacent tissues are all normal.

The site and consistence of the lesion are the features which make one suspect that a parotid swelling is an adenolymphoma.

Carcinoma of the parotid gland

Carcinoma of the parotid gland is uncommon, but not very rare. It can arise de novo, or in a long-standing pleomorphic adenoma.

History

Age The patient is usually over the age of 50 years.

Sex Males and females are equally affected.

Symptoms The common complaint is of a **rapidly enlarging swelling** on the side of the face. The swelling is persistently painful, especially during movements of the jaw. The pain may radiate to the ear and over the side of the face. The patient may

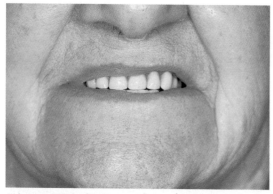

Asymmetry of the mouth.

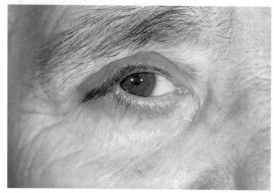

Lateral tarsorrhaphy to protect the cornea from ulceration.

FIG 9.12 FACIAL NERVE WEAKNESS CAUSED BY A CARCINOMA OF THE PAROTID GLAND.

give a history of a preceding painless lump that has been present for many years.

The patient may also complain of asymmetry of the mouth and difficulty in closing the eyes. When this is marked, the patient may require a lateral tarsorrhaphy to protect the cornea from exposure and ulceration.

Examination

Position The swelling is in the site of the parotid gland.

Colour If the overlying skin is being infiltrated by the tumour it may be reddish-blue.

Temperature The skin and the mass are hyperaemic and hot.

Tenderness The mass is not very tender, an important difference from acute parotitis, which also presents with a hot swelling.

Shape The tumour may be of any shape. It is basically a flattened hemisphere but, as it spreads in different directions, its shape becomes irregular.

Size Its size increases inexorably.

Surface The surface is smooth but irregular.

Edge The edge is often indistinct.

Composition The mass has a firm, sometimes hard consistence, is dull to percussion, but is not fluctuant or translucent. Although it may be very vascular, it does not have an audible bruit.

Relations Carcinoma of the parotid becomes fixed to the deep structures early in its growth and may also become fixed to, and infiltrate, the skin.

The thickening of the tissues around the temporo-mandibular joint may restrict jaw movements.

Lymph drainage The cervical lymph glands are likely to be enlarged and hard.

Local tissues If the facial nerve is infiltrated by tumour, the patient will be unable to use the muscles of facial expression. The signs may vary from mild weakness of the lower lip when baring the teeth, to a complete seventh nerve palsy.

If the tumour has infiltrated into the mandible, the jaw may be swollen and tender.

General examination There may be evidence of disseminated blood-borne metastases.

AUTOIMMUNE DISEASE

There are two syndromes of slow, progressive, but relatively painless enlargement of the salivary glands, in which biopsy reveals that the swelling is caused by replacement of the glandular tissue by lymphoid tissue. Both conditions are believed to be autoimmune diseases.

Mikulicz's syndrome

Mikulicz's syndrome is:

- enlargement of the salivary glands: usually both parotid and both submandibular glands enlarge, but the syndrome can begin and remain in one gland for quite a long time;
- enlargement of the lachrymal glands: this causes a bulge at the outer end of the upper

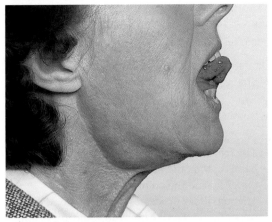

The submandibular swelling in this woman was a lymph gland enlarged by secondary deposits from a carcinoma of the tongue.

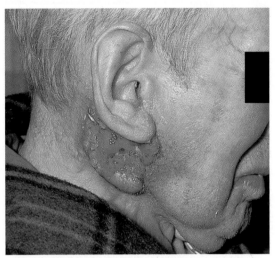

This ulcerating lesion over the parotid gland was initially diagnosed as a parotid carcinoma. However, there was no facial weakness and the lesion was actually in the skin. A biopsy revealed that it was a squamous cell carcinoma of the skin.

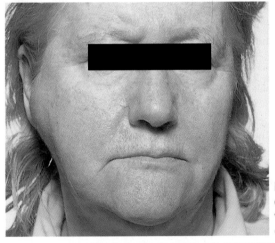

Pre-auricular lymphadenopathy is a condition which is commonly mistaken for parotid gland enlargement. However, this woman's pre-auricular swelling was caused by a secondary deposit of carcinoma in the ascending ramus of the mandible.

FIG 9.13 NOT ALL SWELLINGS IN THE PAROTID AND SUBMANDIBULAR REGIONS ARE CAUSED BY SALIVARY GLAND ENLARGEMENT.

eyelids and narrowing of the palpebral fissures;
■ a dry mouth, which may be the presenting symptom: the patient is not thirsty.

It may be associated with lymphoma, leukaemia, sarcoidosis and tuberculosis.

Sjögren's syndrome

Sjögren's syndrome is all the above conditions, although the degree of salivary gland enlargement is often not so gross, plus:

■ dry eyes
■ generalized arthritis.

Revision panel 9.1
Causes of swelling of a salivary gland

Acute infection
    Viral (e.g. mumps)
    Bacterial (e.g. *Staphylococcus*)
Duct obstruction
Sialectasis (chronic infection)
Tumour
    Benign
    Malignant
Sarcoidosis (Mikulicz's syndrome)
Sjögren's syndrome

10 The mouth

(Lips, teeth, tongue, tonsils, palate and jaw)

Always inspect the mouth with a good light and use a spatula.

- Inspect the external appearance of the lips.
- Retract the lips to see the buccal mucosa.
- Push the cheek outwards to see the buccal side of the gum.
- Push the tongue away from the inside of the gum and the floor of the mouth.
- Push the tongue to one side to see the lateral aspect of its posterior third.
- Depress the tongue to look at the fauces, tonsils and pharynx.

Always remember to **palpate the structures in the mouth bimanually**, one finger inside and one outside. **Always wear a finger cot** or, if there is any possibility that the lesion is contagious, a glove.

CONGENITAL ABNORMALITIES OF THE LIPS AND PALATE

The face, jaw and palate are formed by the fusion of the frontonasal, maxillary and mandibular processes.

- The **frontonasal process** forms the nose, the nasal septum, the nostrils, the philtrum of the upper lip and the premaxilla.
- The **maxillary processes** form the cheek, the upper lip (except the philtrum), the upper jaw and palate.
- The **mandibular processes** form the lower jaw and lip.

Failure of these processes to meet and fuse produces a group of congenital abnormalities: cleft lips, cleft palates and facial clefts.

Half of the infants with a cleft lip also have a cleft palate.

Complete failure of fusion causes a bilateral cleft lip, a cleft palate and a protuberant premaxilla. The diagnosis is apparent from inspection of the lip and palate.

Partial failure of fusion causes unilateral cleft lip and a unilateral cleft of the palate which may be complete or partial.

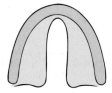

A partial cleft of the hard and soft palates

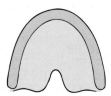

A partial cleft of the soft palate

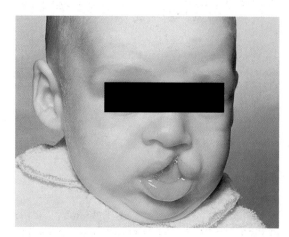

FIG 10.1 A child with a simple cleft lip.

FIG 10.2 The varieties of a simple cleft palate.

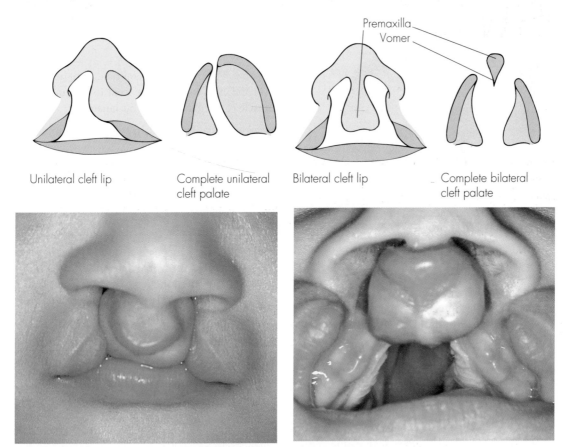

A baby with a bilateral cleft lip and cleft palate. Note the way in which the premaxilla protrudes.

FIG 10.3 CLEFT LIP AND CLEFT PALATE COMBINED.

Rare varieties of failure of fusion may cause a central cleft of the lower lip and jaw, and a facial cleft between the maxilla and the side of the nose.

The symptoms of cleft lip and palate, apart from the **disfigurement**, are an **inability to suckle, interference with speech** (particularly the formation of consonants such as D, T and G) and **distortion of the dental arch.**

THE LIPS, BUCCAL MUCOSA AND TONGUE

Begin by inspecting the external appearance of the lips for any discolouration, pigmentation such as that of Addison's disease or the Peutz–Jegher syndrome or the telangiectasia of Rendu–Osler–Weber syndrome, before looking for any swellings or irregularities in the buccal mucosa lining the inside of the mouth.

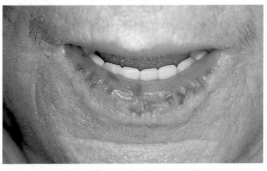

FIG 10.4 The pigmentation of the lips seen in the Peutz–Jegher syndrome.

Mucous retention/extravasation cysts

The inner surface of the lips, and the whole of the inside of the mouth, are covered with an epithelium that contains many small mucus-secreting glands.

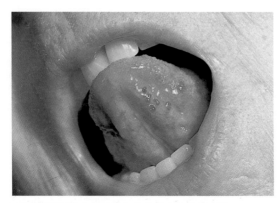

FIG 10.5 Subglossal telangiectasia in a patient with Rendu–Osler–Weber syndrome.

Obstruction of the duct of one of these glands may cause a mucous retention cyst or may cause the gland to rupture and so initiate the formation of a mucous extravasation cyst.

These cysts are common and often rupture spontaneously or get bitten through.

History

Age Mucous retention cysts occur at all ages.

Symptoms The patient complains of a lump on the inner side of the lip or cheek. It is not painful, but grows slowly and may interfere with eating and get bitten.

Examination

Position Mucous retention cysts are most common on the lower lip and in the buccal mucous membrane at the level of the occlusion of the teeth.

Colour Their colour varies according to the state of the overlying epithelium. If the epithelium is healthy, the cyst will be pale pink, with the grey glairy appearance of the mucus in the cyst just visible.

If the epithelium has been frequently damaged by the teeth, it will be white, scarred and slightly boggy, and will obscure the colour of the underlying cyst.

Shape These cysts are spherical.

Size They vary in size from 0.5 to 2 cm in diameter.

Surface Their surface is smooth.

Composition Their consistence varies from soft to hard, depending on the tension of the fluid within them.

Fluctuation and transillumination can be detected if the cyst is large enough to grasp between two fingers.

Relations The mucous membrane can be moved over the cyst, which is not fixed to the underlying muscle (orbicularis oris or buccinator).

Lymph drainage The local lymph glands should not be enlarged.

Local tissues The surrounding tissues should be normal.

Stomatitis

Stomatitis is a general term used to describe an inflammation of the whole lining of the mouth, but the surface of the tongue is also often involved. It can have a variety of clinical appearances and has many causes.

History

Stomatitis occurs in all age groups and equally in both sexes.

Symptoms The patient complains of soreness in the mouth. The mouth may feel dry.

Movements of the tongue and cheeks are painful and individual ulcers are very painful. Mastication is difficult.

The patient may also have the symptoms of a generalized condition that is causing the stomatitis.

Examination

The physical appearances vary according to the cause.

Catarrhal stomatitis

This is often associated with an acute upper respiratory tract infection and acute specific fever. The whole of the mucous membrane of the mouth is oedematous and red. Small ulcers may appear and coalesce to become an ulcerative stomatitis.

Aphthous stomatitis

The inside of the mouth becomes covered with small, tender vesicles which have a thickened hyperaemic base. When a vesicle breaks it leaves a small, white, circular, deep, very painful ulcer. The cause of these ulcers is not known.

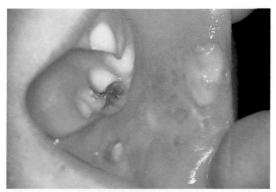

Multiple aphthous ulcers of the buccal mucosa.

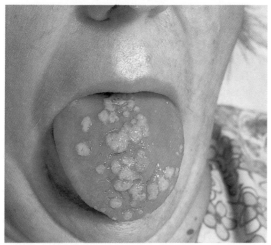

Monilial stomatitis. The colonies of *Monilia* on the tongue and mucous membranes look like patches of cream-coloured paint.

FIG 10.6 STOMATITIS.

Recurrent solitary aphthous ulcers are commonplace in otherwise healthy people. Multiple ulcers are very painful and often associated with a generalized debilitating disease.

Acute monilial stomatitis
(Thrush)

Infection of the alimentary tract by the fungus *Candida albicans* is common in children and in people with debilitating disease, and as a complication of any antibiotic therapy which changes the balance of the bacteria in the alimentary canal.

Small red patches appear on the buccal mucosa and tongue, which then turn **white**. The white appearance is caused by a layer of oedematous desquamating epithelium, heavily contaminated with the fungus.

The mouth is **painful**, and **salivation is excessive**. This induces frequent swallowing, which is also painful if the infection has spread into the pharynx.

Acute ulcerative stomatitis
(Vincent's angina)

This usually follows a severe gingivitis, but may complicate catarrhal stomatitis. It is caused by an

---

Revision panel 10.1
The causes of stomatitis

Local trauma
> Poorly fitting dentures
> Sharp teeth
> Excessive smoking
> Radiotherapy

Local infection
> Herpes
> Monilia
> Vincent's angina
> Glandular fever
> Foot and mouth disease

General conditions
> Stevens–Johnson syndrome
> Behçet's syndrome
> Aphthous ulceration

Vitamin deficiencies
> Vitamin C (scurvy)
> Vitamin B and C (coeliac disease, pellagra, pernicious anaemia, kwashiorkor)

Blood diseases
> Acute leukaemia
> Agranulocytosis
> Aplastic anaemia
> Purpura

Immunosuppression
> Acquired immunodeficiency syndrome (AIDS)
> Chemotherapy

Drugs
> Phenytoin
> Lead, mercury and bismuth poisoning

Debility
> Tuberculosis
> Carcinomatosis

infection (*Borrelia vincenti*) and is often known as **Vincent's angina**.

The **gums are swollen**, inflamed, painful and peppered with small ulcers that are covered by a **yellow slough**. These changes may spread to the tonsils, the fauces and the buccal mucosa.

The gums bleed, there is excessive salivation and a marked foetor oris.

The cervical lymph glands are enlarged and tender.

The patient feels ill, has a fever and loss of appetite.

Gangrenous stomatitis
(Cancrum oris)

Gangrenous stomatitis is now a rare condition except in countries with a high incidence of starvation. It is an uncommon but not rare complication of measles and other specific fevers in malnourished children, and it is occasionally seen in a child with leukaemia.

It begins as an area of **oedema** and **induration** on the lip, which becomes **ischaemic** and **necrotic**. The area of necrosis spreads steadily, and as the dead tissue separates so the contours of the mouth and face are destroyed.

The process is extremely painful, and the patient is very ill with anorexia, prostration and a pyrexia.

Angular stomatitis
(Perlèche)

This term describes inflamed, red-brown fissures at the corners of the mouth. Its common cause is the dribbling of saliva in this area, which follows overclosure of the bite caused by loss of the teeth. Most elderly edentulous patients have some degree of angular stomatitis.

A similar condition occurs in children who rub and lick the corners of their mouth.

The cracks may become infected by *Candida albicans*.

Rhagades is the name given to the small radiating cracks in the corners of the mouth that develop in patients in the **secondary stage of syphilis** (see below). They are sore and uncomfortable, and when they heal they leave fine linear scars.

Syphilis

All three stages of syphilis can cause abnormalities in the mouth.

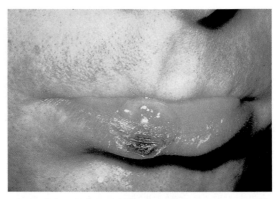

FIG 10.7 Primary chancre of the lower lip.

1. **Primary syphilis**: chancre on the lip or tongue.
2. **Secondary syphilis**: 'snail-track' ulcers, mucous patches, Hutchinson's wart.
3. **Tertiary syphilis**: gummata, chronic superficial glossitis, gummatous parenchymal infiltration.

Primary (Hunterian) chancre

The features of a primary chancre on the lip are similar to those of one on the genitalia (see also page 338).

The initial lesion is an elevated but flat, pink, painless macule. This grows slowly into a hemispherical papule, the mucosal covering of which breaks down to leave a superficial, slightly painful ulcer. The ulcer may be covered with a thick crust.

The papule and its base are rubbery hard and discrete.

The lymph glands in the neck become enlarged and tender 1–2 weeks after the appearance of the lump.

Ultimately, the ulcer heals, the lump dissolves and the only permanent remnant is a fine superficial scar.

Chancres are highly contagious.

The mucous patch

Mucous patches are grey-white or pearl-coloured, raised patches which appear on the inside of the lips and cheeks and on the pillars of the fauces. They vary in size from 3 to 20 mm in diameter. The whiteness is caused by oedema and desquamation of the epithelium. When the grey patch of dead epithelium separates, the underlying mucosa is left raw and bleeding.

Mucous patches are highly contagious.

The patient's main complaint is of a sore throat.

'Snail-track' ulcers

'Snail-track' ulcers are long, narrow ulcers which are covered with transparent glistening mucus or a white boggy epithelium which makes them look like snail tracks. They are commonly seen on the pillars of the fauces.

They form from the coalescence of a number of small mucous patches.

Gummata

Gummatous degeneration may be nodular or infiltrating. A gumma of the tongue presents as a painless, hard, discrete mass, while parenchymal infiltration makes the tongue big, stiff and irregular. Gummata in the hard palate and nasal septum can cause perforation of these structures and collapse of the bridge of the nose. Both varieties affect the tongue. Gummata of the lips and cheeks are uncommon.

Gummata also develop in the hard palate and nasal septum, causing perforations and collapse of the bridge of the nose.

A gumma in the tongue presents as a painless, hard, discrete mass. It usually develops in the anterior two-thirds of the tongue and, unless there is a history of syphilis or other physical signs of the disease, is indistinguishable from an interstitial carcinoma or a secondary deposit.

Gummatous parenchymal infiltration makes the tongue big, stiff, thick and irregular.

Hutchinson's wart

This is a mid-line condyloma of the tongue. A condyloma is an area of hypertrophic epithelium, broad based and flat topped. It is highly contagious.

Chronic superficial glossitis

This condition is commonly caused by syphilis. Its final stage is leukoplakia, which is a pre-cancerous condition. Its other causes are described below.

Chronic superficial glossitis

This is a condition in which a sequence of chronic inflammatory, degenerative and hypertrophic changes occur in the tongue, which terminate in the development of a carcinoma.

The causes of chronic superficial glossitis are usually remembered as six Ss:

- syphilis
- smoking
- sharp tooth
- spirits
- spices
- sepsis.

However, the only conditions which can be definitely incriminated are syphilis and recurrent trauma from a tooth or pipe. The role of the other factors is open to doubt.

History

Age The conditions which predispose to the development of glossitis need to be present for many years before they have any effect. Thus most patients with this disease are over the age of 50 years.

Sex More men are affected than women.

Symptoms The patient has remarkably few symptoms. The condition is not painful and does not interfere with eating. The common complaint is that the tongue has become shiny or white, or developed a lump.

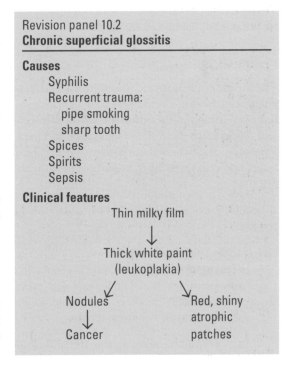

Revision panel 10.2
Chronic superficial glossitis

Causes
Syphilis
Recurrent trauma:
pipe smoking
sharp tooth
Spices
Spirits
Sepsis

Clinical features
Thin milky film
↓
Thick white paint
(leukoplakia)
Nodules ↙   ↘ Red, shiny
↓   atrophic
Cancer   patches

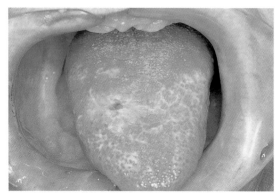

The early stage, when the tongue is covered with a transparent grey film and loses its papillae.

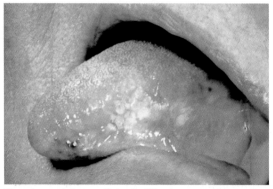

The advanced stage, with hard white plaques, nodules and fissures.

FIG 10.8 CHRONIC SUPERFICIAL GLOSSITIS.

Examination

The surface of the tongue passes through a series of changes as the epithelium thickens. The prickle cell layer hypertrophies (**acanthosis**) and swollen cells with nuclei reach the surface (**spongiosis** and **parakeratosis**). These changes are **patchy**, and all clinical stages may coexist on different parts of the tongue.

First stage The first abnormality is the appearance of a thin, grey, transparent film on a part of the tongue.

Second stage This thin film turns opaque and white. This is **leukoplakia**. Young leukoplakia looks like fresh, soft, semi-matt paint. Old leukoplakia cracks, fissures and gets slightly yellow so that it looks like old, cracking, wrinkled, white gloss paint.

Third stage Beneath the white patches the epithelium becomes hyperplastic. Small nodules and warty

outgrowths appear, which may eventually become overt carcinomata.

The areas of very active cellular division are visible as smooth, red, shiny patches.

Fourth stage The fourth stage is the appearance of clinically detectable carcinomata. The lesions have all the features of a primary carcinoma of the tongue.

Many small cancers may appear together and the cervical lymph glands may be enlarged. Change identical to that of chronic superficial glossitis can occur on the lips and any part of the buccal mucosa – cheek, gums and palate. Leukoplakia of the lips and cheeks is now more common than leukoplakia of the tongue.

Carcinoma of the lip

Carcinoma of the lip is no longer common in Great Britain since the reduction of the incidence of syphilis and leukoplakia of the lip. The factors that produce pre-malignant changes in the epithelium of the lip are leukoplakia and its causes, and recurrent trauma from pipes and prolonged exposure to sunlight.

Since the reduction in the incidence of syphilis, exposure to sunlight, especially the ultraviolet part of sunlight, is the commonest cause of carcinoma of the lip.

History

Age Most of the patients with carcinoma of the lip are over the age of 60 years.

Sex Men are affected more often than women.

Occupation It is particularly common in men with outdoor occupations and is sometimes called 'countryman's lip'; but remember that there are many men with outdoor occupations living in towns.

Ethnic group Negroes are less susceptible but not immune to diseases induced by sunlight.

Geography All sunlight exposure conditions are more common in countries with a tropical or semi-tropical climate and populated by white Caucasians, such as Australia.

Symptoms When the pre-malignant changes are developing in the lip, the patient complains of blistering,

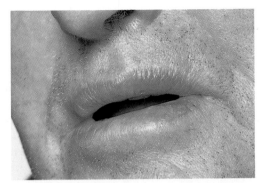

Solar keratoses on the lower lip – a pre-malignant change.

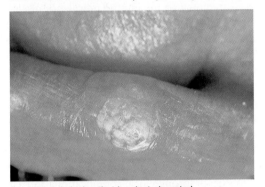

A small, early lesion that has just ulcerated.

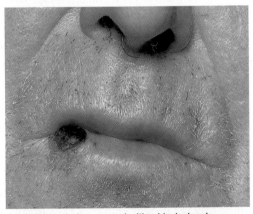

An ulcerating lesion covered with a black slough.

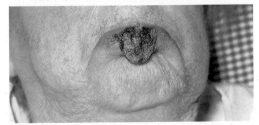

A large proliferating and infiltrating carcinoma distorting the whole lower lip.

FIG 10.9 CARCINOMA OF THE LIP.

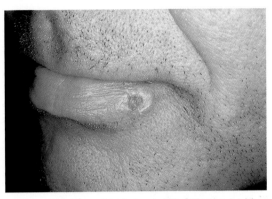

FIG 10.10 Carcinoma of the lip in a habitual pipe smoker. The lesion developed where he used to rest his pipe.

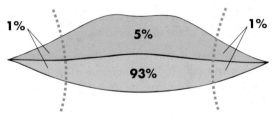

FIG 10.11 The distribution of carcinoma of the lips.

thickening (**keratosis**), and white patches (**leuko-plakia**).

A carcinoma causes a **lump**, or an **ulcer** which fails to heal.

As the ulcer grows it interferes with speech and eating, **bleeds** and produces an **offensive discharge**, but is not always painful.

The patient may notice **lumps under their chin**. Although small lumps and sore spots on the lips are common, be suspicious of any lump that does not heal quickly.

Previous history It is important to ask about previous diseases, especially syphilis and conditions caused by exposure to sunlight.

Habits Ask if the patient smokes a pipe. Carcinoma of the lip was common when clay pipes were popular.

Examination

Position The lower lip is affected over ten times more often than the upper lip. Carcinoma in the angle of the lips is uncommon. The lesion is usually to one side of the mid-line.

Colour The skin over the lump or round the ulcer may show evidence of a pre-malignant condition: blistering, thickening and pigmentation, or white boggy patches.

Tenderness A cancer of the lip, nodular or ulcerative, is **not always tender**. The absence of tenderness should alert your suspicions because most ulcers in the mouth are very painful and tender.

Shape The cancer starts as a small lump or nodule, which ultimately ulcerates in its centre and develops the typical everted edge of a carcinoma.

The initial lesion is small, just a few millimetres across, but can become large if not treated.

Edge Once the lump has ulcerated, the edges proliferate and evert. They are red and, at their junction with the base of the ulcer, bleed easily.

Base The base is covered with a thin, soft, friable, grey-yellow slough. It is a mixture of dying tissue and inflammatory exudate. It is thin because the ulcer is repeatedly rubbed by the tongue.

Depth The ulcer is initially shallow, but can erode deep into the lip, destroying the epithelium and the underlying muscle.

Discharge The discharge is thin, watery and slightly blood stained. It is usually infected but rarely purulent.

Relations The lump is invariably fixed to the subcutaneous structures of the lip but can be moved, with the lip, separately from the jaw. Only very advanced lesions are fixed to the gum and jaw.

Lymph drainage The lymph glands draining the diseased portion of the lip are likely to be enlarged by secondary infection, if not by tumour.

- The lymph draining from the upper lip passes across the face and over the angle of the jaw to the upper deep cervical glands.
- Lymph from the centre of the lower lip drains to the submental glands and then to the lower deep cervical glands.
- Lymph from the lateral third of the lower lip drains to the lymphoid tissue overlying and sometimes within the submandibular gland, and then to the middle deep cervical lymph glands.
- Lymph from the angle of the mouth drains into the lymphatics of both lips.

If the lymph glands contain metastases, they will be hard and discrete. If the enlargement is caused by secondary infection, they will be slightly tender.

Surrounding tissues Away from the ulcer, the rest of the lip is usually normal or mildly affected by the predisposing causes of cancer already mentioned.

General examination Disseminated distant metastases are rare.

Carcinoma of the tongue

Like carcinoma of the lip, the prevalence of carcinoma of the tongue has fallen in parallel with the reduction in the prevalence of syphilis, and there is no longer a high incidence of the disease in males.

The important pre-malignant disease of the tongue is chronic superficial glossitis, especially when it has reached the leukoplakia stage. Thus the causes of chronic superficial glossitis, already described, are the causes of carcinoma of the tongue.

Carcinoma of the tongue spreads locally and causes death through local complications and aspiration or obstructive pneumonia. Distant blood-borne metastases are a late and uncommon event.

History

Age The patients are usually over the age of 50 years. The peak incidence is between 60 and 70 years.

Sex Males were affected far more than females when syphilis and pipe smoking were common. Now there are almost as many women affected as men.

Symptoms The commonest complaint is of a **painless lump** or **irregularity** on the surface of the tongue.

If the early lesion is ignored or not noticed, the patient may not present until they have an enlarging ulcer causing **pain in the tongue** (sometimes **referred to the ear**), **excessive salivation, difficulty with mastication and swallowing**, and **foetor oris**.

If the lesion has spread extensively before it is noticed, it may cause immobility of the tongue (**ankyloglossia**) and difficulty with speech.

Lesions on the back of the tongue may alter the quality of the voice.

Alternatively, the patient may present with a **lump in the neck** (enlarged lymph glands) before they notice any abnormality in the tongue.

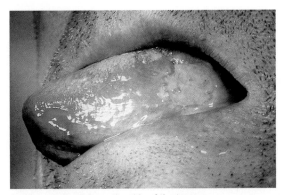

An ulcerated nodule on the side of the tongue.

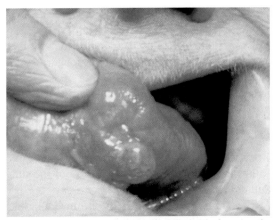

A nodular carcinoma of the tongue.

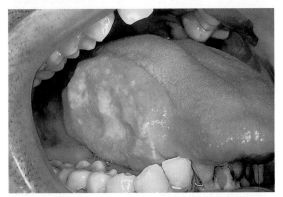

A large ulcer with an everted edge on the side of the tongue.

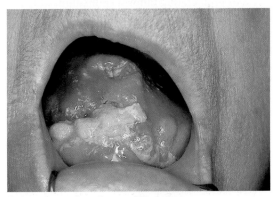

A very advanced carcinoma of the tongue.

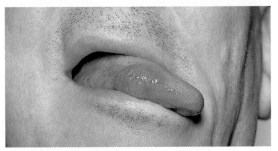

Not all nodules are primary lesions. This one was a metastasis from a carcinoma of the bronchus.

FIG 10.12 CARCINOMA OF THE TONGUE.

Previous history Ask about previous venereal disease, or any trouble with the teeth or dentures that may have caused chronic trauma.

Habits Ask if the patient smokes, or has smoked, a pipe.

Examination

Position Carcinomata of the tongue are most common on the edge and the lateral surface of the tongue, 20 per cent occur in the posterior third, 20 per cent on the dorsum and tip, and 10 per cent on the under-surface.

Colour The epithelium and papillae over a deep-seated lump look normal, but if the lesion is near the surface, the epithelium loses its papillae and looks smooth, shiny and stretched. Ulcers are usually covered with a transparent, yellow-grey slough.

Tenderness The lump, or ulcer, is not tender.

Shape, size and composition Carcinomata of the tongue may present in four forms: an ulcer, a nodule, a papilliferous or warty nodule, or a fissure in an area of induration.

A **carcinomatous lump** tends to be ovoid, with its long axis parallel to the mid-line of the tongue. It may vary in size from a small nodule to a mass 2–5 cm across. It feels hard and has an **indistinct edge** where it is spreading into the rest of the tongue.

A **carcinomatous ulcer** of the tongue usually has the typical features of a carcinoma: a florid, friable, bleeding, everted edge, a sloughing yellow-grey base, a thin serous discharge and induration of the surrounding tissues.

The **papilliferous** or **warty carcinoma** looks like any other papilloma in that it is covered with an excess of proliferating filiform epithelium, which is usually paler than the surrounding pink epithelium, but the **base is broad and firm** and the area of tongue from which it arises is indurated. It may be of any size, but rarely juts out far from the tongue because of the restriction of the mouth.

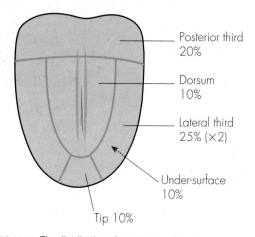

Posterior third 20%

Dorsum 10%

Lateral third 25% (×2)

Under-surface 10%

Tip 10%

FIG 10.13 The distribution of carcinoma of the tongue.

Revision panel 10.3
The causes of ulceration of the tongue

Aphthous ulcer
Trauma (dental)
Non-specific glossitis
Chancre
Gumma
Tuberculosis
Carcinoma

The **fissure in an area of carcinomatous induration** is a rare form of tongue cancer. It is a modified form of the nodule which has spread so diffusely that it does not have a detectable edge. The fissure may be a cleft in the tongue that has deepened and lost its epithelium, or a deep linear ulcer.

Relations It is very important to examine the floor of the mouth, the gums, jaw, tonsils and fauces, because a carcinoma can spread into any of these structures, and once it has done so, its treatment becomes much more difficult.

Lesions on the side or under-surface of the tongue are more likely to spread into the floor of the mouth than lesions on the dorsum.

Spread to the floor of the mouth causes thickening of the tissues and reduces the mobility of the tongue. Infiltration of the gum and jaw fixes the tumour to the bone, and the jaw itself may be swollen. Tumours of the posterior third of the tongue spread into the tonsil and the pillars of the fauces.

Lymph drainage
- The lymph from the tip of the tongue drains to the submental glands and then to either or both jugular lymph chains.
- The lymph from the rest of the anterior two-thirds drains to the glands on the same side of the neck, usually the middle and upper deep cervical glands.
- Lymph from the posterior third drains into the ring of lymph tissues around the oropharynx and into the upper deep cervical lymph glands.

More than half of the patients who present with a cancer of the tongue have palpable cervical lymph glands, but in some cases the enlargement is caused by secondary infection, not tumour.

State of local tissues Involvement of the lingual nerve causes a pain that is referred to the ear, probably through its connections with the auriculotemporal nerve.

Infiltration of the mandible causes pain and swelling of the jaw.

The surface of the tongue around the cancer may be affected by leukoplakia, and there may be other primary tumours.

Differential diagnosis The causes of ulcers on the tongue are given in Revision panel 10.3.

OTHER CONDITIONS OF THE TONGUE

Macroglossia

Macroglossia is a large tongue. The causes of macroglossia are:

- multiple haemangiomata
- multiple lymphangiomata
- plexiform neurofibromatosis
- amyloid infiltration
- infiltrating carcinoma
- muscle hypertrophy (cretins).

Wasting of the tongue

Paralysis of the 12th cranial nerve (the hypoglossal nerve) causes disuse atrophy of one side of the tongue. When the patient is asked to 'put out your tongue', it deviates towards the paralysed side.

Tongue-tie

If the patient has a congenitally shortened frenulum, this can lead to a degree of tongue-tie. This rarely causes any significant impairment of speech, but if it is severe and remains uncorrected into late infancy, it can interfere with speech.

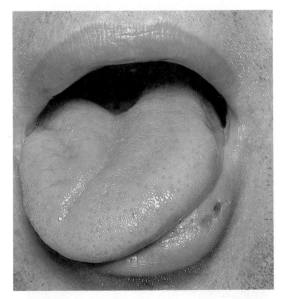

FIG 10.14 A right hypoglossal nerve palsy. When this patient was asked to protrude his tongue, it could be seen to be wasted on the right and deviated to the right.

Mucosal neuromata

In the uncommon condition of multiple endocrine neoplasia type 2b (MEN 2b), multiple mucosal neuromata can be seen, particularly on the tongue.

THE PALATE

The varieties of congenital cleft palate are described on pages 250–1.

Perforation of the palate

A perforation in the palate can be acquired if disease or trauma destroys the bones of the palate.

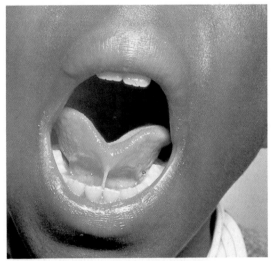

FIG 10.15 Tongue-tie: a congenitally short frenulum. This rarely causes any significant impairment of speech.

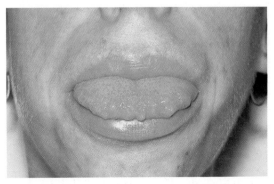

FIG 10.16 Multiple mucosal neuromata on the tongue of a patient with MEN 2b.

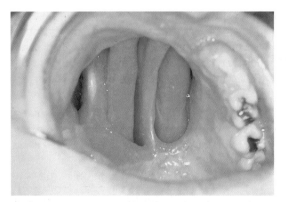

FIG 10.17 Large perforation of the palate. The nasal septum and turbinate bones are clearly visible.

When syphilis was common, perforation of the hard palate following **gummatous destruction** of the bone and mucosa was quite common. Nowadays acquired perforation of the palate is rare. It can be caused by:

- an empyema or tumour of the maxillary antrum bursting through the palate into the mouth,
- repeated trauma from poorly fitting dentures,
- surgical excision of the palate to approach the maxillary antrum.

Tumours of the palate

The mucous membrane covering the hard palate is identical to that of the rest of the buccal mucosa. Retention cysts and carcinoma, similar to those of the lips and buccal mucosa, are not uncommon.

The hard palate also contains many small glands identical in structure and function to the salivary glands.

A **pleomorphic salivary adenoma** (mixed salivary tumour – see Chapter 9) is a common cause of a lump on the palate.

The patient's sole complaint is of a lump on the palate which grows slowly but steadily.

If it is not treated, it can fill the arch of the palate and make speech and eating difficult.

On examination, the lump feels smooth and hard. The overlying mucous membrane is not attached to it and if the lump is small, it can be moved over the underlying palate. As the tumour grows it becomes less mobile and more difficult to distinguish from a tumour growing in or above the palate.

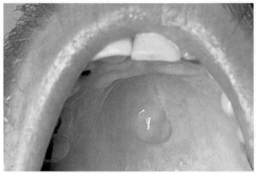

A small pleomorphic adenoma of a salivary gland on the hard palate.

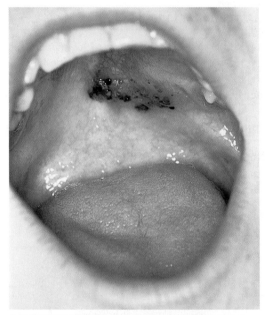

A malignant melanoma of the hard palate. This is a rare condition, but is included as a reminder that malignant melanoma can arise at the mucocutaneous junctions, i.e. around the mouth and anus.

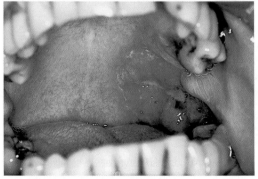

A carcinoma on the side of the hard palate.

FIG 10.18 TUMOURS OF THE HARD PALATE.

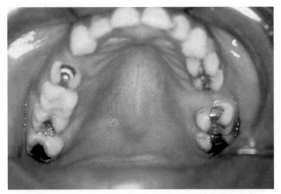

A mid-line bony spur of the hard palate, recognizable by its mid-line cleft, known as a torus palatinus.

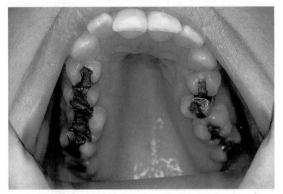

The high-arched palate of Marfan's syndrome.

FIG 10.19

THE TONSILS

Tonsillitis is a condition familiar to all because almost everyone has suffered it. It causes a sore throat and pain during swallowing. On examination, the tonsils are seen to be enlarged and red, with pus exuding from their crypts. The surrounding pillars of the fauces, soft palate and oropharynx are also red and tender, and may be covered with small yellow-based ulcers.

Bilateral enlargement of the tonsils, together with the above signs, is diagnostic of tonsillitis.

Unilateral enlargement of a tonsil, even if it is red and tender, is not always caused by acute tonsillitis. Remember the other causes described below.

Carcinoma of the tonsil

Carcinoma of the tonsil occurs in the elderly. The enlarging tonsil and deep infiltration by the tumour

cells may cause **severe pain** in the throat, which is **referred to the ear**.

The surface of the growth eventually ulcerates to form a deep indolent ulcer, rarely with everted edges, which **bleeds**, causes **severe dysphagia** and a pungent **foetor oris**. The cervical lymph glands often become involved and enlarged at an early stage of the disease.

Lymphoma of the tonsil

Lymphoma of the tonsil occurs in late-middle and old age. In contrast to carcinoma it causes a **painless swelling**. The patient's only complaints are the sensation of a **lump in the back of the mouth and throat** and sometimes mild **dysphagia**.

Gross swelling may interfere with speech and make the words indistinct.

Enlargement of the cervical lymph glands occurs at a late stage of the disease.

Both carcinomatous and lymphomatous tonsils can become infected. Acute tonsillitis in the elderly is not common, so be on your guard and search for an underlying cause.

Peritonsillar abscess
(Quinsy)

This is an abscess, lateral to the tonsil, which pushes the tonsil towards the mid-line and makes it look enlarged. It is a very painful condition. Opening the mouth and swallowing saliva is particularly painful.

The diagnosis rests on observing a red bulge in the anterior pillar of the fauces, tender cervical lymph glands, fever and tachycardia.

THE FLOOR OF THE MOUTH

Ranula

A ranula is a large mucus-containing cyst in the floor of the mouth. The mucus probably comes from acini of the sublingual gland which have ruptured in response to secretory back-pressure secondary to an obstruction of the sublingual duct, or direct injury.

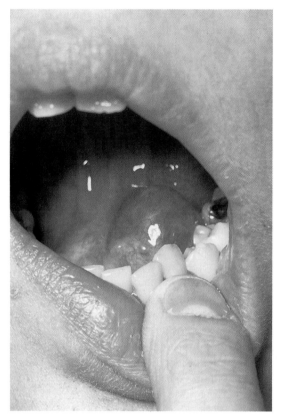

FIG 10.20 A ranula: a tense, translucent, spherical swelling just below the mucosa of the floor of the mouth.

Ranula is the Latin for a small frog. It is said that the swelling was given this name by Hippocrates because he thought it looked like the belly of a frog; but when the patient opens their mouth and the swelling bulges up under the tongue, it looks more like the air-filled swelling under the jaw of a frog when it croaks.

History

Age Ranulata appear most often in children and young adults.

Sex Both sexes are equally affected.

Symptoms The patient complains of a swelling in the floor of the mouth, which has grown gradually over a few weeks.

Some ranulata fluctuate in size, and some swell suddenly and become painful, but they rarely get big enough to interfere with eating or speech.

Examination

Position The swelling lies in the floor of the mouth, between the symphysis menti and the tongue, just to one side of the mid-line.

Colour The lump has a characteristic semi-transparent grey appearance. The colour and the site are the diagnostic features.

Tenderness The swelling is not tender.

Shape Ranulata form spherical cysts, but only the top half is visible.

Size They vary from 1 to 5 cm in diameter.

Surface Their surface is smooth, but their edge is difficult to feel because they are deep within the arch of the mandible.

Composition The swelling is soft, usually fluctuant and transilluminates, but it cannot be compressed or reduced.

Relations The overlying mucosa is not fixed to the wall of the cyst and the cyst is not fixed to the tongue or the jaw.

The swelling is usually closely related to the duct of the submandibular salivary gland (Wharton's duct), which may be seen running over its surface or alongside it.

Ranulata occasionally extend through the mylohyoid muscle into the neck. This variety is called a **plunging** ranula.

Lymph drainage The cervical lymph glands should not be enlarged.

Local tissues These should all be normal.

Sublingual dermoid cyst

When the face and neck are formed by the fusion of the facial processes, a piece of epidermis may get trapped deep in the mid-line just behind the jaw, and later form a sublingual dermoid cyst.

Such cysts are in the mid-line, but may be above or below the mylohyoid muscle.

History

Age The swelling is usually noticed when the patient is between the ages of 10 and 25 years.

Sex Both sexes are equally affected.

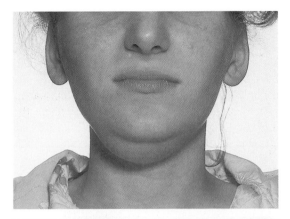

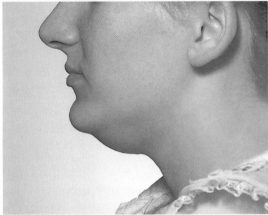

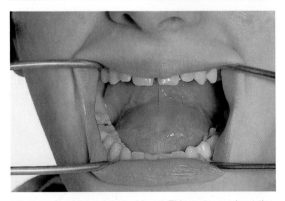

FIG 10.21 A sublingual dermoid cyst. This cyst was above the mylohyoid muscle but large enough to cause a visible swelling below the chin.

Symptoms The patient complains of a swelling under the tongue or just below the point of the chin.

It may appear suddenly, when it is usually painful, or gradually. It is otherwise symptomless. Very rarely, the contents become infected and the cyst becomes tense and painful.

Examination

Position The lump is easily visible, either in the centre of the floor of the mouth between the tongue and the point of the jaw, or bulging down below the chin, looking like a double chin.

Colour The mucous membrane of the mouth and the skin beneath the chin overlying the lump are normal.

Tenderness Sublingual dermoid cysts are not tender.

Shape The cyst is clearly spherical, even though its whole surface cannot be felt.

Size By the time these cysts are noticed they are 2–5 cm across.

Surface The surface is smooth.

Edge The edge is clearly defined.

Composition The lump feels firm, but bimanual palpation reveals that it fluctuates.

These cysts do not usually transilluminate, as their contents are often opaque. They cannot be compressed or reduced.

Relations Sublingual dermoid cysts can be **felt bimanually**, with a finger in the mouth and one beneath the chin.

When the tongue is lifted up, the supramylohyoid variety bulges into the mouth.

If the tongue is pushed against the roof of the mouth with the teeth clenched, the submylohyoid variety bulges out below the chin.

Neither variety is attached to the covering buccal mucosa or skin, or the tongue, but the proximity of the tongue muscles and jaw limits their mobility.

Local tissues The nearby tissues should all be normal.

Lymph drainage The local lymph glands should not be enlarged.

Stone in Wharton's duct

Stones and infection in the submandibular gland and duct are common (see page 239). When such a stone migrates forwards to the mouth of the submandibular duct (Wharton's duct), it forms a lump in the floor of the mouth (see Fig. 9.3, page 241). The lump bulges slightly into the mouth, is tender and, through the surrounding oedema, the centre may feel hard.

Sometimes the surface of the stone can be seen through the open end of the duct.

The submandibular gland is usually swollen and tender.

THE GUMS

Retention cysts, carcinomata and salivary tumours can arise from the mucous membrane that covers the jaw, but there are some swellings which are peculiar to the gum. They are called **epulitides**, but this is just a special name to indicate the site of the lump, not its pathology.

An epulis is a swelling that arises from the alveolar margin of the jaw. It can originate from the bone, the periosteum or the mucous membrane.

Fibroma

The commonest variety of epulis is the **fibrous epulis**. This is a fibroma that arises from the gingival tissues, so forming a firm nodule at the junction of gum and tooth. It may bulge out and become polypoid in shape.

Fibrosarcoma

A **fibrosarcomatous epulis** is the malignant variety of the fibrous epulis. It grows rapidly, is soft and friable, and very rare.

Granuloma

A **granulomatous epulis** is a pyogenic granuloma of the mucosa of the gum. It is usually associated with gingivitis or dental caries.

Bone tumour

A **bony epulis** is usually caused by an osteoclastoma (giant cell tumour). Although the underlying mass is hard, the gum covering the mass becomes hyperaemic and oedematous, and may bleed and ulcerate.

Carcinoma

Carcinoma of the gum presents as a lump or an ulcer. It is usually recognizable as a carcinoma, so the description used in some books – carcinomatous epulis – is confusing and inappropriate.

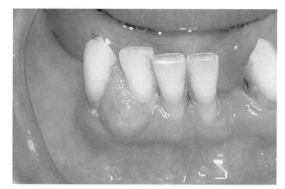

A fibrous epulis.

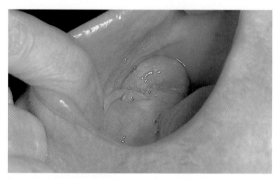

A pyogenic granuloma or granulomatous epulis.

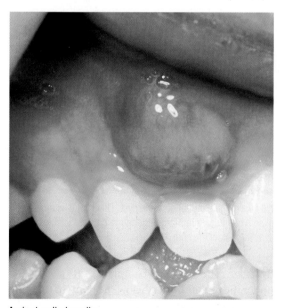

A giant-celled epulis.

FIG 10.22 SWELLINGS OF THE GUM.

SWELLINGS OF THE JAW

Alveolar (dental) abscess

The commonest cause of swelling of the jaw is a dental or alveolar abscess. This is an abscess which forms at the base of the root of a decaying tooth and tracks outwards, through the external surface of the mandible or maxilla, to form an abscess beneath the cheek or jaw.

History

Age An alveolar abscess can develop at any age, with the first or the second dentition.

Symptoms The patient complains of a constant dull ache in the jaw, which gets gradually worse and becomes throbbing in nature.

Soon after the onset of the pain, a swelling appears which is very tender.

There is often sweating, general malaise and loss of appetite.

Previous history The patient may know that they have bad teeth, having had toothache and avoided dental care.

Examination

Position Most alveolar abscesses point to the labial (outer) side of the jaw. Those in the lower jaw also point downwards to the inferior margin of the mandible.

An abscess which points to the lingual (inner) surface causes a swelling on the palate or between the mandible and the tongue.

Colour The overlying skin or mucosa is reddened by the inflammatory hyperaemia.

Temperature and tenderness The swelling is hot and acutely tender.

Shape The abscess takes the form of a flattened hemisphere, but its edges merge into the surrounding tissues, so it does not have a clear-cut shape or edge.

Surface The surface is indistinct.

Composition It is difficult to assess the composition of the swelling because it is so tender.

The deep part of the mass feels firm, but the overlying tissues may be soft and boggy with oedematous fluid. Large abscesses may fluctuate.

Relations The mass is clearly fixed to, and feels as if it is part of, the underlying bone.

The skin and mucosa move freely over the lump until they become involved in the oedema or the inflammatory process. The precise relations depend upon the site of the abscess. The commonest site is

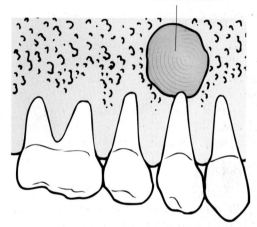

Cyst attached to the root of a tooth

FIG 10.23 The site of origin of a dental cyst.

Revision panel 10.4
The causes of swelling of the jaw

Infections
    Alveolar (dental) abscess
    Acute osteomyelitis
    Actinomycosis
Cysts
    Dental cysts
    Dentigerous cysts
    Other odontogenic cysts and cystic tumours
Neoplasms
Benign
    Fibrous dysplasia
    Giant cell granuloma
    Odontogenic tumours
Locally invasive
    Adamantinoma
Malignant
    Osteogenic sarcoma
    Malignant lymphoma (Burkitt's tumour)
    Secondary tumours (by direct invasion or bloodstream spread)

the posterior part of the lower jaw in relation to caries in the molar teeth or failure of their eruption.

An alveolar abscess in the upper jaw, pointing medially, causes swelling of the palate and fauces.

Lymph drainage The upper cervical lymph glands are usually enlarged and tender.

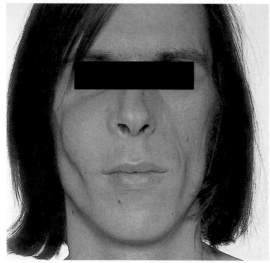

A large dental cyst expanding the maxilla and bulging into the roof of the mouth.

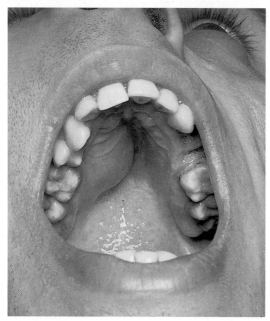

The palate crackled when it was palpated because the bone was so thin.

FIG 10.24

Local tissues The arteries and nerves of the face, jaw and tongue should be normal. There may be visible evidence of neglect of the teeth, such as caries and gingivitis, and there may be unerupted teeth. If an alveolar abscess points and discharges, it may become a chronic discharging sinus.

THE JAW

Cysts of the jaw

Swelling of the whole jaw may be caused by infection, a cyst or a tumour. These are classified in Revision panel 10.4.

There are two common benign cysts of the jaw.

Dental cyst

This is a cyst attached to the root of a normally erupted but usually decayed and infected tooth.

The epithelial cells that form the cyst are thought to be derived from the enamel organ.

These cysts are more common in the upper jaw. They grow steadily, expanding the jaw and filling the maxillary antrum.

Clinical examination can get no further than detecting that the swelling is in the bone. Sometimes the bone is so thin that it 'crackles' when touched, like a broken eggshell.

Dentigerous cyst

A dentigerous cyst is a cyst containing an unerupted tooth.

The cyst can enlarge and cause swelling of the jaw.

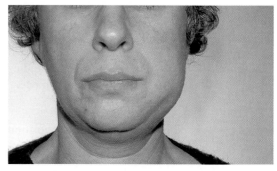

FIG 10.25 A dentigerous cyst causing swelling at the angle of the mandible.

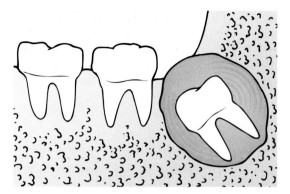

FIG 10.26 A dentigerous cyst.

Tumours of the jaw

Many types of benign and malignant tumours of the jaw are listed in Revision panel 10.4. They all present as a bony swelling that grows steadily, and usually painlessly.

Four neoplastic causes of swelling of the jaw deserve special mention.

Carcinoma of the antrum

Carcinomata of the antrum are much more common than primary bone tumours, and when they invade downwards into the maxilla they cause swelling of the upper jaw and palate.

Adamantinoma

Adamantinoma is a tumour which causes a painless, progressive swelling of the jaw, but it is locally invasive and tends to recur.

Osteosarcoma

Osteosarcomata can occur in both the upper and the lower jaw.

Malignant lymphoma
(Burkitt's lymphoma)

Burkitt's lymphoma is a malignant tumour of B lymphocytes associated with Epstein–Barr virus infection. In 80 per cent of patients it presents as a tumour in the jaw. In its endemic form it affects children below the age of 12 years and occurs in those areas of sub-Saharan Africa and the coastal regions of New Guinea that have a warm, wet climate and endemic malaria. It is believed that the latter causes immune depression of T suppressor cells, which permits the uncontrolled proliferation of Epstein–Barr-virus-infected B cells to form the tumour. Sporadic cases of Burkitt's lymphomata also occur throughout the world.

The child presents with a progressive, painless swelling of the jaw which distorts the face, may displace the eye and partially occludes the mouth.

Lymphomatous tissue may also be present in the retroperitoneal tissues, kidneys, ovaries and spine, where it may cause abdominal and skeletal symptoms.

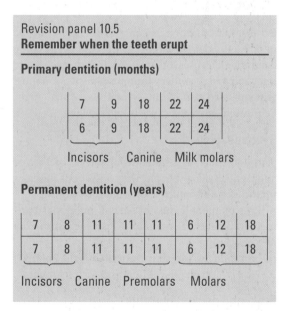

Revision panel 10.5
Remember when the teeth erupt

Primary dentition (months)

7	9	18	22	24
6	9	18	22	24

Incisors   Canine   Milk molars

Permanent dentition (years)

7	8	11	11	11	6	12	18
7	8	11	11	11	6	12	18

Incisors   Canine   Premolars   Molars

THE HISTORY AND EXAMINATION OF SWELLINGS IN THE NECK

The majority of surgical conditions which arise in the neck present as a swelling. Taking the history and performing the physical examination should follow the standard pattern, but there are some important features that deserve special attention.

The history of swellings in the neck

Because the commonest cause of a swelling in the neck is an enlarged lymph gland, and because the commonest causes of enlarged lymph glands are infection and secondary tumour deposits, you must remember to ask about symptoms which might help you identify the cause of the swelling.

Systemic illness

Symptoms such as general malaise, fever and rigors and contact with people with infectious diseases may indicate an infective cause of the swelling.

Loss of appetite, loss of weight, pulmonary, alimentary or skeletal symptoms may suggest the site of a neoplasm.

Irritation of the skin associated with enlarged cervical lymph glands is often seen with lymphoma.

Head and neck symptoms

Ask about: pain in the mouth, sore throats or ulceration; nasal discharge, pain or blockage of the airway; pain in the throat, dysphagia, changes in the voice and difficulty with breathing; and lumps or ulcers on the skin of the head and face that have changed size or begun to bleed.

The skin, mouth, nose, larynx and pharynx are common sites for neoplasms, and although head and neck cancers commonly present with metastases in lymph glands, they are not usually associated with the symptoms of distant metastases such as general malaise and loss of weight.

The examination of swellings in the neck

Site

It is essential to define the site of a lump in the neck.

The neck is divided into two triangles. The **anterior triangle** is bounded by the anterior border of the sternomastoid muscle, the lower edge of the jaw and the mid-line. In clinical practice, the structures deep to the sternomastoid muscle are considered to be inside the anterior triangle.

The upper part of the anterior triangle, below the jaw but above the digastric muscle, is sometimes called the digastric or submandibular triangle.

The **posterior triangle** is bounded by the posterior border of the sternomastoid muscle, the anterior edge of the trapezius muscle and the clavicle.

To define the triangles it is necessary to get the patient to tense the neck muscles.

- The **sternomastoid muscle** is made to contract by putting your hand under the patient's chin

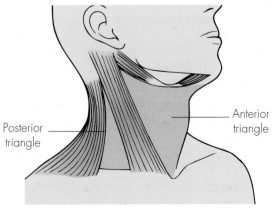

FIG 11.1 The anatomical triangles of the neck.

Posterior triangle

Anterior triangle

and asking them to nod their head against the resistance of your hand. This tightens both sternomastoids.

■ The **trapezius muscle** is made to contract by asking the patient to shrug (elevate) their shoulders against resistance.

Relation to muscles

Always feel lumps in the neck with the muscles relaxed and then with them contracted. If the lump is deep to a muscle, it will become impalpable when the muscle contracts.

Relation to the trachea

Swellings that are fixed to the trachea will move when the trachea moves. The trachea is pulled upwards during swallowing. Assess the relationship to the trachea of every lump in the neck by watching to see if it moves with the trachea during swallowing.

Relation to the hyoid bone

The hyoid bone moves only slightly during swallowing, but ascends when the tongue is protruded. Ask the patient to open their mouth. When the jaw is still, ask them to protrude their tongue. If the swelling in the neck moves as the tongue protrudes, it must be fixed to the hyoid bone.

CERVICAL LYMPHADENOPATHY AND OTHER NECK SWELLINGS

Causes of cervical lymph gland enlargement

Enlargement of the cervical lymph glands is the most common cause of a swelling in the neck. Even when only one gland is palpable, the adjacent glands are invariably diseased.

The four main causes of cervical lymph gland enlargement are as follows.

■ **Infection**: non-specific tonsillitis, glandular fever, toxoplasmosis, tuberculosis, cat scratch fever.
■ **Metastatic tumour** from the head, neck, chest and abdomen.
■ **Primary reticuloses**: lymphoma, lymphosarcoma, reticulosarcoma.
■ **Sarcoidosis**.

The diagnosis of lymphadenopathy caused by systemic illnesses such as glandular fever, toxoplasmosis and sarcoidosis depends upon finding lymphadenopathy elsewhere, other evidence of the underlying disease, and special blood tests.

Non-specific cervical inflammatory lymphadenopathy

Non-specific reactive lymphoid hyperplasia can follow any inflammatory process or be associated with skin conditions, particularly of the scalp, when it is termed dermatopathic lymphadenopathy. However, non-specific inflammatory lymphadenopathy

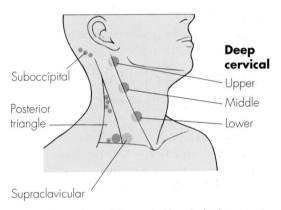

FIG 11.2 The anatomy of the cervical lymph glands.

Suboccipital
Posterior triangle
Supraclavicular
Deep cervical
Upper
Middle
Lower

Revision panel 11.1
Causes of cervical lymphadenopathy

Infection
    Non-specific
    Glandular fever
    Tuberculosis
    Syphilis
    Toxoplasmosis
    Cat-scratch fever (*Rochalimaea henselae*)
Metastatic tumour
    From head, neck, chest and abdomen
Primary reticuloses
    Lymphoma
    Lymphosarcoma
    Reticulosarcoma
Sarcoidosis

commonly follows recurrent bouts of tonsillitis, especially if the attacks have been treated inadequately. The upper deep cervical glands are most often affected.

In a healthy child, small normal lymph glands are often palpable, especially in the posterior triangle.

History

Age When associated with tonsillitis, the majority of patients are below the age of 10 years. Other reactive conditions can occur at any age.

Symptoms The common presenting symptom is a **painful lump** just below the angle of the jaw.

The severity of the pain varies. It is usually a discomfort, which becomes acute when the patient has a **sore throat**.

The lump may be large enough to be **visible** or **felt** by the child's parent when washing the neck.

The child may **snore** at night, have **difficulty in breathing**, have **nasal speech** because of tonsillar and adenoid hyperplasia, and suffer from recurrent **chest infections**.

Cause The child and the parents frequently appreciate the relationship between the appearance of the lump and an episode of tonsillitis.

Systemic effects When the lump is tender the patient often feels ill, has a sore throat and pyrexia and does not want to eat.

Recurrent severe episodes can cause loss of weight and slow down the rate of growth and body maturation.

Social history Recurrent sore throats and upper respiratory tract infections are more common in malnurtured children living in substandard, cold, damp houses.

Examination

Position Lymph from the tonsils drains to the upper deep cervical lymph glands. The gland just below and deep to the angle of the mandible is often called the **tonsillar gland**. This gland and those just below it are likely to be enlarged.

Tenderness If the infection is active, the enlarged glands will be tender.

Shape and size The tonsillar gland is usually spherical and approximately 1–2 cm in diameter. It is rarely bigger than this. The glands below it are usually smaller, even when inflamed.

Composition and relations Each gland is firm in consistence, solid and discrete, not fixed but not very mobile.

Local tissues The tonsils are likely to be enlarged and hyperaemic. Pus may be seen exuding from the surface crypts.

The glands on the other side of the neck are often just as large but may not have been noticed by the parents.

General examination Look for the presence of enlarged lymph glands elsewhere. None should be enlarged.

Recurrent chest infections may have damaged the lungs – look for collapsed lobes, bronchiectasis and lung abscess. However, these are rare complications nowadays.

Tuberculous cervical lymphadenitis and abscess

The **human** tubercle bacillus can enter the body via the tonsils, and from there move to the cervical lymph glands. The upper deep cervical glands are most often affected. There is no generalized infection, so there is little systemic disturbance of health. Infection with bovine tuberculosis ceased in the UK when the control and testing of dairy cattle was introduced.

History

Age and ethnic groups Tuberculous lymphadenitis is common in children and young adults, and in the elderly. In the UK the incidence in the young has diminished since the introduction of *Bacilli*

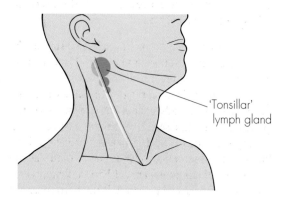

FIG 11.3 The site of the 'tonsillar' lymph gland.

Calmette–Guerin (BCG) vaccination, mass radiography screening and the discovery of effective anti-tuberculosis antibiotics; but the prevalence of cervical lymph gland enlargement caused by anonymous mycobacteria is increasing. In the UK, tuberculous lymphadenitis is found most often in young immigrant adults.

Symptoms The patient complains of a **lump in the neck**. This appears gradually, sometimes with, sometimes without, pain.

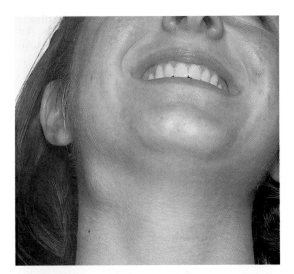

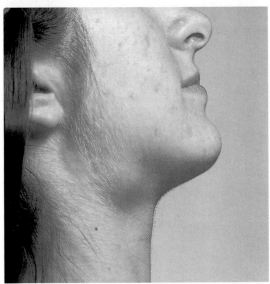

FIG 11.4 Enlargement of the upper deep cervical lymph glands caused by tuberculosis.

The **pain** can be intense if the glands grow rapidly and necrose.

Systemic symptoms are unusual in the young, but the elderly sometimes have anorexia and slight weight loss.

If the glands break down into an abscess, the swelling **increases in size**, becomes more **painful** and the patient notices **discolouration of the overlying skin**.

When the glands are very painful, neck movements and swallowing may be painful.

Previous history Elderly patients often have a history of swollen neck glands when young – sometimes treated at that time by surgical excision.

Immunization Ask whether the patient has been vaccinated with BCG.

Family history Check that no one in the family has had tuberculosis.

Social history Tuberculosis is more common in the poor and socially underprivileged.

Examination
The signs of tuberculous lymphadenitis

Position The upper and middle deep cervical glands are most often involved.

Temperature The mass of glands does *not* feel hot.

Tenderness Although the temperature of the skin is normal and the glands are often slightly tender, pain and tenderness are not prominent features of tuberculous lymphadenitis.

Colour If there is no abscess present, the overlying skin should look normal.

Shape, size and consistence In the early stages, the glands are firm, discrete and between 1 and 2 cm in diameter.

As caseation increases and the glands necrose, the infection spreads beyond the capsules of the glands. This makes the lumps enlarge and coalesce.

A typical patch of tuberculous lymphadenitis is an **indistinct, firm mass** of glands which occupies the upper half of the deep cervical lymph chain, partly beneath and partly in front of the sternomastoid muscle.

The glands are commonly described as **matted together**, but there may be some discrete glands above or below the matted mass.

Local tissues Other cervical lymph glands may be palpable. The tonsils and the other tissues in the neck should be normal.

The signs of a tuberculous abscess

When an infected lymph gland caseates and turns into pus, it becomes, by definition, an abscess. The natural tendency of an abscess is to weaken the overlying tissues until it bursts through them, ultimately to reach and burst through the skin. This is known as **pointing**. At the stage when a tuberculous abscess

has burst through the deep cervical fascia into the subcutaneous tissues, it has two compartments, one on either side of the deep fascia, connected by a small central track. This is called a **collar-stud abscess**.

Position Because a tuberculous abscess forms in tuberculous lymph glands, it is most often found in the upper half of the neck.

Colour When the pus reaches the subcutaneous tissues, the overlying skin turns reddish-purple.

Temperature The skin temperature is normal because the process of caseation and pus formation is slow and does not stimulate excessive hyperaemia – hence the name **cold abscess**.

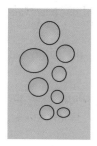 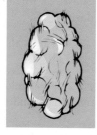 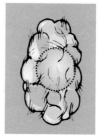 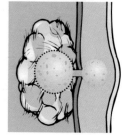

Enlarged discrete glands

'Matted' glands

Abscess forms in the centre of the glands

Abscess bursts through the deep fascia and becomes 'collar-stud' in shape

The development of a 'collar-stud' abscess.

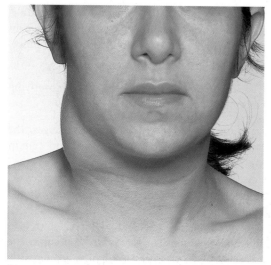 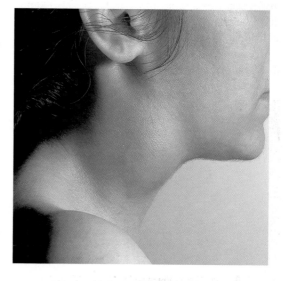

A large tuberculous 'collar-stud' abscess.

FIG 11.5 THE TUBERCULOUS ABSCESS.

Tenderness The mass is tender, sometimes exquisitely so if the abscess is tense.

Shape The deep part of the abscess tends to be sausage shaped, with its long axis parallel to the front edge of the sternomastoid muscle. The superficial pocket of the abscess is usually lower than the deep part.

Size Most tuberculous abscesses are 3–5 cm across, but they can be much larger.

Surface The surface is irregular and indistinct.

Edge The edges are moderately well defined if the abscess is tense, but you will not be able to feel a definite surface or edge if the pocket of pus is lax.

Composition The abscess feels firm and rubbery and if there is sufficient pus present, it will **fluctuate**. This latter sign cannot be elicited if the abscess is small and deep to the sternomastoid muscle.

The subcutaneous part of a collar-stud abscess should be clearly fluctuant, but it is not usually possible to reduce the superficial pocket of pus into the deep pocket.

Relations The original abscess is deep to the deep fascia, partly under the sternomastoid muscle, and fixed to surrounding structures. The superficial part of a collar-stud abscess is immediately below the skin and becomes more prominent when the sternomastoid muscle is contracted. If spontaneous discharge occurs, a chronic sinus may form. Tuberculous sinuses are characterized by minimal erythema and lack of pain, unless secondarily infected.

The other lymph glands in the neck near the abscess may be enlarged.

General examination When the patient has tuberculous lymphadenitis there are often no systemic abnormalities; but when a tuberculous abscess develops there may be tachycardia, pyrexia, anorexia and general malaise.

There may be signs of tuberculosis in the lungs, in other lymph glands and in the urinary tract.

Carcinomatous lymph glands

Metastatic deposits of cancer cells in the cervical lymph glands are the commonest cause of cervical lymphadenopathy in adults.

The primary cancer is most often in the buccal cavity (tongue, lips and mucous membrane) and larynx, but every possible primary site must be examined when cervical glands are thought to be enlarged by secondary deposits.

History

Age Most head and neck cancers occur in patients over the age of 50. Most patients presenting with metastatic deposits in their cervical lymph glands are between 55 and 65 years.

The exception is papillary carcinoma of the thyroid, which occurs in **children** and **young adults**.

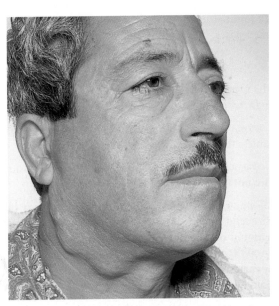

FIG 11.7 This patient presented with hard, enlarged lymph glands in the neck. The primary lesion was the insignificant mole above his right eyebrow.

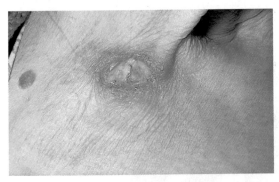

FIG 11.6 A chronic tuberculous sinus that has become secondarily infected.

Sex Most of the head and neck cancers are more common in men than in women.

Local symptoms The patient complains of a **painless lump** in the neck, which they have seen or felt by chance.

It is uncommon for carcinomatous glands to be tender or to become so large that they interfere with neck movements before being noticed.

The lump **grows slowly**, and **new lumps may appear**.

General symptoms The patient may have symptoms from a primary lesion in the head or neck, such as a sore tongue or a hoarse voice. If the primary is in the chest, they may have a cough or haemoptysis; if it is in the abdomen, they may have dyspepsia or abdominal pain.

Generally speaking, head and neck cancers do not cause anorexia and weight loss, whereas cancers in the lungs and intra-abdominal organs do.

Examination

Site The site of the affected glands gives a crude indication of the site of the primary. Lesions above the hyoid bone drain to the upper deep cervical glands. The larynx and thyroid drain to the middle and lower deep cervical glands. An enlarged supra-clavicular lymph gland commonly indicates intra-abdominal or thoracic disease. When enlarged by metastases, this gland is called **Virchow's gland**; its presence is *Troisier's sign*.

Colour The overlying skin is a normal colour unless the mass is so large that it stretches or infiltrates the skin, which makes it pale or blotchy red.

Temperature The skin temperature will be normal unless the tumour is very vascular.

Tenderness Glands containing secondary deposits are **not tender**.

Shape and size Glands containing metastases vary in size and shape. Both features depend upon the amount of tumour within them and the rate of its growth. At first the glands are **smooth, discrete** and a **variety of sizes**. As they grow, they may coalesce into one large mass.

Composition Glands containing tumour are **hard**, often stony hard. Rarely, a very vascular tumour deposit will be soft, pulsatile and compressible.

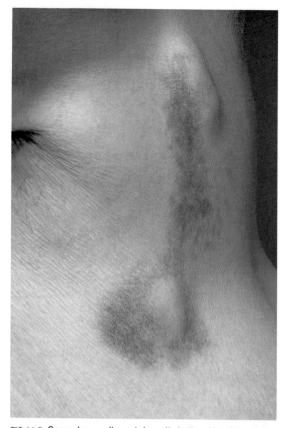

FIG 11.8 Secondary malignant deposits in the skin of the neck.

Relations The glands are tethered to the surrounding structures, so they can usually be moved in a transverse direction, but not vertically.

Their relation to the sternomastoid muscle varies according to the group to which they belong. Secondary cancer is more common in the glands of the anterior than the posterior triangle. These glands are deep to the anterior edge of the sternomastoid.

If the tumour spreads beyond the capsules of the glands, the mass becomes completely fixed.

Local tissues The overlying skin and muscle may be infiltrated with tumour, in which case the tumour must be distinguished from secondary deposits actually in the skin.

Lymph drainage Other lymph glands on the pathway between the primary lesion and the gland complained of by the patient, and beyond it, may be enlarged.

General examination Examine all the sites which might contain the primary lesion, in particular:

- the skin of the scalp, the ear and the external auditory meatus,
- the lips, tongue, buccal mucous membrane and tonsils,
- the nose, maxillary antra and nasopharynx,
- the thyroid gland,
- the skin of the upper limb,
- the breasts,
- the lungs,
- the stomach, pancreas, ovaries and testes.

The symptoms and signs of malignant disease originating in these organs are discussed in the appropriate chapters.

Some of this examination requires special instruments, for example a head mirror and light and a laryngeal mirror.

Primary neoplasms of the lymph glands
(Reticuloses, lymphoma)

The most common primary tumour of lymphoid tissue is the malignant lymphoma. There are many histological varieties of lymphoma, but they are often collectively and loosely divided into **Hodgkin's** and **non-Hodgkin's lymphoma**.

History

Age The reticuloses are common in children and young adults.

Sex Males are affected more often than females.

Symptoms The most common presenting symptom is a **painless lump** in the neck, which is noticed by chance and **grows slowly**.

Malaise, **weight loss** and **pallor** are common symptoms.

Itching of the skin (pruritus) is an unexplained but distinctive complaint.

There may be **fever with rigors**, occurring in a periodic fashion (Pel–Ebstein fever).

Lymphomatous infiltration of the skeleton may cause **pains in the bones**, and there may be **abdominal pain after drinking alcohol**.

If there are large masses of lymph glands in the mediastinum, they may occlude the superior vena

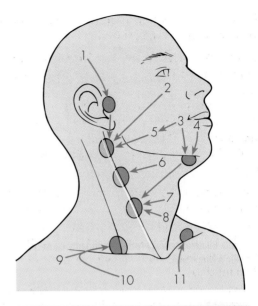

1. Scalp (sometimes via the preauricular node)
   Parotid gland
   Upper face
   Ear
2. Maxillary antrum and other air sinuses
   Nasal cavity and nasopharynx
3. Tongue
   Buccal mucosa
   Floor of mouth
   Mandible
4. Lips
5. Tonsil
   Base of tongue
   Oropharynx
6. Submandibular gland
   Skin of neck
7. Larynx and laryngopharynx
8. Thyroid
   Upper oesophagus
9. Upper limb and both sides of the chest wall
10. Breast
11. Lungs, stomach and all the viscera

FIG 11.9 Sites of primary neoplasms that metastasize to the cervical lymph glands.

cava, causing **venous congestion in the neck** and the development of collateral veins across the chest wall.

Large masses in the abdomen can obstruct the inferior vena cava and cause oedema of both legs.

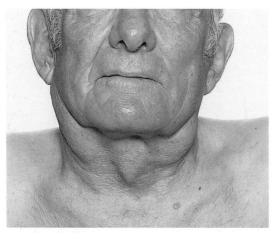

FIG 11.10 Bilateral cervical lymphadenopathy caused by Hodgkin's lymphoma.

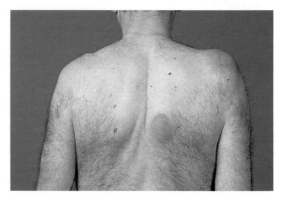

FIG 11.11 Cutaneous deposits of lymphoma.

Examination

Site Any of the cervical lymph glands can be affected. Lymphoma is one of the few conditions, apart from infection, that often causes lympha-denopathy in the **posterior triangle**.

Tenderness The glands are **not tender**.

Shape, size and surface The lymph glands in Hodgkin's disease are ovoid, **smooth** and **discrete**.

It is possible to define individual glands even when they become large. This is the opposite to

---

Revision panel 11.2
Plan of examination for source of secondary cervical lymphadenopathy

(Start at the top and work downwards.)
Examine the **skin** of the scalp, face, ears and neck.
Look in the **nose**.
Look in the **mouth** at the tongue, gums, mucosa and tonsils.
Palpate the parotid, submandibular and thyroid glands.
Examine the arms and the chest wall – including the breast.
Examine the abdomen and genitalia.
Transilluminate the air sinsuses.
Examine the nasopharynx and larynx with mirrors.

---

tuberculosis, in which the lymph glands become matted and indistinct.

Consistence Glands infiltrated by lymphoma are solid and **rubbery** in consistence.

Relations Although tethered to nearby structures, these glands can usually be moved from side to side and rarely become completely fixed.

Local tissues The surrounding tissues should be normal.

General examination **Other groups of lymph glands** may be enlarged. The **liver and spleen** may be palpable. The patient is often **anaemic** and may be **jaundiced**.

Spread to the skin produces elevated, reddened, scaly patches of skin known as **mycosis fungoides**.

Branchial cyst

A branchial cyst is a remnant of a branchial cleft, usually the second cleft. It is therefore lined with squamous epithelium, but there are also patches of lymphoid tissue in the wall which are connected with the other lymph tissue in the neck and which can become infected.

History

Age Although these cysts are present at birth, they may not distend and cause symptoms until adult life. The majority present between the ages of 15 and 25 years, but a number appear in the 40s and 50s.

Sex Males and females are equally affected.

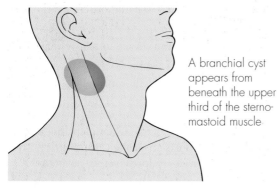

A branchial cyst appears from beneath the upper third of the sterno-mastoid muscle

FIG 11.12 The site of a branchial cyst.

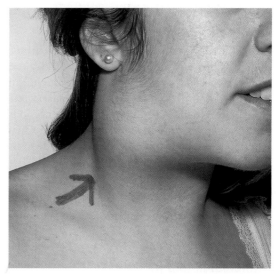

FIG 11.14 A large branchial cyst which had become painful. This commonly follows recurrent bouts of tonsillitis, especially if the infection has been treated inadequately.

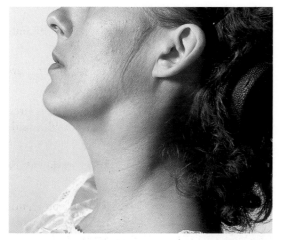

FIG 11.13 A branchial cyst which presented in adult life. The back of the swelling is clearly deep to the sternomastoid muscle.

Symptoms The common presenting complaint is a **painless swelling** in the upper lateral part of the neck.

The lump may be painful when it first appears and later cause attacks of pain associated with an increase in the size of the swelling. The pain is usually caused by infection in the lymphoid tissue in the cyst wall.

A severe throbbing pain, exacerbated by moving the neck and opening the mouth, develops if the contents of the cyst become infected and purulent.

General effects These cysts have no systemic effects and are not associated with any other congenital abnormality.

Examination

Position A branchial cyst lies behind the anterior edge of the upper third of the sternomastoid muscle, and

bulges forwards. Very rarely, the cyst can bulge backwards behind the muscle.

Colour and tenderness The overlying skin may be reddened and the lump may be tender if the cyst is inflamed.

Shape The cyst is usually ovoid, with its long axis running forwards and downwards.

Size Most branchial cysts are between 5 and 10 cm long.

Surface Their surface is smooth and the edge distinct.

Composition The consistence varies with the tension of the cyst. Most cysts are hard, but a lax cyst feels soft. They are dull to percussion.

The lump **fluctuates**. This sign is not always easy to elicit, especially if the cyst is small and the sternomastoid muscle thick.

The lump is usually **opaque** because it contains desquamated epithelial cells that make its contents thick and white. Sometimes the fluid is golden yellow and shimmers with fat globules and cholesterol crystals secreted by the sebaceous glands in the epithelial lining. Such cysts may transilluminate.

The cyst cannot be reduced or compressed.

Relations It is important to ascertain that the bulk of the mass is deep to the upper part of the sternomastoid muscle. It is not very mobile because it is closely tethered to the surrounding structures.

Lymph drainage The local deep cervical lymph glands should not be enlarged. If they are palpable, you should reconsider your diagnosis in favour of an inflammatory process such as a tuberculous abscess rather than a branchial cyst. The other cystic lesions that are often operated upon as presumed branchial cysts are often secondary cystic lymph gland deposits from a papillary carcinoma of the thyroid.

Local tissues The local tissues should be normal.

If the cyst has turned into an abscess, the surrounding tissues will be oedematous and the skin hot and red.

Branchial fistula (or sinus)

This is a rare congenital abnormality. It is the remnant of a branchial cleft, usually the second cleft, which has not closed off.

The patient complains of a small dimple in the skin at the junction of the middle and the lower third of the anterior edge of the sternomastoid muscle, that discharges clear mucus, and sometimes becomes swollen and painful and discharges pus.

When the whole branchial cleft stays patent, the fistula connects the skin with the oropharynx, just behind the tonsil. In most cases the upper end is obliterated and the track should really be called a **branchial sinus**.

Swallowing accentuates the openings on the skin.

Carotid body tumour

This is a rare tumour of the chemoreceptor tissue in the carotid body. It is therefore a **chemodectoma**. It is usually benign, but can become quite large and, occasionally, malignant.

History

Age Chemodectomata commonly appear in patients between the ages of 40 and 60 years.

Symptoms The common presentation is a **painless, slowly growing lump**. The patient may notice that the lump pulsates, and may also suffer from symptoms of **transient cerebral ischaemia** (blackouts, transient paralysis or paraesthesia). These symptoms are unusual because the increasing compression of

the carotid artery by the tumour is a very slow process.

Development The lump grows so slowly that many patients ignore it for many years.

Multiplicity Carotid body tumours may be bilateral.

Examination

Always be especially gentle when palpating a lump close to the bifurcation of the carotid artery. Pressure in this area can induce a vasovagal attack.

Position The carotid bifurcation is at, or just below, the level of the hyoid bone. Carotid body tumours

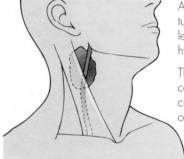

A carotid body tumour should be level with the hyoid cartilage

The external carotid artery may cross the surface of the tumour

FIG 11.15 The site of a carotid body tumour.

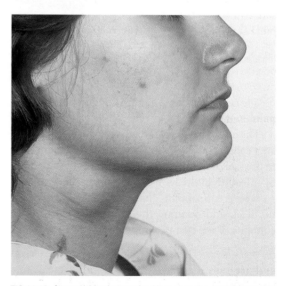

FIG 11.16 A carotid body tumour. Note that the visible mass is lower than that of a branchial cyst (see Fig. 11.13) but indistinguishable on inspection from an enlarged cervical lymph gland. Most carotid body tumours are initially mistaken for enlarged lymph glands.

are therefore found in the upper part of the anterior triangle of the neck, level with the hyoid bone and beneath the anterior edge of the sternomastoid muscle.

Tenderness, colour and temperature These tumours are not tender or hot, and the overlying skin should be normal.

Shape The lump is initially spherical but, as it grows, it becomes irregular in shape, often narrower at its lower end, where it is caught at the bifurcation of the common carotid artery.

Size Carotid body tumours may vary from 2–3 cm to 10 cm in diameter.

Composition The majority of these tumours are **solid** and **hard**. They are dull to percussion and do not fluctuate. They are often called **potato tumours** because of their consistence and shape.

Sometimes these tumours **pulsate**. This is either a transmitted pulsation from the adjacent carotid artery, or a palpable external carotid artery running over the superficial aspect of the lump, or a true expansile pulsation from a soft or very vascular tumour.

It is surprising that in spite of their vascularity most of these tumours are hard. Those which are soft and very vascular not only have an expansile pulsation, but can also be **compressed**.

Relations The lump is deep to the cervical fascia and beneath the anterior edge of the sternomastoid muscle.

The common carotid artery can be felt below the mass, and the external carotid artery may pass over its superficial surface. Without this close relationship to the arteries, this tumour is indistinguishable from an enlarged lymph gland.

Because of their intimate relationship with the carotid arteries, these tumours can be moved from side to side but not up and down.

Cystic hygroma
(Lymph cyst, lymphocele, lymphangioma)

A cystic hygroma is a congenital collection of lymphatic sacs which contain clear, colourless lymph. They are probably derived from clusters of lymph channels that failed, during intra-uterine development, to connect with and become normal lymphatic pathways. Lymph cysts commonly occur near the root of the arm and the leg (i.e. in the anatomical junction between the limbs and head and the trunk).

History

Age The majority of cystic hygromata present at birth or within the first few years of life, but they occasionally stay empty until infection or trauma in adult life causes them to fill up and become visible. Occasionally large lymphoceles can be seen in elderly patients.

Symptoms The only symptom is the complaint about the **lump**, but the parents of an affected child are usually more concerned about the **disfigurement** caused by the cyst.

Family history This condition is not familial.

Examination

Position Cystic hygromata are commonly found around the base of the neck, usually in the posterior

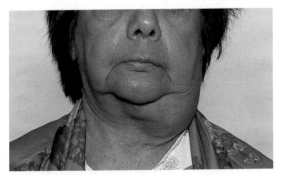

FIG 11.17 A large carotid body tumour. A very large, firm, bosselated carotid body tumour – hence the term 'potato tumour'.

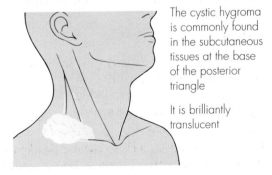

The cystic hygroma is commonly found in the subcutaneous tissues at the base of the posterior triangle

It is brilliantly translucent

FIG 11.18 The site of a cystic hygroma.

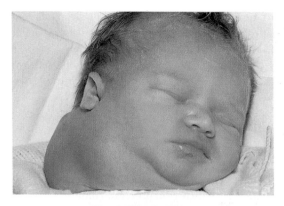

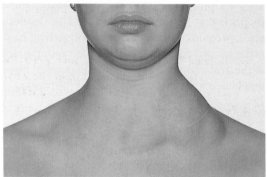

FIG 11.19 TWO EXAMPLES OF CYSTIC HYGROMA. In a very young child – the common age of presentation, and in a young adult.

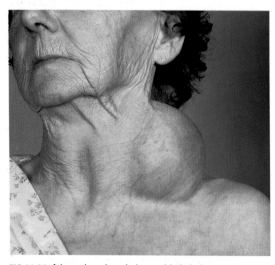

FIG 11.20 A large lymphocele in an elderly lady.

triangle, but they can be very big and occupy the whole of the subcutaneous tissue of one side of the neck.

Temperature and tenderness They are not hot or tender, and the overlying skin is normal.

Shape A cystic hygroma is a mixture of soft unilocular and multilocular cysts, so the whole mass looks **lobulated** and **flattened**.

Size The small cysts are a few centimetres across. Large cysts can extend over the whole of one side of the neck.

Surface If the cysts are close to the skin, it may not be possible to feel a distinct surface. Deep cysts feel smooth, but because they are lax their edges are often indistinct.

Composition Cystic hygromata are soft and dull to percussion. They **fluctuate** easily but, because they are close to the skin and contain clear fluid, their distinctive physical sign is a **brilliant translucence**.

Large cysts will conduct a **fluid thrill**, and in some multilocular swellings the fluid in one loculus can be **compressed** into another.

They cannot be reduced.

Relations Cystic hygromata develop in the **subcutaneous tissues**. Thus they are superficial to the neck muscles and close to the skin but are rarely fixed to the skin. However, it is essential to perform a thorough examination of the oropharynx, as a cyst in the posterior triangle may extend deeply beneath the sternomastoid muscle into the retropharyngeal space.

Lymph glands The local lymph glands should not be enlarged and, as the lymph drainage of the tissues around the cyst is normal, there is no lymphoedema. If there is associated lymphadenopathy, reconsider the diagnosis, as cystic nodal metastases of papillary thyroid carcinoma can present as large, painless cystic swellings in the neck.

Local tissues The local tissues are normal.

Pharyngeal pouch

A pharyngeal pouch is a pulsion diverticulum of the pharynx through the gap between the horizontal fibres of the cricopharyngeus below and the lowermost oblique fibres of the inferior constrictor muscle above. If swallowing is uncoordinated so that the sphincter-like fibres of the cricopharyngeus do not relax, the weak unsupported area just above these fibres (known as **Killian's dehiscence**) bulges out.

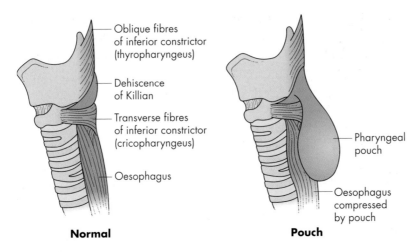

- Oblique fibres of inferior constrictor (thyropharyngeus)
- Dehiscence of Killian
- Transverse fibres of inferior constrictor (cricopharyngeus)
- Oesophagus

Normal

- Pharyngeal pouch
- Oesophagus compressed by pouch

Pouch

FIG 11.21 The anatomy of a pharyngeal pouch.

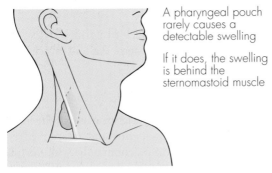

A pharyngeal pouch rarely causes a detectable swelling

If it does, the swelling is behind the sternomastoid muscle

FIG 11.22 The site of a pharyngeal pouch.

Eventually the bulge grows into a sac, which hangs down and presses against the side of the oesophagus.

History

Age Pharyngeal pouches appear in middle and old age.

Sex They are more common in men than in women.

Symptoms Patients often have a long history of halitosis and recurrent sore throats before noticing the common presenting symptom of **regurgitation of froth and food**. The regurgitated food is undigested and comes up into the mouth at any time. There is no bile or acid taste to it.

Regurgitation at night causes **bouts of coughing and choking**, and if pieces of food are inhaled, a **lung abscess** may develop.

As the pouch grows, it presses on the oesophagus and causes **dysphagia**. Patients can sometimes swallow their first few mouthfuls of food (until the pouch is full), but thereafter have difficulty in swallowing.

By the time these symptoms become severe, the patient may have noticed a **swelling in the neck**, and find that pressure on the swelling causes **gurgling sounds** and regurgitation. The swelling changes in size and often disappears.

If the dysphagia continues, the patient may become **malnourished** and **lose weight**.

Examination

Position In most patients there is no palpable swelling, but when a swelling caused by a pharyngeal pouch is apparent, it appears **behind the sternomastoid muscle**, below the level of the thyroid cartilage.

Shape Its shape is indistinct because only part of its surface is palpable. It feels like a bulging deep structure.

Size Most pouches only cause a swelling of 5–10 cm diameter. The pouch is not palpable when it is smaller, so **many patients have symptoms but no abnormal physical signs**.

Surface and edge The surface is smooth, but the edge is not palpable.

Composition The lump is **soft** and sometimes **indentable**. It is dull to percussion and does not fluctuate or transilluminate.

It can be **compressed** and sometimes **emptied**. Compression may cause regurgitation. Although the mass may disappear with compression, not to return until the patient eats again, it cannot be said to have been 'reduced' according to the usual meaning of the word.

Relations A pharyngeal pouch lies deep to the deep fascia, behind the sternomastoid muscle, and is fixed deeply. Its origin from a structure behind the trachea can be appreciated during palpation, but the neck of the pouch and its attachment to the oesophagus cannot be felt.

It cannot be moved about in the neck.

Lymph glands The cervical lymph glands should not be enlarged.

Local tissues The surrounding tissues feel normal. Indeed, when the pouch is empty the whole neck feels normal.

General examination Pay special attention to the chest, as there may be an aspiration pneumonia, collapse of a lobe or a lung abscess.

Sternomastoid 'tumour'
(Ischaemic contracture of a segment of the sternomastoid muscle)

This is a swelling of the middle third of the ster-nomastoid muscle. In neonates it consists of oedema around an infarcted segment of the muscle, caused by the trauma of birth. As the patient grows, the lump disappears and the abnormal segment of muscle becomes fibrotic and contracted.

History

Age The lump is noticed at birth or in the first few weeks of life.

Symptoms The mother may notice the **lump** or that the child keeps their head turned to one side – **torticollis**. Attempts to turn the head straight may cause **pain** or **distress**.

If the muscle is not extensively damaged, the swelling slowly subsides, the muscle spasm relaxes and the torticollis disappears. If the muscle damage becomes an area of permanent fibrosis, the twist and tilt of the head to one side becomes more noticeable as the child grows.

Examination

The lump

Position The swelling lies in the middle of the ster-nomastoid muscle (i.e. in the middle third of the neck on the antero-lateral surface).

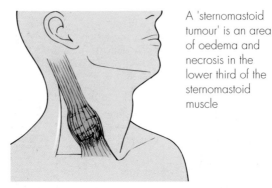

A 'sternomastoid tumour' is an area of oedema and necrosis in the lower third of the sternomastoid muscle

FIG 11.23 The site of a sternomastoid tumour.

Tenderness The lump may be tender in the first few weeks of life.

Shape and size The swelling is fusiform, with its long axis along the line of the sternomastoid muscle. It is usually 1–2 cm across.

Surface The surface is smooth.

Edge The anterior and posterior edges of the lump are distinct but the superior and inferior edges, where the lump becomes continuous with normal muscle, are indistinct.

Composition At first the lump is firm and solid and easy to feel, but as it gradually becomes harder it begins to shrink and may become impalpable.

Surrounding structures and local lymph glands These should be normal.

The neck

Examine the movements of the neck. As the child is too young to obey commands, you must watch how they move their head when lying in their cot, and then manipulate the head and neck very gently.

The sternomastoid muscles rotate and tilt the head. Contraction of the **left** sternomastoid **turns the head towards the right**, but **tilts the head to the left**. Both these deformities may be present. Forced movement to correct the deformity may cause pain and be resisted by the child.

Apart from the restriction of movement caused by spasm of the sternomastoid muscle, the neck movements should be normal.

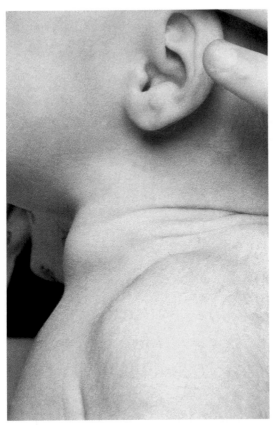

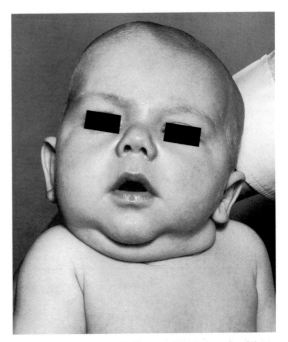

FIG 11.25 An infantile torticollis caused by ischaemia of the sternomastoid muscle.

FIG 11.24 A localized swollen segment of sternomastoid with a slight torticollis in an older child, caused by ischaemia and fibrosis of the muscle after birth. A typical sternomastoid 'tumour'.

The eyes

Look at the eyes and watch their movements to detect any **squint**. Torticollis can be a means of correcting a squint. Move the head into a vertical and central position and watch the eyes. If the torticollis is secondary to a squint and not a sternomastoid tumour, the squint will appear as the head is straightened.

The head

An uncorrected torticollis may affect the growth of the facial bones and cause facial asymmetry.

In adults, recent onset torticollis usually just represents muscle spasm.

Cervical rib

Although the cervical rib can cause serious neurological and vascular symptoms in the upper arm,

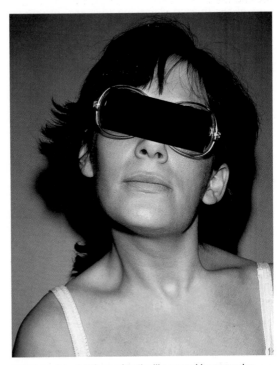

FIG 11.26 An adult form of torticollis caused by muscular spasm.

clinical examination of the neck does not usually reveal any abnormalities. The abnormal rib is usually detected with an X-ray. Sometimes there is a fullness at the root of the neck, but it is rarely distinct enough to justify a firm clinical diagnosis of cervical rib. Occasionally it can be associated with aneurysmal change in the subclavian artery.

The common neurological symptoms caused by a cervical rib are pain in the C8 and T1 dermatomes, and wasting and weakness of the small muscles in the hand. Vascular symptoms such as Raynaud's phenomenon, trophic changes, even rest pain and gangrene, may occur but are uncommon.

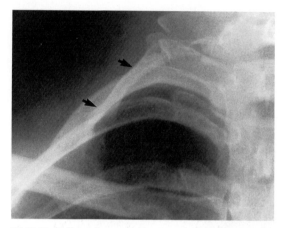

FIG 11.27 An X-ray demonstrating a cervical rib.

Thyroglossal cyst

The thyroid gland develops from the lower portion of the thyroglossal duct, which begins at the foramen caecum at the base of the tongue and passes down to the pyramidal lobe of the isthmus of the thyroid gland. If a portion of this duct remains patent, it can form a thyroglossal cyst.

Theoretically, thyroglossal cysts can occur anywhere between the base of the tongue and the isthmus of the thyroid gland, but they are commonly found in two sites: between the isthmus of the thyroid gland and the hyoid bone, and just above the hyoid bone. Thyroglossal cysts within the tongue and in the floor of the mouth are rare.

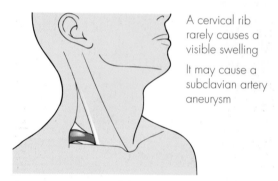

A cervical rib rarely causes a visible swelling

It may cause a subclavian artery aneurysm

FIG 11.28 The site of a cervical rib.

History

Age Thyroglossal cysts appear at any age, but the majority are seen in patients between 15 and 30 years old.

Sex They are more common in women than in men.

Symptoms The commonest symptom is a **painless lump** in a prominent and noticeable part of the neck. **Pain, tenderness** and an **increase in size** occur only if the cyst becomes infected.

Duration of symptoms The lump may have been present for many years before an increase in its size causes the patient to complain.

Systemic symptoms There are no systemic symptoms associated with this condition.

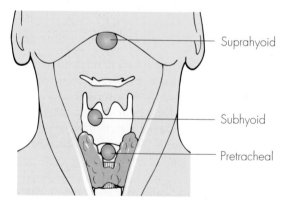

Suprahyoid

Subhyoid

Pretracheal

FIG 11.29 The sites of a thyroglossal cyst.

Examination

Position Thyroglossal cysts lie close to the mid-line, somewhere between the chin and second tracheal ring. In the fetus the thyroglossal duct is in the

Composition Thyroglossal cysts have a firm or hard consistence, depending upon the tension within the cyst. Some cysts are too tense and others too small to fluctuate, but the majority of thyroglossal cysts are between these extremes and **fluctuate** with ease. Some cysts transilluminate but many do not, either because the contents have become thickened by desquamated epithelial cells or the debris of past infection, or because they are too small.

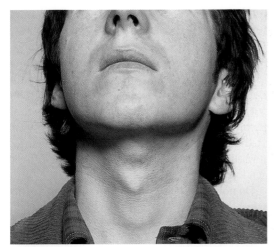

Subhyoid cyst.

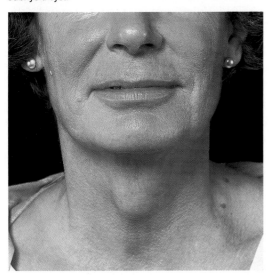

Pretracheal cyst.

FIG 11.30 TWO THYROGLOSSAL CYSTS.

mid-line, but when a cyst forms in adult life it often slips to one side of the mid-line, especially if it develops in front of the thyroid cartilage.

Colour, temperature and tenderness If the cyst is infected, the overlying skin will be red, hot and tender. When there is no infection, the overlying skin is normal.

Shape and surface Thyroglossal cysts are spherical and smooth, with a clearly defined edge.

Size They vary from 0.5 to 5 cm in diameter. Because a lump in the front of the neck is so noticeable, patients often complain of these cysts when they are very small.

Revision panel 11.3
A scheme for the diagnosis of swellings in the neck (deep to the deep fascia)

After your examination you should be able to answer four critical questions:
1. Is there one or more than one lump?
2. Where is the lump?
3. Is it solid or cystic?
4. Does it move with swallowing?

Multiple lumps are invariably *lymph glands*

A single lump

In the anterior triangle that does not move with swallowing

Solid:
- a lymph gland
- carotid body tumour

Cystic:
- cold abscess
- branchial cyst

In the posterior triangle that does not move with swallowing

Solid:
- a lymph gland

Cystic:
- cystic hygroma
- pharyngeal pouch
- occasionally a secondary deposit of a papillary thyroid carcinoma

Pulsatile:
- subclavian aneurysm

In the anterior triangle that moves with swallowing

Solid:
- thyroid gland
- thyroid isthmus lymph gland

Cystic:
- thyroglossal cyst

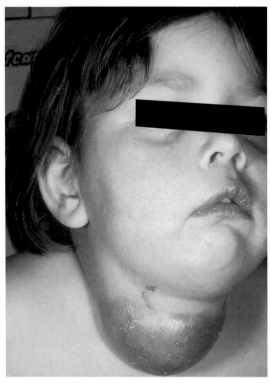

FIG 11.31 An infected thyroglossal cyst.

Relations Thyroglossal cysts are tethered by the remnant of the thyroglossal duct. This means that they can be moved sideways, but not up and down.

The thyroglossal duct is always closely related, usually fixed, to the hyoid bone. When the hyoid bone moves the cyst also moves.

The hyoid bone moves upwards when the tongue is protruded. First, ask the patient to open their mouth and keep the lower jaw still; next hold the cyst with your thumb and forefinger, and then ask the patient to protrude their tongue. If the cyst is fixed to the hyoid bone, you will feel it **tugged** upwards as the tongue goes out. This is a difficult sign to elicit.

Do not expect to see much movement. It is easier to feel the tugging sensation than to actually see the movement. Although this test is diagnostic of attachment to the hyoid cartilage, the absence of movement does not exclude the diagnosis. Indeed, this sign is absent from most cysts that are below the level of the thyroid cartilage.

Lymph glands The local lymph glands should not be enlarged unless there is secondary infection of the cyst.

Local tissues Whenever there is an abnormality of thyroid gland development, **examine the base of the tongue** for ectopic (lingual) thyroid tissue. A lingual thyroid looks like a flattened strawberry sitting on the base of the tongue.

THE THYROID GLAND

SYMPTOMS OF THYROID DISEASE

The thyroid gland can cause two groups of symptoms and signs: those connected with the swelling in the neck, and those related to the endocrine activity of the gland. Therefore, in order to appreciate fully the symptoms and signs that may be produced by diseases of the thyroid, a clear understanding of the physiology of the gland is essential. The history and examination should be directed towards detecting both local and general symptoms and signs that may be produced, either by any physical abnormality in the configuration of the thyroid or by any pathophysiological abnormality of its endocrine activity.

Neck symptoms

A lump in the neck

The majority of thyroid swellings grow slowly and painlessly. Quite often the patient will come across a swelling coincidentally when washing, or a member of their family or a close friend will point it out to them. Other swellings may have been there for some years before the patient suddenly decides to seek advice concerning their nature and management. In a few patients, a lump will appear suddenly and may be painful, or a long-standing lump may enlarge quickly.

A rapid change in the size of part of the gland, or of an existing lump, may be caused by haemorrhage into a necrotic nodule, a fast-growing carcinoma,

PHYSIOLOGY OF THE THYROID GLAND.

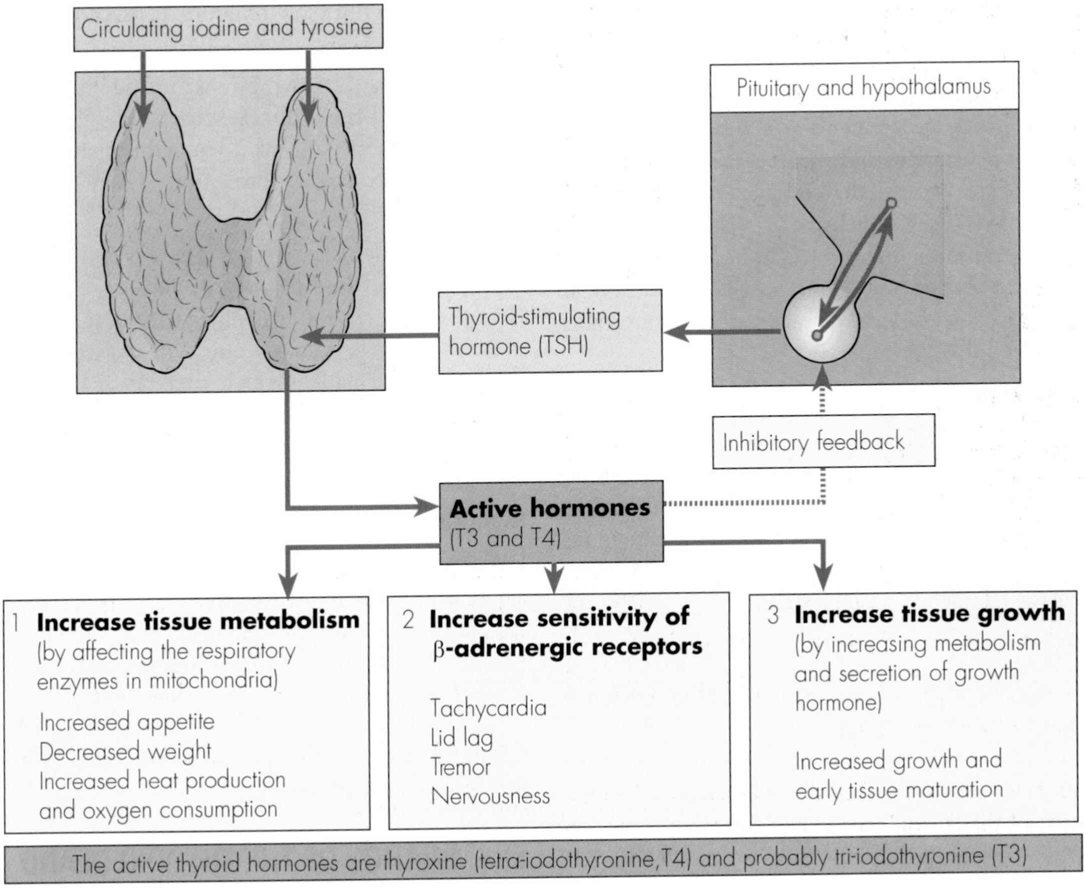

FIG 11.32

or subacute thyroiditis. The sudden enlargement of a lump caused by haemorrhage is usually painful, whereas a fast-growing anaplastic carcinoma is not usually painful until it invades nearby structures.

A special feature of papillary and follicular carcinomata of the thyroid gland is their very slow growth. They may exist as a lump in the neck for many years before metastasizing. Thus the length of

Revision panel 11.4
Physiology of the thyroid gland

Changes in hormone activity can be assessed by:
- clinical examination
- measuring circulating tri-iodothyronine (T3) and thyroxine (T4)
- measuring the rate and quantity of radioactive iodine taken up by the gland.

Hormone secretion can be suppressed by:
- iodine, which inhibits hormone release
- potassium perchlorate, which interferes with iodine trapping
- carbimazole and thiouracil, which inhibit the iodination of tyrosine and the coupling of tyrosines to make thyronines
- destroying the gland surgically or with radiotherapy.

time that a lump has been present is no indication as to its underlying nature.

Discomfort during swallowing

Large swellings may give the patient a tugging sensation in the neck when they swallow. This is not true dysphagia. Thyroid swellings rarely obstruct the oesophagus because the oesophagus is a muscular tube that is easily stretched and pushed aside. However, because the thyroid has to be pulled upwards with the trachea in the first stage of deglutition, an enlarged gland can make swallowing uncomfortable, or even difficult.

Dyspnoea

Deviation or compression of the trachea by a mass in the thyroid may cause difficulty in breathing. This symptom is often worse when the neck is flexed laterally or forwards and when the patient lies down. The whistling sound of air rushing through a narrowed trachea is called **stridor**.

Pain

Pain is not a common feature of thyroid swellings. Acute and subacute thyroiditis can present with a painful gland, and Hashimoto's disease often causes an uncomfortable ache in the neck.

Anaplastic carcinoma can cause local pain and pain referred to the ear if it infiltrates surrounding structures.

Hoarseness

A change in the quality of the voice of a patient with a lump in the neck is a very significant symptom because it is probably caused by a paralysis of one of the recurrent laryngeal nerves, which means that the lump is likely to be malignant and infiltrating the nerve.

Symptoms and signs of endocrine dysfunction

Every patient with any thyroid disorder should be a carefully questioned and examined for any symptoms or signs of endocrine dysfunction.

Symptoms and signs of thyrotoxicosis
(see also pages 299–301)

Nervous system Symptoms include nervousness, irritability, insomnia and nervous instability, and examination may reveal a tremor of the hands. Occasionally a full-blown thyrotoxic psychosis may be apparent.

Cardiovascular system Symptoms include **palpitations**, breathlessness on exertion, swelling of the ankles and chest pain, which may be manifest as tachycardia, auricular fibrillation dyspnoea and peripheral swelling.

Metabolic and alimentary systems There is an **increase in appetite but loss of weight**, and sometimes a change of bowel habit, usually diarrhoea. Proximal muscle myopathies may occur with **wasting** and **weakness**. The patient has a **preference for cold weather**, and often complains of excessive **sweating** and an intolerance of hot weather. Some women have a change of menstruation, usually **amenorrhoea**.

Symptoms and signs of myxoedema
(see also pages 301–3)

There is an **increase of weight**, with deposition of fat across the back of the neck and shoulders. Symptoms also include: **slow thought, speech and action; intolerance of cold weather; loss of hair**, especially the outer third of the eyebrows; **muscle fatigue**; a **dry skin** and 'peaches and cream' complexion; and **constipation**.

EXAMINATION OF THE THYROID GLAND

Although this should be part of the general examination, the method of examining the neck is described in detail because it is so important. The important features of the general and eye examination are also reiterated.

Concentrate upon both the nature of any gland enlargement or abnormal configuration, as well as any change in endocrine activity. It is best to assess both aspects in a combined approach, rather than try to assess each separately.

Look at the whole patient

First confirm that the swelling in the neck is in the thyroid gland by watching to see if it **moves when the patient swallows**. Then **look at the whole patient**.

Are they sitting still and composed, or fidgeting about, constantly moving their fingers and looking nervous and agitated, or are they slow and ponderous in their movements?

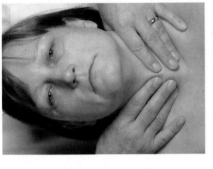

Palpate both lobes and the isthmus with the fingers flat.

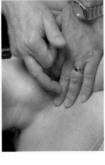

Percuss the lower limit of the gland.

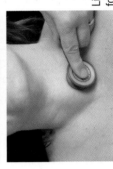

Listen over the gland for a systolic bruit.

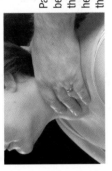

Palpate the neck from behind, with the thumbs pushing the head forwards to flex the neck slightly.

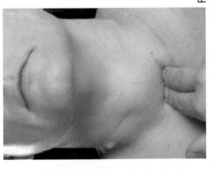

Feel the trachea.

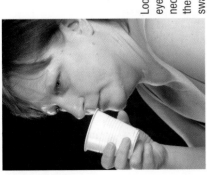

Look at the eyes and the neck and ask the patient to swallow.

If one lobe is difficult to feel, make it more prominent by pressing firmly on the opposite side.

Try to decide if there is:
- one lump
- two lumps
- diffuse enlargement

FIG 11.33 EXAMINATION OF THE THYROID GLAND.

Are they thin or fat? Where is the wasting or the fattening? Patients with thyrotoxicosis have a generalized loss of weight, especially about the face, but may also have localized wasting of their hands, face and shoulder muscles.

Are they under-clothed and sweaty, or wrapped up in a large number of jumpers but still cold?

Look at the hands

- **Feel the pulse** Tachycardia suggests thyrotoxicosis; bradycardia suggests myxoedema. In middle-aged and elderly patients thyrotoxicosis may cause atrial fibrillation.
- **Are the palms moist and sweaty?**
- **Is there a tremor?** Test for a tremor by asking the patient to hold their arms out in front of them, elbows and wrists straight, fingers straight and separated. Thyrotoxicosis causes a fine, fast tremor. If in doubt, hold out your own hand beside the patient's for comparison. A fine tremor may be accentuated by placing a sheet of paper over the fingers.

Examine the eyes

Eye symptoms

Patients who suffer from thyrotoxicosis may complain of **staring** or **protruding eyes** and **difficulty closing their eyelids** (exophthalmos), **double vision** caused by muscle weakness (ophthalmoplegia) and swelling of the conjunctiva (chemosis). They may get pain in the eye if the cornea ulcerates.

There are four important underlying changes that can occur in the eyes of patients with hyperthyroidism that produce the above effects (Figs 11.34 and 11.35). Each one may be unilateral or bilateral.

Lid retraction and lid lag

This sign is caused by over-activity of the involuntary (smooth muscle) part of the levator palpebrae superioris muscle. If the upper eyelid is higher than normal and the lower lid is in its correct position, the patient has **lid retraction**. Do not be deceived into thinking this abnormality is caused by exophthalmos.

When the upper lid does not keep pace with the eyeball as it follows a finger moving from above downwards, the patient has **lid lag**.

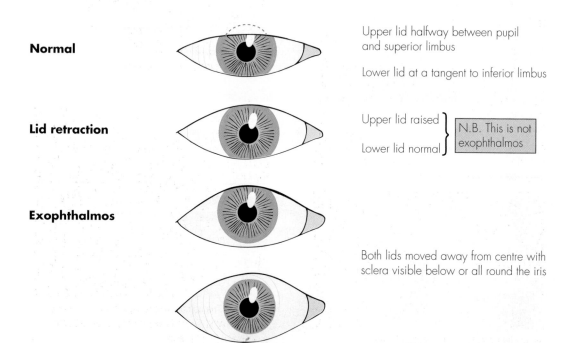

Normal

Upper lid halfway between pupil and superior limbus

Lower lid at a tangent to inferior limbus

Lid retraction

Upper lid raised
Lower lid normal
} N.B. This is not exophthalmos

Exophthalmos

Both lids moved away from centre with sclera visible below or all round the iris

FIG 11.34 The relations of the eyelids to the iris.

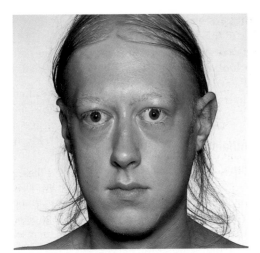

Exophthalmos.

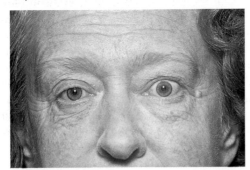

Unilateral lid retraction.

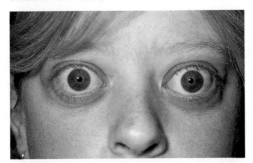

Exophthalmos and lid retraction.

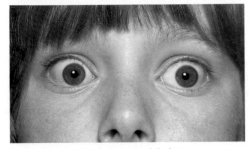

Severe lid retraction but no exophthalmos.

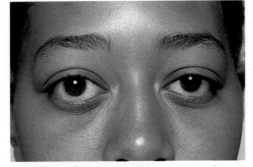

Exophthalmos but no lid retraction.

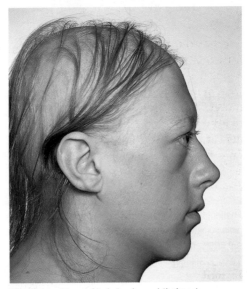

Wasting and loss of hair (and exophthalmos).

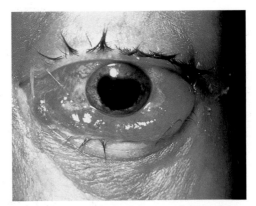

Chemosis. The conjunctiva is hyperaemic and bulging over the eyelid. There is exophthalmos, lid retraction and peri-orbital oedema.

FIG 11.35 SOME EYE SIGNS ASSOCIATED WITH THYROTOXICOSIS.

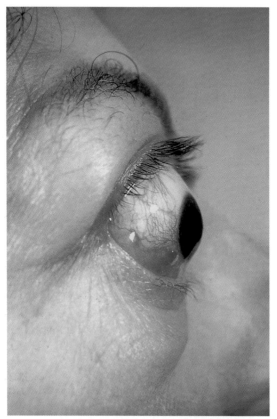

This patient had gross chemosis and exophthalmos but the eye was pulsating. The cause of these abnormalities was a carotid artery–cavernous sinus fistula.

FIG 11.35 continued

Exophthalmos

If the eyeball is pushed forwards by an increase in retro-orbital fat, oedema and cellular infiltration, the normal relationship of the eyelids to the iris is

---

Revision panel 11.5
The eye signs of thyrotoxicosis

Lid retraction and lid lag
Exophthalmos, which also causes difficulty with convergence and absent forehead wrinkling when looking upwards
Ophthalmoplegia, particularly of the superior rectus and inferior oblique muscles (cannot look 'up and out')
Chemosis

---

changed. Sclera becomes visible below the lower edge of the iris (the inferior limbus).

Because the eyes are pushed forwards, the patient can **look up without wrinkling the forehead**, but will have **difficulty converging**. In severe exophthalmos the patient cannot close their eyelids and may develop corneal ulceration.

Ophthalmoplegia

Although exophthalmos stretches the eye muscles, it does not usually affect their function. The cause of the weakness of the ocular muscles (ophthalmoplegia) associated with severe exophthalmos is oedema and cellular infiltration of the muscles themselves and of the oculomotor nerves. The muscles most often affected are the superior and lateral rectus and inferior oblique muscles. Paralysis of these muscles prevents the patient looking upwards and outwards.

Chemosis

Chemosis is oedema of the conjunctiva. The normal conjunctiva is smooth and invisible. A thickened, crinkled, oedematous and slightly opaque conjunctiva is easy to recognize.

Chemosis is caused by the obstruction of normal venous and lymphatic drainage of the conjunctiva by the increased retro-orbital pressure.

Inspect the neck

After checking that the lump is in the anatomical site of the thyroid gland, **ask the patient to swallow**. The patient may need a sip of water to help deglutition. **All thyroid swellings ascend during swallowing.**

Observe the general contours and surface of the swelling. The skin may also be puckered and pulled up by swallowing if the patient has a thyroid carcinoma which has infiltrated into the skin, although this is uncommon.

Ask the patient to open their mouth and then to **put out their tongue**. If the lump moves up as the tongue comes out, it must be attached to the hyoid bone, and is likely to be a thyroglossal cyst.

The neck veins will be distended if there is a mass obstructing the thoracic inlet.

Look at the position of the thyroid cartilage. Is it in the centre of the neck or deviated to one side?

Palpate the neck from the front

The most important part of palpation is done from behind (see below), but it is worthwhile placing your hand on any visible swelling while standing in front of the patient, to confirm your visual impression of its size, shape and surface, and to find out if it is tender. It is sometimes helpful to measure and record the circumference of the neck with a tape measure.

Check the **position of the trachea**. This is best done by feeling with the tip of two fingers in the suprasternal notch. The trachea should be exactly central at this point. When a thyroid mass extends below the suprasternal notch and obscures the trachea, you must examine the thyroid cartilage. A mass that is displacing the trachea will tilt the thyroid cartilage laterally.

Palpate the neck from behind the patient

Stand behind the patient. Place your thumbs on the ligamentum nuchae and tilt the patient's head slightly forwards to relax the anterior neck muscles. Let the palmar surface of your fingers rest on each side of the neck. They will be resting on the lateral lobes of the thyroid gland. A small lobe can be made prominent and easier to feel by pressing firmly on the opposite side of the neck.

Ask the patient to swallow while you are palpating the gland to confirm that any swelling moves with swallowing and is actually part of the thyroid. This manoeuvre also lifts up lumps that are lying behind the sternum into the reach of your fingers.

At the end of palpation you should know the following facts about the gland and/or the lump: tenderness, shape, size, surface and consistence.

A normal thyroid gland is not palpable.

Palpate the whole of the neck for any cervical and supraclavicular lymphadenopathy.

Percussion

Percussion is used to define the lower extent of a swelling that extends below the suprasternal notch by percussing along the clavicles and over the sternum and upper chest wall. This can be done when standing in front of or behind the patient. Percussion of the lump in the neck itself is rarely helpful.

Auscultation

Listen over the swelling. Thyrotoxic and vascular glands and lumps may have a systolic bruit.

General examination

Pay particular attention to the cardiovascular and nervous systems for any evidence of hyperthyroidism or hypothyroidism, the signs and symptoms of which are described on pages 299–303.

DIFFERENT FORMS OF GOITRE

Simple hyperplastic goitre

Simple enlargement of the thyroid gland is invariably caused by excess stimulation by thyroid-stimulating hormone (TSH), the production of which is stimulated by low levels of circulating thyroid hormone. Relative iodine deficiency is the commonest pathological cause for a low level of thyroid hormone production. Physiological states that require increased activity of the thyroid gland, such as puberty and pregnancy, are also associated with enlargement of the gland.

The term **colloid goitre** is used to describe the late stage of diffuse hyperplasia, when all the acini are distended with colloid which has not been released because the stimulation by TSH has dropped off.

History

Age In areas where goitre is endemic (i.e. prevalent in the local population), hyperplastic goitres appear in **childhood**.

Revision panel 11.6
Plan for the examination of a patient with a goitre

Look at the *whole patient* for agitation, nervousness or lethargy.
Examine the *hands* for sweating, tremor, tachycardia.
Examine the *eyes* for exophthalmos, lid lag, ophthalmoplegia, chemosis.
Examine the *neck*: always check that the lump moves with swallowing.
Palpate the *cervical lymph glands*.

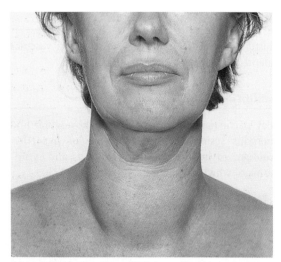

A large colloid goitre. The patient was euthyroid.

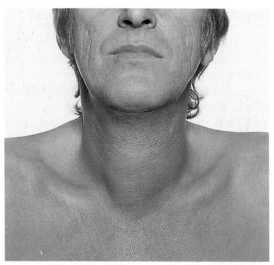

A large central solitary nodule.

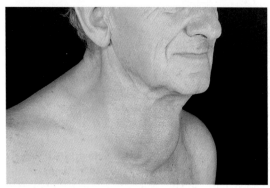

A nodular goitre extending below the sternum and causing venous obstruction. Distended veins are visible above the right clavicle. The patient was euthyroid.

Beware! Not all lumps in the neck are thyroid swellings. This mass was soft and did not move with swallowing. It was a lipoma. Never make a spot diagnosis. Examine every lump carefully and thoroughly.

FIG 11.36 VARIOUS GOITRES.

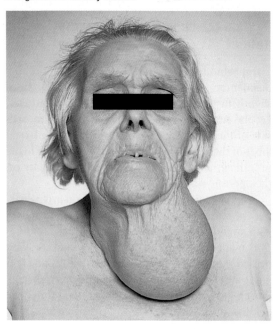

Sporadic physiological hyperplastic goitres appear at puberty, during pregnancy, and during severe illnesses and emotional disturbances, and so they are commonly seen in **puberty** and **young adult life**.

Sex Hyperplastic goitres are five times more common in women than in men.

Geography Endemic goitre is common in places where the drinking water has a low iodine content, such as the habitable valleys of the Alps, Andes, Himalayas and Rocky Mountains, and the lowland areas that depend upon water from mountain ranges, such as the Nile Valley, Congo Delta and Great Lakes of the USA. The rain that falls on the mountains has a normal iodine content, but it is filtered out by the time it reaches the springs and streams of the highland valleys.

Diet Some vegetables contain chemicals which are **goitrogens** (i.e. they interfere with hormone synthesis). An excess dietary intake of the brassica family of

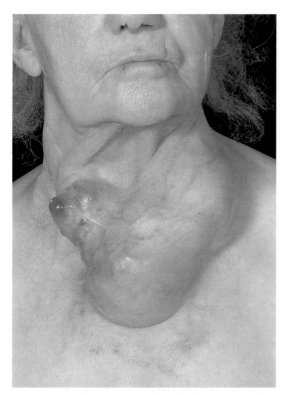

FIG 11.37 A large goitre causing skin changes and imminent ulceration.

foods (e.g. cabbage, sprouts and kale) can cause a goitre.

Local symptoms The principal complaint is of a **swelling in the neck**. This appears slowly and without pain.

If it becomes large – especially if it remains as a colloid goitre after the initial stimulus has gone – it can cause pressure symptoms such as **dyspnoea**, **venous engorgement** and mild **discomfort during swallowing**.

General symptoms Diffuse hyperplastic goitres are not usually associated with clinically significant hyperfunction or hypofunction of the gland.

Long-standing colloid goitres often become nodular goitres and occasionally secondary thyrotoxicosis (Plummer's syndrome) or myxoedema may develop.

Examination

Position The swelling occupies the anatomical site of the thyroid gland.

Tenderness It is not tender.

Shape The swelling usually follows the configuration of the gland and can be seen to have two lobes and an isthmus.

Size Physiological goitres are only two or three times larger than a normal gland, but iodine-deficiency goitres can become very large.

Surface The surface of a hyperplastic goitre is **smooth**. If it turns into a colloid goitre, its surface becomes **bosselated** and, in time, **nodular**.

Composition The gland feels **firm** and is **dull** to percussion. Hyperaemic physiological goitres may have a very soft systolic bruit.

Relations The gland **moves upon swallowing**. The other tissues in the neck should be normal.

Lymph glands The deep cervical lymph glands should not be palpable.

The eyes The eyes should be normal.

General examination The patient is usually euthyroid.

Multinodular goitre

Multinodular goitres develop spontaneously and in glands subjected to prolonged stimulation (i.e. hyperplastic glands). They can therefore be **endemic** (in iodine-deficient areas) or **sporadic** (occurring haphazardly).

A nodular goitre results from a disorganized response of the gland to stimulation, and contains areas of **hyperplasia** and **hypoplasia**, side by side.

The cut surface of a nodular goitre reveals nodules with haemorrhagic, necrotic centres, separated by normal tissue. The normal tissue contains normally active follicles; the nodules contain both hyperactive and degenerate, involuting, follicles.

When the nodules are hyperplastic the patient may develop secondary thyrotoxicosis.

In long-standing nodular goitres, most of the nodules are inactive and the quantity of normally active follicles may be so reduced that thyroid hormone production is inadequate and myxoedema develops.

History

Age In **endemic** areas, nodular goitres appear in **early adult life** (15–30 years). **Sporadic** nodular goitres appear later, between the ages of 25 and 40 years.

Sex Nodular goitres are six times more common in women than in men.

Geography These goitres are common in areas where the drinking water is deficient in iodine (see hyper-plastic goitre).

Symptoms The commonest presenting symptom is an **enlarging, painless swelling** in the neck, which may cause **dyspnoea, discomfort when swallowing, stridor** and **engorged neck veins**.

Sudden enlargement and **pain** can occur if there is haemorrhage into a necrotic nodule. Necrotic nodules are not cysts, and it is wrong to call this event a haemorrhage into a cyst.

Thyrotoxicosis occurs in a significant proportion (maybe as high as 25 per cent) of patients with long-standing nodular goitres. The symptoms of thyrotoxicosis are listed on pages 299–300.

Myxoedema: as the follicular hyperplasia and its stimulation subside, the patient is left with a devastated gland that has little normal tissue. Ultimately, its endocrine secretions are inadequate and the patient has a considerable chance of becoming myxoedematous by the time they reach 60 or 70 years of age. The symptoms of myxoedema are described on pages 301–2.

Examination

Position The swelling is in the lower third of the neck in the anatomical site of the thyroid gland and is usually asymmetrical.

Tenderness A nodular goitre is only tender when there has been a recent haemorrhage into a nodule.

Shape and size The nodules are asymmetrical and the gland can become any shape. Nodules in the isthmus are prominent. The nodules may extend below the clavicles and the sternal notch, into the superior mediastinum.

Surface The surface of a nodular goitre is **smooth** but **nodular**. Frequently, **only one nodule may be**

Revision panel 11.7
Causes of a 'solitary' nodule in the thyroid gland

A dominant nodule in a multinodular goitre
Haemorrhage into a nodule
Adenoma
Carcinoma (papillary or follicular)
Enlargement of the whole of one lobe (usually Hashimoto's disease)

---

palpable, even though the rest of the gland is grossly diseased. This is termed a 'dominant nodule' and malignancy must be excluded.

Composition The consistence of the nodules varies: some feel hard, others feel soft. There is an old saying that 'Solid lumps in the thyroid feel cystic, whereas cystic lumps feel solid'. The explanation is that a nodule composed of thyroid tissue is soft, whereas a nodule full of blood and liquefied necrotic tissue becomes tense and feels hard.

The nodules of a nodular goitre do not fluctuate, or transilluminate, and are dull to percussion.

There should be **no bruit** over the gland.

Relations The lump will **move upwards during swallowing**, indicating that it is fixed to the trachea. It should not be fixed to any other nearby structures.

Lymph drainage The cervical lymph glands should not be palpable.

State of local tissues The trachea may be **compressed** and/or **deviated**, depending on the site of the nodules. Bilateral nodules will compress the trachea into a narrow slit, causing dyspnoea and stridor – especially during lateral flexion of the neck. Large unilateral nodules will push the trachea laterally.

When the trachea is pushed to one side, the 'keel' of the **larynx is tilted away from the mid-line**.

If the gland is jammed in the thoracic inlet, it may obstruct and distend the jugular veins.

Rarely, the goitre is so large that it starts to cause pressure on the overlying skin, and on occasions may even start to ulcerate through.

The eyes The eyes should be normal. It is unusual to get neurological or eye changes with secondary thyrotoxicosis associated with a nodular goitre. These systems are affected more often in primary thyrotoxicosis.

General examination There may be the general signs of thyrotoxicosis – especially the **cardiovascular** signs or, in elderly patients with very long-standing nodular goitres, the signs of **myxoedema**.

The solitary nodule

Although only one nodule may be palpable, **approximately one-half of the patients who present with a solitary nodule actually have a multinodular goitre, i.e. a clinically dominant nodule in a macroscopical multinodular goitre.**

It is unusual to be able to determine the pathology of a solitary nodule by clinical examination. Thus, although the majority of solitary nodules are benign, they must all be investigated, as many well-differentiated carcinomata of the thyroid present as solitary nodules. Fine-needle aspiration (FNA) to determine the cytology of the nodule has become part of the routine of clinical examination in many clinics.

Thyrotoxicosis caused by a solitary toxic/autonomous adenoma is uncommon and is never (well, hardly ever) caused by a solitary malignant nodule.

The causes of a solitary nodule in the thyroid gland are:

- dominant nodule in a multinodular goitre,
- haemorrhage into, or necrosis of, a hyperplastic nodule,
- adenoma,
- carcinoma (papillary or follicular),
- enlargement of the whole of one lobe by thyroiditis.

THYROTOXICOSIS AND MYXOEDEMA
(Hyperthyroidism and hypothyroidism)

Thyrotoxicosis

Thyrotoxicosis is caused by an excess of circulating thyroid hormone. The gland may be diffusely hyperplastic (Graves' thyroiditis), nodular, or the site of disease such as thyroiditis or an adenoma, but rarely a carcinoma.

The terms 'primary' and 'secondary' are used to describe thyrotoxicosis arising in a previously normal or previously abnormal gland, respectively. They can be confusing terms, but usually primary thyrotoxicosis (Graves' disease) is caused by a form of autoimmune thyroiditis, whereas secondary thyrotoxicosis (Plummer's syndrome) usually occurs in a long-standing multinodular goitre.

The thyroid hormones tri-iodothyronine (T3) and thyroxine (T4) have three effects.

1. They increase the metabolic rate of all cells.
2. They increase the sensitivity of beta-adrenergic receptors.
3. They stimulate all cells to grow, but the effect on growth is only significant before natural growth has finished.

The increased tissue metabolism causes an increased appetite, a decrease in weight and an increased heat production.

The increased adrenergic receptor sensitivity causes tachycardia, extrasystoles, atrial fibrillation, tremor and nervousness, and lid retraction and lid lag.

Stimulation of growth during childhood produces early maturation and a slight increase in the rate of growth.

In myxoedema (hypothyroidism), all of these symptoms are reversed. The lack of growth stimulation in a child causes dwarfism.

History

Age Primary thyrotoxicosis occurs most often in young women, between 15 and 45 years of age. Toxic autonomous nodules can occur at any age.

Secondary thyrotoxicosis (from a nodular goitre) occurs in middle age – between 45 and 65 years.

Sex Primary thyrotoxicosis is ten times more common in women than in men.

Geography Secondary thyrotoxicosis is more common in those areas where simple hyperplastic goitre (and nodular goiter) is endemic.

Metabolic symptoms The patient complains of a **ravenous appetite**, but in spite of eating excessively, tends to **lose weight**. Patients may also find that they always feel warm, and therefore **like cold weather** and **dislike hot weather**. There may be **excessive sweating**.

Cardiovascular symptoms The patient complains of **palpitations**, **shortness of breath** during exertion, missed and irregular heart beats (extrasystoles and atrial fibrillation) and **tiredness**. Cardiovascular symptoms are often the presenting symptoms of secondary thyrotoxicosis, whereas atrial fibrillation may be the only sign of thyrotoxicosis in an elderly patient.

Neurological symptoms Symptoms such as **nervousness**, **irritability**, **insomnia**, depression and excitement, even mania and melancholia, may be noticed by close relatives long before the patient is aware of them.

There may be hyperaesthesia, headaches, vertigo and tremors of the hands and tongue.

The patient may complain that their eyes have become more protuberant and that some eye movements are difficult.

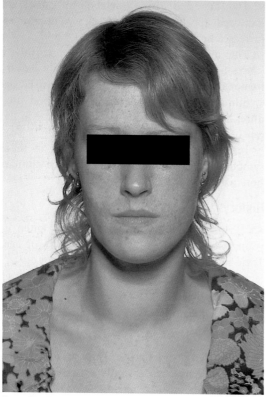

A small goitre, nervousness and agitation, beginning to lose weight, left lid retraction and very early exophthalmos (sclera visible below right inferior limbus).

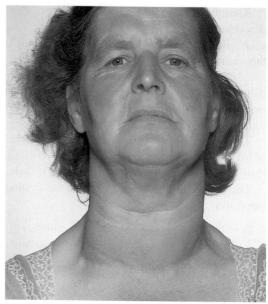

A nodular goitre. No eye or nervous system signs, but palpitations, breathlessness and atrial fibrillation.

Alimentary symptoms The changes in appetite and weight have been mentioned under metabolic symptoms. There is often a slight change in bowel habit – usually mild diarrhoea.

Genital tract symptoms Most women have a reduction in the quantity of their menses; some have amenorrhoea.

Musculoskeletal symptoms In addition to generalized weight loss, there may be specific wasting and weakness of the small muscles of the hand, shoulder and face. These muscles rarely become completely paralysed.

Cause Patients with primary thyrotoxicosis may relate the onset of their symptoms to puberty, pregnancy, an illness or a sudden emotional upset. Although it is difficult to be certain that events of this sort are the prime cause of hypersecretion of the thyroid gland, they undoubtedly exacerbate any hidden or developing abnormality. They are sometimes remembered as the three Ss – **sex** (puberty and pregnancy), **sepsis** and **psyche**!

Examination

Signs in the neck

The thyroid gland is usually enlarged, but thyrotoxicosis can be present without any enlargement of the gland.

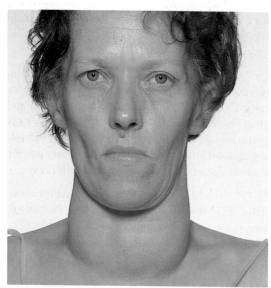

A large goitre, increasing appetite but weight loss – particularly of the face and shoulder girdle – no eye signs.

FIG 11.38 THE FACIES OF THYROTOXICOSIS.

The enlargement may be diffuse, nodular or tender, depending on the local pathology.

A diffusely enlarged hyperaemic gland usually has a **systolic bruit** audible over its lateral lobes.

Signs in the eye

Thyrotoxicosis is associated with four groups of physical signs in the eyes.

LID RETRACTION AND LID LAG

These are common signs. In lid retraction the upper eyelid crosses the eye above its usual level (mid-way between the pupil and the superior limbus of the iris) because the autonomic part of the levator palpebrae superioris muscle is hypertonic.

Ask the patient to follow your finger as you move it slowly from above downwards. If the upper eyelid does not keep pace with the eye, the patient has **lid lag**. This is also caused by the increased tone of the levator palpebrae superioris muscle.

The patient may blink less frequently than normal.

EXOPHTHALMOS

Oedema of the retro-orbital tissues pushes the eye forwards. The first abnormality is the appearance of sclera **below the inferior limbus**, but when the condition is extreme, the eye appears to be popping out and the eyelids cannot be completely closed.

Exophthalmos **makes convergence difficult** and allows the patient to look up without raising their eyebrows or wrinkling their forehead. **Corneal ulceration** may complicate severe exophthalmos.

OPHTHALMOPLEGIA

Infiltration of the ocular muscles weakens the eye muscles and diminishes the eye movements. The muscles most often affected are the superior rectus and inferior oblique muscles. As these muscles normally turn the eye upwards and outwards, this is the first movement to become weak.

CHEMOSIS

This is oedema of the conjunctiva. The conjunctiva becomes thick, boggy and crinkled and may bulge over the eyelids. The eyes water excessively.

General signs

These are best described in bodily systems.

METABOLIC SIGNS

The patient looks thin and their face and hands may be particularly wasted. They may look hot and be sweating, even in a cold room.

CARDIOVASCULAR SIGNS

There is usually a **tachycardia** of 90 beats/minute or more **at rest**, which **persists during sleep**.

If there are **extrasystoles** or **atrial fibrillation**, the pulse will be irregular.

If there is mild heart failure, there may be râles at the bases of the lungs and oedema of the ankles.

NEUROLOGICAL SIGNS

The patient looks worried and nervous and moves about in an agitated, jerky way. They will often twist and twine a handkerchief between their fingers.

A **fine tremor** may be demonstrated when they stretch out their hands with their fingers spread. A similar tremor may be present in the protruded tongue.

MUSCULOSKELETAL SIGNS

The muscles of the hands, shoulders and face may be wasted and weak and the finger tips enlarged.

SKIN

In certain patients with Graves' disease, red, blotchy, raised areas may be seen over the shins. This is termed **pretibial myxoedema** and is caused by deposits of myxoid tissue within the skin.

Myxoedema

History

Myxoedema is the clinical state which follows a severe lack of thyroid hormone (hypothyroidism). The term means 'mucous swelling' and is used because when it was first described it was believed that the increase in weight and body swelling was caused by a new form of oedema.

Age Myxoedema tends to occur in middle and old age.

Sex It is more common in women than in men.

Metabolic symptoms The patient complains of **tiredness** and **weakness**, which become intense physical and mental **lethargy**.

The patient always **feels cold**, and therefore **likes hot weather and dislikes cold weather**. They gain weight but have a poor appetite.

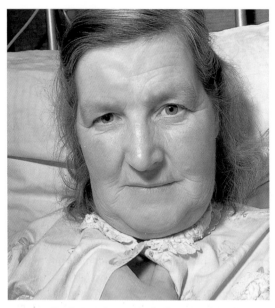

FIG 11.39 The facies of myxoedema. Thinning of the hair, loss of the outer third of the eyebrows, 'peaches and cream' complexion, thickening and heaviness of the eyelids.

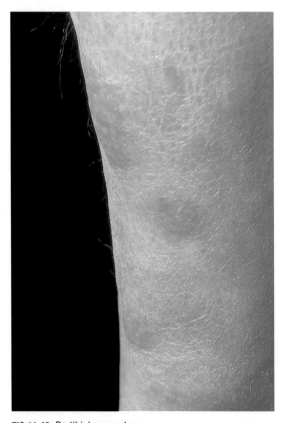

FIG 11.40 Pretibial myxoedema.

Cardiovascular symptoms **Breathlessness** and **ankle swelling** indicate the onset of cardiac failure.

Neurological symptoms The patient finds it difficult to think and to speak quickly and clearly. Hallucinations, dementia ('myxoedema madness') and, in severe cases, 'myxoedema coma' can occur.

Alimentary symptoms Progressive and obdurate **constipation** is common.

Genital tract symptoms Menorrhagia is common when myxoedema occurs before the menopause.

Examination

Signs in the neck

The thyroid gland may be enlarged by long-standing disease such as a nodular goitre, but in many cases the neck is normal.

Signs in the eyes

The eyes are normal but the eyelids become swollen and heavy, making the patient look sleepy and lethargic.

The hair of the outer third of the eyebrows falls out.

General signs

General appearance and metabolic signs The complexion of a white-skinned patient with myxoedema is said to resemble **peaches and cream**. The skin is **smooth** and has a **pale-yellow** (the cream) **colour**. The cheeks are often slightly flushed and have a pink-orange tinge (the peaches).

The skin is **dry and inelastic** and does not sweat. Although it may look oedematous, it does not pit after prolonged pressure.

The patient is overweight, with excess connective tissue and fat in the supraclavicular fossae, across the back of the neck and over the shoulders.

The hair looks thin and ragged and falls out.

The hands are **puffy** and **spade-like**.

The tongue **enlarges** and seems to fill the mouth during speech and interfere with the articulation of words. The voice becomes **deep** and **hoarse**.

Cardiovascular signs The pulse rate is slow (40–60 beats/minute) and the blood pressure is low. Both these changes may be reversed if heart failure develops.

The **hands are cold** and the finger tips blue.

Neurological signs Mental alertness and the ability to respond to questions and solve problems are noticeably retarded. Conversation is also hampered by the difficulty in articulation caused by enlargement of the tongue.

All movements are slow and deliberate.

The reflexes are sluggish and their relaxation period prolonged.

Cretinism

A cretin is a child whose mental and physical development has been retarded by a lack of thyroid hormone. Nowadays cretins are rare because the hormone deficiency can be replaced.

Cretinism is likely to occur in those places where goitre is endemic. The child may have a goitre.

The cretin has an underdeveloped skeleton (a dwarf) and a large protruding tongue, the eyes are wide apart, and the skull is also wide. The limbs and neck are short and the hands spade-like.

The skin is dry and there are supraclavicular pads of fat.

The abdomen is distended and protuberant and there is often an umbilical hernia.

There is mental retardation, even imbecility.

When hypothyroidism occurs in older children, they develop a mixture of the symptoms of cretinism and myxoedema.

CARCINOMA OF THE THYROID GLAND

The thyroid gland is a very vascular organ, and secondary tumour deposits from primary lesions in the breast, stomach, colon and lung are often found at autopsy. However, these secondary deposits rarely become large and noticeable and rarely present

Revision panel 11.8
Correlation between clinical state of the thyroid gland, endocrine function and pathological diagnosis

	Hypothyroid	**Euthyroid**	**Hyperthyroid**
Diffuse enlargement	Thyroiditis	Iodine deficiency Enzyme defects Goitrogens Thyroiditis Amyloid Physiological (pregnancy, puberty)	Primary hyperthyroidism (Graves' disease)
Multinodular enlargement	Multinodular goitre with gross degeneration	Multinodular goitre Lymphoma Anaplastic carcinoma Medullary carcinoma	Secondary hyperthyroidism (Plummer's syndrome)
Solitary nodule	Coincidental nodule with myxoedema	Cyst Dominant nodule Adenoma Follicular or papillary carcinoma	Autonomous toxic nodule
No palpable goitre	Thyroiditis Primary myxoedema Post-thyroidectomy or post-radioactive iodine	Normal gland	Primary hyperthyroidism Thyroxine overdose

primarily as a thyroid swelling. The majority of the neoplasms in the thyroid gland that present as a lump in the neck are primary thyroid tumours.

There are three varieties of carcinoma of the thyroid follicles:

- papillary carcinoma
- follicular carcinoma
- anaplastic carcinoma.

The parafollicular (C) cells can also undergo malignant change, and this cancer is called:

- medullary carcinoma.

The lymphoid tissue in the gland can also undergo malignant change to become a lymphoma, but this is not a true thyroid tissue neoplasm. Lymphoma is more common in patients with Hashimoto's disease.

Papillary carcinoma

This tumour contains a few formed follicles, but its bulk consists of hyperplastic follicular epithelium with a papilliferous configuration which sometimes produces a small quantity of colloid. This tumour spreads in the lymphatics. The cervical lymph glands may be palpable long before the primary lesion in the thyroid gland becomes palpable.

History

Age Papillary carcinoma is a tumour of **children** and **young adults**. Because it occurs in young children, the metastases in the lymph glands were once thought to be clusters of aberrant normal thyroid tissue. They are not. They are true metastases and may often be the presenting feature. Often these enlarged nodes can present as large cystic swellings and mimic a branchial cyst.

Sex Females are affected three to four times more often than males.

Symptoms The common presenting symptom is a **lump in the neck**. The lump may be in the region of the thyroid gland or, if it is caused by secondary deposits in the lymph glands, in the antero-lateral part of the neck.

Distant secondary deposits or a change in thyroid function are very uncommon with papillary carcinomata.

Duration of symptoms The lump may have been present for many years before the patient seeks advice, because these tumours are slow growing and slow to spread beyond the thyroid gland and its draining lymph glands.

Cause The patient will have no idea of the cause of the lump, but it is important to ask them if they have had any **radiation** to the neck or mediastinum. There is a greater incidence of papillary carcinoma in children who have had their neck or chest intentionally irradiated for conditions such as asthma, tuberculosis, enlargement of the thymus, tonsillitis and acne (a form of treatment no longer practised), and unintentionally following a nuclear reactor accident.

Examination

The principal, and usually the only, abnormality is the lump or lumps in the neck.

Position The lump may be in the region of the thyroid gland or deep to the sternomastoid muscle.

Temperature and tenderness The skin of the neck should be normal, provided the tumour has not infiltrated into it. The lumps are usually **not tender**.

Shape and size The primary nodule in the thyroid gland may vary in size from a minute, impalpable nodule to a nodule 3–5 cm in diameter. When palpable, it is usually spherical, smooth and clearly defined, but its surface may be bosselated.

Lymph glands containing thyroid carcinoma metastases are ovoid or nodular, and usually smooth and clearly defined. Occasionally they can be cystic, providing a diagnostic dilemma. The thyroid gland lymph first drains to the pretracheal and paratracheal lymph glands and then to the lower deep cervical lymph glands which lie beneath the anterior edge of the lower third of the sternomastoid muscle.

Composition The consistence of both the primary nodule and the secondary lymph glands is hard or firm. Both are dull to percussion, do not fluctuate and do not cause a bruit.

Relations The primary nodule in the thyroid gland will move upon swallowing and is not usually fixed to superficial structures.

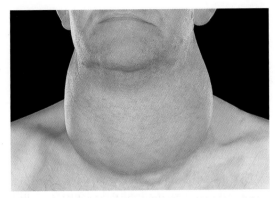

FIG 11.41 A poorly differentiated follicular carcinoma arising in a long-standing multinodular goitre.

Enlarged lymph glands move more easily in a transverse than in a vertical plane and do *not* move with swallowing. They are not usually attached to the skin.

Lymph drainage If you feel a nodule in the thyroid gland, examine all the lymph glands in the neck with care.

General examination The patient usually appears fit and well, without any of the systemic signs which suggest a disseminated neoplasm or thyroid dysfunction.

Follicular carcinoma

The cells in this well-differentiated thyroid cancer retain their normal follicular configuration. Most of the follicles contain a small amount of colloid, which implies that the cells are synthesizing hormone. This has an important bearing on treatment, because the tumour cells will often take up radioactive iodine. This tumour spreads by the bloodstream.

History

Age Follicular carcinomata occur in adults between the ages of 20 and 50 years.

Sex Women are affected more often than men.

Symptoms The common presenting symptom is a **lump in the neck**, which may have been present for many years.

If the tumour has spread beyond the thyroid, the patient may complain of breathlessness, chest pain or **pain or swelling in a bone**, caused by lung and bone metastases, respectively. In these circumstances the pathologist usually finds that the tumour has a thin capsule and has spread into the substance of the gland – the 'invasive' variety of follicular carcinoma.

Multiple lumps in the neck caused by metastases in lymph glands do occur, but not as frequently as with papillary carcinoma.

Systemic effects These patients are euthyroid.

Examination

The principal, and often the only, abnormality is the **lump in the neck**.

Position Follicular carcinoma usually arises in one of the lateral lobes of the thyroid gland.

Temperature and tenderness The overlying skin is not hot and the lump is not tender.

Shape and size The lump is usually **spherical** and **smooth**, with distinct edges. Even the invasive variety feels as if it has a distinct surface.

Composition The lump is firm to hard, does not fluctuate, is dull to percussion and has no bruit.

Relations The lump moves with swallowing, but is not attached to overlying structures.

Lymph glands The deep cervical lymph glands may be enlarged and hard.

Local tissues The local tissues are usually normal.

General examination Examine the **chest** carefully for any evidence of consolidation or collapse. Pulmonary secondary deposits are quite common but may not cause any abnormal physical signs.

Metastases in the **skeleton** are often painful and tender. A bone near to the skin containing a metastasis may be visibly deformed, swollen and hot. Some thyroid cancer metastases are so vascular that they are **soft** and **pulsatile** and have an audible **bruit**.

Anaplastic carcinoma

This is the worst variety of thyroid cancer because it spreads rapidly. Most patients with this disease are dead within 1 year of diagnosis. Its cells do not synthesize thyroid hormone.

History

Age Anaplastic carcinoma of the thyroid gland appears between the ages of 60 and 80 years.

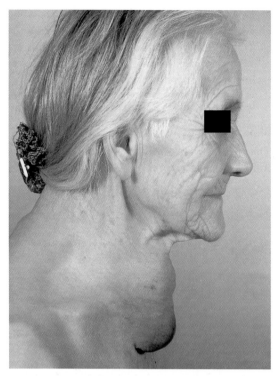

FIG 11.42 An anaplastic carcinoma of the thyroid.

Sex Females are affected more often than males.

Symptoms The common complaint is a **swelling of the neck** rather than 'a lump', which may be rapidly growing. The patient complains of swelling because the tumour is diffuse and infiltrating, not localized.

A dull **aching pain** in the neck is quite common.

Dyspnoea occurs when the tumour begins to compress the trachea, especially when the neck is flexed. It may also occur if there are multiple pulmonary metastases.

Hoarseness or a **change in the quality of the voice** is a diagnostic symptom because it implies infiltration of the recurrent laryngeal nerve.

Pain in the ear, caused by infiltration of the vagus nerve, is not uncommon.

There may be **bone pain**. Any bone can be the site of a secondary deposit, and **pathological fractures** can occur.

General malaise and **weight loss** appear when there is disseminated disease.

Duration of symptoms The symptoms of an anaplastic carcinoma often develop rapidly as this carcinoma grows quickly and is highly invasive. Local invasion and compression of the trachea can lead to death from asphyxia or precipitate a fatal pneumonia.

Examination

Position The swelling in the neck is in the region of the thyroid gland. At first this is in one lobe, but in advanced cases the whole gland may be enlarged and irregular.

Colour The overlying skin often has a red-blue tinge because the underlying infiltration interferes with its venous drainage.

Temperature The skin temperature is normal, or slightly raised.

Tenderness The mass often becomes tender as the tumour infiltrates beyond the thyroid gland.

Shape The mass in the neck has no definable shape once it has spread beyond the thyroid gland, and before this stage it is not easy to define because the surface is so indistinct.

Size The mass may become so big that it interferes with neck movements.

Surface and edge The surface is irregular and indistinct and the lump often has no palpable edge.

Composition The mass is hard and solid. It does not fluctuate, is dull to percussion and has no bruit.

Relations Provided the mass is not infiltrating the whole neck, it will move during swallowing.

It may be fixed to one or both sternomastoid muscles and the overlying skin as well as to the trachea. When the sternomastoid muscle is contracted, the movement of the lump during swallowing is limited and the skin becomes puckered.

The skin may be infiltrated with tumour, making it thick, nodular and a reddish-brown colour.

Lymph glands Although the deep cervical lymph glands are invariably involved in the disease, their enlargement may be obscured by the primary mass in the gland.

If the local lymph glands are palpable, they feel hard and fixed. At first they are smooth and discrete, but they become irregular and indistinct when the tumour begins to spread through their capsules.

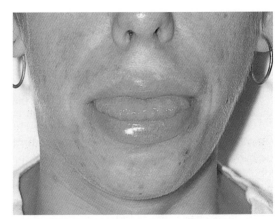

FIG 11.43 Tongue neuromata in a patient with MEN 2b and medullary carcinoma of the thyroid.

State of local tissues The skin of the neck may be tethered or fixed to the lump or even infiltrated with tumour.

The **trachea is often compressed** and deviated, causing **stridor**.

One vocal cord may be paralysed by infiltration of the recurrent laryngeal nerve. This may be suspected if the patient has a hoarse voice, but must be confirmed by indirect laryngoscopy.

All the soft tissues of the neck may be fixed and hardened by infiltrating tumour.

General examination Patients often breathe with difficulty and have stridor. There may be basal pneumonia or collapse caused by pulmonary secondary deposits or the restriction of lung expansion by the narrowed trachea.

There is often **wasting** and **anaemia**.

There may be evidence of skeletal metastases – even **pathological fractures**.

In advanced cases the **liver may be enlarged**, and secondary deposits occasionally appear in the skin.

Medullary carcinoma

This is a rare condition but is mentioned because it can sometimes be diagnosed before operation. It is a neoplasm of the parafollicular (C) cells.

The common presentation is a firm, smooth and distinct lump in the neck, indistinguishable from any other form of thyroid solitary nodule.

The majority of patients are between the ages of 50 and 70 years when the tumour is sporadic in

nature. When the condition occurs in young adults (20–30 years), often with a family history, it may be a manifestation of the multiple endocrine neoplasia syndrome (MEN) types 2a or 2b.

In these cases, the medullary thyroid carcinoma may be accompanied by associated conditions such as:

- phaeochromocytoma ⎫ MEN 2a
- parathyroid tumours ⎭

or

- phaeochromocytoma ⎫
- neuromata of the tongue, lips and conjuctiva
- pale-brown birthmarks ⎬ MEN 2b
- megacolon
- marfanoid habitus. ⎭

The symptoms which should make you think of medullary tumour, apart from a lump in the neck and the presence of the above lesions in the patient or their family, are **diarrhoea** and **flushing**. Diarrhoea occurs in one-third of the patients. The fluidity of the stool and the frequency of defaecation are both increased.

If this tumour is suspected, it is important to measure the serum calcitonin level.

THYROIDITIS

There are three varieties of thyroiditis which can be diagnosed clinically: Hashimoto's disease, de Quervain's thyroiditis and Riedel's thyroiditis.

The term thyroiditis is a non-specific description of the histological changes occurring in the gland. Although the aetiology of these conditions is only partly understood, the eponyms are useful because they do not imply an aetiology but rather a clinical description (provided you ignore the aetiologies proposed by the three gentlemen who made the original descriptions!).

Hashimoto's disease

This is an autoimmune thyroiditis. The body fails to recognize part of itself – in this case both the mitochondria of the thyroid cells and the thyroglobulin they produce – and sets up an immune response against its own tissues. The result is lymphocyte and plasma cell infiltration of the gland that ultimately destroys the thyroid cells. In the first instance the thyroid cells respond by becoming hyperplastic, causing a degree of thyrotoxicosis, but eventually and inevitably the gradual destruction of the thyroid cells causes myxoedema (hypothyroidism).

History

Age and sex Hashimoto's disease is most common in middle-aged women, especially those near the menopause; but it can occur in men, and at any age.

Symptoms in the neck The patient usually complains of a **swelling** or **lump in the neck**. This lump may appear gradually or rapidly, and is often **painful**, particularly when it appears rapidly.

The swelling, or lump, fluctuates in size, and the pain is often intermittent. The symptoms are worse when the patient is tired, or run down, or has an intercurrent illness.

The voice should not alter.

Systemic effects The symptoms of mild **thyrotoxicosis** or **myxoedema** may be present.

The common course of events is for the mild symptoms of thyrotoxicosis, which appear at the onset of the disease, to die out gradually and become replaced by the opposite symptoms of myxoedema.

The majority of patients are euthyroid when they complain of the lump, having ignored or not had any symptoms of thyrotoxicosis, and not reached the myxoedematous phase.

This variability of the local and systemic effects of the disease makes the diagnosis difficult.

Family history Other members of the family may have suffered from the same or other forms of autoimmune disease, such as pernicious anaemia and autoimmune gastritis.

Examination

The main complaint is usually the lump in the neck.

Position The swelling is in the region of the thyroid gland and may be unilateral or bilateral.

Temperature In the initial acute phase – if it occurs – the overlying skin may feel warm.

Tenderness The swelling is often slightly tender.

Shape The swelling may be any shape – a solitary nodule, the whole of one lobe, or the whole gland.

When one lobe or more is involved, the swelling is usually lobulated.

Size Hashimoto's disease usually causes a moderate swelling of the gland, easily visible but rarely gross.

Surface The swelling has a smooth surface and the edge is distinct.

Composition The swelling has the texture of firm rubber. This texture is homogeneous, in spite of the lobulated shape, which helps distinguish the swelling from a nodular or colloid goitre.

There is no bruit.

The composition and mild tenderness are the features most likely to alert you to the possibility of the diagnosis.

Relations The swelling moves with swallowing but is not fixed to any other structures.

Local tissues All the local tissues should be normal.

Lymph glands The nearby lymph glands should not be enlarged.

General examination The majority of patients are euthyroid, but some will have the signs of mild thyrotoxicosis and others of early myxoedema.

De Quervain's thyroiditis

This condition is a true subacute inflammation of the thyroid gland, often associated with mild hyperthyroidism. It may be caused by a virus infection, and sometimes occurs in epidemics.

History

De Quervain's thyroiditis occurs in adults. The main complaint is of the sudden appearance of a painful swelling in the neck. The patient feels ill and may notice that they are anxious, sweaty and hungry and have palpitations.

Examination

Examination reveals a diffuse, firm, **tender** swelling of the whole of the thyroid gland.

There may be signs of **mild thyrotoxicosis** – nervousness and agitation, lid lag and tachycardia.

De Quervain's thyroiditis is self-limiting. It disappears in 1–3 months.

Riedel's thyroiditis

This is a very rare condition but is mentioned because the changes in the gland can be mistaken for the signs of a carcinoma.

It is a condition in which the gland is gradually replaced by dense fibrous tissue, which may even infiltrate beyond the gland into the nearby strap muscles.

The patient complains of a **lump in the neck** or, very rarely, increasing **dyspnoea** caused by compression of the trachea.

Examination reveals a **stony hard swelling** of the thyroid gland, at first of one lobe, but eventually of both lobes and the isthmus.

The lump moves with swallowing but may be fixed to the surrounding tissues, which are otherwise normal.

When both lobes are involved, the smooth, discrete surface usually excludes the diagnosis of carcinoma, but when one lobe is involved it is impossible to make a firm clinical diagnosis.

Note

A scheme for diagnosing thyroid swellings is shown in Figure 11.44 on pages 310–11.

A SCHEME FOR THE DIAGNOSIS OF THYROID SWELLINGS

Once you have examined the patient you should be able to draw conclusions as to the nature and texture of the gland and as to its endocrine activity.

The gland

1. Solitary palpable nodule
2. Multinodular goitre
3. Diffusely enlarged gland

Activity of the gland

1. Normal (euthyroid)
2. Hypersecretion (hyperthyroidism/thyrotoxicosis)
3. Hyposecretion (hypothyroidism/myxoedema)

Having established the configuration of the gland and its endocrine activity, a table can be drawn up as to possible differential diagnoses (see Revision panel 11.8 on page 303). This allows a degree of clarity in interpreting the presenting clinical features and in arriving at a working diagnosis.

If only one lump is palpable it may be:

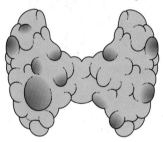

The only palpable nodule of a multinodular goitre

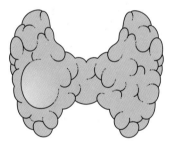

A cyst

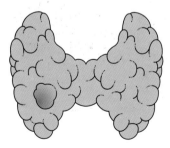

A benign adenoma

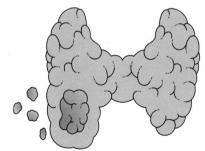

Carcinoma (papillary, follicula or medullary). The lymph glands may be palpable, especially with the papillary type

FIG 11.44

If more than one lump is palpable the swelling may be:

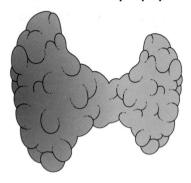

The whole of one lobe involved by
Hashimoto's thyroiditis

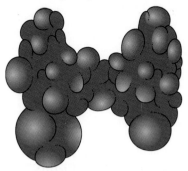

A multinodular goitre

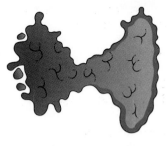

An anaplastic carcinoma
especially if the voice is
hoarse and the mass is fixed
to the surrounding tissues

If there is diffuse, homogeneous enlargement of the whole gland the swelling may be:

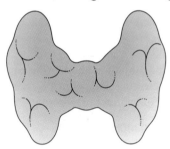

Grave's disease. Primary thyrotoxicosis.
Slight to moderate enlargement.
Soft, smooth with a bruit

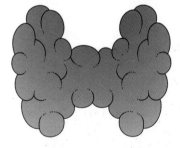

Hyperplastic (colloid) goitre.
Moderate to gross enlargement.
Bosselated. No bruit

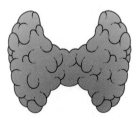

Thyroiditis. Hashimoto's,
de Quervain's or Riedel's.
Moderate or small. Hard, tender

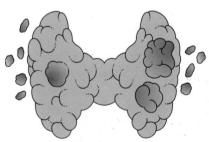

Multifocal carcinoma

FIG 11.44 continued

12 The breast

More than a quarter of general surgical outpatient referrals are females with breast symptoms, only a small proportion of whom will have breast cancer. Less than ten per cent of general surgical operations are for breast disease.

Breast cancer has by far the best prognosis of the common solid organ malignancies and, with constantly improving treatments, up to 80 per cent of sufferers are alive and well 10 years after diagnosis. Nevertheless, public perception and constant media attention ensure that women with breast symptoms are significantly more anxious than other surgical patients.

At first, students find the assessment of the breast difficult but, with practice, a carefully taken history and painstaking examination will yield an accurate diagnosis in most cases. Most patients require no more than reassurance, but rapid identification of those few with malignant disease remains a challenge.

Development and physiology of the breast

Breast development is occasionally seen in neonates as a consequence of maternal oestrogens crossing the placenta. Babies of both sexes may be affected and lactation can occur ('witches' milk'), sometimes complicated by abscess formation.

Normally the female breast develops shortly before the menarche. Occasionally, the enlargement is asymmetrical and causes great parental anxiety.

The breasts increase in size in the second half of each menstrual cycle, following ovulation. Mild pain and tenderness during this phase are common.

In pregnancy, the size and texture of the breasts change profoundly in preparation for lactation. At this time and during lactation, clinical assessment is much more difficult.

HISTORY AND EXAMINATION OF BREAST DISEASE

History

Age

Age is a simple but very important piece of diagnostic information.

Young women will only very rarely have cancer, but over the age of 70 most breast lumps turn out to be malignant.

After taking the past medical history and the history of the presenting complaint, it is essential to ask specific questions about the following.

Previous pregnancies

How many children has the patient had?

Were the children breast-fed and, if so, for how long?

Parity and breast-feeding reduce the incidence of breast cancer: a mother of five who fed all her children is less likely to have breast cancer than a nulliparous woman of the same age.

Menstrual pattern

What is the menstrual pattern? (Regularity, duration and quantity of bleeding.)

Breast symptoms which alter with the menstrual cycle are highly likely to be associated with benign disease.

Medication

Is the patient taking drugs containing female sex hormones? Oral contraceptives commonly reduce the severity of cyclical change in the breasts. Hormone replacement therapy taken by menopausal and post-menopausal patients extends the age at which they are likely to suffer from benign conditions such as breast cysts.

Mental attitude

When taking a detailed history of the presenting complaint, remember that patients are often fearful of the consequences of breast lumps and hide their symptoms with an impressive degree of self-delusion. One may be told that a fungating cancer was only noticed last week when it has clearly been present for much, much longer. Never be censorious about this facet of human nature – you do not know how you would react in similar circumstances!

Your assessment of the way in which the patient is reacting to her symptoms will help you decide how to guide her through her subsequent treatment and management.

Examination

Position

The patient must be fully undressed to the waist, resting comfortably on an examination couch with her upper body raised at 45° to the legs. This position is the best compromise between lying flat, which makes the breasts fall sideways, and sitting upright, which makes the breasts pendulous. Patients sometimes say that their lump can only be felt when they adopt a certain posture, e.g. standing or lying on one side, and they should therefore be examined in this position as well.

Inspection

Stand or sit directly in front of the patient, inspect both breasts and look for the following features.

Size There is enormous variation, with individual sensitivities at each extreme.

Symmetry It is quite normal for there to be a difference between the sides. However, any marked size difference of recent onset is likely to be caused by significant pathology.

Skin The skin may be pulled in or puckered by an underlying cancer. There may be oedema caused by obstruction of skin lymphatics by cancer cells, which is commonly referred to as **peau d'orange**, an accurate description. Other skin changes include nodules of tumour or a malignant ulcer due to direct invasion of the skin by a cancer.

The nipples and areolae The colour of the nipples and areolae changes with age, and there is darkening during pregnancy. The areolar skin is naturally corrugated with small nodules known as *Montgomery's tubercles*.

The nipple may be inverted. Is this bilateral, and does it display the transverse slit pattern seen in duct ectasia? There may be evidence of fluid leaking from the nipple, or there may be eczematous skin changes as in Paget's disease.

Duplication There may be accessory nipples along the mammary line from axilla to groin, or visible ectopic breast tissue in the anterior axillary fold.

Revision panel 12.1
Points to remember when examining the breast

History
  Menarche, development, menopause, changes during menstrual cycle, pregnancies, lactation, family and drug history.
Examination
  Expose all of the top half of the trunk.
  Inspect the breasts at rest and ask the patient to raise her arms above her head.
Look at:
  size
  symmetry
  skin:
  ■ puckering
  ■ peau d'orange
  ■ nodules
  ■ discolouration
  ■ ulceration
  nipples and areolae
  axillae, arms and neck.
Feel the normal side first.
Examine the axillae and arms.
Examine the supraclavicular fossae.
Palpate the abdomen for:
  hepatomegaly
  ascites
  nodules in the pouch of Douglas.
Examine the lumbar spine:
  percussion
  movements
  straight-leg raising
  ankle jerks.

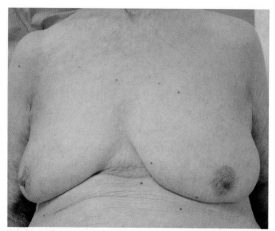

Look at the breast for asymmetry and for changes in the skin and nipple.

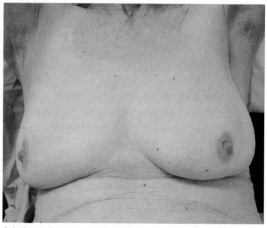

Ask the patient to raise her hands above her head. This exaggerates asymmetry and skin tethering.

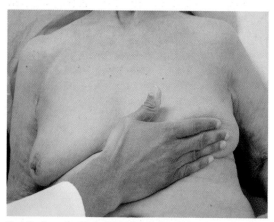

Feel the breast with the flat of your fingers.

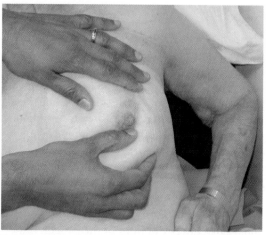

Test the mobility of every lump in two directions, with the pectoralis muscles relaxed and tense. Tense the muscles by asking the patient to place her hands on her hips and press in.

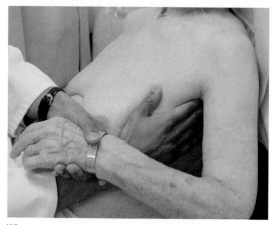

When you palpate the axilla, hold the patient's arm to relax the muscles that form the axillary folds.

FIG 12.1 THE EXAMINATION OF THE BREAST.

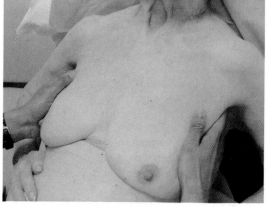

If necessary, compare the axillae simultaneously.

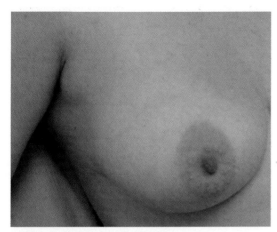

An ectopic mass of breast tissue in the axilla. This is easily mistaken for a pathological abnormality.

FIG 12.1 continued

Ask the patient to slowly raise her arms above her head. Skin changes may then become more apparent, particularly tethering to a carcinoma. Exposure of the underside of the breasts in an obese patient with large breasts may reveal intertrigo.

Ask the patient to press her hands against her hips to tense the pectoral muscles. This may reveal a previously invisible swelling.

Inspect the axillae, arms and supraclavicular fossae. Grossly enlarged lymph glands may be visible, and distended veins or arm lymphoedema may be obvious.

Palpation

The breast should be palpated with the flat of the fingers and not with the palm of the hand. Surgical mythology says that the breast should be felt with 'the flat of the hand' – this is wrong: use the fingers, which are far more sensitive.

With the patient sitting up at 45°, either begin with the normal side or face the patient and feel both breasts together. The texture of the breast is enormously variable, more so than any other organ, depending on age, parity, body mass and hormonal activity. It may be quite soft and apparently feature-less, or it may be firm and fibrous, with easily palp-able nodules, which are in fact normal lobules. In a menstruating woman and at the end of the second half of the menstrual cycle, the breasts may be engorged and tender. In a patient with pendulous breasts and firm breast tissue, the edge of the breast may be readily felt at its upper margin.

Do not forget to feel the axillary tail, which lies over the anterior axillary fold. This may be very obvious in a slim woman with firm breast tissue. Occasionally this part of the breast seems to be separate from the main breast and so presents as an apparently axillary swelling.

Do not be discouraged by your initial difficulty in differentiating normal from abnormal breast tissue. Clinical examination remains an art, not a science, and requires frequent practice.

If you find a lump, ascertain its *site*, *shape*, *size*, *surface*, *edge* and *consistence*, as with a lump in any other area of the body. This may require bimanual examination, controlling movement of the lump with one hand and feeling it with the other.

Not infrequently, even after a thorough palpation, you may fail to find swelling. If so, ask the patient to find it. Often she will then demonstrate to you a very obvious abnormality! Do not consider this a personal affront – it happens to the most experienced! Even if you still cannot feel the lump that the patient can feel, take the symptom seriously and arrange further investigations or a re-examination. Believe the patient and not your inexperienced fingers.

Relations to skin

There is a difference between **skin fixation** and **skin tethering**.

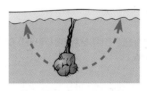

Most lumps can be moved anywhere within the arc depicted, without moving the skin.

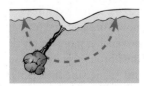

If when a lump is pulled outside the arc the skin indents, it is **tethered**.

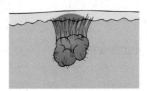

If a lump cannot be moved without moving the skin, it is **fixed**.

FIG 12.2 Tethering and fixation.

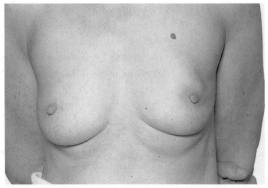

Displacement and deviation. The left nipple is elevated (displaced) and pointing downwards and inwards, not downwards and outwards (deviation). The tumour can be seen just above the areola.

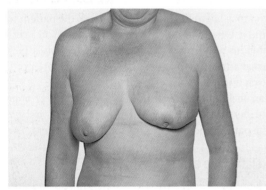

Retraction and displacement. The left nipple has been pulled into the breast (retraction) and pulled upwards (displacement) by the underlying carcinoma.

FIG 12.3 CHANGES IN THE NIPPLE THAT MAY BE CAUSED BY AN UNDERLYING CARCINOMA.

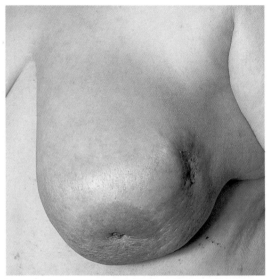

Retraction and peau d'orange. This carcinoma has invaded the skin and ulcerated. The skin of the lower part of the breast is oedematous and looks like the skin of an orange.

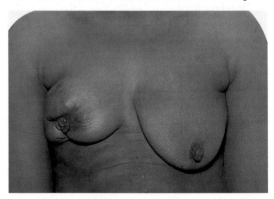

Destruction. The right nipple and areola have been invaded and destroyed by the underlying carcinoma.

When a lesion is fixed to the skin it has spread into the skin and cannot be moved or separated from it.

A tethered lesion is one which is more deeply situated and, by distorting the fibrous septa which separate the lobules of breast tissue (the ligaments of Astley Cooper), puckers and pulls the skin inwards, but remains separate from the skin and can be moved independently.

Relations to the structures beneath the breast

The difference between fixation and tethering to deep structures is less obvious because the muscles beneath the breast are invisible, soft and mobile. If there is a deep-seated lump, ask the patient to press her hand against her hip, thereby tensing the pectoral muscles. If the lesion becomes less mobile, it is either fixed or tethered. The less the movement, the more likely it is to be fixed.

The nipple

If there is nipple inversion, it may be possible to evert it by gentle squeezing its base or by asking the patient do it for you.

Nipple inversion that is easily everted is not an abnormality.

If the nipple will not evert, there is likely to be underlying disease.

Unilateral inversion is more significant than bilateral inversion.

If there is said to be a **discharge**, it may be possible to express it by gently pressing the areola around the base of the nipple and observing whether any fluid comes from one or many duct orifices. The character of the fluid should be noted. Nipple discharges may be red, white, creamy yellow or watery (see page 326).

The axilla

Clinical assessment of the axilla in the absence of gross pathology is difficult. Small, firm, 'shotty' glands can often be felt in thin patients, but this finding is usually symmetrical. In the obese, it may be virtually impossible to feel even significantly enlarged glands.

The axillary lymph glands form a three-sided pyramid whose apex is in the narrow gap between the first rib and the axillary vessels.

Stand on the patient's right side. Take hold of her right elbow with your right hand and let her forearm rest on your right forearm. Persuade her to allow you to hold the weight of her arm. (Patients always want to help by holding their arm away from their side, but this tenses the muscles in the anterior and posterior axillary folds and makes palpation of the lymph glands impossible.) Place your left hand flat against the chest wall and feel for any glands that may lie in the central or medial aspects of the right axilla by sweeping the tips of your fingers across and from the top to the base of the axilla to catch the glands against the chest wall.

To reach the apex of the axilla you will have to push the tips of your fingers upwards and inwards. Explain to the patient that you must push firmly to examine the axilla thoroughly and that this may cause discomfort. (Some patients find this ticklish!)

Next move your left hand anteriorly over the edge of the pectoralis minor muscle and downwards into the axillary tail and behind the edge of the pectoralis major muscle. Turn your hand (or change hands) to feel the subscapular glands on the posterior wall of the axilla, and finally feel the lateral aspect of the axilla in case there are any brachial glands level with the neck of the humerus.

To palpate the left axilla, lean across the patient, hold her left elbow with your left hand and use your right hand to feel the axilla. If it is difficult to feel the axilla in this way, move round to her left side.

With a cooperative patient who is able to relax (and is not ticklish!), you may be able to obtain good access to the axillae by asking her to place her hands on her iliac crests and slacken her muscles, and then approach from in front. This position is particularly useful for comparing the two sides when glands are palpated but may not be pathological.

Finally, palpate the supraclavicular fossa and the neck.

Record the number, size and consistence of any glands that you feel.

General examination

Check the arms for swelling or any neurological or vascular abnormalities, palpate the abdomen looking for hepatomegaly or ascites, and examine the lumbar spine for pain or restricted movements.

Triple assessment

In the UK, most patients with breast problems are seen in dedicated breast clinics. Those with suspected

---

Revision panel 12.2
The changes that can occur in the nipple

Destruction
Depression (retraction or inversion)
Discolouration
Displacement
Deviation
Discharge
Duplication

Revision panel 12.3
The types of discharge from the nipple

Colour	Cause
Red (blood)	Duct papilloma
Pink (serum + blood)	Duct carcinoma
Clear pale yellow (serum)	Duct ectasia
Brown ⎫ (breast	Duct ectasia
Green ⎬ secretions	Cysts
Black ⎭ and debris)	
Creamy white or yellow (pus)	Duct ectasia
Thin white (milk)	Lactation

cancer receive a *triple assessment*, which consists of:

1. history and examination,
2. diagnostic imaging by mammography and/or ultrasound scanning,
3. cytology or histology.

Cytological examination looks at smears obtained by aspiration of a lump with a fine needle (FNA).

Histological examination is based on biopsy specimens obtained with special core-cutting needles, often with radiological guidance.

PRESENTATION OF BREAST DISEASE

Breast disease presents in three main ways:

- a lump, which may or may not be painful,
- pain, which or may not be cyclical,
- nipple discharge or change in appearance.

The common conditions which cause these symptoms are described individually in the rest of this chapter, but the *likely* diagnoses when the patient presents with one or more of the above are as follows.

A painless lump

- Carcinoma
- Cyst
- Fibroadenoma
- An area of fibroadenosis

A painful lump

- An area of fibroadenosis
- Cyst
- Periductal mastitis
- Abscess (usually postpartum or lactational)
- Sometimes a carcinoma

Pain and tenderness but no lump

- Cyclical breast pain
- Non-cyclical breast pain
- Very rarely, a carcinoma

Nipple discharge

- Duct ectasia
- Intraduct papilloma
- Ductal carcinoma-in-situ
- Associated with a cyst

Changes in the nipple and/or areola

- Duct ectasia
- Carcinoma

- Paget's disease
- Eczema

Changes in breast size and shape

- Pregnancy
- Carcinoma
- Benign hypertrophy
- Rare large tumours

The fact that many diagnoses are repeated in different sections explains why it is often difficult to make a definite clinical diagnosis. Note carefully that carcinoma, the only life-threatening disease of the breast, can present in almost any way, to which must be added, in recent years, cases discovered in asymptomatic women by screening mammography.

CARCINOMA OF THE FEMALE BREAST

Cancer of the breast is an adenocarcinoma and the commonest cancer in women. There are many macroscopic varieties and histological types. A particular feature is the variable quantity of fibrous tissue that surrounds the cancer cells. Sometimes 90 per cent of the mass is fibrous stroma, with just a few cancer cells scattered through it, while at the other end of the spectrum is the cancer with no fibrous reaction. This variety may be so cellular, vascular and fast growing that it is clinically indistinguishable from acute inflammation.

The cut surface of a carcinoma is classically concave, rough, gritty and pale grey with prominent yellow and white flecks, and is said to cut like 'an unripe pear'. The cut surface of a benign lesion bulges out to become convex, is white rather than grey, and feels smooth and rubbery, not gritty.

The designation 'cancer' for malignant tumours originates from the Latin word for a crab. Certainly the cut surface of some breast carcinomata, with an indefinite edge and extending, infiltrating tentacles, rather like crab claws, fits this description.

In a proportion of cases, the malignant cells remain inside the ducts and there is no invasive element. This is termed 'ductal carcinoma-in-situ' (DCIS). It may present as a lump in a manner similar to invasive cancer, or with nipple discharge, or be picked up on screening because it is often associated with microcalcification, which is visible on mammography.

When carcinoma cells migrate along the ducts to the nipple, they produce the skin changes known as **Paget's disease**.

History

Age Carcinoma of the breast is extremely rare in teenagers and rare in the twenties. From the thirties onwards there is a progressively increasing incidence to which peaks in the late fifties. It remains common into old age. There are unexplained geographical variations in its incidence, but it is predominantly a disease of Western civilizations.

Symptoms The presenting symptoms may be related to the primary lesion or, rarely, to the effects of secondary deposits.

Classically the patient notices a painless lump, often when washing or looking into a mirror. The size of the lump when first noticed does not give an accurate indication of how long it has been present. Occasionally there is a pricking sensation in the breast and the patient finds a lump when feeling the symptomatic area. A lump may be found in the axilla if there are lymph gland metastases.

The patient may notice a skin dimple caused by tethering.

The nipple may become retracted, or even destroyed.

The breast may be noticed to be harder or to have changed shape.

Swelling of the arm, caused by lymphatic or venous obstruction in the axilla, is an uncommon but significant presentation.

Backache, caused by secondary infiltration and collapse of lumbar vertebrae, with nerve root pains radiating down the back of the legs, is a common symptom of advanced disseminated disease, but an uncommon mode of presentation, as are respiratory symptoms from pleural effusions or malignant infiltration.

A cerebral metastasis may cause a fit.

A pathological fracture may be the first indication of the presence of the disease.

Curiously, the general symptoms commonly associated with cancer, such as malaise, weight loss and cachexia, are rare in patients with breast cancer. Even those with disseminated fatal disease usually feel well in themselves (apart from bone pain) until the final stages.

Family history Two per cent of women with breast cancer have the *BRCA* gene. This declares itself before the age of 40, and other members of the family will have been affected, some of them with ovarian cancer as well.

Breast cancer is a common disease and so finding several sufferers in one family is not unusual. Whether there is a significantly increased risk in those with a strong family history but without the specific gene is not yet clear.

Parity Carcinoma of the breast is more common in nulliparous women, and less common in women who have had many children and breast-fed them.

Examination

A technique for examining the breast is described earlier in this chapter.

Site Half of carcinomata of the breast occur in the upper outer quadrant, which includes the axillary tail, so do not forget to feel this when palpating the breast.

Colour If the tumour is close to the surface, the overlying skin may be discoloured. Tumours fixed to the skin first give the skin a smooth, reddened appearance, but as the process advances and ulceration is imminent, the skin becomes paler.

Tenderness Most carcinomata are not tender, but palpation may produce a mild discomfort, often because of the patient's fear of the consequences of the surgeon finding a lump.

Temperature Only the very rare 'inflammatory' type of breast cancer feels warm.

Shape A carcinoma of the breast may grow into any shape but in the early stages it is roughly spherical. The disease may also be **multifocal**, and it is not that unusual to find two separate primary tumours.

Surface The surface is usually indistinct, which makes it difficult to define the shape except when the lesion is small. However, a few cancers are

---

Revision panel 12.4
The cardinal signs of a late cancer of the breast

Hard, non-tender, irregular lump
Tethering or fixation of the lump
Palpable axillary lymph glands

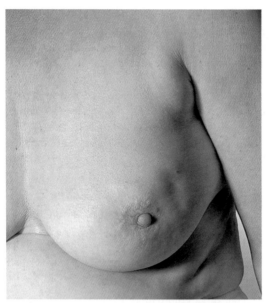

Retraction, deviation and displacement of the nipple.
Puckering and tethering of the skin.

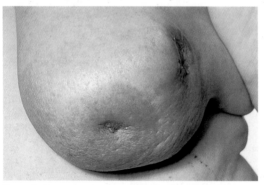

Peau d'orange.

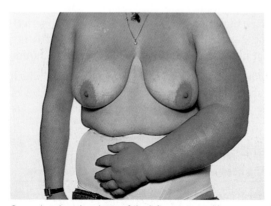

Secondary lymphoedema of the left arm caused by
metastases in the lymph glands.

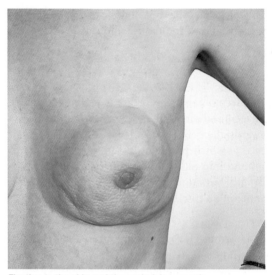

Fixation to the skin and the underlying muscle.

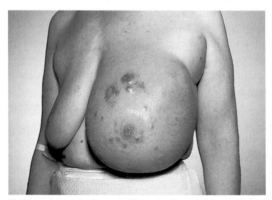

Enlargement of the breast with secondary nodules of tumour
in the skin.

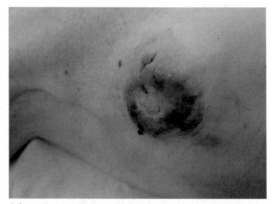

A fungating carcinoma with local secondary tumour nodules
in the surrounding skin. The axillary lymphadenopathy is
visible as well as palpable.

FIG 12.4 SOME DIAGNOSTIC FEATURES OF ADVANCED CARCINOMA OF THE BREAST.

encapsulated and have a smooth surface, mimicking cysts and fibroadenomata.

Composition Carcinomata are solid, so they do not fluctuate, transilluminate or have a fluid thrill. Their consistence is normally quite firm. However, some tumours are soft, almost as soft as a lipoma, so do not attribute too much significance to the absence of a textbook 'stony hard' consistence.

Relations to surrounding structures The terms fixation and tethering have already been defined. If a lump is tethered to the skin, it behaves as if it is tied to it by a piece of string. It can move freely and independently of the skin within the limits determined by the length of the string, but pulls the skin when moved beyond these limits. If a lump is fixed, it cannot be moved independently.

Fixation of a lump to the skin is almost diagnostic of a carcinoma. The only other condition producing fixation is traumatic fat necrosis (or, of course, a pointing abscess, which should be obvious).

A cancer may also infiltrate through the underlying muscle into the chest wall. Such a lesion will be fixed. If neglected, the tumour will invade and consume the whole breast, leaving only a large malignant ulcer on the chest wall. Such lesions are still seen.

When a tumour spreads along the fibrous septae of the breast it blocks the lymphatics which run alongside them. This causes oedema of the overlying skin between the many small pits which mark the openings of the hair follicles and sweat glands. The result is an orange-peel appearance known as **peau d'orange**.

Lymph drainage The axillary lymph glands are often palpable, but this does not necessarily indicate tumour involvement except when the glands are very large. They may sometimes be visible.

Lymph glands containing metastases are usually hard and discrete. As they enlarge, they may mat together and become adherent to nearby structures such as the skin, axillary vessels and nerves. They may eventually become tethered or fixed to the skin, but by this stage the primary tumour is usually obvious. Ulceration in the axilla is rare.

Glands may become fixed to the chest wall, particularly at the apex of the axilla where there is less space for gland enlargement.

Nearby tissues Extensive (but not necessarily palpable) involvement of the axillary lymph glands may cause lymphoedema of the arm or venous thrombosis and oedema.

The other breast may contain a lump, which the patient has not noticed. It may be a secondary deposit or another primary lesion. Do not forget to examine the axilla on the non-symptomatic side, both to make a comparison and to look for separate pathology.

General examination A full general examination is essential to detect the presence of metastases, which commonly occur at the following sites.

- **The skeleton** – especially the lumbar spine, causing back pain and reduced spinal movements, and pathological fractures in long bones. There may even be paraplegia from cord compression.
- **The lungs** – causing pleural effusions. Lung parenchymal involvement, in the form of diffuse

---

The International TNM classification

T = Tumour

T_1	2 cm diameter or less. No fixation or tethering
T_2	2–5 cm diameter (or less than 2 cm) with tethering or nipple retraction
T_3	5–10 cm diameter (or less than 5 cm) with infiltration, ulceration or peau d'orange over the tumour, or deep fixation
T_4	Any tumour with infiltration or ulceration wider than its diameter. Tumours larger than 10 cm

N = Nodes

N_0 No palpable axillary nodes
N_1 Mobile palpable axillary nodes
N_2 Fixed axillary nodes
N_3 Palpable supraclavicular nodes. Oedema of the arm

M = Metastases

M_0 No evidence of distant metastases
M_1 Distant metastases

FIG 12.5 The TNM classification.

lymphatic involvement known as **lymphangitis carcinomatosa**, may cause severe dyspnoea.

- **The liver** – making it palpable and causing jaundice and ascites.
- **The skin** – producing multiple hard nodules within the skin. These are usually in the skin of the breast containing the cancer, but may be seen in the neck, trunk and further away.
- **The brain** – producing any variety of neurological symptoms and signs.

Conditions mimicking breast cancer

Fat necrosis Fat necrosis occurs in the elderly. After an injury, not necessarily noticed by the patient, there may be a focal necrosis of subcutaneous fat with local scarring which causes skin tethering. There may be a history of trauma or of bruising. The condition resolves spontaneously.

Mondor's disease Mondor's disease is a thrombophlebitis of the lateral thoracic vein which produces a cord-like, linear skin puckering that can alarm patient and clinician. It resolves spontaneously.

BENIGN BREAST TUMOURS

Fibroadenoma

A fibroadenoma is a benign neoplasm of the breast in which the fibromatous element is the dominant feature. The cut surface of a fibroadenoma reveals lobules of whorled, white fibrous tissue which bulge out of their capsules.

There are two histological varieties of fibroadenomata, **pericanalicular**, which mainly consist of fibrous tissue, and **intracanalicular**, which contain more glands. The former tend to be harder and more discrete. Clinically the distinction is unimportant.

Most fibroadenomata present in young women, aged between 15 and the late twenties. They are seen, however, into the forties and occasionally even later, but not in the elderly. They grow slowly and may become quite large. They are then termed 'giant fibroadenoma', but the histological appearance does not change.

History

The patient presents with a painless lump in the breast, usually noticed by accident. Occasionally there is more than one lesion.

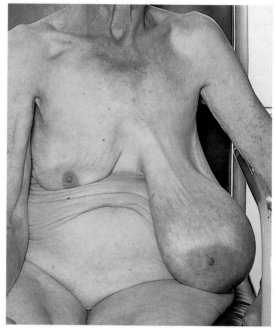

A giant fibroadenoma of the left breast.

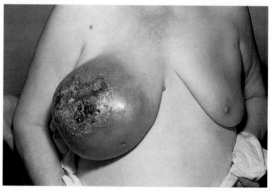

A large phylloides tumour (Brodie's tumour) causing necrosis of the overlying skin.

FIG 12.6

Examination

Look out for a mobile, very discrete lump.

Position It may be anywhere in the breast.

Shape and size Fibroadenomata are usually spherical or ovoid, but sometimes lobulated, and may be any size.

Surface The surface is smooth, the edge definite and the consistence like firm rubber.

Mobility Classically the fibroadenoma is the most mobile of all breast lesions and fully merits the description of 'breast mouse'.

The breast swelling most like a fibroadenoma is a breast cyst, but cysts are found in a different age group and are not usually mobile.

Phylloides tumour

This is a rare lesion, first described as *cystosarcoma phylloides* or *Brodie's sarcoma*. It is not a sarcoma but may recur locally after simple excision. It does not metastasize.

It presents as a slow-growing, smooth swelling in the middle aged, rather like a large fibroadenoma, from which it is usually only distinguished on histology. It can be big enough to cause skin necrosis.

Intraduct papilloma

This uncommon condition is a papillary neoplasm arising from duct epithelium and enlarging into the duct system. It usually presents with a bloodstained discharge from the nipple, although there may be a soft swelling near the areola.

Lipoma of the breast

Lipomata may occur anywhere in the body where there is fat, which includes the breast, both subcutaneously and more deeply seated between the lobules.

Subcutaneous lipomata are just like lipomata elsewhere, and there may be others on the trunk or limbs. If more deeply seated, they may have clinical features similar to those of cysts and fibroadenomata.

BENIGN BREAST DISEASE

Most of the conditions which lead women of reproductive age to seek medical advice in relation to their breasts are not truly a disease process, but reflect or are exaggerations of the normal pattern of life in Western civilizations, where women have relatively few children, relatively late in life, and frequently do not put their breasts to the purpose for which they are designed, namely feeding babies.

Biologically, women are able to have children at regular intervals from the menarche onwards and could be almost constantly breast-feeding until the menopause (should they survive that long!). In these circumstances it is unlikely that so-called benign breast disease would occur, or perhaps be noticed.

For many years the term *chronic mastitis* was used to describe the various symptom complexes seen in benign breast disease. This is an inappropriate name because there is no clinical or microscopic evidence of an inflammatory process; but the term is still heard. The same is true for many other names used for the same condition, such as fibroadenosis, fibrocystic disease and cystic hyperplasia. These names are derived from the histological features of breast biopsies, such as fibrosis, adenosis, microcyst formation, epithelial hyperplasia and lymphocytic infiltration. Studies of normal breasts have shown that all these changes are non-specific and are commonly present in women without breast complaints. They are the histological manifestations of the dynamic changes that occur throughout normal reproductive life during breast development, cyclical menstrual change, pregnancy and menopausal involution.

It is best when considering the manifestations of so-called benign breast disease not to apply a histopathological label to the various symptom patterns seen in clinical practice, but to use simple clinical descriptions.

Most patients' symptoms fall, with considerable overlap, into three categories:

- lumps and nodularity
- pain
- cysts.

Lumps and nodularity

History

The symptoms of lumps and nodularity occur during the years of ovarian activity, from menarche to menopause, beginning in the early twenties and reaching a peak in the thirties.

Revision panel 12.5
The causes of massive enlargement of the breast

Benign hypertrophy (usually bilateral)
Giant fibroadenoma
Phylloides tumour (Brodie's disease)
Sarcoma
Colloid carcinoma
Filarial elephantiasis

Most patients present complaining of **more than one** lump in the breast, which are commonly **tender**. It is often the tenderness that draws the patient's attention to the lump. The swelling may be **intermittent** and clearly related to the menstrual cycle, usually being more obvious in the premenstrual phase and resolving when the menses begins. The history is often quite long, as patients are not unduly concerned by an intermittent swelling which they correctly conclude is unlikely to be malignant.

Examination

Benign breast lumps can vary from a **diffuse nodularity** to quite **discrete lesions** which mimic a cancer.

Begin by assessing the asymptomatic breast to get some idea of its consistence. There is enormous variability. In thin women, the lobular structure is often clearly discernible and the breast tissue may be picked up and palpated. In women with large breasts, gravity stretches the breast downwards and outwards, and the axillary tail may be readily palpable as a nodular ridge on each side. Sometimes the upper border of the firm breast tissue is easily felt separate from the subcutaneous fat.

Nodular benign lumps tend to be in the **upper outer quadrants** and have a moderate hardness, sometimes described as **rubbery**. Sometimes the nodularity is so obvious as to resemble a bunch of small grapes.

They are **not fixed or tethered** to skin or muscle.

Comment Experience is needed to differentiate discrete lesions which might be malignant and require further investigation, from diffuse swellings which only require reassurance and perhaps re-assessment at a different phase of the menstrual cycle. Do not become discouraged by this difficulty, but try to see patients with obvious real pathology before attempting to interpret the more subtle physical signs of benign breast disease.

Breast pain

Breast pain falls into various patterns and may be cyclical or non-cyclical.

Cyclical breast pain

Cyclical breast pain is very common. Almost all women experience it to some degree during their

---

Revision panel 12.6
A comparison of the clinical features of four common breast lumps

Type of lump	Age (years)	Pain	Surface	Consistence	Axilla
Solitary cyst	35–55	Occasionally	Smooth	Soft to hard	Normal
Nodularity	20–55	Occasionally	Indistinct	Mixed	Normal
Fibroadenoma	15–55	No	Smooth and bosselated	Rubbery	Normal
Carcinoma	35+	No	Irregular	Stony hard	Glands may be palpable

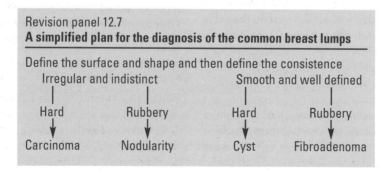

Revision panel 12.7
A simplified plan for the diagnosis of the common breast lumps

Define the surface and shape and then define the consistence

Irregular and indistinct   Smooth and well defined

Hard   Rubbery   Hard   Rubbery

Carcinoma   Nodularity   Cyst   Fibroadenoma

reproductive life. It comes on during the second half of the cycle and is relieved, sometimes dramatically, when menstruation commences. It is unusual before the age of 30 and resolves spontaneously in the forties.

Curiously, as it is clearly of hormonal origin, it is quite commonly unilateral. It may be felt throughout the breast, or more in the upper outer quadrants. There may be associated tenderness, sometimes to the extent that the sufferer cannot bear any pressure on the breasts at that time in the cycle, even from a brassiere. The pain is usually reduced by the use of oral contraceptives.

On examination, there may be **tenderness** but **no discrete lump**. Diffuse nodularity is common, particularly in the upper outer quadrants.

It is important to appreciate that cyclical breast pain is never a symptom of cancer. Several large studies have shown that women with breast pain are no more likely to have an impalpable carcinoma than women who do not complain of it, and so no special investigations are necessary.

Non-cyclical breast pain

Non-cyclical breast pain is less common than cyclical breast pain and has many causes.

Girls at the menarche sometimes experience discomfort during very early breast development.

Women in their twenties may present with a persistently painful, tender area in one breast, but this usually resolves spontaneously.

Non-cyclical breast pain without any physical signs is also seen around the menopause and again resolves on its own.

Elderly women sometimes complain of unilateral breast pain, many years after hormonal activity has ceased. Careful examination is essential, as very occasionally there is an underlying cancer, especially when the pain is described as 'prickling'.

Breast pain in the elderly is often skeletal in origin, arising from conditions such as frozen shoulder and osteoporosis of the spine.

Conversely, very large painful breasts may produce skeletal symptoms in the neck and shoulder region, from both abnormal posture and pressure from brassiere straps.

Tietze's syndrome is an uncommon condition in which pain and tenderness arise from a costochondral junction lateral to the sternum. The patient complains of pain that is exacerbated by movement and finds what she thinks is a breast lump. Careful examination will demonstrate that the lump noticed by the patient is in fact behind the breast and is part of the chest wall.

Breast cyst

Breast cyst is probably the commonest of the discrete breast swellings.

In pathological terms, a fluid-filled cavity appears in the breast, without a demonstrable endothelial lining or a capsule. The condition is age related and occurs at times when the patient's hormone environment is changing, usually around the menopause. Cysts may be multiple and recurrent.

History

Age Breast cysts are unusual before the age of 40. The peak incidence is in the forties and early fifties. Hormone replacement therapy has extended the age range, and cysts are sometimes seen in women in their seventies.

Presentation They may develop suddenly, the patient, to their surprise, finding a large swelling that was not there the day before, and naturally assumes the worst if this is the first cyst she has had. Moderate pain and tenderness are common.

Past history Many patients have had previous cysts and will be aware that it is worth waiting for a while before consulting their doctor, as most cysts will eventually resolve.

Examination

Shape and surface A solitary cyst is smooth, spherical and of variable consistence, from soft and cystic to a hardness equal to cancer. The clinical diagnosis of a cyst usually rests upon its smooth, spherical shape, but the swelling may be more diffuse.

Size Large breast cysts may be visible and even appear blue or green through the skin, but there will never be tethering or fixation to skin or muscles.

Consistence It is rarely possible to elicit fluctuation or a fluid thrill or to transilluminate the lesion.

Comment The experienced clinician, having made a confident clinical diagnosis of a cyst, will proceed immediately to needle aspiration, the appropriate treatment. The fluid that emerges is variable in colour and clarity, varying from very dark green,

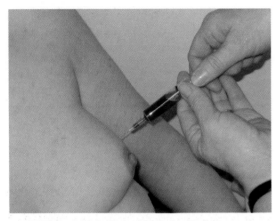

FIG 12.7 Aspiration of a breast cyst, a simple clinic procedure. The aspirant has the typical green colour of a benign cyst.

almost black, to clear yellow. There are few more rewarding (or simpler) surgical procedures than the aspiration of a breast cyst in a concerned woman.

Occasionally a breast cyst communicates with the duct system and there is concomitant nipple discharge. This resolves when the cyst is aspirated or settles spontaneously.

A **galactocele** is a milk-containing cyst and occurs during or shortly after lactation. It presents as above and the physical signs are similar. Aspiration produces milk, but the cyst rapidly refills and resolution must await cessation of breast-feeding.

THE NIPPLE

The symptoms associated with the nipple are discharge, inversion and skin changes.

Revision panel 12.8 **The differences between eczema and Paget's disease of the nipple**	
Eczema	**Paget's disease**
Bilateral	Unilateral
Commonly occurs at lactation	Occurs at menopause
Itches	Does not itch
Vesicles	No vesicles
Nipple intact	Nipple may be destroyed
No lumps	May be an underlying lump

Nipple discharge

Considering that the breast is designed to produce milk, it is hardly surprising that a fluid discharge is a common symptom.

It may occur in any age group, but is commonest during reproductive life. Most women who have breast-fed can express fluid on request for some time afterwards, and in most patients seen with this symptom no cause is ever demonstrated.

The fluid may be thick or thin, cloudy or clear, or bloodstained. The discharge may be unilateral or bilateral.

Endocrine causes of nipple discharge are very rare.

Significant causes of nipple discharge include ductal carcinoma-in-situ (DCIS), duct papilloma and, most commonly, duct ectasia.

Nipple discharge is rarely associated with invasive cancer.

Nipple inversion

Unlike nipple discharge, this condition is frequently associated with significant disease and always merits full assessment. The commonest cause by far is duct ectasia, but it is a regular presentation of breast cancer, with or without a palpable lump.

Nipple skin changes

It is fixed in the minds of the public and the profession that an eczematous rash on the nipple indicates the presence of a cancer. In fact most patients with a rash on or around the nipple have a skin disease, not Paget's disease of the nipple.

Paget's disease of the nipple

Paget's disease of the nipple is caused by cancer cells migrating or spreading along the duct system from a carcinoma situated deeply in the breast, which in the early stages is usually confined to the epithelium (DCIS).

The presence of carcinoma cells in the skin of the nipple produces a clinical appearance similar to that of eczema. Patches of skin first become **red** and then **encrusted** and **oozy**. The edges of these lesions are distinct, unlike eczema, and they **do not itch**, although the patient may complain of abnormal

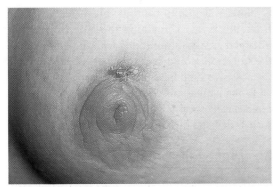

FIG 12.8 A mammillary duct fistula. This tract connects with a mammary duct. Recurrent infection causes recurrent acute breast abscesses.

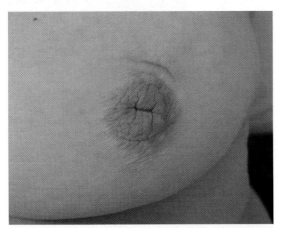

FIG 12.9 The typical appearance of the nipple in duct ectasia. Note the transverse slit. The scar above the areola is the aftermath of an incision made to drain an abscess caused by periductal mastitis.

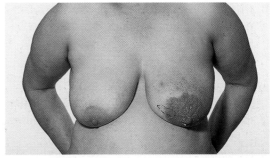

Florid exudative eczema of the left nipple and areola.

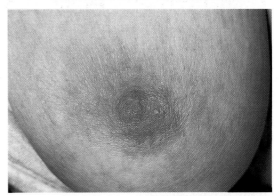

Paget's disease of the left nipple. The skin of the outer lower quadrant of the areola is red and slightly thickened. Careful palpation revealed the mass of a small underlying carcinoma.

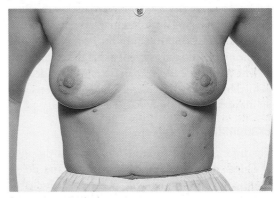

Supernumerary nipples.

FIG 12.10 THE NIPPLE.

sensations and prickling. In time the nipple is destroyed, and replaced by a malignant ulcer.

In the early stages of the disease there may be no palpable abnormality in the breast, but ultimately the in-situ carcinoma becomes invasive and a lump appears.

Never forget that **Paget's disease of the nipple always indicates an underlying malignant process in the breast itself**.

Duct ectasia

This is a common condition of unknown aetiology and, as the name implies, the characteristic pathological feature is dilatation of the mammary ducts, which are full of inspissated material containing macrophages and chronic inflammatory debris. It has the following presenting features.

- **Nipple inversion**, which is at first mild and readily everted. There is a characteristic transverse slit appearance. In many patients this is the only feature, and as it is mild and long-standing, it is ignored.

- **Difficulty in breast-feeding** because the infant is unable to apply suction to the partly inverted nipple.
- **Nipple discharge** of sometimes purulent material from the dilated ducts.
- **Chronic low-grade infection of the peri-areolar area**, with tender thickening around the nipple, going on to abscess formation, known as **periductal mastitis**. This is genuine inflammation and merits the description mastitis (unlike the outdated expression 'chronic mastitis' mistakenly applied to the changes of benign breast disease).
- **A periductal abscess** that may rupture (or be drained externally) and stay in communication with the duct system. This results in a **mammillary fistula** and the pathogenesis is identical to that of the analogous anal fistula and requires similar principles of treatment.

BREAST ABSCESS

Acute breast abscess

History

Acute breast abscess is often associated with lactation. Bacteria may gain access to the engorged breast lobules, an excellent medium for bacterial culture, via the nipple and duct system or via the circulation.

The patient develops **malaise** and **fever** accompanied by an ache in the breast which progresses to an inexorable **throbbing pain**.

Examination

The infected breast prominently displays the *signs of Celsus*, namely rubor, calor, tumour and dolor. Eventually the abscess will point and discharge through the skin. There may be very obvious tender lymphadenopathy in the ipsilateral axilla.

Revision panel 12.9
The varieties of true mastitis

Neonatal (caused by maternal hormones)
Milk engorgement during lactation
Diffuse infection during lactation
Mumps

Note: it is safe to continue breast-feeding, even from the breast containing the abscess. Had the inflamed area communicated with the duct system, the infection would have discharged this way and the abscess would have not have formed.

When a breast abscess occurs in a women who is not lactating there is often a predisposing risk factor such as diabetes mellitus or immunocompromise.

Recurrent and chronic breast abscess

Recurrent and chronic breast abscess is usually associated with duct ectasia, described above.

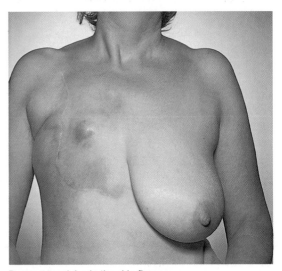

Recurrent nodules in the skin flaps.

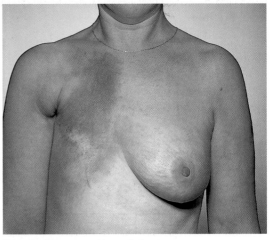

Telangiectases caused by radiotherapy.

FIG 12.11 TWO COMMON APPEARANCES AFTER MASTECTOMY.

Tuberculosis of the breast remains common in some parts of the world and is occasionally seen in the UK in immigrants.

Granulomatous infections of the breast caused by atypical mycobacteria are rare but on the increase.

Both forms of infection present with a painless mass and mimic carcinoma.

PREGNANCY

Pregnancy is always associated with changes in the breast.

Within a few weeks of the ovum being fertilized, the breasts become tense, heavy and slightly uncomfortable. Many women notice pricking sensations deep inside the breast.

By 2 months the breasts are enlarged and feel granular – even 'lumpy' – in texture. The subcutaneous veins dilate and become prominent, and the skin of the breasts is warm. The nipples enlarge and the areolae become darker. The skin around the areolae may also become slightly pigmented. The sebaceous glands of the areolae become larger and the skin over them appears stretched and pale. The lumps they form are called Montgomery's tubercles.

By the fourth month, a thin, clear secretion may sometimes exude from the nipple.

THE MALE BREAST

There are two causes of enlargement of the male breast: gynaecomastia, which is benign and common, and carcinoma, which is malignant and rare.

Gynaecomastia

All males have rudimentary breasts. Gynaecomastia is an abnormal development of both ductal and stromal elements, with the following patterns of presentation.

- **Transient breast enlargement in male infants** due to ingestion of maternal oestrogens.
- **Early breast development in adolescents**, presumably caused by a temporary imbalance of adrenal and testicular steroid hormones. Testicular atrophy and hormone-secreting testicular tumours are rare causes.
- **Breast enlargement in middle-aged adults** is usually **idiopathic**, but in some cases is caused

by repeated minor trauma from belts and harnesses. It is usually bilateral.
- **Breast enlargement in elderly men**, almost invariably **caused by drugs**. This is often an expected part of the action of the drug, as in the

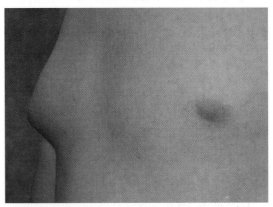

Unilateral gynaecomastia in a young man.

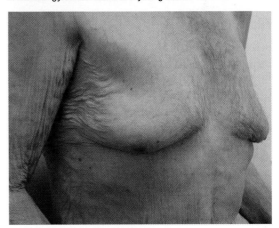

Bilateral gynaecomastia in an old man.

FIG 12.12 GYNAECOMASTIA.

Revision panel 12.10
The breast changes of pregnancy

Fullness and pricking sensations
Enlargement
Distended subcutaneous veins
Increased nipple and areolar pigmentation
Circumareolar pigmentation
Hypertrophy of subareolar sebaceous glands
(Montgomery's tubercles)
A clear, expressible secretion (colostrum)

use of oestrogens for prostatic carcinoma. (A similar effect occurs in younger males abusing anabolic steroids.)

Gynaecomastia may also be a true side-effect of histamine antagonists, diuretics and cardiac drugs. Curiously, it tends to resolve without the offending agent having to be stopped.

- A few cases are caused by **inappropriate hormone secretion or metabolism**, as may occur in **cirrhosis of the liver** and **bronchial carcinoma**.

History

The patient complains of painless, or slightly tender, enlargement of one or both breasts. Schoolboys with gynaecomastia are often teased by their (so-called) friends.

There may be a history of a recent illness.

Taking a drug history is essential.

Examination

Sometimes there is a clearly palpable disc of firm breast tissue behind and attached to the areola and this is the usual form of gynaecomastia seen in younger men. Drug-induced breast enlargement tends to be more diffuse, with a fatty element. Tenderness is unusual and the axillary lymph glands will not be enlarged.

A general examination, especially of the abdomen (liver) and scrotum (testes), may yield information that indicates the likely cause.

CARCINOMA OF THE MALE BREAST

This is an uncommon condition, usually of elderly men. Its symptoms and physical signs are identical to those of carcinoma of the female breast except that there is little public awareness of the condition and presentation may be late.

Because the male breast is small and not covered by a thick layer of subcutaneous fat, the disease spreads rapidly. Physical signs such as skin and muscle fixation, ulceration and axillary lymphadenopathy are often present by the time of presentation.

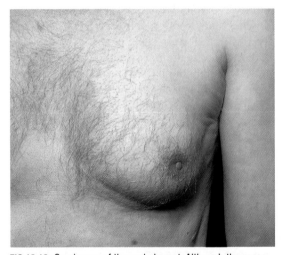

FIG 12.13 Carcinoma of the male breast. Although the mass of tumour is relatively small, it has already caused retraction of the nipple and is fixed to, and dimpling, the skin.

13

The external genitalia

The penis and testes are sensitive organs and difficult to examine when they are tender. This is especially true of the testes. You must be very gentle and careful when examining a tender testis if you wish to gain your patient's confidence and elicit all the abnormal physical signs.

EXAMINATION OF THE MALE GENITALIA

Always put on protective gloves, especially if there is any urethral discharge or if you have any suspicion that the patient is suffering from a communicable disease.

The penis

Inspection

Note the size and shape of the penis, the colour of the skin, the presence or absence of the foreskin and any discharge, scaling or scabbing around its distal edge.

Palpation

Assess the texture of the body of the penis and the whole length of the urethra right down to the perineal membrane.

Always ask the patient to retract the prepuce to examine the skin on its inner aspect, the glans penis and the external urethral meatus. Some patients are

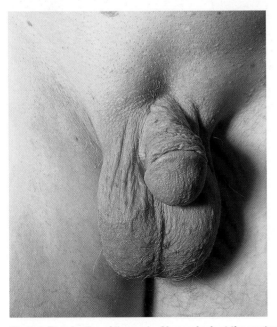
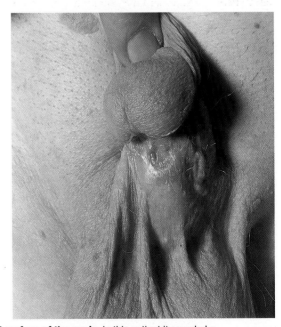

FIG 13.1 Examination of the penis. **Always look at the ventral surface of the penis.** In this patient it revealed a hypospadias.

unable or unwilling to do this and the examiner must take over. This is commonly the case with children.

At birth the foreskin is tethered to the glans penis with only a small meatus. Do not expect, therefore, to be able to retract the foreskin of a small child.

Phimosis is a narrowing of the distal rim of the prepuce, which also prevents retraction. It is seen in all age groups and, when tight, prevents proper examination.

The scrotal skin

The skin of the scrotum is usually wrinkled and freely mobile over the testes. If it is reddened, tethered or fixed, there is probably a deep abnormality, but do not forget that the conditions which affect hair-bearing skin on any other part of the body – sebaceous cyst, infected hair follicle, and squamous carcinoma – may affect the scrotal skin.

The scrotum is two-thirds of a sphere. Remember it has a back and front and do not forget to examine its posterior aspect.

Should you find a lesion in the scrotal skin, proceed methodically through your examination of any lump or ulcer found elsewhere.

The scrotal contents

The shape of the scrotum and the position of the testes within it can only be observed properly when the patient is standing up, but it is more comfortable for patient and student to perform the major part of the examination with the patient lying supine.

Inspection

Note the size and shape of the scrotum, particularly any asymmetry.

Palpation

The scrotal contents are examined by gently supporting the scrotum on the fingers of one or both hands, while feeling the testis and any other lumps between your index finger, which is behind the scrotum, and your thumb, which is in front. Do not squeeze the testis or a lump between your thumb and index finger – let it slip from side to side so that you can feel its shape and surface.

First, check that the scrotum contains two testes.

Next, decide the position and nature of the body of each testis, epididymis and spermatic cords.

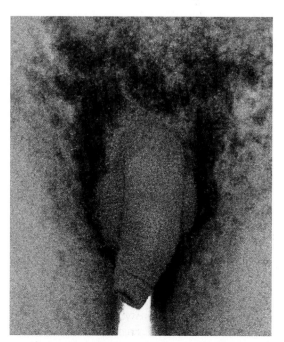
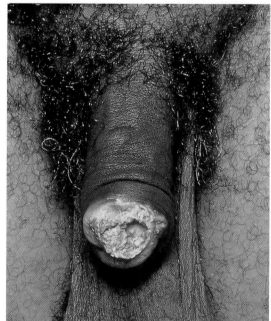

FIG 13.2 Examination of the penis. **Always retract the prepuce** and inspect its inner surface, and the glans penis. In this patient it revealed a carcinoma.

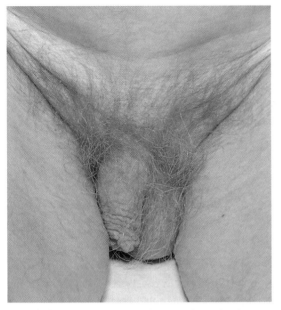
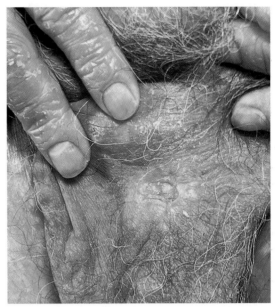

FIG 13.3 Examination of the scrotum. **Always look at the posterior surface** of the srotum. In this patient it revealed a carcinoma.

If you are unsure that what you are feeling is indeed the testis, ask the patient. The testis has unique sensation and, even with gentle palpation, the patient will know when you are holding the testis rather than a similarly sized and shaped swelling.

Assessment of the scrotal contents is one of the last refuges of clinical assessment alone, without investigation. Armed with knowledge of the anatomy and the pathology of the scrotal conditions, it is possible to make an accurate diagnosis in nearly every case.

There are three main characteristics of any scrotal lump which you must determine, and which will be mentioned time and time again in the descriptions of individual diseases.

1. **Is the lump confined to the scrotum?** (Can you get above it?)
2. **Does the lump transilluminate?**
3. **Does the lump have an expansile cough impulse?**

If you have established the answers to these three questions and have defined the physical characteristics of the lump and its relations to each testis and epididymis, you will have no difficulty making the diagnosis. Record your findings on a diagram similar to that in Figure 13.4.

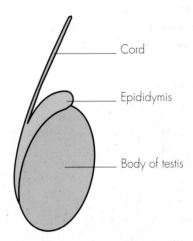

FIG 13.4 If you think of the way in which you will draw the testes, and any abnormality you find, in your notes, it will help you define the anatomy. Do not stop your examination until you have defined the position and condition of the cord, the epididymis and the body of the testes.

The perineum and rectum

Examination of the perineum is an essential part of the examination of the genitalia. Rectal examination to feel the prostate and seminal vesicles is obligatory.

Lymph drainage
(Fig. 13.5)

The skin of the external genitalia drains to the inguinal lymph glands. The scrotal contents, however, develop in the para-aortic area in the back wall of the abdomen. During descent into the scrotum, the arterial blood supply and venous and lymphatic drainage follow the testicle. In consequence:

- lymph from the skin of the penis and scrotum drains to the inguinal glands,
- lymph from the coverings of the testis and spermatic cord (i.e. the tunica vaginalis and the cremasteric and spermatic fasciae) drains to the internal and then to the common iliac glands,
- lymph from the body of the testis drains to the para-aortic glands.

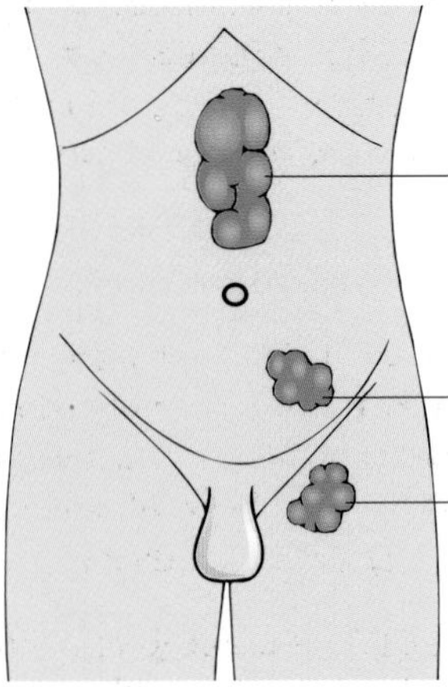

The testis drains to the **para-aortic** lymph glands

The coverings of the testis and the vas drain to the **iliac** lymph glands

The scrotal skin drains to the **inguinal** lymph glands

FIG 13.5 The lymph drainage of the testis, its coverings and the scrotum.

Revision panel 13.1
Age-related incidence of separation/retractability of the foreskin

At birth	4%
At 1 year	50%
At 5 years	90%

Note that the majority of non-retractable foreskins in children do not have a phimosis.

The aortic bifurcation is at the level of the umbilicus; therefore, the abdominal aorta is above the level of the umbilicus. Thus, enlarged para-aortic glands are felt in the upper half of the abdomen, in the epigastrium.

THE PENIS

Phimosis

Phimosis is a narrowing of the end of the prepuce (foreskin), which prevents its retraction over the glans penis. It may be congenital, or it may develop due to scarring of the skin following infection or trauma.

Natural history of the foreskin

At birth, the foreskin covers and is adherent to the glans penis. The opening may initially be very narrow, like a pinhole. In the first few years of life, the foreskin gradually separates and widens so that by the age of 5 approximately 90 per cent of boys are able to retract it freely and easily. The mechanism by which this happens is uncertain. Certainly the normal skin secretions that build up between foreskin and glans (smegma) play a part, and there is also stretching from erections and patient curiosity.

It is normal to have a non-retractile foreskin in early childhood. Even when the foreskin retracts, adhesions between the foreskin and glans may persist into the early teens. There is no 'normal' age beyond which failure to be able to retract the prepuce may be termed abnormal and require treatment, but full retraction should be possible in all adults.

It could therefore be said that phimosis is the normal state of affairs in infants but not in adults; so when does failure to be able to retract become a disease? This is a grey area, and can cause considerable parental concern.

There is one variety of phimosis that is clearly pathological from the beginning, and that is **balanitis xerotica obliterans** (BXO). In this condition, there is scarring of the tip of the foreskin, presumably due to minor tearing and healing with scarring, perhaps with some element of low-grade infection caused by skin organisms. The appearance is characteristic. On gently attempting retraction, whitish, irregular scarring is seen. The process begins at the tip of the foreskin but may spread on to the glans and even narrow the urinary meatus.

Symptoms **Ballooning of the prepuce** on micturition may not be abnormal in a young child. It can only occur when there are no preputial adhesions. Therefore ballooning is only a sign of phimosis when there are no preputial adhesions.

Recurrent balanitis (see below) causing **pain** and a **purulent discharge** is a common complication, but actual urinary tract infection is uncommon, although sometimes attributed to phimosis.

Similar symptoms may occur in the adult, but the commonest complaint is of **discomfort with erection** and **during sexual intercourse**. If a tight foreskin does get retracted, it may not be possible to pull it forwards again; the patient then has a **paraphimosis** (see below).

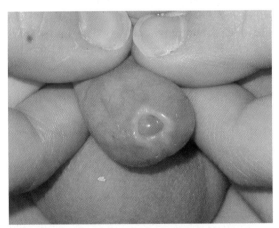

Phimosis in a child with a ring of BXO. Note the white scar tissue made prominent as the patient tries to retract his foreskin.

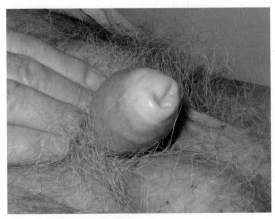

Phimosis and BXO in an adult.

FIG 13.6 TWO EXAMPLES OF BALANITIS XEROTICA OBLITERANS (BXO) AND PHIMOSIS.

Examination

In a child, gently draw back the foreskin and look at the tip. In a normal but narrow foreskin in a small child, the orifice will be small but the skin will appear normal. Sometimes as you continue to retract, the foreskin will not come back completely but skin on the inside of the prepuce will appear. It is pinker and more delicate than the skin on the outside, which has been exposed to friction from clothing. If there is any balanitis xerotica obliterans (BXO), you will see a narrow ring of white scar tissue and will be unable to retract the skin at all.

In children, **smegma** may build up as yellow masses visible and palpable through the foreskin. This appearance may alarm parents and referring physicians.

Paraphimosis

This occurs when the narrowing of the prepuce is just sufficiently tight to get stuck behind the glans penis during an erection, although not necessarily at other times. In this position it impedes venous blood flow and causes oedema and congestion of the glans, which in turn makes reduction of the prepuce more difficult.

History

Age Paraphimosis usually occurs in young men and is very rare in children. It is a common complication of urethral catheterization at any age. It is always preventable by the simple expedient of always pulling the foreskin forwards over the catheter.

Symptoms Shortly after the failure of the foreskin to return to its normal position, there is **swelling** and **discomfort** of the glans penis with a tender, tight band in the coronal sulcus. It is uncommon for the urethra to be so compressed that micturition is obstructed.

Past history The patient will not usually have been circumcized, but note that some religious circumcisions do not involve removal of the whole of the prepuce, so recurrent phimosis and hence paraphimosis may occur.

Examination

The diagnosis is usually obvious. The glans penis is swollen and oedematous and there is a deep groove

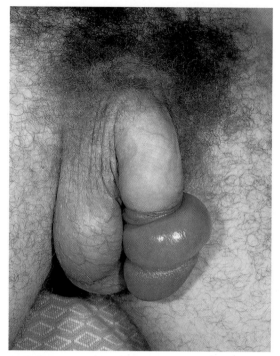

FIG 13.7 Paraphimosis. The retracted, tight, constricting ring of preputial skin is causing oedema of the skin distal to it and congestion of the glans penis.

just below the corona where the skin looks tight, and may be split and ulcerated.

The condition may be chronic, in which case there may be superficial ulceration and infection of the skin of the glans penis.

Hypospadias

Hypospadias is a congenital abnormality in which the urethra opens on the ventral surface of the penis (i.e. proximal to its usual position at the tip of the glans penis).

The opening may be anywhere along the line of the urethra, from a few millimetres from the usual position at the tip of the penis, to the perineum. If the urethral opening is in the perineum, the scrotum is bifid. The site of the opening may be classified as **glandular** (on the glans), **penile** (on the shaft) or **perineal**.

Glandular hypospadias is easy to miss because it causes no symptoms and there is a deceptive vertical slit at the normal site of the urethral opening. The

actual meatus may be quite small and a common site is in the coronal sulcus. Sometimes the parents notice that during micturition, urine is coming from this ectopic opening and not the end of the penis, but quite commonly they do not.

The prepuce has a hooded appearance in hypospadias, because it is deficient ventrally where the urethra emerges. It is vital never to carry out circumcision in a child with any degree of hypospadias, as the preputial skin may be needed for corrective plastic surgery.

Chordee is commonly associated with hypospadias. It is a descriptive term for a curved penis. The curvature is convex dorsally and is more pronounced the further the urethral meatus is away from the end of the organ. It is caused by the corpus spongiosum being shorter than the corpora cavernosa when the urethral opening fails to reach the end of the penis. It may only be visible on erection.

Chordee in the other direction, convex ventrally, is seen in adults with Peyronie's disease.

Epispadias

Epispadias is the opposite of hypospadias. The urethral opening is on the dorsal surface of the glans penis. This condition is extremely rare.

Balanitis

Strictly speaking, balanitis is inflammation of the prepuce, and the correct term for inflammation of the glans is **posthitis**. Many patients have inflammation of both prepuce and glans, and therefore have **balanoposthitis**, but in practice the only term used is balanitis.

Symptoms The patient may complain of itching, pain or discharge, almost invariably with difficulty in retracting the foreskin.

Examination

The foreskin appears reddened and there may be a purulent discharge. In children there will usually be collections of smegma, which may be visible. Look for signs of BXO.

In elderly males, remember the possibility that balanitis may be caused by a carcinoma hidden beneath the prepuce, so retract it if possible.

Palpate the glans and the inguinal lymph glands.

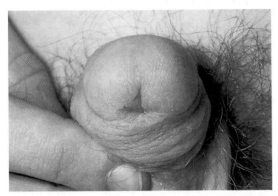

Glandular hypospadias. The urethral opening is on the edge of the glans penis. The pit where the opening should be is also visible.

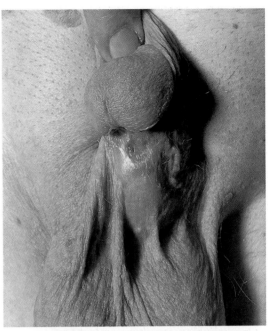

Penile hypospadias. The urethral opening is 1 cm below the edge of the glans.

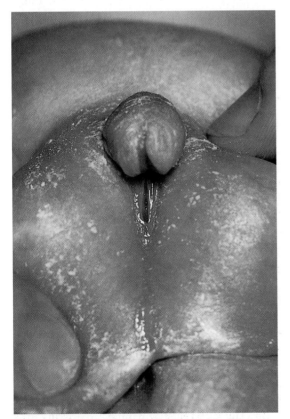

Penoscrotal hypospadias. The urethral opening is at the junction between the shaft of the penis and the scrotum.

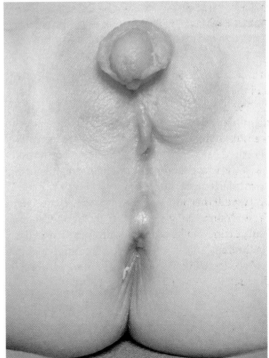

Perineal hypospadias. The urethral opening is in the perineum. The scrotum is bifid.

FIG 13.8 HYPOSPADIAS. Note that the external urethral meatus may be on the glans penis, the shaft of the penis or the perineum.

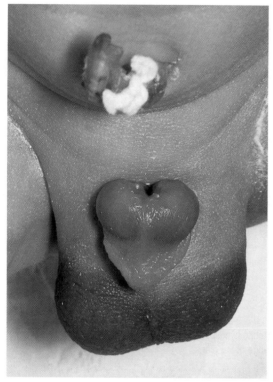

FIG 13.9 Epispadias. The urethra opens on the dorsum of the glans penis, almost on the dorsal aspect of the shaft of the penis.

Special types of balanitis

Candidal balanitis is seen in diabetics and in immunosuppressed patients. The glans penis will show red patches, which may be itchy. The foreskin has a white appearance with longitudinal fissuring, particularly at the tip.

Genital herpes can involve the shaft, glans or foreskin. The vesicles, initially itchy, are soon replaced by shallow, painful erosions. Particularly in the first attack, there may be painful inguinal lymphadenopathy.

Reactions to drugs Drug eruptions are usually painless discolourations, most often seen on the glans penis, and are sometimes the only manifestation of drug hypersensitivity.

Dirt Poor personal hygiene with failure to wash behind the foreskin, particularly in surroundings with a high concentration of dust and dirt, can encourage the accumulation of debris beneath the prepuce. The resulting irritation may cause non-specific inflammation. Coexisting diseases, such as **diabetes**, which render patients more susceptible to infection, increase the risk of secondary infection.

Syphilitic chancre

In many parts of the developed world, syphilis is now rare.

The primary sore, known as a **chancre**, is **solitary** and always **painless**. It usually occurs in the coronal sinus, the prepuce or the frenulum, and produces a serosanguinous discharge.

Beneath an area of **superficial ulceration** is an indistinct, indurated lump, 5–10 mm in diameter. The ulcer is covered with a slough and has a sloping, indolent edge. It is not fixed to deeper structures.

The inguinal lymph glands are invariably enlarged, often mainly on one side. They are rubbery and discrete, but **not tender**.

General examination may reveal no other abnormalities, but a primary sore may still be present should the patient present with the secondary manifestations of the disease 4–6 weeks after the appearance of the chancre.

Carcinoma of the penis

Carcinoma of the penis is a squamous cell carcinoma. It is exceedingly rare in men who have been circumcized at birth or in adolescence, as is common in Jewish and Muslim communities.

It may be preceded by a number of pre-malignant conditions described below. It invades from the penile skin into the tissues of the shaft of the penis and spreads via the lymphatics.

History

Age Carcinoma of the penis commonly presents in middle or old age, but can, rarely, occur in young men.

Ethnic group Carcinoma of the penis is more common in cultures that do not practise ritual circumcision.

Symptoms Most patients present with a **lump** or an **ulcer**. The lesion may be **painful**, especially if it is infected.

There is usually a **purulent discharge**, which may be blood stained.

The patient may also complain of **phimosis**. In these circumstances the primary lesion can become quite advanced before it is detected.

The inguinal lymph glands may be enlarged by secondary infection or secondary deposits and may be the first abnormality noticed by the patient. Presentation with distant metastases is rare.

The occasional patient ignores his symptoms until the tumour compresses or invades the urethra and urinary retention occurs.

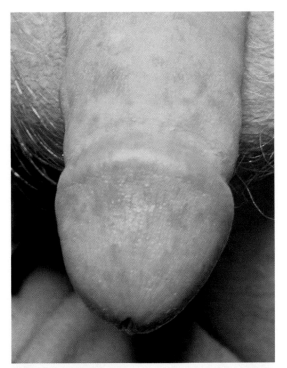

Monilial balanoposthitis.

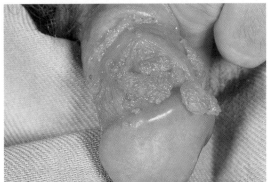

Penile warts.

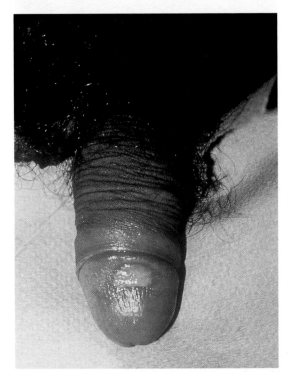

A drug eruption. This ulcer was part of a reaction to Septrin.

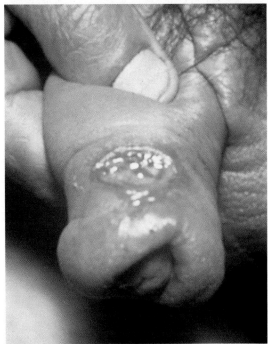

A syphilitic chancre on the inner surface of the prepuce. (The ungloved hand is that of the patient.)

FIG 13.10 FOUR COMMON PENILE CONDITIONS.

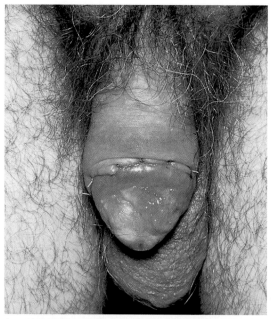

An early carcinomatous ulcer on the glans penis, exposed by a circumcision.

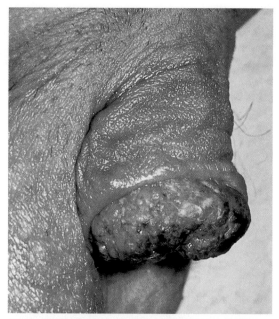

An advanced infiltrating carcinoma which has invaded the whole thickness of the prepuce.

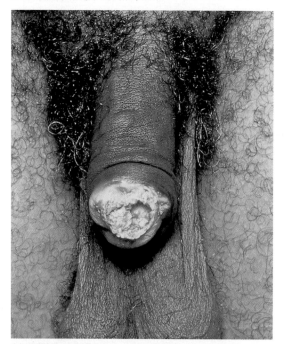

A papilliferous carcinoma arising in the coronal sulcus.

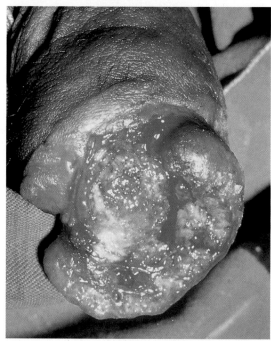

An ulcerating carcinoma that has destroyed half of the glans penis.

FIG 13.11 CARCINOMA OF THE PENIS.

Examination

Prepuce The patient is most unlikely to have been circumcized, and in the UK is commonly elderly and self-neglected. There may be a serous, purulent or sanguinous **discharge** coming from beneath the prepuce. If the foreskin cannot be retracted, full examination of its inner surface and the glans penis may require a surgical slit.

Deformity The penis may be swollen at its tip owing to the mass beneath the prepuce. In the advanced stages the tumour may appear through the opening in the prepuce or erode through the preputial skin.

Position The lesion may be anywhere on the skin of the prepuce or the glans penis.

Tenderness The lump or ulcer is not usually tender, except when secondarily infected.

Shape Carcinoma of the penis tends to adopt one of two macroscopic forms: a classic carcinomatous **ulcer** with a raised everted edge and necrotic base, or a **papilliferous** tumour with a wide sessile pedicle and an indurated base. The microscopic pathology is the same.

The shape simply reflects the degree of tumour necrosis.

Size Most patients appear early in the course of the disease provided they can retract their foreskin. If they have phimosis, and have grown accustomed to an occasional discharge, they may not present until the tumour is large or visible.

Composition The tumour has a hard consistence, especially at its base. Any part of the penis that is infiltrated also feels hard. The surface of the papilliferous variety is soft and friable. It often looks like granulation tissue, and bleeds easily.

Relations In the early stages the tumour is confined to the skin, but it may invade and spread through the whole corpus cavernosum, making it indurated and hard, and if it begins on the inner side of the prepuce, it may spread to and through the outer layer of skin.

Lymph drainage The inguinal lymph glands of both groins are likely to be enlarged, by infection or secondary deposits.

Skin conditions of the penis

Various skin conditions are associated with an increased incidence of carcinoma of the penis, and the underlying pathological condition is called **intraepithelial neoplasia**. This is the same as that seen in the female genital tract in the cervix and vulva, and also in the peri-anal skin.

It is now appreciated that various clinical appearances, often classified by their colour (e.g. leukoplakia) or the name of the physician who fist described them (e.g. Paget's disease or the erythroplasia of Querat), have essentially the same pathology. The student needs to remember that any chronic skin eruption on the penis might be penile intraepithelial neoplasia (PIN) and should be assessed and treated accordingly.

Clinical diagnosis is difficult because any skin disease may occur on the skin of the penis. Lichen sclerosis particularly mimics intraepithelial neoplasia.

Viral warts are common and behave as they do elsewhere in the body.

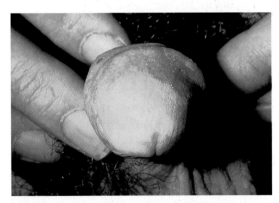

FIG 13.12 An example of penile intraepithelial neoplasia (PIN). This variety is commonly called leukoplakia.

Priapism

Priapism is a persistent, usually painful erection. There are two varieties, **primary** and **secondary**.

Secondary priapism is caused by a haematological disorder which triggers thrombosis of the corpora cavernosa, such as **leukaemia** or **sickle-cell disease**, or by obstruction to the venous and lymphatic drainage of the penis by pelvic malignancy. Presentation is part of a generalized advanced illness.

Primary idiopathic priapism is seen in previously fit men after sexual activity. It is usually caused by a failure of the venular spasm that sustains the erection to relax. Because of embarrassment, presentation may be late.

The erection seen in priapism is not of the normal pattern and shape. It is confined to the corpora cavernosa and may affect only one side, producing a lateral chordee. The corpus spongiosum remains soft.

Without immediate surgical treatment, impotence will result.

Peyronie's disease

This is an idiopathic plaque of fibrosis in one of the corpora cavernosa, usually on the dorsal side. It occurs in middle-aged men. The symptoms are pain and a curvature of the penis when erect. It rarely interferes with sexual intercourse. The plaque may be palpable when the penis is flaccid.

The differential diagnosis includes metastatic tumour deposits, but this is a rare event and the patient will usually be clearly unwell.

THE SCROTAL SKIN

Sebaceous cysts

Sebaceous cysts are common in the scrotal skin and are often multiple. They have all the features described in Chapter 3 but are mentioned here because it is surprising how often they are misdiagnosed.

Occasionally they can become infected, discharge and produce so much granulation tissue that they look like a carcinoma.

Carcinoma of the scrotal skin

This is a squamous carcinoma. It can be caused by frequent contact with soot (chimney sweep's cancer), tar or oil (mule spinner's cancer). The skin must be exposed to these irritants for many years before a cancer develops.

History

Age Carcinoma of the skin of the scrotum is uncommon below the age of 50 years.

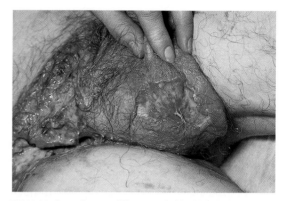

FIG 13.13 A carcinoma of the scrotal skin. Note that it is on the postero-medial surface of the scrotum.

Occupation The patient's occupation may be responsible for frequent soiling of the scrotal skin with oil and other carcinogenic hydrocarbons. Even today, the clothes of garage mechanics and machine operators become soaked in oil, which percolates through to their underclothes.

Symptoms Most patients present with a **lump** or an **ulcer** or a **lump**. A **purulent discharge** may appear, and if the ulcer is hidden in the cleft between the scrotum and leg, the discharge may be noticed before the ulcer.

The patient may notice **lumps in the groin** if the inguinal lymph glands are involved.

Examination

Position A carcinomatous ulcer can occur on any part of the scrotal skin, but industrial cancers are often high up in the cleft between the leg and the scrotum, where there is repeated friction and persistent traces of oil.

Tenderness The ulcer is usually painless and not tender.

Shape In its early stages the ulcer is small and circular, but it usually enlarges in an irregular fashion and develops an irregular outline.

Edge The edge is reddish, friable and typically everted.

Base The base is covered with yellow-grey, infected, necrotic tumour.

Discharge There is often a purulent, bloody, offensive discharge.

Relations In the early stages the skin and ulcer are freely mobile, but if the tumour cells spread deep to the skin, the ulcer may become tethered to the underlying testicle.

Lymph drainage The inguinal lymph glands may be enlarged by tumour metastases or secondary infection.

General examination Distant metastases are unusual with scrotal cancer.

Tinea cruris

Common conditions present in diverse clinics. Tinea cruris is a fungal infection of the skin of the upper medial aspect of the thigh and the adjacent scrotal skin.

The first symptom is **itching**, but this is soon followed by the appearance of a dry **erythematous rash** with a sharply defined edge **on the thigh and scrotum**.

If the patient perspires heavily, the rash may become macerated and ooze serum, which forms pale-brown crusts.

The patient may present to a surgical clinic because of the changes in the scrotal skin, or you may notice the distinctive skin changes when examining the patient's scrotum for another complaint, such as a hernia.

Lymphoedema

Swelling of the penis and scrotum caused by excess fluid in the subcutaneous tissue (oedema) is seen commonly in patients confined to bed with heart failure or fluid retention. It may also occur after surgery in the groin.

True lymphoedema of the genitalia – oedema caused by retention of protein-rich lymph in the subcutaneous tissues – is uncommon. It may be associated with lymphoedema of one or both limbs. The usual cause is obstruction of the inguinal and iliac lymph pathways by secondary or primary malignant disease or, in tropical areas, by worms (*Wuchereria bancrofti*, **filariasis**).

Primary genital lymphoedema is very rare and caused by hypoplastic lymphatics. It is not known if it is a congenital or an acquired condition.

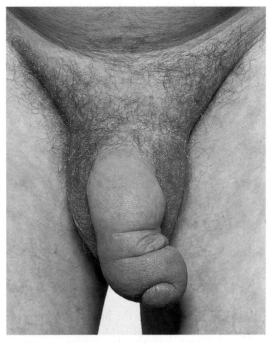

FIG 13.14 Lymphoedema of the penis.

Sinuses of the scrotum

Disease of the testis or epididymis may occasionally spread to, and through, the scrotal skin to create a sinus between the primary lesion and the skin surface.

Provided the testis is lying in the normal position, disease of the body of the testis tends to spread to the antero-lateral surface of the scrotum, whereas disease of the epididymis spreads to the posterior surface. Both are rare occurrences requiring gross intrascrotal pathology. Most sinuses in the scrotal skin are discharging **sebaceous cysts**.

THE TESTES

Failure of normal testicular descent

The testis develops in utero in the posterior abdominal wall from nephric tissue. Its blood supply comes from the aorta and its veins drain into the inferior vena cava, on the left via the renal vein. Lymph drainage is to the para-aortic glands.

Guided by the gubernaculum, the testicle descends into the scrotum, the left before the right. Most testicles have reached the scrotum by the time of birth

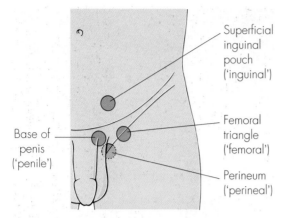

FIG 13.15 The sites where you may find an ectopic testis.

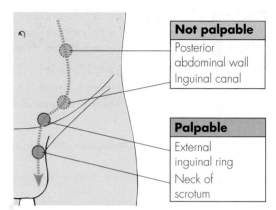

FIG 13.16 The line of normal testicular descent. An incompletely descended testis may be found anywhere on this line. If it is above the external inguinal ring, it will be impalpable.

and it is unlikely that any natural descent occurs thereafter.

Examination of the scrotum and groin can be difficult in small babies.

You can only confirm the presence or absence of the testes by careful palpation. A quick glance at the scrotum is not good enough.

By 3 months, only 1–2 per cent of testicles cannot be found by an experienced examiner.

If a testis has never descended into the scrotum, the scrotal skin on that side will be underdeveloped.

If a testis is not in the scrotum, it may either have stopped somewhere along its line of normal descent or have found its way to an abnormal site. The aetiology of these two abnormalities is different and there is no standardization of the names used to describe them. A simple classification is as follows.

- **A testis which has descended to an abnormal site is an *ectopic testis*.** There is no confusion about this term. The testis may be in the superficial inguinal pouch, the femoral triangle or the perineum. The mechanism causing descent is normal but the guidance system has gone wrong. The testicle itself is normal.
- **A testis which is in its correct anatomical path but has failed to reach the scrotum is best called a *truly undescended testis*.** Although this is a cumbersome name, it is better than 'undescended' or 'maldescended' because both these names could reasonably be used to describe the two sorts of missing testicle.

The truly undescended testicle is small and abnormal, with a separated epididymis and often an associated indirect inguinal hernial sac. We do not know whether the testicle is abnormal because it fails to descend, or fails to descend because it is abnormal.

Absence of both testes from the scrotum caused by a failure of descent is known as **cryptorchism**.

True congenital absence of a testicle is rare and is usually on the left. The testicle is sometimes missing because it has met with a vascular accident, usually torsion (see below) in early or even intrauterine life.

Examination of a child with a missing testicle

This can be difficult with a child who does not want to be examined and frequently anxious parents. Make sure the room and your hands are warm. The child has to be persuaded to lie down. Do not be downhearted if you cannot persuade the child to let you carry out the necessary careful examination. Try again later, or accept that more experienced help on another occasion will be needed.

Inspection The child must be undressed from the waist downwards in a good light. An empty scrotum, with very little development of the scrotal skin because it has never had the testicle within it, is usually obvious. However, a prominent gubernaculum may look like a testis but it will not feel like one.

If the testicle is in the superficial pouch, it may be visible in the inguinal region in a thin patient.

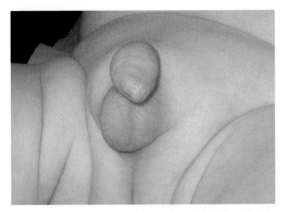

FIG 13.17 This baby has a truly undescended and impalpable left testis. The scrotal skin is very poorly developed compared to the right side, where the testis has fully descended.

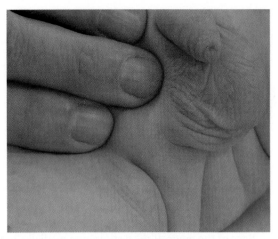

FIG 13.18 A perineal ectopic testis. As the testicle was milked downwards and medially, it did not enter the scrotum, but passed backwards into the perineum.

Palpation You must try to get the child to relax, as muscular activity makes the dartos muscle contract and draw the testicle up towards the groin.

Examine the groin before palpating the scrotum. If you cannot see or feel the testis in the subcutaneous tissues, find out if it is in the inguinal canal by gently sweeping your fingers from the anterior superior iliac spine obliquely across the groin to the pubis, along the line of the inguinal canal, towards the neck of the scrotum, to 'milk' the testis, if present, through the external ring. If the testis becomes palpable, catch it gently with the thumb and index finger of your other hand and draw it down to the scrotum. If it is a retractile testis, it will move down easily.

Should you get the testicle down into the scrotum, show it to the parents before you remove your fingers and the testicle retracts!

Ectopic testis

History

Age Children in developed countries will usually be routinely examined at birth and again in the first year of life. Examination requires experience. An ectopic testis may readily be missed, a prominent gubernaculum being mistaken for the testicle. Not all parents notice that their infant child has one or both testes missing from his scrotum.

The patient may not discover the abnormality himself until adolescence.

Symptoms **Absence of a testis** is the common presenting symptom, but the patient may also complain of pain or discomfort if the testis is in a site, such as the superficial inguinal pouch, likely to be rubbed or compressed during normal physical activity. Note that the pain pathway is via autonomic afferent nerves and for developmental reasons may be experienced in the groin or even loin.

Systemic effects If both testes are ectopic, the patient may be subfertile but rarely lacks secondary sex characteristics.

Examination

The side of the scrotum without the testis may be poorly developed, but not so obviously as with a truly undescended testicle.

Site An ectopic testis is nearly always palpable, although with difficulty in a fat child. A truly undescended testis lying in the inguinal canal or abdomen is not palpable. If the testis is not in the scrotum, you must search for a smooth, sensitive, ovoid swelling in those sites where ectopic testes are known to settle.

- **Superficial inguinal pouch.** This is by far the commonest site in which to find an ectopic testicle. It is also the place to which the retractile testicle retreats. An ectopic testicle in this site has emerged through the external ring but, having failed to enter the scrotum, turns upwards and laterally to lie in a pouch deep to the superficial fascia. This may be caused by some obstruction at the neck of the scrotum from tight fascia. The testis can be palpated in the subcutaneous tissue just above and lateral to the crest of the pubis and the pubic tubercle.

- **Femoral triangle.** If the testis moves laterally after leaving the external inguinal ring, it can come to rest in the upper medial corner of the femoral triangle. A testis in this site is easy to feel and easily misdiagnosed as a lymph gland or even a femoral hernia, although the latter is very rare in children. This variety is sometimes termed **crural**, as it lies in the thigh.
- **Base of the penis.** If the testis moves medially, it will lie at the base of the penis, where it can be easily felt against the underlying pubic bone.
- **Perineum.** Occasionally, the testis passes over the pubis and then backwards, instead of downwards, to lie in the perineum just to one side of the corpus cavernosum of the penis. An ectopic testis cannot be manipulated into the scrotum.

The lump An absent scrotal testis and a lump in one of the four sites described above make the diagnosis of ectopic testis very probable, but it is important to confirm that the lump has the features of a testis.

It should be ovoid, smooth, slightly tender and soft-solid in consistence. It should be mobile within the subcutaneous tissues, and gentle pressure should cause the mild sickening sensation recognized by most males as testicular sensation.

It is unusual to be able to define the separate features of the body of the testis and the epididymis.

Any enlargement, irregularity or immobility should make you suspect the presence of malignant change in the testis, or make you look for another diagnosis.

Truly undescended testis

History

Truly undescended testes are usually noticed in early life but occasionally not until adolescence.

Symptoms An **absence of one or both testes from the scrotum** is the presenting symptom. The parents may first notice that the **scrotum has not developed** – unaware of the absence of the testes. A

small proportion of patients present in adult life with **infertility**. Although failure of testicular descent is invariably associated with abnormal spermatogenesis, the hormone-producing cells are usually normal so the boy has a normal puberty and secondary sex characteristics.

All truly undescended testes are associated with an **indirect inguinal hernia**, and a groin swelling may be the presenting complaint.

Examination

The scrotum When both testes are undescended the scrotum is small and hypoplastic. If only one testis has descended, it is markedly asymmetrical.

Site A truly undescended testis lies somewhere in the line of normal descent (i.e. at the neck of the scrotum, in the external inguinal ring, in the inguinal canal or in the posterior abdominal wall).

The testis only becomes palpable when it reaches, or is outside, the external inguinal ring.

Within the inguinal canal it cannot be felt because the tense overlying external oblique aponeurosis conceals it and it tends to slip back through the internal ring into the abdomen. Thus, if you can feel a testis lateral to the external inguinal ring, it must be superficial to the external oblique and is therefore an ectopic testis not a truly undescended testis.

Some testes which lie in the inguinal canal can be milked down to the external ring by gently stroking along the line of the canal as described above.

The lump A truly undescended testis is usually smaller than normal but otherwise has all the expected characteristics of a testis.

In an adult, the appearance of a mass in the line of testicular descent, whether within the abdomen or the inguinal canal, and an empty scrotum should make you suspect malignant change in a truly undescended testicle. The risk of malignant change is many times greater than in a normally descended or ectopic testis. Fixing the testis in the scrotum (orchidopexy) does not eliminate this risk.

The truly undescended testis is also more likely to undergo torsion than a normally descended testis.

Retractile testes

The cremaster is a strong active muscle during childhood, and the testes of many young children move freely up and down between the scrotum and the inguinal canal or the superficial inguinal pouch. A cold examining hand may be sufficient stimulus to cause retraction. If the patient is seen when the testis is retracted, it may be misdiagnosed as a truly undescended testis and surgical treatment advised. This will be an unnecessary operation because all retractile testes ultimately descend properly, before or at puberty.

History

The parents notice that the testicle (frequently both) is absent from the scrotum. This situation is often intermittent, and it may be noticed that everything appears normal when the child is warm and relaxed, typically in the bath.

The testicles may have been reported in the scrotum at previous routine examinations.

Examination

When the testes are retractile, the scrotum is normally developed.

You should always attempt to manipulate the testis into the scrotum, as described above. If the testicle can be persuaded into the scrotum and it rests there when you let go, it is a retractile testicle. A testis should only be classified as truly undescended or ectopic if you cannot manipulate it into the scrotum.

However, experience is required to be certain of this physical finding.

The ascending testicle

Many boys are referred to the surgical clinic with a missing or intermittently absent testicle, a normal scrotum, and a testicle that is palpable in the superficial inguinal pouch. On examination, the testicle may or may not be placed in the scrotum. However, a single assessment is not reliable. A testicle that cannot be placed in the scrotum one day may be persuaded to go there on another, perhaps by a different examiner.

There is also a group of patients in whom the testicle has been found and placed in the scrotum to the satisfaction of all, but, some while later, the parents notice that the testicle is no longer visible and seek further advice. On this occasion, the testicle may be palpable in the superficial inguinal pouch and cannot be persuaded into the scrotum, even by the examiner who was successful on the previous occasion.

The testicle has, on our clinical criteria, changed from being retractile to ectopic. This is termed the 'ascending testicle' or sometimes 'acquired undescended testicle', a confusing term.

Thus there is often uncertainty in differentiating between superficial pouch ectopic and superficial pouch retractile testicles. The only solution to the dilemma is to repeat the assessment until puberty is attained, when any testicle not resting in the scrotum should be considered to be abnormal and in need of surgical treatment. Note, however, that the truly undescended testicle may be diagnosed definitively because it is impalpable and the scrotum is poorly developed.

Hydrocele

A hydrocele is an abnormal quantity of fluid within the tunica vaginalis. There are two varieties:

- **primary**, of unknown cause,
- **secondary**, caused by trauma, infection or neoplasm.

Most secondary hydroceles appear rapidly in the presence of other symptoms associated with their cause, are not tense, and contain some altered blood. They are much less common than primary (idiopathic) hydroceles, which develop slowly and progressively and become large and tense.

History

Age Primary hydroceles are most common over the age of 40 years. In children, although the physical signs are the same as in adults, the condition is always associated with a patent processus vaginalis and is a variety of inguinal hernia.

Secondary hydroceles are more common between 20 and 40 years because trauma, infection and testicular neoplasms are more common in this period.

Symptoms The patient complains of an increase in the size of the testis, or a **swelling** in the scrotum. There may be pain and discomfort if there is underlying testicular disease, but idiopathic hydroceles reach a considerable size without causing pain. The patient may complain of the social embarrassment of his large scrotum, which shows through his trousers.

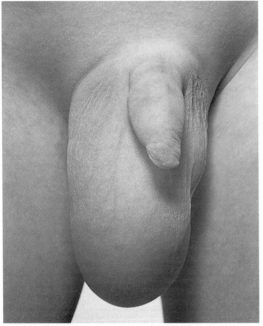

A large hydrocele. The swelling is confined to the scrotum, not tender, fluctuant, translucent, and the testis is not palpable.

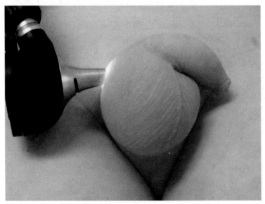

A transilluminated hydrocele.

FIG 13.19 HYDROCELE.

Revision panel 13.2
The causes of hydrocele

Primary
    Idiopathic
Secondary
    Trauma
    Epididymo-orchitis
    Tumour
    Lymphatic obstruction

Hydroceles do not affect fertility, although a large one may cause problems during sexual intercourse.

Examination

Position The swelling fills one side of the scrotum but is within the scrotum and you can feel the spermatic cord above the lump. The testis cannot be palpated separately because it is within the swelling. This is the cardinal physical sign that distinguishes a hydrocele from an epididymal cyst.

Hydroceles may be bilateral.

Colour and temperature The colour and temperature of the overlying scrotal skin are normal.

Tenderness Primary hydroceles are not tender. Secondary hydroceles may be tender if the underlying testis is tender.

Shape and size When the tunica vaginalis first fills with fluid, the resulting hydrocele is just a little larger than the testis. As time passes, the volume of fluid increases.

Hydroceles can become 10–20 cm in diameter and contain as much as 500 mL of fluid. They are ovoid in shape.

Surface The surface is always smooth and well defined. Occasionally a weak spot in the wall gives way to form a small fluctuant bump, a hernia of the hydrocele fluid through its coverings.

Composition Hydroceles contain a clear yellow fluid which is protein rich. They are therefore **fluctuant**, have a **fluid thrill** if they are large enough, are **dull to percussion** and usually **transilluminate**.

They do not pulsate and are not compressible.

They may be **tense or lax**, depending on the pressure of the contained fluid.

The wall of a long-standing hydrocele may become calcified, making the mass hard and opaque.

Reducibility Hydroceles cannot be reduced.

Relations The **fluid** of a hydrocele **surrounds the body of the testis**, making the **testis impalpable**. This is its most important relationship. If you can feel the testis separate from a scrotal swelling, the swelling cannot be a hydrocele.

When a hydrocele is lax, a feature almost invariably seen only in secondary hydroceles, it may be possible to feel the surface of the testis through the fluid.

The testis produces an opaque area in an otherwise highly translucent swelling, but it is usually too small to see clearly.

The spermatic cord can be felt coming down to and running into the swelling. The skin of the scrotum is freely mobile over the swelling.

Lymph drainage The para-aortic lymph glands, which receive lymph from the testis, should be carefully palpated if you think the swelling is a secondary hydrocele, because they may be enlarged if there is an underlying testicular tumour.

Epididymal cyst

Epididymal cysts are fluid-filled swellings arising from the epididymis. Their aetiology has not been satisfactorily explained, but they are derived from the collecting tubules of the epididymis.

An epididymal cyst usually contains clear fluid. The variety that contains slightly grey, opaque, 'barley water'-like fluid and a few spermatozoa is sometimes termed a **spermatocele**. This distinction can only be made after aspiration, and there is no clinical way of differentiating between the two types. As the large majority of cysts connected with the epididymis contain clear fluid, it is best to call them all epididymal cysts and not use the term spermatocele.

History

Age Most epididymal cysts occur in men over the age of 40 years, but they are occasionally seen in children and adolescents.

Symptoms The main complaint is of **swelling** in the scrotum, with the occasional patient believing that he has developed a third testis.

In older age groups the swelling is usually painless. Small epididymal cysts in men in their thirties and forties may be painful and tender.

Development Epididymal cysts enlarge very slowly, over many years, but rarely become gigantic. A really big, fluid-filled scrotal swelling is likely to be a hydrocele.

Multiplicity They are often **multiple** or **multilocular**, and are frequently **bilateral**.

Fertility Epididymal cysts do not interfere with fertility. However, surgery to remove such cysts may have an effect equivalent to that of a vasectomy.

Examination

Position The swelling lies within the scrotum, usually above and slightly behind the testis. **The testis can be felt separately from the swelling.** If the swelling is similar in size to a testicle, ask the patient which of the lumps is which. He will always be able to tell you!

The spermatic cord can be felt above it.

Tenderness Small cysts of the epididymis in younger men may be tender, but larger cysts in older men are not.

Shape Because the cysts are usually multilocular, the swelling is rarely a perfect sphere. It is usually elongated and bosselated, and individual loculi may be palpable.

Size Epididymal cysts may vary in size from a few millimetres to 5–10 cm in diameter. They rarely reach the size of the large hydroceles.

Surface The surface is smooth but the contours of individual loculi may be palpable.

Composition These swellings are **fluctuant**, have a **fluid thrill**, are **translucent** if large enough to transilluminate, and are **dull** to percussion.

Epididymal cysts cannot be reduced.

All the signs mentioned in this section on composition are identical to those for hydrocele. The difference between a hydrocele and an epididymal cyst lies in the relation of the swelling to the testis.

Relations Epididymal cysts are separate from the testis, therefore the **testis remains palpable**.

Most epididymal cysts are connected to the head of the epididymis and so lie above the testis with the spermatic cord descending into or behind them. They occasionally lie at the lower pole.

Lymph drainage The regional lymph glands should not be palpable.

General examination This should be quite normal.

Differential diagnosis The normal epididymis is usually palpable and may be noticed by concerned young men who think they have a testicular tumour. It may on occasion be difficult to say if a swelling is a normal palpable organ or a small cyst. A period of observation will provide the answer.

Tumours of the epididymis itself are so rare as to be virtually non-existent. Any swelling that is clearly in the epididymis is therefore benign.

Varicocele

A varicocele is a bunch of dilated and tortuous veins in the pampiniform plexus. The condition could be renamed varicose veins of the spermatic cord. It is almost invariably on the left. The right testicular veins drain into the inferior vena cava, but on the left they drain into the left renal vein. The left testicular vein (or veins) is thus a long vessel and it is hardly surprising that its valves often fail and produce a varicocele.

Small **symptomless varicoceles occur in 25 per cent of normal men**, on the left side. When the veins become large, they may cause a vague, dragging sensation and aching pain in the scrotum or groin. The appearance may embarrass adolescents and young men.

The sudden appearance of a varicocele in middle or old age may be caused by a renal neoplasm spreading along the renal vein and obstructing the testicular vein. This is a very rare presentation of carcinoma of the kidney but should not be forgotten, particularly if there are other urinary tract symptoms.

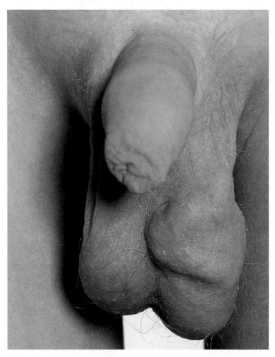

FIG 13.20 A varicocele. When standing, the tense, tortuous, distended veins are said to feel like a 'bag of worms'. When supine, they collapse and are almost impalpable.

You cannot feel a varicocele when the patient is lying down because the veins are empty. This is one of the reasons why you must always examine the scrotum with the patient standing up. The dilated, compressible veins above the testis are then palpable and often visible. They feel like a 'bag of worms', an accurate description.

The testis below a large varicocele may be smaller and softer than the testis on the normal side. The effect of a varicocele on spermatogenesis is controversial.

Haematocele

A haematocele is a collection of blood within the tunica vaginalis. The bleeding is usually caused by trauma or underlying malignant disease.

In the acute phase the mass has the same physical signs as a hydrocele, except that it is **not translucent** and may be **tender**. When the blood clots, it contracts and forms a small, hard mass, which can cause diagnostic problems.

Acute haematocele

The patient usually but not always gives a clear history of an injury, or of vague discomfort in the testis, followed by a painful, rapid swelling of the scrotum. It is a condition particularly associated with cycling.

The swelling, which is in one side of the scrotum, is **tense**, **tender** and **fluctuant**, but does not transilluminate. **The testis cannot be felt separate from the swelling.**

Chronic haematocele

If the acute episode is ignored and not treated, or if the bleeding occurs without the patient's knowledge, the blood in the tunica vaginalis will clot. As time passes, the clot that surrounds the testis contracts and hardens. The result is a hard mass, which is no longer tender and is not fluctuant. Normal testicular sensation may be lost if the contracting clot causes ischaemic necrosis of the testis.

These changes make a chronic haematocele difficult to distinguish from a testicular tumour, and the testis may need to be explored before the final diagnosis can be made.

Torsion of the testicle

The tunica vaginalis covers the sides and anterior aspect of the testis. The back of the epididymis and the posterior surface of the testis covered by the epididymis are not covered by the tunica vaginalis. A normal testis is, therefore, fixed within the tunica and cannot twist.

However, there is variability in the extent to which the tunica vaginalis covers the body of the testis. In one variation, the testicle is suspended in the tunica like the clapper in a bell, and is thus able to twist on its attachment. This process can be aided by contraction of the spiral fibres of the cremaster muscle.

In another variety, the testis is separated from the epididymis by a long mesorchium, long enough to allow a twist to occur between the testis and the epididymis. This is less common.

Extravaginal torsion – torsion of the spermatic cord itself – is another rarer possibility.

The anatomical abnormality that allows torsion is invariably bilateral.

The condition may resolve spontaneously or progress to testicular infarction.

History

Age Torsion presents most commonly in teenagers, but as the cause is a congenital abnormality, it can occur in young children, neonates and even in utero. It is very uncommon in men over 25 years of age and unknown over 40.

Symptoms The initial symptom is an uncomfortable, poorly localized pain, which may initially be felt in the abdomen or loin because it is autonomically modulated and so referred to the embryological site

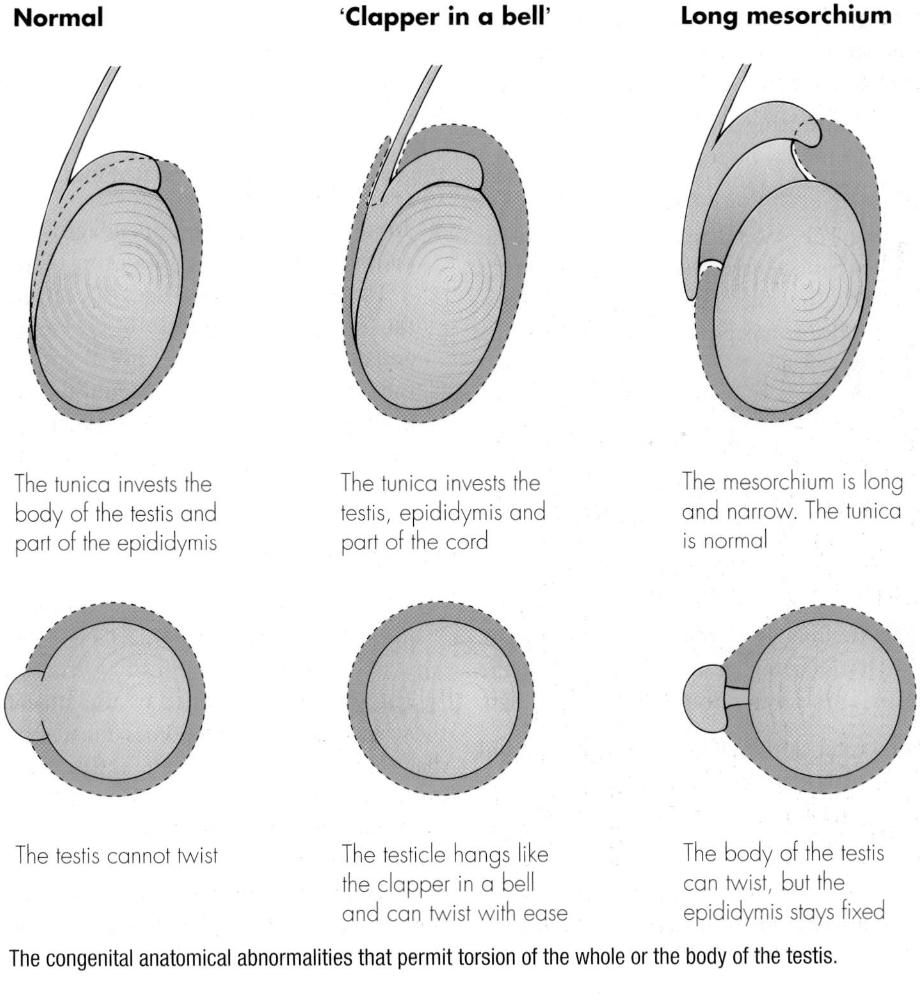

Normal	**'Clapper in a bell'**	**Long mesorchium**

The tunica invests the body of the testis and part of the epididymis

The tunica invests the testis, epididymis and part of the cord

The mesorchium is long and narrow. The tunica is normal

The testis cannot twist

The testicle hangs like the clapper in a bell and can twist with ease

The body of the testis can twist, but the epididymis stays fixed

FIG 13.21 The congenital anatomical abnormalities that permit torsion of the whole or the body of the testis.

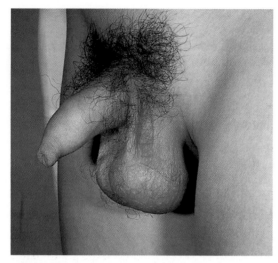

FIG 13.22 A testis hanging horizontally and susceptible to torsion.

of origin of the testis. **Severe pain and tenderness in the testicle** follow the abdominal pain, but the abdominal component may be absent or forgotten.

Nausea and **vomiting** are common.

In a baby there may be restlessness and a failure to eat.

Previous attacks The patient may have had similar mild attacks of pain, which subsided spontaneously, or an episode on the other side which required surgery. Recurrent torsion is possible if the testicle has not been securely fixed.

Cause Although the majority of torsions seem to occur spontaneously, often in the early hours of the morning, some follow minor trauma, one of the commonest being a blow on the scrotum as the boy jumps on to his bicycle.

Examination

Position The swelling is confined to the scrotum. The affected testis lies higher in the scrotum than the normal testis. This is a most important physical sign.

Colour The scrotal skin may be normal, or red and oedematous. Although the latter changes are more commonly associated with epididymo-orchitis, their presence must not dissuade you from making a diagnosis of torsion.

Temperature The skin will feel hot if it is red and hyperaemic.

Tenderness The **testis is exquisitely tender**, making palpation very difficult.

Shape The whole of the testis is swollen and it is usually impossible to distinguish the contours of the epididymis from those of the body of the testis.

Surface The surface of the testis is smooth, but it may be obscured by scrotal oedema.

Composition It is usually impossible to elicit the signs which will reveal the composition of the mass in the scrotum because of tenderness. The mass may be the testicle, or the testicle surrounded by an acute secondary hydrocele.

Surrounding tissues Apart from the scrotal skin, which may be red and oedematous, the other nearby tissues, including the other testis, will be normal.

Differential diagnosis Torsion of a testis within the scrotum may be indistinguishable from acute **epididymo-orchitis**, particularly if there are no urinary symptoms. However, epididymo-orchitis usually occurs in an older age group. Torsion of a truly undescended testicle in the groin may be indistinguishable from a **strangulated inguinal hernia**.

- **Torsion of a testicular appendage** is the commonest condition mimicking torsion.

  There are two appendages (the appendix of the testis and the appendix of the epididymis) and either may tort. Their initial symptom (abdominal pain) may be identical. The testicle is not usually so tender, and sometimes the torted appendage is palpable as a tender nodule. However, a secondary hydrocele may obscure this.
- **Idiopathic scrotal oedema** is a condition in which the skin and subcutaneous tissues of the scrotum become oedematous, red and inflamed, in most cases as a result of a streptococcal infection.

The swelling is confined by the attachments of the scrotal fascia and sometimes unilateral. A clinical diagnosis can usually be made, as the testicle itself is not tender.

Warning: when in doubt about a painful scrotal/testicular swelling, make a diagnosis of torsion, because failure to explore the scrotum and reduce the torsion will result in death of the testicle. The window of opportunity during which the testicle

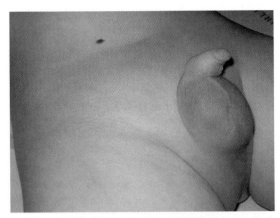

FIG 13.23 A very severe case of idiopathic scrotal oedema. The scrotal skin has lost its wrinkled appearance. Unusually, the oedema has tracked into the groin, perineum and the other side of the scrotum. The attachment of Scarpa's fascia in the thigh is clearly visible.

can be saved is only a few hours. If the diagnosis turns out to be wrong and the patient has an epididymo-orchitis, the surgical exploration will have done no harm and the decompression of the tunica vaginalis will have relieved painful pressure from the secondary hydrocele.

There are reports from experienced school medical officers describing manipulative reduction of testicular torsion. While undoubtedly successful at times, this is for experts only.

Gumma

This is now a very rare condition in Europe. Congenital syphilis causes testicular atrophy, but in adult life the same interstitial inflammation turns the testis into a round, hard and insensitive mass – the 'billiard ball testis'.

A gumma of the testis is **painless** and therefore presents either as a lump felt by chance on the surface of the organ or as an enlargement of the whole organ. It is usually indistinguishable from a tumour.

Orchitis

Acute orchitis, in the absence of epididymitis, is invariably due to a virus infection, commonly the mumps virus. The damage caused by a bilateral orchitis may leave the patient with a painful testis or, rarely, make him subfertile. Mumps orchitis may occur without enlargement of the salivary glands, but there is usually a history of contact with mumps.

Acute epididymo-orchitis

This is primarily an infection of the epididymis, but some oedema and inflammatory changes spread into the testis. There is usually an associated urinary tract infection, often prostatitis.

The common infecting organism in patients under 40 years old is *Chlamydia trachomatis*, and in older patients *Escherichia coli*, and do not forget the possibility of **gonorrhoea**.

History

Age This condition can affect all age groups but is commonest in young and middle-aged men. It is rare in children.

Symptoms There is often an initial flu-like illness, with **malaise** and **fever**, and sometimes deep-seated pelvic pain caused by inflammation of the prostate. The patient then develops **severe pain** and **swelling** in one side of the scrotum, which usually come on quite quickly over 30–60 minutes and are sometimes relieved by supporting the scrotum. **Frequency of micturition** and **painful micturition** may indicate the presence of a urinary tract infection.

Examination

Position The swelling is confined to one side of the scrotum.

Colour The scrotal skin is red and shiny. After a few days it turns a bronze colour and the superficial layers of skin desquamate.

Temperature The scrotal skin is hot.

Revision panel 13.3
The causes of a solid single mass in one side of the scrotum

Tumour
Orchitis (mumps)
Haematocele
Gumma
Epididymo-orchitis (when the epididymis is large and the testis is small)

Tenderness The scrotal skin is not tender but the testis and epididymis beneath it are extremely tender.

You must be patient and gentle. Careful palpation will reveal that the tenderness is in the swollen epididymis and that the body of the testis itself is not so tender.

Shape and size The whole testicle may be enlarged and tender and you may be unable to distinguish epididymis from testis. This is more likely in the presence of a small secondary hydrocele. If a hydrocele does not form, you should be able to distinguish the testis from the epididymis, which is commonly enlarged to about 1 cm or so in width.

In mild cases the inflammation may be localized to the head or tail of the epididymis.

Surface The surface of the epididymis remains smooth but will probably be too tender for this to be obvious.

Composition If there is a small hydrocele, the swelling may be fluctuant, with the testis palpable through the fluid.

If there is no hydrocele, you may be able to detect that the body of the testis feels a little more tense than normal. Initially the epididymis is soft, but as the inflammation subsides, it becomes hard and craggy.

Relations and local tissues The skin over the involved testicle is oedematous and mobile. Should there be no antibiotic treatment, the infection may spread beyond the epididymis to the surrounding tissues and the skin becomes fixed. If an abscess develops in the epididymis, nowadays a rare event, it may point and discharge through the area of skin fixation. As the epididymis normally lies behind the testis, epididymal disease involves the skin of the back of the scrotum, so always remember to look at its posterior aspect.

The spermatic cord is always thickened and tender because epididymal infection spreads distally from the urinary tract along the vas deferens.

The other testis should feel normal.

General examination Pay particular attention to the lower urinary tract. Rectal examination may reveal tenderness of the prostate and seminal vesicles.

There may also be a fever and a tachycardia.

The para-aortic glands will not be tender.

Tuberculous epididymo-orchitis

History

This condition is now uncommon in the UK, but is still seen in many other parts of the world. The tubercle bacillus reaches the epididymis via the bloodstream or by travelling along the vas from the lower urinary tract. The infection develops slowly without causing severe or acute pain or tenderness. There may be systemic symptoms of tuberculosis, or only the urinary tract may be involved.

Most patients complain of a **lump in the scrotum**, and an associated **dull, aching pain**.

Examination

On examination, the **epididymis is hard, knobbly** and two or three times its normal size. A secondary hydrocele is unusual. The spermatic cord is thickened as far as you can feel. The **vas deferens** is often irregular and swollen and **feels like a string of beads**. This physical sign is rare but is diagnostic of tuberculosis.

Tumours of the testis

There are two main varieties of testicular tumour:

- **seminoma** – a carcinoma of the seminiferous tubules,
- **teratoma** – a malignant germ cell tumour.

There are some clinical features which help differentiate between the two types, but usually the diagnosis is made by the histopathologist.

History

Age Teratoma commonly occurs between the ages of 20 and 30 years but seminoma may occur a few years later. Both are very rare in childhood and the teenage years.

There is now high public awareness of this quite uncommon condition, and the anxiety engendered by a recently noticed scrotal swelling, particularly in younger men, approaches that found in women with a breast lump. The chance of malignancy in these circumstances is substantially lower than with the breast, and the swelling found is usually a normal epididymis.

Symptoms The commonest presentation is a **swelling** of the testicle, which is not usually painful.

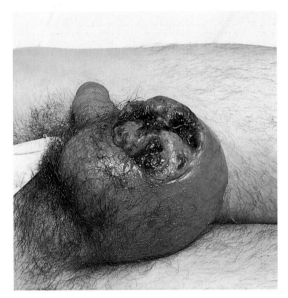

FIG 13.24 A testicular tumour fungating through the anterior surface of the scrotum. Note that the edge of the scrotal skin is sloping and trying to heal.

However, the occasional patient presents acutely with a painful, tender testicle, and diagnosis is not always straightforward.

Dull, aching, dragging pains in the scrotum and groin occur in some patients, particularly if the testis becomes significantly enlarged. An important symptom to enquire about is whether the **testicle feels heavy**. This is almost diagnostic of a testicular tumour.

Presentation with distant metastases may occur in many different ways, such as general malaise, loss of appetite, wasting, abdominal pains and dyspnoea.

Cause Many patients will state that their scrotal symptoms followed an injury. Ignore this view unless there is an obvious haematocele. It is better to explore a testis for benign disease than to miss a tumour.

There is a considerably higher incidence of malignant change in the incompletely descended testis. As an incompletely descended testis will not, by definition, be in the scrotum, diagnosis will be difficult.

Examination

Position The swelling is confined to the scrotum.

Temperature and colour The scrotal skin should be normal, except in the rare circumstance in which the tumour has invaded and ulcerated through it.

Tenderness Testicular tumours are not tender except in the unusual acute presentation.

In many instances, **normal testicular sensation is lost**. Ask the patient about this, as it is an important symptom of a testicular tumour, rarely associated with other conditions.

Shape The majority of testicular tumours are not noticed until they occupy the whole testis. Rarely, you may be able to feel a nodule that is clearly in the testis and not in the epididymis. A nodule that is in the epididymis is never a tumour.

Testicular tumours are irregular and variable in shape but are basically spherical.

Size Tumours are noticed by the patient when the testicle is clearly larger than its companion. Large swellings are now uncommon in the UK because of heightened public awareness.

Surface This is usually smooth, but can be irregular or nodular.

Composition Testicular tumours feel harder than a normal testis, are dull to percussion, not fluctuant and not translucent.

Heaviness is an important physical sign. With the patient lying on his back, place your fingers underneath the testicle and lift it up. Compare it with the normal side. A feeling of heaviness is characteristic of a tumour.

Relations to surrounding tissues The other testis should be normal, but bilateral tumours occur in 2 per cent of cases. The spermatic cord and the vas deferens should be normal. Once the tumour breaks through the tunica albuginea, it infiltrates the skin of the scrotum.

Lymph drainage Lymph from the testis drains to the para-aortic lymph glands. Remember that these glands lie in the centre of the abdomen above the level of the umbilicus.

Seminomata commonly metastasize to the para-aortic lymph glands, sometimes producing a palpable abdominal mass. The inguinal glands will only be enlarged if the tumour has spread to the scrotal skin, a rare event.

General examination Pay particular attention to all the lymph glands, especially the para-aortic and supraclavicular groups.

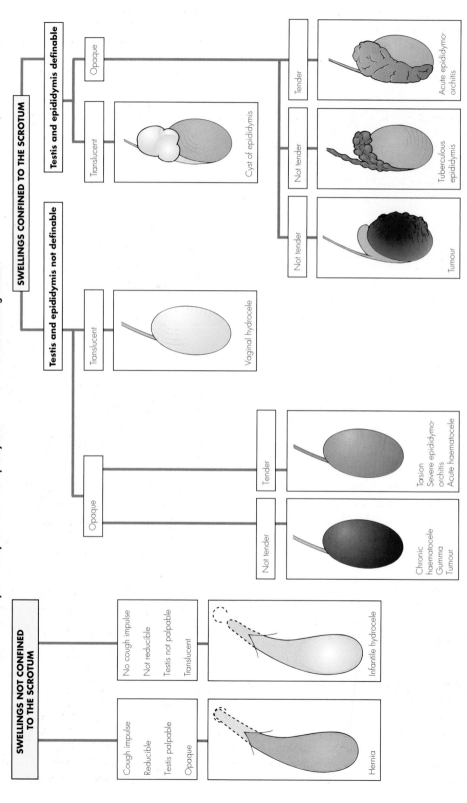

FIG 13.25 A plan for the diagnosis of scrotal swellings.

Testicular tumours may metastasize to any tissue in the body. Unusual swellings may be detected on general examination. Lung metastases are usually peripheral and not detectable on clinical examination, but are readily visible on a chest X-ray.

Differential diagnosis The testicular swellings likely to be confused with tumours are acute and chronic epididymo-orchitis, and haematocele. However, if the patient tells you that his testicle feels heavy, you find that testicular sensation is lost, and the enlarged testis feels, to you, heavier than the other side, the diagnosis of testicular tumour is almost certain.

Chronic testicular pain

This is a common reason for referral to a surgical clinic. The patient is a young or middle-aged man. The pain may be localized to the testicle or it may radiate to the groin. It may be associated with exercise and movement, or sitting in certain positions.

Common findings are:

- a mildly tender but otherwise normal epididymis, occasionally associated with a chlamydial urinary tract infection;
- a small epididymal cyst: differentiation from a normal epididymis may be difficult;
- an inguinal hernia: the skin of the scrotum is supplied by the genito-femoral nerve, which may be compressed in the groin by a hernia, causing discomfort referred to the testicle;
- rarely, but significantly, a testicular tumour;
- nothing abnormal.

The possibilities are many, but frustratingly for both patient and doctor, there may be no physical signs and a diagnosis cannot be made. In this case, the symptom usually settles with time.

THE FEMALE EXTERNAL GENITALIA

Most complaints about the external genitalia are referred to gynaecologists and are described in detail in their textbooks, but there are three common conditions that quite often appear in a general surgical clinic.

Bartholin cyst

Bartholin's glands are a pair of small glands that lie at the sides of the lower end of the vagina, and whose ducts open on to the inner side of the posterior part of the labium minus. They are normally impalpable. When the duct of a gland is distended by obstruction or infection, it forms a cystic swelling in the posterior part of the labium majus. The site betrays the diagnosis.

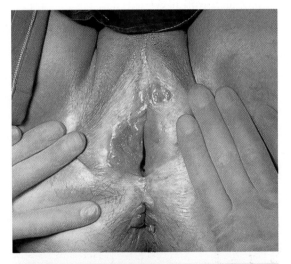

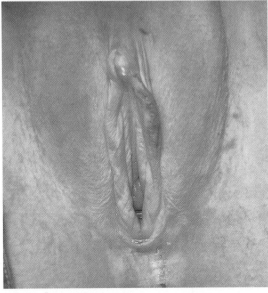

FIG 13.26 Two examples of carcinoma of the vulva.

Urethral caruncle

This is a bright-red, polypoid granuloma that arises from the mucosa of the urethral orifice in post-menopausal women. It is very **tender** and causes **painful micturition**, **dyspareunia** and occasional **bleeding**.

The differential diagnosis is urethral prolapse, which is purple in colour and not so tender.

Carcinoma of the vulva

Carcinoma of the vulva usually takes the form of a chronic ulcer with an everted edge.

The patient complains of **pain**, a purulent or **bloody discharge** and sometimes of a lump in the labia. Very small carcinomata can metastasize early and present with enlargement of the inguinal glands. The primary ulcer can be small and hidden in the folds of the labia.

There will usually be evidence of pre-malignant changes in the surrounding skin (vulval intra-epithelial neoplasia).

The abdominal wall, herniae and the umbilicus

14

The abdominal wall has a complex structure and many of the surgical conditions affecting it are embryological in origin. It develops laterally from the vertebral column, later than the intestinal tract, and ultimately fuses in the mid-line to form a seam-like fibrous cord, the linea alba. This is pierced at the umbilicus by the umbilical cord, which in early embryonic life contains the yolk sac and the entire mid-gut. The testes develop in the peritoneum of the posterior abdominal wall and migrate through the muscles just above the inguinal ligament into the scrotum followed by the spermatic cord. It is thus hardly surprising that there are many weak areas in the abdominal wall.

The abdominal wall is also afflicted by many of the common skin, subcutaneous, fascial and muscle tissue lesions described elsewhere, which can be just as difficult to diagnose as when they appear in other sites.

It is important to decide whether any abdominal swelling is deep to, or part of, the abdominal wall. This may be established by palpating the lump with the abdominal wall relaxed and then with it tense. A lump deep to the abdominal wall becomes impalpable when the abdominal muscles contract. A lump superficial to the muscles becomes more prominent. Do not forget to apply this simple reliable test to all abdominal swellings.

Contracting the abdominal muscles

If you ask a patient to lift their head and shoulders off the couch, they will contract their abdominal muscles – provided they do not lever themselves up with their elbows, which the elderly tend to do. Another way to achieve contraction of the abdominal muscles is to lift the patient's heels yourself and then ask the patient to hold them in that position. This tenses the rectus abdominis muscle very effectively and any mass deep to it will become impalpable unless it is huge. However, frail elderly patients may be unable to maintain a sustained contraction of their abdominal muscles, whatever method you try.

Swellings in the rectus sheath

Acute

The inferior and superior epigastric arteries lie deep to, or within, the rectus abdominis muscles. If these muscles contract suddenly and violently, the epigastric arteries may be torn. The haematoma which then develops within the muscle causes pain and swelling.

Rupture of the *inferior* epigastric artery occurs in athletes and during coughing in elderly patients with chronic obstructive airways disease, especially if they are taking steroid medication. The blood spreads within the muscle, but as there is no posterior rectus sheath below the arcuate line (the lower edge of the posterior rectus sheath, mid-way between the pubis and the umbilicus), the blood spreads out into the extraperitoneal area of the iliac fossa.

The patient complains of pain and tenderness in the iliac fossa, right or left, which is made worse by contracting the abdominal muscles. Examination reveals a diffuse, tender mass in the iliac fossa, deep to the abdominal wall. Skin discolouration may appear a few hours after the onset of the pain. If the pain is not made worse by contracting the rectus abdominis muscle, and if there is no bruise in the skin, the condition may be confused with acute appendicitis, but there will be none of the systemic features of the latter.

Rupture of the *superior* epigastric artery may follow a bout of violent coughing, and cause pain and tenderness in the upper abdomen, made worse by tensing the abdominal muscles and by deep breathing. A bruise may appear below the costal margin 12–24 hours later. When this condition occurs on the right-hand side it can be confused with cholecystitis.

Tears of the muscle fibres alone, with no major vessel disruption, may also cause rectus sheath haematomata.

Chronic

Chronic haematomata Patients occasionally present with a painless mass which examination reveals to be in the rectus sheath. The most likely cause is a **chronic rectus sheath haematoma** with the acute phase forgotten or not noticed. Discrete swellings are more likely to occur in the upper abdomen, confined by the fibrous intersections in the upper part of the muscle.

The swelling will be firm to hard, clearly in the abdominal wall and without a definite edge because it is deep seated.

Sarcomata The rare **desmoid tumour** and other **sarcomata** may arise in the rectus sheath.

Lipomata The most common swelling found in the anterior abdominal wall, superficial to the rectus sheath, is the subcutaneous lipoma. This is clearly in the subcutaneous fat and displays the smooth surface, rolled edge and pseudo-fluctuant consistence characteristic of the condition. Such lipomata are either solitary or multiple. Multiple lipomata are rarely bigger than 2–3 cm across and are also found in the chest wall and limbs (but never below the knee). They may be familial and tender, a condition sometimes called **Dercum's syndrome**.

ABDOMINAL HERNIAE

A hernia is the protrusion of an organ through its containing wall. The term can be applied to the herniation of a muscle through its fascial covering, to the herniation of brain through a fracture of the skull or through the foramen magnum into the spinal canal, as well as to the protrusion of an intra-abdominal organ through a defect in the abdominal wall, pelvis or diaphragm.

Before an organ can herniate through its retaining wall there must be a weakness in that wall. This may be a normal weakness, found in everyone, and

related to the anatomical configuration of the area such as a place where a vessel or viscus enters or leaves the abdomen. Alternatively, the weakness may be due to a congenital abnormality, or acquired as a result of trauma or disease.

This chapter deals with abdominal herniae, excluding those through and around the oesophageal hiatus. There are a few common varieties and a larger number of rarities. The common ones in order of frequency in adult life are:

- inguinal
- umbilical
- incisional
- femoral
- epigastric.

In childhood, umbilical hernia is more common than inguinal hernia.

You seldom need to remember rarities, but it is important to have some knowledge of the rare types of abdominal herniae, because failure to diagnose any type of strangulated hernia, common or rare, may lead to the patient's death. They are:

- spigelian
- obturator
- lumbar
- gluteal

Herniae occur frequently in both sexes. Inguinal hernia affects 9 per cent of men at some time in their lives and 1 per cent of women.

Although the femoral hernia is found more often in women than in men, the commonest hernia in women is the inguinal hernia.

Certain physical signs are common to all herniae but are not always present:

- they occur at congenital or acquired weak spots in the abdominal wall;
- most herniae can be reduced;
- most herniae have an expansile cough impulse.

The last two signs may be absent, especially if the hernia is tightly constricted at its neck, so their absence does not exclude the diagnosis of hernia.

The diagnosis of a hernia is therefore made initially by the site and confirmed by the presence of reducibility and an expansile cough impulse. It may also be made when these signs are absent, by the exclusion of other causes of a lump.

The common herniae

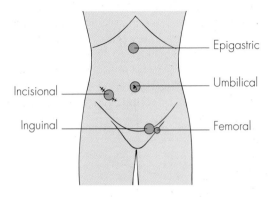

Epigastric

Umbilical

Incisional

Femoral

Inguinal

The rare herniae

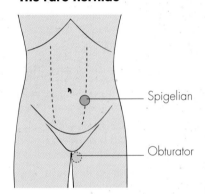

Spigelian

Obturator

Lumbar

Gluteal

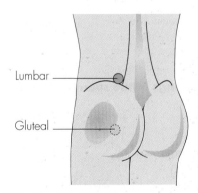

FIG 14.1 The sites of herniae.

INGUINAL HERNIA

An inguinal hernia is the protrusion of part of the contents of the abdomen through the inguinal region of the abdominal wall. To understand inguinal herniae it is necessary to understand the anatomy of the inguinal canal (Fig. 14.2).

Surface anatomy

The inguinal ligament stretches between the anterior superior iliac spine, which is easy to see and feel, and the pubic tubercle, which is not. A skin crease runs across the lower abdomen, convex downwards, separating the abdomen from the triangle known as the mons veneris. The centre of this crease lies over the upper edge of the pubic bones. The pubic tubercles lie beneath this crease, approximately 2–3 cm either side of the mid-line. To find a pubic tubercle, put your finger on the centre of this skin crease, push gently inwards until you feel the crest of the pubis, and then slide your finger sideways until you reach the tubercle. You can practise this on yourself.

Muscles

Beneath the skin and subcutaneous tissue lies the aponeurosis (a word meaning a flat tendon) of the external oblique muscle. The lower inwardly folded edge of this aponeurosis, which runs between the anterior superior iliac spine and pubic tubercle, forms the inguinal ligament. The fibres of the aponeurosis run parallel to the inguinal ligament in the direction taken by a hand when placed in a trouser pocket,

---

Revision panel 14.1
The basic features of all herniae

They occur at a weak spot
They reduce on lying down, or with direct pressure
They have an expansile cough impulse

Revision panel 14.2
The causes of abdominal herniae

An anatomical weakness where:
- structures pass through the abdominal wall
- muscles fail to overlap
- there are no muscles, only scar tissue (e.g. umbilicus)

An acquired weakness following trauma
High intra-abdominal pressure from:
- coughing
- straining
- abdominal distension

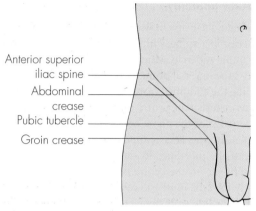

Anterior superior iliac spine

Abdominal crease

Pubic tubercle

Groin crease

Surface landmarks

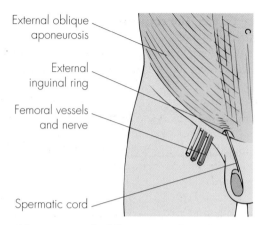

External oblique aponeurosis

External inguinal ring

Femoral vessels and nerve

Spermatic cord

The external oblique muscle

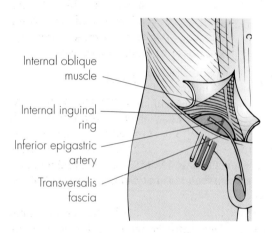

Internal oblique muscle

Internal inguinal ring

Inferior epigastric artery

Transversalis fascia

The internal oblique muscle

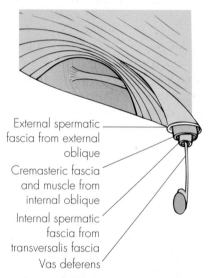

External spermatic fascia from external oblique

Cremasteric fascia and muscle from internal oblique

Internal spermatic fascia from transversalis fascia

Vas deferens

The coverings of the spermatic cord

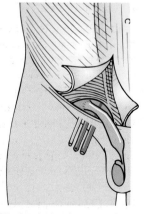

An indirect inguinal hernia

Sac begins at the internal ring and is inside the spermatic cord

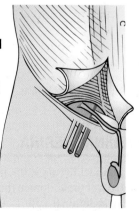

A direct inguinal hernia

Sac appears medial to the inferior epigastric artery and is outside the spermatic cord

FIG 14.2 The anatomy of the inguinal region.

and separate above the crest of the pubis to form the external inguinal ring.

Deep to the external oblique aponeurosis are the lowermost fibres of the internal oblique muscle arising from the lateral half of the inguinal ligament. They run medially in an arch, convex upwards, to the edge of the rectus abdominis muscle, where they join the aponeurosis of the transverse abdominal muscle to form the anterior rectus sheath. At this point the fused aponeuroses are known as the *conjoined tendon*.

The half-moon gap beneath the arch of the internal oblique muscle is the weak spot of the inguinal region. The tissue filling the gap is not very strong and is called the transversalis fascia. This area is crossed by the inferior epigastric artery as it runs upwards (from the femoral artery), curving medially towards the rectus sheath. The point where the vas deferens and testicular artery pierce the transversalis fascia is *lateral* to the inferior epigastric artery and known as the internal inguinal ring. Indirect inguinal hernial sacs leave the abdomen at this point. Direct inguinal herniae push through the weak area of the posterior wall *medial* to the inferior epigastric artery. Remember that the exit point of an indirect hernia is lateral to this artery and that of a direct hernia medial to it. You cannot palpate the inferior epigastric artery, but the femoral pulse, which can be felt at the mid-inguinal point (halfway between the anterior superior iliac spine and the mid-line pubic symphysis), will tell you where it begins. The important clinical point is that the exit point of an indirect hernia is lateral to that of a direct hernia.

As the vas deferens enters the inguinal canal it takes with it a thin layer of fascia derived from the transversalis fascia called the internal spermatic fascia. Further down the canal it collects a covering of muscle fibres and fascia from the internal oblique muscle. These coverings are called the cremaster muscle and cremasteric fascia. Finally, as the vas passes through the external ring, it acquires another thin layer of fascia derived from the external oblique aponeurosis called the external spermatic fascia.

Because the sac of an indirect inguinal hernia comes down obliquely alongside the vas deferens inside the spermatic cord, it has an easy path of little resistance down into the scrotum. The three fascial layers of the cord funnel the peritoneal sac towards the scrotum. By contrast, the sac of a direct inguinal hernia begins medial to the epigastric artery, outside the spermatic cord with its three external layers of tissue, and so has no easy path to the scrotum, which in consequence it rarely enters.

Technique for the examination of an inguinal hernia

Ask the patient to stand up

It is not possible to see the true size of a hernia, examine it properly or even detect it at all when the patient is lying down. If you suspect the diagnosis from the history, start the examination with the patient standing. If, during a routine supine abdominal examination, you discover a lump that looks like a hernia, complete the routine examination and then ask the patient to stand up in order to examine it properly.

Always examine both inguinal regions.

Look at the lump from in front

It is essential to see the exact site and shape of the lump. With practice you will be able to distinguish an inguinal from a femoral hernia at sight because the bulge of an inguinal hernia begins well above the crease of the groin, whereas a femoral hernia is more medial and related to the medial end of the groin crease.

Inspection will also reveal whether the lump extends down into the scrotum, if there are any other scrotal swellings and if there are any swellings on the 'normal' side.

Feel from the front

1. Examine the scrotum and its contents. It is not unusual to find an epididymal cyst or a hydrocele as well as a hernia because they are all common conditions.
2. In men, first decide if the lump is a hernia or a true scrotal lump by examining its upper edge. If you can 'get above it' (i.e. feel its upper edge between your thumb and index finger and a normal spermatic cord above it), it must be a scrotal swelling and not a hernia. If you cannot feel the upper edge of the lump because it passes into the inguinal canal, it is likely to be a hernia, except in children, when it might be an encysted hydrocele of the cord (page 372).

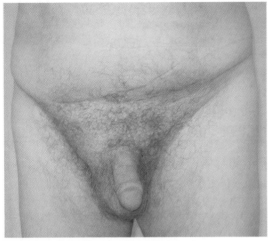

Ask the patient to stand up. When palpating the groin, stand at the patient's side.

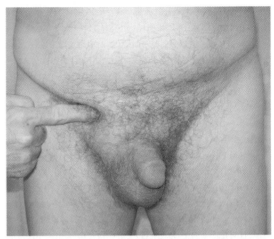

The upper crease of the mons veneris indicates the crest of the pubis and the level of the pubic tubercle. Note that it is not low down in the crease of the groin.

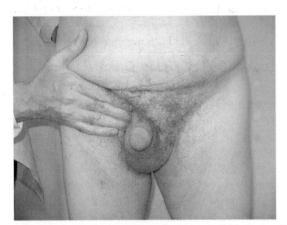

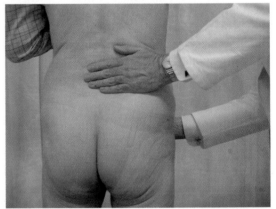

Place your examining hand flat on the groin parallel to the inguinal ligament and your other hand on the patient's back to stop you pushing him over. You will then be able to manipulate and probably reduce the hernia with ease.

FIG 14.3 TECHNIQUES FOR THE EXAMINATION OF AN INGUINAL HERNIA.

3. Do not examine the external ring or palpate the pubic tubercle by pushing a finger up along the spermatic cord into the neck of the scrotum. This is a painful, unnecessary method of examination that very rarely yields useful information.

Feel from the side

Having examined the scrotal contents and decided that you cannot get above the lump, you can make a provisional diagnosis of inguinal hernia and proceed to examine the lump itself.

Stand at the side of the patient, on the same side as the hernia. Place one hand in the small of the patient's back to support him, and your examining hand on the lump with your fingers and arm roughly parallel to the inguinal ligament.

You must now ascertain the following facts about the lump:

■ position
■ temperature
■ tenderness
■ shape
■ size

- tension
- composition (solid, fluid, or gaseous)
- reducibility.

Expansile cough impulse

Compress the lump firmly with your fingers, then ask the patient to turn his head towards the opposite side, and then to cough. If the swelling becomes tense and **expands** with coughing, it has a 'cough impulse'. Movement of the swelling without expansion or an increase in tension is not a cough impulse. A localized swelling in the spermatic cord or an undescended testis will sometimes *move* down the inguinal canal and come out through the external ring during coughing, and *look* exactly like a hernia, but neither will get bigger or more tense during coughing. The presence of an expansile cough impulse is diagnostic of a hernia, but its absence does not exclude a diagnosis of hernia because the neck of the sac may be blocked by adhesions, which prevent the movement of additional viscera into the sac during coughing.

Is the swelling reducible?

The main reason for standing at the side of the patient is to be able to place your hand in exactly the same position as the patient places his own hand when he is reducing or supporting the hernia. He puts his hand on the lump and lifts it upwards and backwards. You must do the same. You can only do this if your arm comes from a position above and behind the hernia.

First, press firmly to reduce the tension of the lump. Then gently compress the lower part of the swelling. As the lump gets softer, lift it up towards the external ring. Once it has all passed in through this point, slide your fingers upwards and laterally towards the internal ring to see if the hernia can be controlled (kept inside) by pressure at this point.

If the lump reduces into or through the abdominal wall at a point above and medial to the pubic tubercle, it is an inguinal hernia. If the point of reduction is below and lateral to the pubic tubercle, it is a femoral hernia.

Note that this method of differentiation refers to the point where the lump reduces, not the position of the unreduced hernia, because once a hernia reaches the subcutaneous tissue it can expand and spread in any direction.

If the hernia can be held reduced only by pressure over the external inguinal ring, it is a direct inguinal hernia. If it can be controlled by pressure over the internal ring, it is an indirect inguinal hernia.

If there is any difficulty in reducing the hernia, ask the patient to lie down and try again. This will also allow you to examine the abdomen (see below).

Remove your hand and watch the hernia reappear

The direction of movement of the swelling and the way in which it reappears will help to confirm your deductions about its site of origin.

A reappearing indirect hernia will seem to slide obliquely downwards along the line of the canal, whereas a direct hernia will project directly forwards.

Comment. It may be impossible, particularly in the obese, to differentiate between these two types of hernia with any certainty, but attempting to do so ensures that you conduct a thorough examination.

Percuss and auscultate the lump

If there is gut in the sac, it may be resonant and there may be audible bowel sounds.

Feel the other side

Move to the other side of the patient and examine that inguinal region. Inguinal herniae are commonly bilateral, particularly when they are direct. Even when you cannot see or feel a lump, ask the patient to cough whilst you are palpating the inguinal canal. There may be a small bulge that is only made detectable by the raised intra-abdominal pressure produced by coughing.

Examine the abdomen

Look particularly for anything that may be raising the intra-abdominal pressure, such as a large bladder, an enlarged prostate, ascites, chronic intestinal obstruction or pregnancy.

With the patient lying flat, ask the patient to cough as you observe the groin. Particularly in a slim adult, you may see the contents entering the sac, which will help you to decide if the hernia is direct or indirect. With a direct hernia, the swelling will advance directly upwards towards you. With an indirect hernia, you may be able to see oblique motion from the internal ring to the neck of the scrotum. Indirect herniae are sometimes referred to as *oblique herniae*.

With the patient in this position, it is easier to decide if a hernia is femoral. Femoral herniae rarely reduce into the abdomen on lying down, and will be found to be below the inguinal ligament and rather more lateral than an inguinal sac extending downwards to the same level.

Cardiovascular and respiratory assessment

Assess the cardiovascular and respiratory systems with the patient's fitness for operation in mind.

Symptoms and signs of an inguinal hernia

History (elective presentation)

Age Inguinal herniae may appear at any age. They may be present at birth or appear suddenly in an 80 year old. The peak times of presentation are in the first few months of life, in the late teens and early twenties, and between 40 and 60.

Occupation Heavy work, especially lifting, puts a great strain on the abdominal muscles. If there is an underlying weakness, the appearance of a hernia may coincide with strenuous physical effort, or it may be first noticed at such a time. Despite the fact that herniae are no more common in manual workers than in office workers, compensation law in many countries accepts that a hernia may be an industrial injury.

Local symptoms The commonest symptoms are **discomfort** and **pain**. The patient complains of a dragging, aching sensation in the groin, which gets worse as the day goes on.

If the hernia becomes very painful and tender, it is probably strangulated. There may be pain long before a lump is noticed.

On the other hand, many herniae cause no pain and the patient presents having noticed a swelling in the groin or in the scrotum. The lump gets smaller on lying down and the patient may have noticed that the swelling can be pushed back into the abdomen. Symptoms may be bilateral.

Other abdominal symptoms A loop of bowel in the sac of a hernia may become obstructed. Obstruction is associated with a colicky pain caused by bowel distension because bowel pain is mediated via sympathetic afferent nerves and hence felt, not in the groin, but in the mid-line of the abdomen, at a level which depends on which part of the intestine is involved. The pain occurs when the bowel is trapped in the sac of the hernia and resolves when the bowel is reduced into the abdomen.

Large herniae may interfere with bowel activity and cause a change in bowel habit.

However, beware: patients with a carcinoma of the left colon, or diverticular disease, may experience progressive constipation and hence increased straining during defaecation. The increase in abdominal pressure that accompanies straining may make a coincidental hernia more prominent, and lead the patient to attribute their symptoms to the hernia. Therefore you must enquire of all patients presenting with a hernia whether their bowel action has recently changed and **investigate any significant bowel symptoms in their own right** before dealing with the hernia.

It is also usual to ask about other diseases which may have cause increased abdominal pressure, such as chronic bronchitis with persistent coughing, and difficulty with micturition.

History (emergency presentation)

Herniae, pre-existing or just discovered, often present as a surgical emergency. The patient may notice that the groin swelling will not reduce or that it is painful and tender. This may be associated with the cardinal symptoms of intestinal obstruction – colicky abdominal pain, vomiting, distension and absolute constipation. The hernial orifices of any patient with intestinal obstruction must always be carefully examined, as the patient may not have noticed a small lump in their groin. This is particularly common with femoral herniae.

The definitions of the terms irreducible, incarcerated, obstructed and strangulated, which are freely used in the description of herniae, must be understood.

Irreducible means simply what it states, that the contents of the hernia sac cannot be replaced into the abdomen. An irreducible hernia may be associated with three other categories of complication – incarceration, obstruction and strangulation.

Incarcerated means that contents are literally imprisoned in the sac of the hernia (usually by adhesions) but are alive and functioning normally. An incarcerated hernia is not tender.

Obstructed means that a loop of bowel is kinked or trapped within the sac of the hernia in such a way that its lumen but not its blood supply is obstructed. The bowel is therefore alive and the patient has the signs and symptoms of intestinal obstruction but not of strangulation. The hernia will not be unduly tender.

Strangulation means that the blood supply to the contents of the sac has been cut off and they are dead or dying. The patient will usually be obviously unwell and the swelling will be acutely tender. An entrapment that interferes with the blood supply to the bowel wall will usually obstruct its lumen, so most strangulated herniae containing bowel have intestinal obstruction.

However, there is variety of strangulated hernia in which only a segment of the bowel wall is trapped and the lumen remains patent. The strangulation makes the hernia very tender but there are no symptoms or signs of intestinal obstruction. This is called **Richter's hernia**.

Examination

The principal features to be determined are the site, size and constituents of the lump, together with the two diagnostic signs, reducibility and the presence of an expansile cough impulse.

Position An inguinal hernia will be visible in the groin in all but the obese. The anatomical landmarks and the site and line of direction of indirect and direct hernias are described above.

Note that once a hernia has passed through the external inguinal ring it can spread out into the loose subcutaneous tissue under the membranous layer of the superficial fascia and, if it is indirect, descend to fill the scrotum. The oft-quoted description that the inguinal hernia is found 'above and medial to the pubic tubercle' refers *not* to the position of the whole hernia, but to the point at which the hernia reduces into the abdominal wall (the external inguinal ring).

Colour The skin colour over an inguinal hernia should be normal. If the hernia is strangulated, the skin may be reddened. If the patient has worn a truss for many years, the skin over the external inguinal ring may be scarred and pigmented.

Temperature The temperature of the skin overlying a hernia will be the same as the surrounding skin except when the hernia is strangulated. In this event the skin may be warm.

Tenderness A hernia may contain any viscus and, as all abdominal structures have a visceral sensory innervation, manual pressure is uncomfortable but not truly painful. By contrast, a strangulated hernia is very tender. An irreducible, non-strangulated hernia is not tender to light pressure, but any attempt at reduction by excessive pressing and squeezing can cause considerable pain.

Shape An indirect hernia moving obliquely along the inguinal canal towards the scrotum is sausage

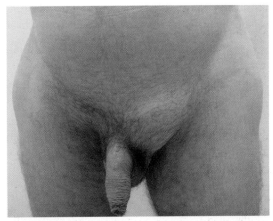

A left indirect inguinal hernia, moving obliquely down towards the scrotum.

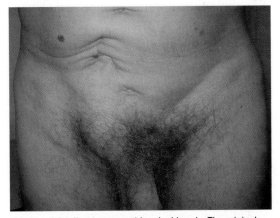

This is a right direct recurrent inguinal hernia. The original inguinal hernia probably developed because of the disruption and distortion of the abdominal wall caused by the previous abdominal operation. Always look for a scar in the groin. The bulge is coming out directly towards you.

FIG 14.4 INGUINAL HERNIAE.

shaped, but when it extends beyond the external inguinal ring it widens out to become pear shaped. A direct hernia is usually round, like a plum in the groin.

Size Inguinal herniae vary from very small bulges which are just detectable, to large masses descending almost to knee level. The larger a hernia is, the more likely it is to be irreducible.

Surface The surface will vary according to the nature of the contents but is usually smooth. In a large hernia it is sometimes possible to palpate indentable faeces inside an incarcerated segment of colon.

Composition Herniae that contain gut should be soft, resonant and fluctuant, and you may be able to hear bowel sounds. If the contents within the sac are tense, the hernia will feel hard, but if it contains bowel, it should still be resonant and fluctuant. Visible peristalsis may be observed with a large scrotal hernia containing small intestine.

Many herniae contain omentum, which makes them feel firm (rubbery), non-fluctuant and dull to percussion.

Cough impulse A hernia will nearly always become larger and more tense in all directions during coughing, which is referred to as an **expansile** cough impulse. Most lumps in the groin move up and down with coughing, an impulse transmitted from the abdominal wall. Only herniae and vascular tumours expand in all directions.

Compressibility A hernia can be compressed by steady pressure but, unlike vascular tumours displaying the same physical sign, it will not expand immediately the compression is released unless some force, such as gravity or coughing, forces it out.

Reducibility A cardinal physical sign of a hernia is reducibility. This means that it is possible to return the contents of the hernia to their normal anatomical site – the abdomen.

Unlike a compressible swelling, a hernia which has been reduced does not immediately reappear when the pressure is removed, unless forced to do so by gravity or muscle tone. When you reduce a hernia you move all parts of it to another place. When you compress a lump you just move its fluid contents to another place.

Relations The relations of the lump will have already been defined when deciding the site and nature of the hernia.

State of local tissues As acquired inguinal herniae are caused by weakness of the tissues of the inguinal canal, bulging of both inguinal regions with coughing is common. Minor bilateral bulging of the inguinal canal in slim individuals is normal and known as **Malgaigne's bulges**.

Look carefully for any scars near the hernia. It may have been repaired in the past.

There is an increased incidence of direct right inguinal hernia in patients who have had an appendicectomy through a right iliac fossa incision because this incision weakens the adjacent muscles and occasionally divides the iliohypogastric or ilioinguinal nerves.

General examination Look for the common causes of a raised intra-abdominal pressure, namely chronic bronchitis and coughing, chronic retention of urine, difficulty in micturition, ascites and intra-abdominal masses. These factors may have exacerbated or even caused the hernia.

Look for any signs of intestinal obstruction, such as distension, increased bowel sounds and visible peristalsis.

Special varieties of inguinal hernia

The differences between a *direct* and an *indirect* inguinal hernia are listed in Revision panel 14.3. Distinction between the two is not totally irrelevant. When an inguinal hernia strangulates, the usual site of constriction is the external ring. Hence a direct hernia, which does not pass through this ring, is much less likely to place the patient's life at risk by becoming strangulated. This may influence management in a poor-risk patient.

It is important to try to differentiate between the two varieties because it makes you examine the hernia more carefully.

Bilateral herniae are more likely to be direct than indirect.

It is not uncommon to find both a direct and an indirect hernia in the same groin. When this does occur, the two sacs are straddled by the inferior epigastric artery and the hernia is sometimes called a **pantaloon hernia**.

A **sliding hernia** is a hernia of a piece of extraperitoneal bowel (the caecum or terminal ileum on the right and the sigmoid colon on the left), which slides down into the inguinal canal, pulling a sac of peritoneum on its surface. The viscus involved is part of the wall of the sac. It is sometimes possible to guess that a hernia is of the sliding variety by the slow way in which it reappears after reduction and the manner in which it slithers down into the scrotum. The clinical differentiation of this variety is never certain, but it is far more common on the left, and involvement of the sigmoid colon may produce disproportionate pain and even symptoms of bowel dysfunction. Sliding herniae are occasionally diagnosed during the investigation of bowel symptoms when contrast X-rays demonstrate colon in a hernial sac.

Maydl's hernia (hernia-en-W) is a rare condition in which there are two loops of bowel in the sac, with strangulation of the loop of bowel in the abdomen which connects them. Diagnosis is made at operation.

Recurrent herniae

Inguinal hernia is a common condition and not all of the many surgical repairs that are performed are successful.

Recurrent herniae are more likely to present with local pain than new herniae. They tend to be direct and, because of the scarring from the previous surgery, are unlikely to be large. They are very rarely scrotal. The hernia may consist of extraperitoneal fat without a peritoneal sac, infiltrating itself into the defects that have arisen in the previous repair. Recognition is important because strangulation is more likely than with a new hernia.

Differential diagnosis

There are very few conditions which can be mistaken for an inguinal hernia provided you remember to check the scrotum, feel for a cough impulse and test reducibility.

Confusion may occasionally be caused by swellings which occur in the line of the spermatic cord that can pop in and out of the external ring, such as an undescended testis and a hydrocele of the cord. In the former event, routine examination of the scrotum should reveal an absent testis. Neither has an expansile cough impulse.

Inguinal herniae in women

In females there is a rudimentary testicular analogue which descends through the muscles of the groin as in males. The equivalent of the spermatic cord is the round ligament, which, inside the abdomen, joins the uterus just as the vas deferens joins the prostate. Herniae in women nearly always follow the

---

Revision panel 14.3
The features of inguinal herniae

Features of an indirect inguinal hernia
Can (and often does) descend into the scrotum
Reduces upwards, then laterally and backwards
Controlled, after reduction, by pressure over the internal inguinal ring
The defect is not palpable, as it is behind the fibres of the external oblique muscle
After reduction, the bulge reappears in the middle of the inguinal region and then flows medially before turning down to the neck of the scrotum

Features of a direct inguinal hernia
Does not (hardly ever) go down into the scrotum
Reduces upwards and then straight backwards
Not controlled, after reduction, by pressure over the internal inguinal ring
The defect may be felt in the abdominal wall above the pubic tubercle
After reduction, the bulge reappears exactly where it was before
Uncommon in children and young adults

Revision panel 14.4
The differential diagnosis of inguinal hernia

Femoral hernia
Vaginal hydrocele
Hydrocele of the cord or the canal of Nuck
Undescended testis
Lipoma of the cord

SOME DEFINITIONS

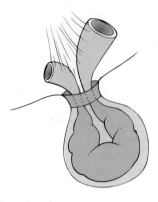

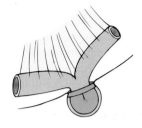

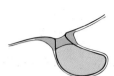

Neck of sac
This tight ring of peritoneum is usually the site of any strangulation.

A strangulated hernia
The blood supply of the contents of the hernia is cut off. When a loop of gut is strangulated there will also be intestinal obstruction.

A strangulated hernia
If the sac is small, a knuckle of bowel can be caught in the sac and strangled without causing intestinal obstruction. This is called a *Richter's hernia*.

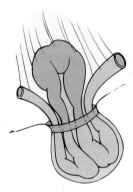

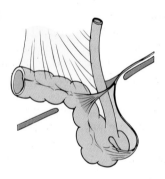

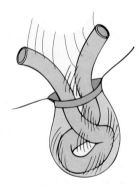

Maydl's hernia
When two adjacent loops of bowel are in the sac, the intervening portion in the abdomen is the first to suffer if the neck of the sac is tight, because it is the centre of the whole loop involved. Thus the strangulated piece is intra-abdominal. This is a rare variety of strangulation.

Sliding hernia
If bowel which is normally extraperitoneal forms one side of the sac, it is thought to have slid down the canal pulling peritoneum with it, hence the name *hernia-en-glissade*. The sac can contain other loops of bowel, and the gut forming the wall of the sac can be strangled by the external ring.

Incarceration
The contents are fixed in the sac because of their size and adhesions. The hernia is irreducible but the bowel is not strangulated or obstructed.

FIG 14.5

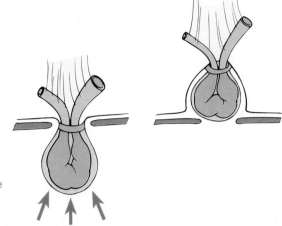

Reduction-en-masse

It is possible to push a hernia back through the abdominal wall, so apparently reducing it, without actually pushing the contents out of the sac. If they were strangulated in the first position they will still be strangulated in the second. Never push hard when trying to reduce a hernia.

FIG 14.5 continued

round ligament and are therefore indirect. The sac passes obliquely towards the labium in the same way as it would pass towards the scrotum in the male.

There are two conditions of the groin peculiar to women.

Hydrocele of the canal of Nuck is a fluid-filled distal part of the sac of an indirect hernia. The proximal part of the sac is too narrow to admit bowel or other abdominal contents. It is analogous to the encysted hydrocele of the cord seen in children. It presents with a smooth, fluctuant swelling without a cough impulse, which will transilluminate.

Haematocele of the round ligament is a curious condition in which the round ligament becomes distended with multiple small sacs containing blood-stained fluid. It presents in pregnancy with a soft, sausage-like swelling in the groin extending into the labium. This may have a weak cough impulse and when gently squeezed it feels spongy and reduces in size. It is commonly confused with a hernia, but it resolves when the pregnancy is over, which herniae certainly do not.

Inguinal herniae in children

Groin herniae in male children are, for practical purposes, always indirect and are caused by failure of the processus vaginalis to obliterate after the testicle enters the scrotum. There are three clinical manifestations of this abnormality, but it is important to appreciate that the pathological process in all three is identical, namely a **patent processus vaginalis**. The three clinical manifestations are:

- an infantile hydrocele,
- an obvious hernia,
- an encysted hydrocele of the cord.

An **infantile hydrocele** is a fully patent processus vaginalis (i.e. one extending right down to the scrotum) which is too narrow to admit bowel but which allows fluid from the peritoneal cavity to accumulate within it. The condition may present at birth or shortly afterwards as a scrotal swelling which is usually large, tense, brilliantly translucent and often bilateral. It is should be possible to get above the swelling, i.e. to feel or see that its upper limit is at or below the external inguinal ring. It is rarely possible to squeeze the fluid back into the abdomen, as the narrow neck of the processus acts as a non-return valve. It does not have an expansile cough impulse.

When the child cries, intra-abdominal pressure is raised and the scrotal swelling may become harder. It is important to reassure the parents that the child is not crying because the hydrocele is tense, but that the swelling is tense because the child is crying.

The usual natural history is spontaneous resolution during the first year of life as the processus slowly obliterates, but once the child begins to walk this is less likely. In ambulant children the swelling often increases in size during the day, presumably exacerbated by gravity.

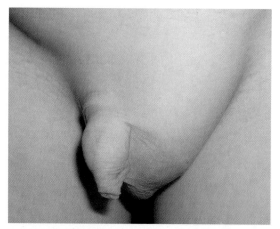

FIG 14.6 A large left inguinal hernia in a child.

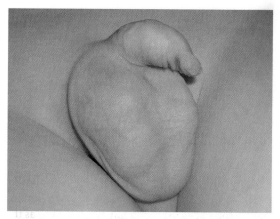

FIG 14.8 A right encysted hydrocele of the cord. It is clearly separate from the testicle. You can get above it and there is no cough impulse in the swelling or in the groin above it.

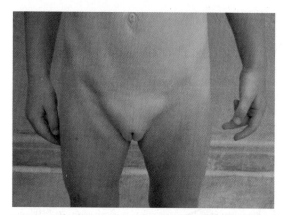

FIG 14.7 This young lady's parents gave a history of an intermittent left groin swelling and pointed to the inguinal canal, but nothing was visible when she came to the clinic. Nevertheless, the history was good enough for an operation to be planned. But, when on holiday in Spain, a lump appeared in the other groin and the parents took this photograph confirming the presence of bilateral inguinal herniae.

An **inguinal hernia in a child** displays the physical signs listed above for an indirect inguinal hernia. The contents reduce easily and the swelling does not transilluminate.

Children's groin herniae occasionally become irreducible, but strangulation is rare. If strangulation does occur, the gonadal vessels are more likely to be damaged than the vessels of the bowel, so testicular infarction is more common than bowel infarction.

Direct herniae do occur in children but are very rare.

Children's herniae may only appear intermittently. The swelling that the parents have definitely seen obstinately refuses to appear in the presence of the examining physician. If the site of the swelling indicated by the parents is the inguinal canal, exploration is justified on the history alone and an indirect sac is invariably found.

In girls, the wall of the sac may include the ovary and Fallopian tube. When the contents are reduced, there may remain a small mass, which is tender to touch. The child may also complain of pain in the area.

An **encysted hydrocele of the cord** is the least common variety of patent processus vaginalis in which a narrow patent processus, which extends down to a level just above the testis and becomes dilated and filled with fluid. It presents as a discrete swelling in the spermatic cord below the external inguinal ring, above or near the top of the scrotum, separate from the testicle, which transilluminates brilliantly and has no cough impulse.

Comment. Do not confuse the infantile with the adult hydrocele.

In children the condition is really a fluid-filled congenital inguinal hernia with a narrow sac which communicates with the peritoneal cavity on every occasion.

The adult hydrocele is an acquired condition in which fluid accumulates around the testicle, within the tunica vaginalis, in response to a local abnormality. It has no communication with the peritoneum.

FEMORAL HERNIA

Anatomy

A femoral hernia is a protrusion of extraperitoneal fat, a peritoneal sac and sometimes abdominal contents through the femoral canal. The anatomical margins of this canal are the inguinal ligament anteriorly, the pubic ramus and pectineus muscle posteriorly, the lacunar ligament and pubic bone medially, and the femoral vein laterally.

The femoral canal provides a space into which the femoral vein can expand. It normally contains loose areolar tissue and a lymph gland known as the gland of Cloquet. With bone or ligament on three sides and a major vessel on the fourth, the femoral canal cannot distend easily. A peritoneal sac coming through it therefore has a stiff, narrow neck and any contents are at risk of strangulation.

A characteristic but not invariable feature of the sac of a femoral hernia is that it is thick walled with layers of fat and connective tissue, which when cut across looks like an onion. This means that the sac remains palpable even when empty and so seems to be irreducible.

History

Age Femoral herniae are rare in children and do not become common until over the age of 50, with no upper age limit.

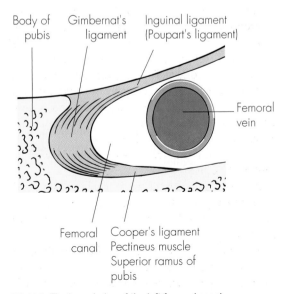

Body of pubis   Gimbernat's ligament   Inguinal ligament (Poupart's ligament)

Femoral vein

Femoral canal   Cooper's ligament
Pectineus muscle
Superior ramus of pubis

FIG 14.9 The boundaries of the left femoral canal.

Sex Femoral herniae are much more common in women than in men. Nevertheless, do not forget that even in women the commonest hernia in the groin region is the inguinal hernia, and that a man can have a femoral hernia.

Symptoms The symptoms of this variety of hernia are similar to those described above for inguinal hernia:

- local – lump in the groin, pain and discomfort,
- general – if causing obstruction: colic, distension, vomiting and constipation.

The femoral hernia is able to strangle a part of the wall of the bowel without occluding the lumen and causing intestinal obstruction – Richter's hernia.

Femoral herniae are occasionally bilateral.

Examination

All the comments made about the examination of inguinal herniae apply to femoral herniae. Ask the

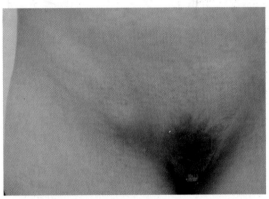

A right femoral hernia. Note that the femoral hernia bulges into the crease of the groin.

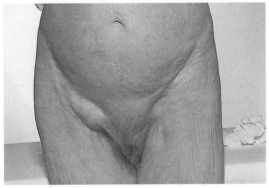

A larger femoral hernia, in an elderly woman, with a wide neck stretching laterally over the femoral vein.

FIG 14.10 FEMORAL HERNIA.

patient to stand up, try to determine the exact anatomical relations of the lump to the inguinal ligament and pubic tubercle, and then decide if the lump has a cough impulse and whether it is reducible.

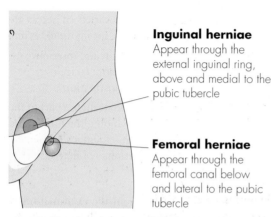

Inguinal herniae
Appear through the external inguinal ring, above and medial to the pubic tubercle

Femoral herniae
Appear through the femoral canal below and lateral to the pubic tubercle

FIG 14.11 The sites of appearance of inguinal and femoral herniae.

Revision panel 14.5
The differential diagnosis of femoral hernia

Inguinal hernia
Enlarged lymph gland
Sapheno-varix
Ectopic testis
Psoas abscess
Psoas bursa
Lipoma

Revision panel 14.6
The differential diagnosis of a lump in the groin

Inguinal hernia
Femoral hernia
Enlarged lymph glands
Sapheno-varix
Ectopic testis
Femoral aneurysm
Hydrocele of the cord or hydrocele of the canal of Nuck
Lipoma of the cord
Psoas bursa
Psoas abscess

The easiest way to confirm that a hernia is coming through the femoral canal is to examine the patient lying down, because it is easier in that position to find the pubic tubercles and other related anatomical landmarks.

Most femoral sacs are thick walled and remain palpable, even when empty – a diagnostic clue in itself.

Position The femoral canal is lateral to the body of the pubis and inferior to the tip of the pubic tubercle. Therefore, the neck of a femoral hernia, or the point at which it disappears into the abdomen, is below and lateral to the pubic tubercle. The main sac of the hernia may expand in any direction. It usually points downwards and laterally, but it can pass medially and may bulge up and over the inguinal ligament. Normally the bulge appears to be directly behind the skin crease of the groin, whereas the inguinal hernia bulges out above the groin crease. With experience, this feature allows correct spot diagnosis.

Feel the lump and, if it appears to have a neck tethered deeply, palpate around this area very carefully to determine its exact position.

A small hernia in a fat person is very difficult to feel, so take great care when examining this region in a patient with intestinal obstruction.

Colour The overlying skin should be of normal colour. The skin may become red and oedematous if the hernia is strangulated.

Temperature The skin temperature is normal unless there is hyperaemia caused by an underlying inflammatory response to strangulation.

Tenderness Femoral herniae are not usually tender unless strangulated, but you may cause pain if your attempts at reduction are too vigorous.

Shape and size The lump is almost spherical, with an area above and deep to it which is difficult to define, corresponding to the site of the neck in the femoral canal.

Most femoral herniae are small. If they do enlarge, they tend to flatten and spread upwards towards the fold of the groin because downward extension is limited by the attachment of the membranous layer of the superficial fascia (Scarpa's fascia) to the deep fascia of the upper thigh.

Surface The surface of the sac is usually smooth.

Composition The majority of femoral herniae feel firm and are dull to percussion because they consist of a small, empty sac surrounded by a lot of extraperitoneal fat and usually just contain omentum. They occasionally contain bladder.

Reducibility The size of most femoral herniae can be reduced by firm pressure but can rarely be completely reduced, for the reasons given above.

Cough impulse For the same reason that many femoral herniae do not reduce easily – adherence of the contents and a thick-walled sac – many do not have a cough impulse. This may make the diagnosis difficult.

Relations Because many femoral herniae do not have the two signs diagnostic of herniae – reducibility and a cough impulse – the diagnosis depends primarily upon the site of the lump, hence the importance of clearly defining its relations to surrounding structures.

State of local tissues Femoral herniae develop because the femoral canal is a naturally weak spot in the abdominal wall, but the region may have been weakened by injury, the commonest of which is the surgical repair of an adjacent inguinal hernia. Look out for other scars near the hernia and always examine the other groin.

General examination Look for causes of raised intra-abdominal pressure, namely chronic bronchitis, retention of urine and constipation, and for signs of intestinal obstruction.

Prevascular femoral hernia

This is the only special variety of femoral hernia that you need remember. It is rare, but usually easy to diagnose. Instead of the sac coming through the narrow femoral canal, it bulges down underneath the whole inguinal ligament, in front of the femoral artery and vein. This means that it has a wide neck and a flattened wide sac, which bulges downwards and laterally.

Prevascular herniae are usually easy to reduce, and have a cough impulse. They rarely strangulate. They are difficult to repair by open techniques because the femoral vessels form the posterior wall of the defect.

UMBILICAL HERNIA

All herniae which appear to be closely related to the umbilicus may be called umbilical herniae. They may be congenital or acquired. All congenital umbilical herniae come through the umbilical defect itself. In adults, most umbilical herniae are acquired and come through a defect adjacent to the umbilical cicatrix, and not through the umbilical scar itself, and should be termed para-umbilical. In practice, the distinction is academic and the simple expression 'umbilical hernia' is commonly used for both varieties.

Congenital umbilical hernia

In early fetal life the whole of the mid-gut protrudes through the umbilicus. As it returns into the abdomen, the gap in the abdominal wall gradually closes, leaving a small central defect through which the umbilical vessels connect the fetus with the placenta.

Congenital umbilical herniae appear at this site if the process by which scar tissue closes the gap, once the umbilical vessels have atrophied after birth, fails.

A congenital persisting protrusion of bowel through the umbilical defect without a covering of skin is called an **exomphalos**. This is not a true hernia and is discussed below.

History

Age Although the weakness is present at birth, the hernia may not be noticed until the umbilical cord has separated and healed. Even then, it may be very small and not noticed until it enlarges months later.

Ethnicity Congenital umbilical herniae are more common in the Afro-Caribbean races.

Symptoms The swelling rarely causes any symptoms for the patient, but parental anxiety is common. Intestinal obstruction is extremely rare.

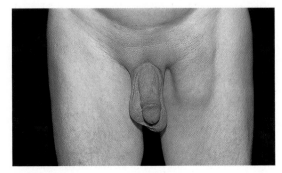

FIG 14.12 A prevascular femoral hernia.

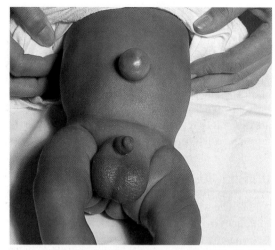

This baby also has a left inguinal hernia and a right hydrocele.

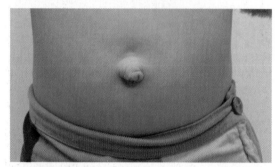

An umbilical hernia in a 3-year-old girl.

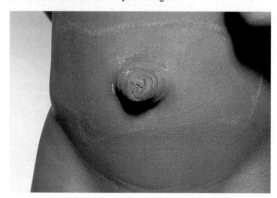

A regressing congenital umbilical hernia. The defect has almost closed and the overlying skin is collapsing inwards to become a normal umbilicus.

FIG 14.13 CONGENITAL UMBILICAL HERNIAE.

ANATOMY OF UMBILICAL HERNIA

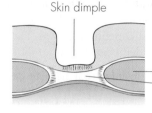

Skin dimple

The normal umbilicus

Rectus abdominis muscle
Scar in linea alba tethered to the skin

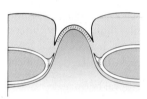

A congenital umbilical hernia

The umbilical scar fails to form or is weak. The abdominal contents bulge through the weak spot and evert the umbilicus.

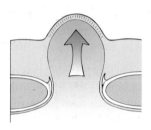

An acquired true umbilical hernia

The umbilical scar is stretched by a raised intra-abdominal pressure and the umbilicus everts.

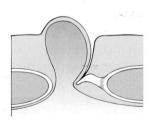

A paraumbilical hernia

The hernial orifice is at the side of the umbilical scar so the sac bulges out beside the umbilicus, turning it into a crescent-shaped slit.

FIG 14.14

A visible hernia may be embarrassing to a child, when noticed by others.

'Tummy ache' in children may be attributed to the hernia, but it is unlikely that there is ever a genuine association.

Natural history The vast majority of congenital umbilical herniae disappear spontaneously during the first few years of life. It is difficult to believe that a large defect will close over in an active child, but this is the usual course of events. The hernia becomes gradually smaller, and then disappears. If there is still a defect at the age of 4, it is unlikely to seal itself and operation is required.

Examination

Shape and size Congenital umbilical herniae are usually hemispherical and overlie an easily palpable defect in the abdominal wall. The size of the lump can vary from very small (0.5 cm diameter) to very large (10 cm diameter). Very small herniae can only be diagnosed by carefully exploring the depth of the umbilicus with the tip of a finger to find the defect in the abdominal wall.

Although there may be quite a large visible hernia, the palpable defect is often very small. Sometimes, however, it is easy to insert a finger into the hole.

In neonates, the remnants of the umbilical cord, and sometimes a chronic granuloma, may be visible.

Composition Congenital umbilical herniae are soft, compressible and easy to reduce. They usually contain bowel and so may be resonant to percussion, if you can elicit this sign in a small child. They reduce spontaneously when the child lies down and become tense when the child cries.

Cough impulse An expansile cough impulse is invariably present.

UMBILICAL HERNIA IN ADULTS

A true umbilical hernia comes through the umbilical scar and has the umbilical skin tethered to it. It is not common in adults and usually secondary to raised intra-abdominal pressure, so clinical examination should concentrate on finding the cause of the raised intra-abdominal pressure.

The causes of abdominal distension are discussed in detail in Chapter 15, but the common causes of an acquired umbilical hernia are pregnancy and ascites. The local physical signs of the hernia are identical to those described for the congenital variety.

Para-umbilical hernia

This is the common acquired umbilical hernia. It appears through a defect that is adjacent to the

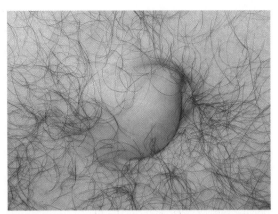

Note that the hernia is clearly coming out alongside the true umbilical scar.

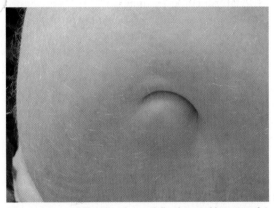

A large para-umbilical hernia, partially obscured by a very fat abdominal wall. Note the classical crescentic shape of the umbilicus.

FIG 14.15 PARA-UMBILICAL HERNIAE.

umbilical scar. That it is beside the umbilicus (para-umbilical) rather than coming through the umbilicus is clinically apparent because it does not bulge into the centre of the umbilicus, and the umbilical skin is not attached to the centre of the sac. Why the linea alba should give way so often just adjacent to the umbilical scar is not known.

History

Age Para-umbilical herniae usually develop in middle and old age. They are more common in women than in men, especially parous and obese women.

Symptoms The commonest symptoms are discomfort and a swelling. Sometimes the swelling is so small that it is not noticed by the patient, even when they present complaining of pain or discomfort and tenderness around the umbilicus, made worse by prolonged standing or strenuous exercise.

Strangulation of an umbilical hernia, whether or not it has been previously noticed by the patient, is common. The usual contents in this case are extraperitoneal fat or omentum, so even though the hernial contents may be strangulated, the bowel is not obstructed.

Examination

Position The main bulge of the hernia is beside the umbilicus, which is pushed to one side and stretched into a crescent shape. With a large hernia in a fat patient there may be a crescent-shaped pit, with the attachment of the skin to the umbilicus at the bottom. This pit may be so deep that it cannot be cleansed, and in consequence there may be a foul-smelling discharge and even a collection of dried-up sebaceous secretions, an **ompholith** (see below).

Surface and edge The surface is smooth and the edge easy to define, except when the patient's abdominal wall is very fat.

Composition The lump is firm as it usually contains omentum. If it contains bowel, it is soft and resonant to percussion. It will be reducible unless the contents are adherent to the sac or the defect is very narrow.

Cough impulse Most of these herniae have an expansile cough impulse.

Relations The skin at the centre of the umbilicus is not attached to the centre of the sac as in the true umbilical hernia, but the umbilical skin is usually firmly applied to the side of the sac and may be fixed to it.

If the hernia can be reduced, the firm fibrous edge of the defect in the linea alba is easy to feel. It may vary in size from a few millimetres in diameter to a defect big enough to admit your hand.

General examination The patient is quite likely to be obese and may have other herniae and generalized abdominal wall laxity. There may be an apron of pendulous fat across the lower abdomen.

Although abdominal distension usually causes a true umbilical hernia, it can cause a para-umbilical

hernia, so examine the contents of the abdomen with care.

EPIGASTRIC HERNIA

An epigastric hernia is a protrusion of extraperitoneal fat, and sometimes a small peritoneal sac, through a defect in the linea alba somewhere between the xiphisternum and umbilicus.

The patient complains of epigastric pain which is localized exactly to the site of the hernia, but often does not notice the underlying lump.

The pain is often associated with eating, so the patient calls it 'indigestion' and makes a self-diagnosis of peptic ulceration. A likely explanation for this is that the fatty hernia is 'nipped' by the linea alba on leaning forward in the sitting position adopted at the dining table. Thus when a patient complains of epigastric discomfort, palpate the abdominal wall very carefully before concentrating on deep palpation, because all the symptoms may be caused by a small, fatty, epigastric hernia.

On examination, these herniae feel firm, do not usually have a cough impulse and cannot be reduced. It is sometimes impossible to distinguish them from lipomata, only the typical position suggesting the correct diagnosis. However, although the defect is always exactly in the mid-line, the sac and hence the palpable swelling may lie to the side of the mid-line.

Epigastric hernia in children

This condition is reasonably common in childhood, sometimes associated with divarication of the rectus abdominis muscles. A small hernia may only be visible intermittently, leading to diagnostic uncertainty. As strangulation of such a sac in a child rarely, if ever, occurs, it is safe to wait until the hernia is seen before recommending surgery, unlike inguinal herniae in children, for which an operation may be indicated on the history alone.

INCISIONAL HERNIA

An abdominal incisional hernia is a hernia through an acquired scar in the abdominal wall, caused by a

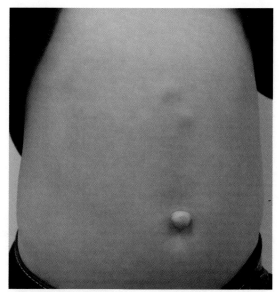

A 3-year-old boy with two epigastric herniae and an umbilical hernia. These small herniae can be the source of epigastric pain.

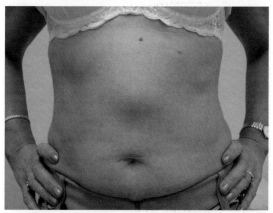

A lady with a large epigastric hernia, which was misdiagnosed as a lipoma and ignored for 5 years.

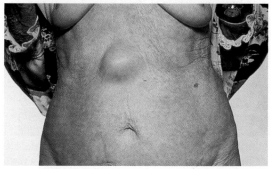

An elderly lady with an epigastric hernia. This reduced easily and caused no symptoms.

FIG 14.16 THREE PATIENTS WITH EPIGASTRIC HERNIAE.

previous surgical operation or injury. Scar tissue is inelastic and stretches progressively if subjected to constant stress.

History

Patients usually remember the operation or wound that caused the scar, but may not recall any complications in the original wound such as a haematoma or infection, which weakened it and made it more susceptible to the development of a hernia.

There may be a history of factors likely to weaken the abdominal musculature, such as chronic cough, obesity or steroid therapy.

Age Incisional herniae occur at all ages but are more common in the elderly.

Symptoms The commonest symptoms are a **lump** and **pain**. Intestinal obstruction can occur, causing distension, colic, vomiting, constipation and severe pain in the lump.

Examination

The common findings are a lump with an expansile cough impulse, beneath an old scar. The defect in the abdominal wall may be palpable. Incisional herniae are not infrequently irreducible, the defect being plugged with adherent omentum.

If the lump does not reduce and does not have a cough impulse, it may not be a hernia, but rather a deposit of tumour, a chronic abscess or haematoma, or a foreign-body granuloma. All these lesions, except recurrent tumour, appear shortly after the initial surgery.

Incisional herniae usually appear in the first year after surgery but may develop many years later.

The local tissues may be thin and weak because of local damage or general cachexia.

DIVARICATION OF THE RECTI

This is separation of the rectus abdominis muscles with extenuation of the linea alba, from xiphisternum to umbilicus and occasionally below.

It may be seen **in children** in the first few years of life. It is only noticeable when the abdominal wall is tensed. Children have a relatively larger abdominal

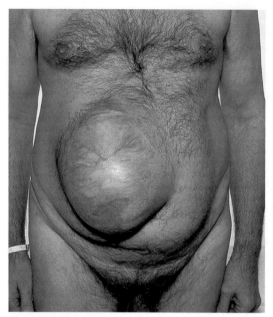

A large incisional hernia.

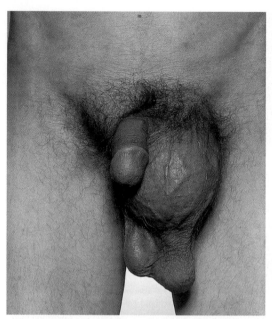

Is this a hernia? No, because it was possible to feel the spermatic cord above the lump and it had no cough impulse. It was a hydrocele of the cord.

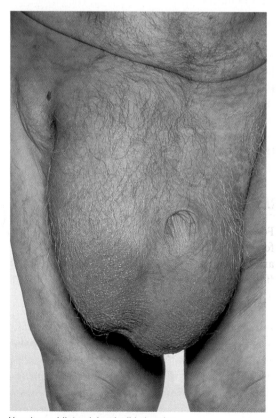

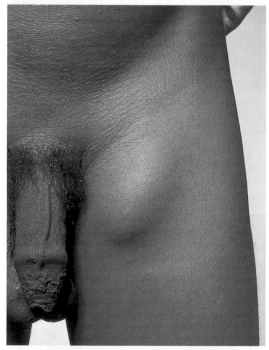

Is this a hernia? No, because it was firm, tender, not reducible and distant from both the inguinal and femoral canals. It was a mass of enlarged inguinal lymph glands caused by lymphogranuloma.

Very large, bilateral, irreducible herniae.

FIG 14.17 HERNIAE: THE OBVIOUS AND THE DECEPTIVE.

cavity than adults; even the slimmest appear somewhat 'pot bellied'.

The condition usually improves and eventually disappears as the child grows, but occasionally persists into adult life. There may be a coincidental umbilical hernia or an epigastric hernia.

The only clinical concern is the cosmetic disfigurement, as strangulation is impossible with such a wide-necked bulge.

Divarication of the recti is also seen **in adults**, in women during and immediately after childbirth. There may be a wide separation of the muscles, with stretched overlying abdominal skin. The examiner may be able to push a hand into the abdominal cavity. (Ask permission to do this!)

As abdominal tone recovers, the defect closes, although it may become permanent after multiple pregnancies.

Although strictly speaking an incisional hernia, iatrogenic divarication may follow repeated surgery through a long mid-line incision.

Divarication is best observed with the patient lying supine. If asked to raise the head and legs together, the recti are fully tensed and the abdominal pressure rises. The thinned-out linea alba then bulges, producing a visible swelling. Patients of all ages learn the best way to produce the swelling.

RARE ABDOMINAL HERNIAE

Spigelian herniae occur at the edge of the rectus sheath, below the umbilicus and above the inguinal area. They are seen in obese patients and may be difficult to diagnose.

Obturator herniae come through the obturator foramen, and the small sac is concealed among the adductor muscles of the thigh. Only on very rare occasions will there be a palpable mass. The usual presentation is small bowel obstruction of unknown cause. The sac may compress the obturator nerve and cause pain in the medial side of the thigh.

Lumbar and gluteal herniae are extremely rare. They are commonly associated with previous surgery near to the defect, such as a loin incision or an excision of the rectum. Diagnosis is difficult and often requires imaging by magnetic resonance imaging (MRI) scanning.

An **interstitial hernia** is a variety of inguinal hernia in which the sac of the hernia spreads between the muscles that form the inguinal canal, above the groin, and emerges through a defect in the internal oblique and transverse muscles rather than the external inguinal ring. It may be suspected when the sac, though clearly in the groin, appears more laterally and looks flatter than usual.

THE UMBILICUS

The commonest abnormality of the umbilicus is an umbilical hernia, described above.

The important congenital abnormalities of the umbilicus are exomphalos and fistula, and the common acquired conditions (apart from herniae) are inflammation and invasion by tumour.

Exomphalos

This condition, which is present at birth, represents an intrauterine failure of the intestines to return to the abdomen combined with a failure of the two sides of the laterally developing abdominal wall to unite to cover the embryonic defect.

The intestines protrude through a central defect of all layers of the abdominal wall. Their only covering is a thin, transparent membrane formed from the remnant of the coverings of the yolk sac. Once this membrane is exposed to the air, it rapidly loses its thin, transparent appearance, becoming thicker and covered with an opaque, fibrinous exudate. If this membrane ruptures, death from peritonitis may follow.

Umbilical fistulae

Four structures pass through the umbilicus during fetal development: the umbilical vein, the umbilical arteries, the vitello-intestinal duct and the urachus. If either of the last two tubes fails to close properly, there will be an intestinal or a urinary fistula.

A **patent vitello-intestinal duct** produces an intermittent discharge of mucus and sometimes faeces from the umbilicus in the neonate. It is a rare abnormality. Sometimes there is visible small intestinal mucosa lining an obvious fistula, but on other occasions there may only be a small fluid leak and the condition mimics an umbilical granuloma. The duct connects to the ileum at the site of a Meckel's diverticulum.

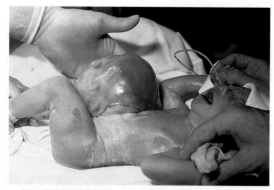

The bowel can be seen through the thin membrane.

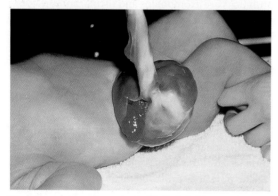

The thin membrane is covered with fibrin but has, nevertheless, ruptured. The umbilical cord is still present.

FIG 14.18 TWO EXAMPLES OF EXOMPHALOS.

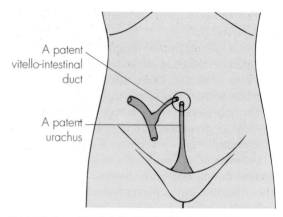

A patent vitello-intestinal duct

A patent urachus

FIG 14.19 A persistent vitello-intestinal duct or patent urachus can become an intestinal or urinary fistula, respectively.

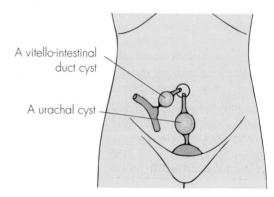

A vitello-intestinal duct cyst

A urachal cyst

FIG 14.20 If the vitello-intestinal duct or urachus are not completely obliterated, they may turn into cysts.

A **patent urachus** can become a track through which urine can leak onto the external surface of the abdomen through the umbilicus. This rare condition occasionally presents in childhood, but more commonly in adult life in association with chronic retention of urine caused by disease of the prostate.

The patient complains of a watery discharge from the umbilicus.

A watery umbilical discharge is nearly always caused by infection in the umbilicus; nevertheless, remember the possibility of a urachal fistula, particularly if there are symptoms of urinary obstruction or a palpable bladder.

Both these embryonic tracts may partially close, leaving a patent segment that becomes a cyst.

A **vitello-intestinal duct cyst** is a small, spherical, mobile swelling deep to the umbilicus that is tethered to the umbilicus and to the small bowel by a fibrous cord. It is usually impalpable.

A **urachal cyst** is an immobile swelling below the umbilicus deep to the abdominal muscles. It may become large enough to fluctuate and have a fluid thrill. If it is still connected to the bladder, it may vary in size and be difficult to distinguish from a chronically distended bladder.

Umbilical granuloma

After the umbilical cord has been severed and tied, the proximal remnant shrivels and separates spontaneously. This leaves an area of chronic inflammation at the line of demarcation, which is quickly covered by epithelium. If the inflammatory process becomes florid, with associated infection, excess granulation tissue is formed which prevents the raw area becoming epithelialized.

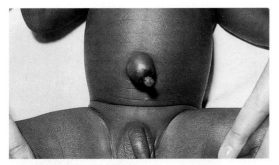

FIG 14.21 An umbilical granuloma. This is an excessive amount of granulation tissue at the point where the umbilical cord separated. These granulomata are often associated with an umbilical hernia.

The baby presents with a pouting umbilicus surmounted by a bright-red, moist, friable, sometimes hemispherical mass of bleeding granulation tissue. This condition is similar to the pyogenic granuloma seen in other parts of the skin. It usually regresses spontaneously in the first month or so of life. If the condition persists longer than this, the possibility of a patent vitello-intestinal duct or an umbilical adenoma should be considered.

Umbilical adenoma

An umbilical adenoma is a patch of intestinal epithelium left behind when the vitello-intestinal duct closes. It may produce a discharge from the depths of the umbilicus, but more often protrudes from the umbilicus and looks like a raspberry. Although it resembles an umbilical granuloma, the cause is quite different. It will not resolve spontaneously.

The mother complains that the baby has a lump at the umbilicus and a mucous discharge.

Omphalitis

Infection within the umbilicus is not uncommon in adults. It is usually associated with inadequate hygiene and a sunken umbilicus caused by obesity. The condition is similar to the intertrigo that occurs between the folds of skin associated with obesity and sweating, which frequently becomes secondarily infected with skin organisms that produce an unpleasant smell.

The patient complains of umbilical discharge, pain and soreness.

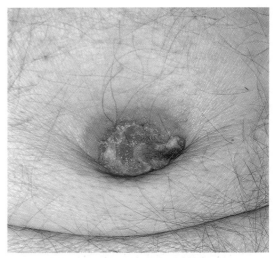

FIG 14.22 Omphalitis. A protruding mass of infected granulation tissue caused by a large ompholith, the brown tip of which is just visible.

On examination, the skin within and around the umbilicus is red and tender, and exuding a seropurulent discharge with a characteristic foul smell.

The whole umbilicus may feel indurated, especially if there is an ompholith or a tumour deposit.

Although simple dermatitis or skin infection is by far the commonest cause of a discharge from the umbilicus, it is essential to exclude the other causes of an umbilical discharge, which are listed in Revision panel 14.7.

True omphalitis is infection of the stump of the umbilical cord following inadequate post-natal care and cleanliness.

Revision panel 14.7
The causes of a discharge from the umbilicus

Congenital
  Intestinal fistula
  Patent urachus
  Umbilical adenoma
Acquired
  Umbilical granuloma
  Dermatitis (intertrigo)
  Ompholith (umbilical concretion)
  Fistula (intestinal)
  Secondary carcinoma
  Endometriosis

Ompholith

When the sebaceous secretions which accumulate in the umbilicus are mixed with the broken hairs and fluff from clothing that become sucked into the umbilicus, the mixture can form a firm lump, worthy of the name **umbilical stone** or **ompholith**. The outside tip of the concretions dries out and may protrude like a sebaceous horn. In certain parts of the UK there is an old wives' tale that if this stone is removed, the sufferer will bleed to death!

Routine personal hygiene will usually prevent the formation of an ompholith, but this is not always as simple as it sounds, for the umbilicus can be deep and narrow, particularly in the obese.

Small concretions are common and uncomplicated. Occasionally an abscess will develop in a narrow-necked umbilicus containing an ompholith. The patient feels unwell and has a very painful, throbbing, swollen umbilicus which may be difficult to distinguish from a strangulated umbilical hernia.

Pus tracking from an intra-abdominal abscess may occasionally point at the umbilicus, the commonest cause being diverticular disease.

Secondary carcinoma
(Sister Joseph's nodule)

A firm or hard nodule bulging into the umbilicus, underneath the skin or eroding through it, in a patient who is losing weight and looks unwell is likely to be a nodule of metastatic cancer. This presentation always indicates advanced, widespread intra-abdominal disease, and the primary tumour is usually in the abdomen.

The tumour cells reach the umbilicus via lymphatics that run in the edge of the falciform ligament alongside the obliterated umbilical vein, or by trans-peritoneal spread.

Nodules of secondary carcinoma may ulcerate, bleed and become infected. Rarely, the tumour deposit is in continuity with bowel and there may be an acquired intestinal fistula.

Endometrioma

If, in a female patient, the umbilicus enlarges, becomes painful and discharges blood during menstruation, it may contain a patch of ectopic endometrial tissue.

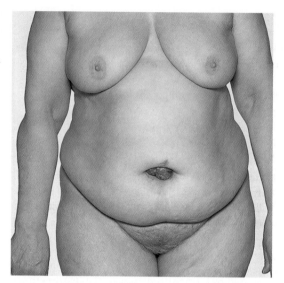

FIG 14.23 A nodule of metastatic carcinoma bulging through the umbilicus causing a serosanguinous discharge. This is known as Sister Joseph's nodule.

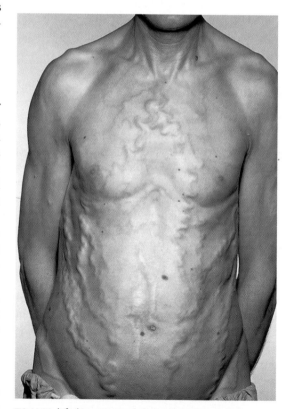

FIG 14.24 Inferior vena caval obstruction may present with dilated subcutaneous veins in the abdominal and chest walls.

Discolouration of the umbilicus

The following physical signs are rare, but the diseases that cause them are common and serious.

A **blue tinge** around the umbilicus, caused by dilated, tortuous, sometimes visible, veins, is called a **caput medusae**, after Medusa, the mythical Gorgon who had small snakes on her scalp instead of hair. The dilated veins are collateral vessels that have developed to circumvent portal vein obstruction. There will be other signs of portal hypertension and liver failure.

Yellow-blue bruising around the umbilicus (*Cullen's sign*) and in the flank (*Grey Turner's sign*) may be caused by pancreatic enzymes which have tracked along the falciform ligament to the umbilicus or across the retroperitoneal space to the loin and digested the subcutaneous tissues following an attack of severe acute pancreatitis. Both appear a few days after the beginning of the acute symptoms.

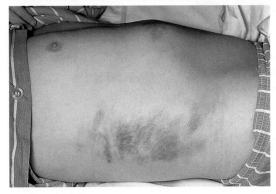

FIG 14.25 Grey Turner's sign. Bruising in the left flank caused by acute haemorrhagic pancreatitis.

Bruising at the umbilicus can also be associated with intra-abdominal bleeding, particularly when it is extraperitoneal. Causes include ruptured ectopic pregnancy and accidental peri-uterine bleeding in pregnancy.

THE EXAMINATION OF THE ABDOMEN

The abdomen contains the stomach, duodenum, small and large bowel, liver, gallbladder, spleen, pancreas, kidneys, uterus, bladder, aorta and vena cava and, in women, the uterus, ovaries and Fallopian tubes. This relatively small cavity therefore contains a number of vital organs, all of which are susceptible to disease or malfunction but many are inaccessible to palpation, being hidden behind the lower ribs or inside the bony pelvis (Fig. 15.1).

Because the abdominal organs are so close together, the brain is often incapable of distinguishing which of them is the source of a pain, but other symptoms and signs may help to distinguish the likely organ and the pathology responsible for the pain.

Preparation

The environment

The examination room must be warm and private if the patient is to lie undressed and relaxed. A cold couch placed in a draught or in the view of other patients makes proper examination impossible. A good light is essential, with, ideally, daylight coming obliquely from the side of the patient to emphasize the shadows. Artificial light obliterates the soft shadows that often give the first indication of asymmetry, and many neon lights falsify colours, particularly the yellows and blues.

The examination couch or bed

A hard, flat couch makes the patient lie absolutely flat and opens the gap between the pubis and the xiphisternum, but unfortunately stretches and tightens

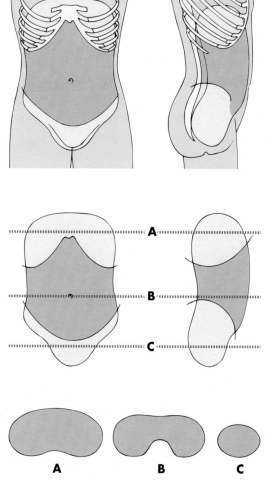

FIG 15.1 These drawings show the extent of the abdominal cavity. The paler lavender areas indicate the parts of the abdomen protected by the ribs and the pelvis. The levels of the three cross-sections are indicated on the central diagram.

the abdominal muscles. A soft bed lets the lumbar spine sink into a deep curve and closes the gap between the pubis and the ribs. The best compromise in the office or outpatients is a hard couch with a backrest that can be raised by 15–20°. The hard couch ensures that patients retain their lumbar lordosis, opening access to the abdomen and pushing the central contents anteriorly. The elevation of the thoracic cage relaxes the anterior abdominal wall muscles.

Exposure

The full extent of the abdomen must be visible and, ideally, patients should be uncovered from nipples to knees. Many find this embarrassing and a compromise is to cover the lower abdomen with a sheet or blanket while palpating the abdomen, but never forget to examine the genitalia and the hernial orifices.

Getting the patient to relax

It is not possible to feel anything within the abdomen if the patient is tense. There are several ways in which relaxation can be encouraged.

- Ask the patient to rest their head on the couch or a pillow to avoid tensing the rectus abdominis muscles.

- Ask the patient to place their arms by their sides, not behind their head.
- Encourage the patient to sink their back into the couch and breathe regularly and slowly.
- Only press your hands into the abdomen during expiration as the abdominal muscles relax.

If these manoeuvres do not work, ask the patient to flex their hips to 45° and their knees to 90° and place an extra pillow behind their head. Although these manoeuvres tilt up the pelvis and reduce access to the abdomen, they usually relax the abdominal muscles.

The position of the examiner

The examiner's hands should be clean and warm with short nails. It is impossible to palpate deeply with long nails and it is an insult to the patient to have dirty hands.

The whole hand should rest on the abdomen by keeping the hand and forearm horizontal, in the same plane as the front of the abdomen. To achieve this the examiner must sit or kneel beside the bed. Do not examine the patient from a standing position by leaning forwards and dorsi-flexing your wrist.

Sitting or kneeling beside the patient with your forearm level with the front of the abdomen puts your

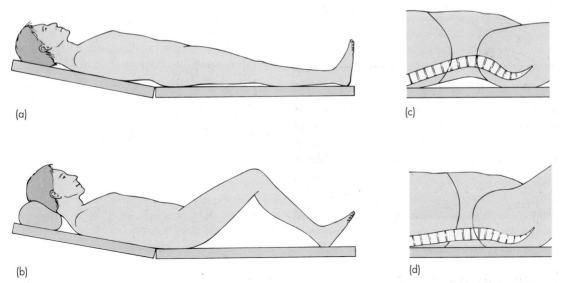

(a)

(b)

(c)

(d)

FIG 15.2 EXAMINATION OF THE ABDOMEN. (a) Examine the abdomen with the patient on a firm couch or bed with just sufficient support beneath the shoulders and head to stop the anterior abdominal wall being stretched tight. (b) If the abdominal wall is tight, raise the head and flex the hips. (c) and (d) These figures show the reduction in the area of abdomen available for palpation if the patient lies on a soft bed that allows the lumbar lordosis to straighten.

eyes about 50 cm above your hand, an ideal level for seeing any soft shadows caused by lumps and bumps.

Examination

This should follow the standard routine of inspection, palpation, percussion and auscultation.

Inspection

Look at the whole patient. Look for any general abnormality indicative of intra-abdominal pathology such as cachexia, pallor or jaundice.

Inspection of the abdomen from the end of the bed will reveal if there is any asymmetry or distension.

Note the position, shape and size of any bulge, any changes in its shape, and whether it moves with respiration or increases with coughing.

Observe the reaction of the patient to coughing or moving. Patients with peritonitis find movement extremely painful and, consequently, tend to lie very still, whilst patients with colic roll around with each bout of pain.

Record the presence of any scars, sinuses or fistulae.

Dilated surface veins may indicate the possibility of portal hypertension or inferior vena caval occlusion (see Fig. 14.24, page 384).

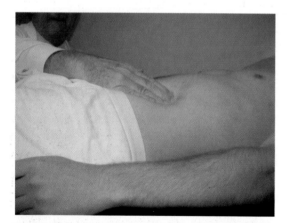

FIG 15.3 When you palpate the abdomen, sit or kneel so that your forearm is horizontal and level with the anterior abdominal wall, and your eyes are 50 cm above this level. If you are higher, your wrist will be extended and you will not be able to palpate comfortably and firmly. In this illustration the abdomen is inadequately exposed. The patient's pants should have been removed or lowered down to the level of the pubis.

Palpation

Palpate gently but deliberately, firmly and with purpose. Rapid, jerky or circular movements reminiscent of kneading dough are distressing for the patient and cause them to lose confidence. Keeping your hands still and feeling the intra-abdominal structures moving beneath them gives more information than rapid and thoughtless palpation.

Finish (or begin) by feeling the areas that might otherwise be forgotten.

1. Feel the supraclavicular fossae and neck for lymph glands.
2. Feel the hernial orifices at rest and when the patient coughs.
3. Feel the femoral pulses.
4. Examine the external genitalia.
5. Look at the hands, nails and facies.

General light palpation for tenderness

This should be done by gently resting a hand on the patient's abdomen and pressing lightly. The hand should be systematically moved over the whole of the abdomen. If you are right handed, start in the left iliac fossa and move round in an anti-clockwise direction to finish in the right iliac fossa.

When a patient complains of pain, asked them to indicate its site before you begin your palpation, so that you can start over a non-tender area and move towards the tender spot. Carefully define the area of tenderness so that you can depict it as a hatched area on a drawing of the abdomen (Fig. 15.4).

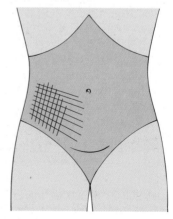

FIG 15.4 Indicate areas of tenderness by oblique lines on a sketch like this. Masses are depicted by outlining their shape.

Assess the degree of tenderness. Palpation over an area of mild tenderness just causes pain. **Guarding**, the tightening of the patient's abdominal muscles in response to pressure, indicates severe tenderness.

The sudden withdrawal of manual pressure may cause a sharp exacerbation of the pain, which is known as **rebound** or **release tenderness**. This test may be distressing for the patient and it is preferable to assess rebound tenderness by the patient's response to light percussion.

Sometimes, release of pressure on a distant non-tender part of the abdomen may cause pain in a tender area.

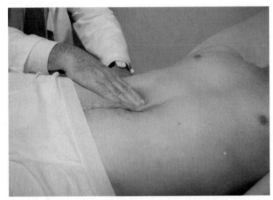

Palpate the **liver** by resting your fingers on the abdomen almost parallel to the right costal margin and asking the patient to breathe in. The liver edge can be made more prominent by putting your left hand under the lower ribs and lifting them forwards.

General palpation for tenderness

When no pain is elicited by systematic light palpation over the whole abdomen, repeat the process, pressing more firmly and deeply to see if there is any deep tenderness.

Palpation for masses

The whole abdomen must be carefully palpated for the presence, position, shape, size, surface, edge, consistence, fluid thrill, resonance and pulsatility of any masses.

Tender masses in the abdomen are very difficult to feel because of the protective guarding of the abdominal wall muscles. A good idea of the surface and size of a tender mass may be obtained by resting your hand gently on the tender area and pressing a little deeper during each exploration and feeling the mass as it moves beneath your hand.

Rapid, hard pressure achieves nothing under these circumstances because the patient just tightens their abdominal muscles.

Palpation of the normal solid viscera

The liver To feel the liver, place your right hand transversely and flat on the right side of the abdomen at the level of the umbilicus, parallel with the right costal margin. Then ask the patient to take a deep breath. If the liver is grossly enlarged, its lower edge will move downwards and bump against the

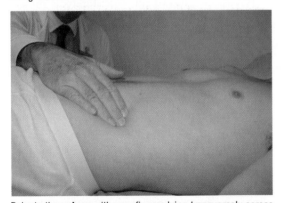

Palpate the **spleen** with your fingers lying transversely across the abdomen so that its tip will hit the tips of your index and middle fingers when the patient breathes in. You can make the spleen more prominent by lifting the lower ribs forwards with your left hand as you do when palpating the left kidney.

FIG 15.5 PALPATING THE ABDOMEN.

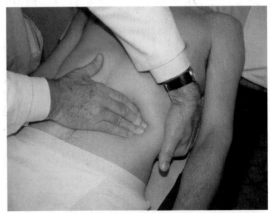

Palpate the **kidneys** by pressing firmly into the lumbar region during inspiration while lifting the kidney forwards with your other hand in the loin. (The exposure is inadequate for a proper examination of the whole abdomen in these three illustrations.).

radial side of your index finger. If nothing abnormal is felt, repeat the process after moving your hand upwards, inch by inch, until the costal margin is reached.

The liver edge may be straight or irregular, thin and sharp, or thick and rounded. Palpation beginning just below the costal margin can easily miss a large liver. Gross hepatomegaly may fill the whole abdomen so, if in doubt, begin your palpation in the left iliac fossa.

The spleen An enlarged spleen appears below the tip of the tenth rib along a line heading towards the umbilicus and, if really large, may extend into the right iliac fossa. A normal spleen is not palpable.

To feel the spleen, place the fingertips of your right hand on the right iliac fossa just below the umbilicus. Ask the patient to take a deep breath. If nothing abnormal is felt, move your hand in stages towards the tip of the left tenth rib. When the costal margin is reached, place your left hand around the lower left rib cage and lift the lower ribs and the spleen forwards as the patient inspires. This manoeuvre occasionally lifts a slightly enlarged spleen far enough forward to make it palpable.

The spleen is recognized by its shape and site and, when present, the notch on its supero-medial edge. It is dull to percussion as it lies immediately beneath the abdominal wall with no bowel in front of it, unlike a renal mass (see below).

The kidneys Normal kidneys are usually impalpable, except in very thin people, but both lumbar regions should always be carefully examined.

To feel the patient's right kidney, place your left hand behind the patient's right loin between the twelfth rib and the iliac crest, so that you can lift the loin and kidney forwards. Then place your right hand on the right side of the abdomen just below the level of the anterior superior iliac spine. As the patient breathes in and out, palpate the loin between both hands. The lower pole of a normal kidney may be felt at the height of inspiration in a very thin person. If the kidney is very easy to feel, it is either enlarged or abnormally low. To feel the left kidney, lean across the patient, place your left hand around the flank into the left loin to lift it forwards, then place your right hand on the abdomen and feel any masses between the two hands.

An enlarged kidney can be pushed back and forth between the anterior and posterior hands. This is called **balloting**. It feels like patting a ball back and forth in a pool of water. Balloting is also used to palpate a fetus in a pregnant uterus.

Percussion

The whole abdomen must be percussed, particularly over any masses. A dull area may draw your attention to a mass that was missed on palpation and indicate a more detailed and careful palpation of the area of dullness. When there is a circumscribed mass, a tap on one side while feeling the opposite side with the other hand may reveal that it conducts a **fluid thrill**. Any area of dullness should be outlined by percussion with the abdomen in two positions to see if it moves or changes shape. Free fluid (ascites) changes shape and moves (**shifting dullness**, see pages 433–4).

Percussion causes pain if peritonitis is present and is a useful method for mapping out a tender area (see above).

If a part or the whole of the abdomen is distended, the patient should be held at the hips and the abdomen shaken from side to side. Splashing sounds, a **succussion splash**, indicate that there is an intra-abdominal viscus, usually the stomach, distended with a mixture of fluid and gas.

Auscultation

Listen to the bowel sounds. Peristalsis produces gurgling noises because the bowel contains a mixture of fluid and gas. The pitch of the noise depends upon the distension of the bowel and the proportions of gas and fluid. Normal bowel sounds are low-pitched gurgles which occur every few seconds. The absence of bowel sounds indicates that peristalsis has ceased.

Revision panel 15.1
Never forget to examine

Supraclavicular lymph glands
Hernia orifices
Femoral pulses
Genitalia
Bowel sounds
Anal canal and rectum

This may be either a primary or secondary phenomenon. If you can hear the heart and breath sounds but no bowel sounds over a 30-second period, the patient probably has a paralytic ileus.

Increased peristalsis increases the volume and frequency of the bowel sounds. Distension of the bowel caused by a mechanical intestinal obstruction is associated not only with increased bowel sounds but also with a change in the character of the sounds. They become amphoric in nature with runs of high-frequency gurgles, sounding like sea water entering a large cave through a narrow entrance, often described as 'tinkling'.

Having assessed the quality of the bowel sounds, it is important to listen for any systolic vascular bruits.

ABDOMINAL PAIN

Time spent taking a careful history is never wasted, as abdominal pain is the only symptom of many intra-abdominal diseases. The two most significant properties of an abdominal pain are its *site* and its *character*.

The significance of the site of abdominal pain

The abdomen can be divided into three horizontal zones – upper, central and lower – by two horizontal lines. These are the transpyloric plane (a line circling the body mid-way between the suprasternal notch and the symphysis pubis) and the transtubercular plane (a line circling the body that passes through the two tubercles of the iliac crest) as shown in Figure 15.6. Each of these three zones can be further vertically subdivided into three regions – central, right and left – by the two mid-clavicular lines.

The anatomical names of these nine regions are:

- the epigastrium
- the right hypochondrium
- the left hypochondrium
- the umbilical region
- the right lumbar region
- the left lumbar region
- the hypogastrium or suprapubic region
- the right iliac fossa
- the left iliac fossa.

Sometimes patients are only capable of localizing pain to the upper or lower half of the abdomen and/or to the left or right side.

Colicky pain is referred to the centre of the abdomen whatever its source, as it is a visceral sensation, whereas the pain from the parietal peritoneum is felt over the inflamed area (somatic sensation).

Pain in the upper abdomen is most likely to arise from the biliary tree, stomach, duodenum or pancreas. These structures produce right-sided, central and left-sided pain respectively. The pain from these three organs radiates in different directions.

- Gallbladder pain may radiate through to the back and to the right to reach the tip of the

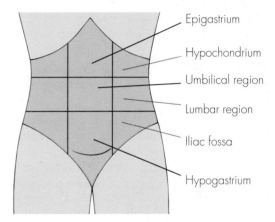

FIG 15.6 The names of the regions of the abdomen.

> Revision panel 15.2
> **The features of a pain that must be elicited**
>
> Time and nature of onset
> Site
> Character (burning, throbbing, stabbing, constricting, colicky, aching)
> Severity
> Progression
> Duration
> End
> Radiation
> Relieving factors
> Exacerbating factors
> Associated symptoms, e.g. vomiting, diarrhoea, painful micturition, missed or absent periods

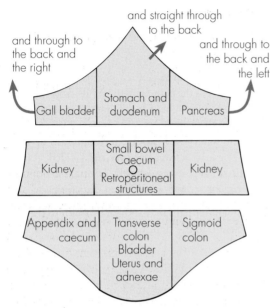

and straight through
to the back

and through to
the back and
the right

and through to
the back and
the left

Gall bladder	Stomach and duodenum	Pancreas
Kidney	Small bowel Caecum ○ Retroperitoneal structures	Kidney
Appendix and caecum	Transverse colon Bladder Uterus and adnexae	Sigmoid colon

FIG 15.7 The structures that commonly cause pain in the nine anatomical regions of the abdomen and often radiate through to the back.

scapula. When felt in this area, it often seems to the patient to be a separate, independent pain.

- Ulcers in the posterior wall of the stomach or duodenum cause a pain that radiates through to the back.
- Pancreatic pain also tends to go through to the back and sometimes to the left.

Pain in the centre of the abdomen is most likely to arise from the small bowel, caecum and mid-line retroperitoneal structures such as the aorta. Pain from retroperitoneal structures often radiates through to the back. Pain in the lateral zones of the central region is most likely to come from the kidneys. Pain

Revision panel 15.3
The principal causes of abdominal pain

Inflammation/infection
Perforation of a viscus
Obstruction of a viscus
Infarction/strangulation
Intraperitoneal/retroperitoneal haemorrhage
Injury
Extra-abdominal and medical causes

from the kidney is also felt in the loin and may radiate down to the groin. All visceral pain may move and become localized if the inflammatory process in the viscus involves the parietal peritoneum.

Pain in the lower abdomen is most likely to come from the appendix, caecum, colon, bladder, uterus, ovaries and Fallopian tubes. Pain in the hypogastric region usually arises from the bladder, rectum, uterus and its adnexae. Pain in the right iliac fossa usually comes from the caecum and the appendix. Pain in the left iliac fossa usually comes from the sigmoid colon.

Lower abdominal pains rarely radiate, but pain from pelvic structures may be referred to the lower back or perineum.

The significance of the character of abdominal pain

It is possible to subdivide the character of the pain of the majority of the painful conditions that occur within the abdomen into two large categories: a **constant pain** associated with inflammation and neoplasic infiltration, and a **colicky pain** associated with obstruction of a muscular conducting tube such as the bowel or the ureter (colic).

The constant pain caused by inflammation or infiltration, whether it is the mild inflammatory response around a chronic peptic ulcer or the acute response to a perforated appendix, is made worse by any local or general movement and persists until the underlying cause subsides. Inflammation within the abdomen does not throb or burn in the same way that inflammatory pains do elsewhere.

The colic caused by obstruction to a muscular conducting viscus is a pain which fluctuates in severity at frequent intervals and feels griping in nature. The source of bowel colic can be suspected from the time interval between the peaks of the pain – short in the jejunum, longer in the ileum, and longer still in the colon. In biliary colic and renal colic, the peaks of pain are short and the pain seldom goes away completely between exacerbations. Prolonged obstruction to the outflow of any hollow viscus ultimately causes it to distend. This produces a constant 'stretching' pain, which is different from the ache of inflammation but not colicky in nature. A similar pain can come from conditions that stretch the retroperitoneal tissues.

Colic can also be caused by muscular dysfunction, i.e. disorders of gastrointestinal mobility such as the irritable bowel syndrome, as opposed to true colic which is secondary to obstruction.

The significance of radiation

Radiation of a pain signifies that other structures are becoming involved. For example, when the pain from a duodenal ulcer radiates through to the back, it indicates that the inflammation has spread beyond the duodenum into adjacent structures in the posterior abdominal wall, such as the pancreas. Radiation, therefore, not only indicates the source of the pain, but may also hint at the extent of the disease.

The significance of the rate of onset and severity

Patients with severe abdominal pain of acute onset are usually collectively grouped as having an 'acute abdomen'. These patients usually consult their general practitioner or seek emergency medical help once their pain has persisted for more than an hour or so. However, many will have had chronic symptoms over the preceding months or years caused by the condition currently causing their acute symptoms, i.e. the same condition can present acutely or chronically.

Therefore, although the rate and severity of presentation may indicate the urgency of the problem, they do not always indicate the nature of the underlying pathology.

Whatever the urgency and underlying pathology, a full history and clinical examination (as described above) must be carried out so that a working diagnosis or differential diagnosis can be made and the patient assigned to one of the following management categories.

- An acute abdomen, e.g. peritonitis, with a known or unknown underlying cause requiring urgent treatment.
- An abdominal pain of known or unknown cause requiring pain palliation pending further investigation and treatment.
- An abdominal pain with no evidence of any clinically detectable intra-abdominal pathology that can be observed and investigated later if necessary, i.e. time to wait and see.

Put another way:

- I may or may not know the diagnosis but the problem needs urgent management.
- I understand the problem but not necessarily its cause and have time to investigate further in order to decide what to do.
- I do not think there is anything wrong and can wait and see whether further investigations will be required.

In almost every case, additional investigations are likely to be required to refine the diagnosis and plan treatment but, when the diagnosis is 'uncertain', **careful monitoring and repeated re-examination are essential to detect any progression or resolution of the problem and ensure that important new physical signs are not missed**. Acute physical signs often develop over several hours and become clear cut, often diagnostic, by the time of a later examination. In contrast, the signs of chronic conditions may take months to develop.

UPPER ABDOMINAL PAIN – ACUTE AND/OR CHRONIC – CAUSED BY INFLAMMATORY AND MALIGNANT CONDITIONS

The common sites of inflammation and malignant disease in the upper abdomen causing upper abdominal pain are in the stomach and duodenum, gallbladder and pancreas.

The conditions causing acute and/or chronic upper abdominal pain are summarized in Revision panels 15.4 and 15.5.

Revision panel 15.4
The common conditions that present with acute upper abdominal pain

Oesophagitis
Boerhaave's syndrome
Acute gastritis
Perforated peptic ulcer
Acute cholecystitis
Gallstone and biliary colic
Acute pancreatitis

Oesophagitis

This occurs when acid pepsin refluxes up out of the stomach into the oesophagus through the lower oesophageal sphincter onto the squamous epithelium lining the oesophagus, which is not able to resist these powerful chemicals. In many instances the reflux occurs because of gastro-oesophageal junction incompetence caused by a hiatus hernia.

Patients complain of **heartburn**, which is a severe burning discomfort felt in the centre of the chest behind the heart, often at night. The frequency and severity of the heartburn is made worse by lying flat, so patients sleep propped up on pillows to try to reduce its occurrence. Heartburn is often initiated by bending, stooping or heavy lifting. When reflux occurs, patients may experience a bitter taste developing in the mouth, which is often accompanied by flatulence and coughing if any of the refluxing acid spills over into the lungs. Sometimes the burning pain may only be experienced in the epigastrium.

After many years, patients may complain of difficulty with swallowing and of food sticking in their gullet. Although the presence of **dysphagia** suggests the development of a stricture caused by the acid reflux, achalasia or a carcinoma of the oesophagus or cardia must be excluded.

Examination

This rarely reveals any diagnostic signs. The diagnosis relies on endoscopy and other investigations.

Boerhaave's syndrome

This syndrome is caused by a full-thickness tear at the oesophago-gastric junction, perhaps as a consequence of attempting to suppress a vomit.

Revision panel 15.5
The common conditions that present with chronic upper abdominal pain

Chronic peptic ulceration
Carcinoma of the stomach
Chronic cholecystitis
Chronic pancreatitis
Liver metastases
Splenomegaly

The patient complains of the **sudden onset of a severe pain** in the upper abdomen or lower chest after a bout of vomiting. The condition should be suspected if, in addition to tenderness, guarding and rigidity in the upper abdomen, there is **supraclavicular subcutaneous emphysema**.

Subcutaneous bubbles of air – emphysema – feel like the little plastic air pockets in 'bubble wrap' which compress, crackle and pop beneath the fingers during gentle palpation.

Acute gastritis/duodenitis/peptic ulceration

Benign gastric and duodenal ulcers are classified together as peptic ulceration. Mucosal infection with *Helicobacter pylorides* is a major factor in the development of both these conditions.

Gastric ulcers are now rare in the UK, so any patient presenting with indigestion, non-specific upper abdominal pain and the recent onset of weight loss should be suspected of having a gastric cancer.

Duodenal ulcers are still common everywhere and affect both sexes in equal numbers. They can occur at any age, but do so most often in middle-aged patients.

History

Symptoms Patients with acute peptic ulceration present with acute pain of short duration but may have had previous similar episodes interspersed with periods of relief lasting for many months or even years.

The main symptom of acute peptic ulceration is an **epigastric discomfort or pain**, which is related to meals and described as indigestion. It can vary from a mild discomfort to a very severe pain that forces the patient to lie down. The severity and tenderness may equal those of a perforated peptic ulcer.

Patients with **acute gastric ulcers** are typically **afraid to eat** because the pain is induced by food. **Vomiting often relieves the pain.**

Patients with **duodenal ulcers** typically have a **good appetite** and rarely lose weight because they **eat frequently to relieve their pain**. Acid brash, water brash and heartburn are rare symptoms. They are more frequent in patients with duodenal than gastric ulceration.

Haematemesis and **melaena** may complicate all forms of peptic ulceration.

Drugs Many drugs, but especially aspirin and the non-steroidal anti-inflammatory drugs that are used to treat arthritis, irritate the gastric mucosa and cause ulceration, even perforation, so it is essential to ascertain the precise details of any drug ingestion.

Social history Cigarette smoking and periods of stress may be important risk factors.

Examination

Abdominal examination usually reveals epigastric tenderness, with guarding if the pain is severe. The patient may be anaemic if there has been chronic silent bleeding before the acute episode.

Chronic peptic ulceration, gastritis and duodenitis

History

Age Peptic ulceration tends to occur between the ages of 20 and 60 years.

Sex Both gastric and duodenal ulcers are more common in men than in women.

Occupation There is a higher incidence amongst the professional and executive classes.

Symptoms Although a few patients present to hospital with an acute, sometimes very severe upper abdominal pain of short duration as described above, the great majority of patients with chronic peptic ulceration present with a **chronic,** less severe and more **intermittent pain,** which they usually call '**indigestion' or dyspepsia** because it is directly related to the ingestion of food. Nevertheless, some experience continuous pain over many hours or days which is unaffected by food.

Night pain, which wakes the patient and seems to be unrelated to food, is a common symptom of duodenal ulceration. This is thought to be caused by the drop of pH in the stomach at night, when the acid secretions are no longer buffered by the presence of food. The pain is usually experienced in the **epigastrium** and **may radiate into either the back or the right hypochondrium** if the ulcer is situated in the posterior part of the stomach or the second part of the duodenum. The pain is usually described as a continuous gnawing or boring ache and is

rarely very severe. It is usually **episodic**, occurring for two or three weeks at a time before resolving spontaneously, only to recur a few months later – a feature known as periodicity. The rapid onset of pain after food, causing food fear and loss of weight, suggests the presence of a gastric ulcer. Pain that is relieved by eating indicates the probability of a duodenal ulcer.

The pain is usually relieved by the commercially available antacids, H2 receptor blockers and proton pump inhibitors.

Peptic ulcers commonly arise in middle-aged smokers, but are also common in middle-aged and elderly patients on long-term non-steroidal anti-inflammatory drugs.

Vomiting is rare unless a pyloric stenosis has developed.

Excessive salivation (water brash) and acid brash are highly suggestive of duodenal ulceration. Some patients develop heartburn.

Haematemesis and melaena are important complications which occur in a small proportion of patients with chronic, and acute, peptic ulceration. Chronic blood loss may cause an iron deficiency anaemia, which presents with tiredness and shortness of breath.

Chronic peptic ulceration must be differentiated from other causes of chronic abdominal pain. A clear history of weight loss suggests a gastric carcinoma, whereas acid heartburn and reflux (see below) suggest oesophagitis. Gallstones and chronic cholecystitis may coexist and are important differential diagnoses (see below).

Examination

General Anaemia and cervical lymphadenopathy with obvious cachexia should suggest the possibility of carcinoma of the stomach rather than peptic ulceration.

Abdomen

Inspection. Epigastric distension and visible peristalsis may be present if pyloric stenosis has developed.

Palpation. Minor tenderness in the epigastrium is often the only abnormality. The presence of a succussion splash indicates the presence of pyloric stenosis.

The diagnosis of chronic peptic ulcer is now almost exclusively made on flexible endoscopy and biopsy. The importance of *Helicobacter pylorides* as a cause has already been described, and a breath test is available to confirm its involvement.

Percussion and auscultation. These should be normal.

Perforated peptic ulcer

Acid gastric juice will enter the peritoneal cavity if a peptic ulcer erodes the wall of the stomach or duodenum at a point where it is only covered by visceral peritoneum. This causes a chemical peritonitis, which later becomes infected with bacteria.

History

Age and sex Perforated peptic ulcers are most common between the ages of 40 and 60 years but also occur in the very old because many old people are given non-steroidal anti-inflammatory drugs. Men and women are equally affected.

Symptoms The perforation causes **sudden severe and constant pain**. This usually begins in the epigastrium, reaches its maximum intensity quickly and remains severe for many hours. It gradually extends to involve the whole of the abdomen. All movement, including respiration, makes the pain worse, causing the patient to lie immobile on the bed. Many patients give no history of previous dyspepsia, but it is important to ask if they have ever suffered from indigestion in the past.

Drug history It is important to enquire whether the patient has taken steroids, non-steroidal anti-inflammatory drugs or salicylates, because these dispose to perforation.

Examination

General appearance The patient looks ill and is obviously in pain, lying completely still. A tachycardia is common and respiration is shallow, but the temperature is usually normal.

Abdomen

Inspection. The abdomen is flat and does not rise and fall with respiration. The abdominal muscles can be seen to be tightly contracted.

Palpation. In the early stages, tenderness and guarding may be confined to the epigastrium and right side, but eventually, when the whole peritoneal cavity is contaminated, the whole abdomen becomes **very tender**, with **intense guarding**, often described

as **board-like rigidity**. No intra-abdominal viscus or masses can be felt because the abdominal musculature is permanently contracted.

Percussion. This is usually painful. If a large quantity of air has escaped into the peritoneal cavity, the liver dullness may be diminished or completely absent.

Auscultation. The bowel sounds disappear once generalized peritonitis is established.

Beware: after 4–6 hours, the acid in the peritoneal cavity becomes diluted and the pain and guarding decrease. Patients think they are improving but they are in fact getting worse. The peritonitis is progressing and hypervolaemia is developing. An increasing tachycardia and absent bowel sounds associated with increasing abdominal distension and sunken eyes indicate that the patient is becoming extremely ill.

Carcinoma of the stomach

Carcinoma of the stomach is a common cause of death in men. Pernicious anaemia, gastric polyps and chronic gastric ulcers are known to be premalignant conditions, but the majority of gastric ulcers arise spontaneously. *Helicobacter pylorides* is an important predisposing factor.

History

Age The incidence of gastric carcinoma reaches its peak between 50 and 70 years but can arise at an earlier age.

Sex Gastric cancer is two to three times more common in men than in women.

Geography There are unexplained variations in the incidence of this disease. It is very common in Japan, closely followed by Chile, Austria and Finland. In the United Kingdom, it affects approximately 20–30 per 100 000 of the population. Genetic and dietary factors may be important, as may be the ingestion of nitrites.

Symptoms The onset of **indigestion** or **epigastric pain** in a patient over 40 years of age, however vague, should be treated very seriously. The pain may be mild and related to food but, unlike the indigestion associated with peptic ulcer, the pain of a gastric ulcer is constant and not solely brought on by eating. When patients have had symptoms of a

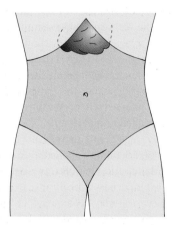

FIG 15.8 Some cancers of the stomach may present as a palpable mass in the epigastrium, but the majority are impalpable.

peptic ulcer for many years, they are usually aware that the nature of the pain has changed. Often their periodic pain becomes constant.

Patients with stomach cancer do not want to eat, and **loss of appetite** is a cardinal symptom. The inevitable consequence of a loss of appetite is **loss of weight**. The patient may lose 10–20 kg in 1 or 2 months. The loss of appetite and weight often occur long before any other symptoms.

Tumours near the cardia may cause oesophago-gastric junction obstruction and cause the patient to complain of difficulty in swallowing (dysphagia). As the dysphagia increases, undigested food may be regurgitated from the oesophagus.

Cancers in the pyloric region often obstruct the outflow of food from the stomach. If so, the patient may vomit large quantities of undigested food (undigested because of the low acid production associated with the accompanying atrophic gastritis) and notice epigastric discomfort and distension. Some cancers grow to a considerable size without producing symptoms, apart from mild weight loss.

Systematic questions A systematic review of the other systems may reveal symptoms that suggest that the tumour has metastasized, such as weakness, tiredness or dyspnoea.

Previous history The patient may have a long history of peptic ulceration or have had an ulcer some years previously which was cured with medicine. Pernicious anaemia and atrophic gastritis predispose to gastric cancers. The patient may have been taking vitamin B12 supplements for their anaemia.

Examination

General appearance The most noticeable features are **wasting** and **pallor**. The wasting is often most apparent in the face and hands. The pallor is usually caused by an iron deficiency anaemia that is the result of chronic bleeding and lack of iron in the diet. Many patients present at an advanced stage with multiple hepatic metastases or metastases in the lymph glands around the porta hepatis. Mild jaundice suggests the latter.

The neck The supraclavicular fossa must be carefully examined, as secondary deposits in the supraclavicular lymph glands are common. A palpable supraclavicular gland in a patient with a carcinoma of the stomach is called **Virchow's gland** and its presence is referred to as *Troisier's sign*.

The lungs The presence of a pleural effusion suggests pulmonary metastases.

Abdomen

Inspection. The abdomen is often scaphoid as a consequence of weight loss but, paradoxically, there may be generalized abdominal distension if ascites is present. Pyloric obstruction causes epigastric distension and visible peristalsis. These physical signs can only be seen in thin patients. In the majority the primary tumour is too small, too high or too deep to be seen.

Palpation. In the majority of patients, the only physical sign is epigastric tenderness. Deep palpation on full inspiration may reveal an epigastric mass. In a thin patient with advanced disease, there may be a hard, irregular, dull epigastric mass which moves with respiration. The liver may be palpable and its edge and surface knobbly and irregular. The epigastrium may be distended and there may be a succussion splash if there is pyloric obstruction.

Percussion. Shifting dullness may be present if there is an associated ascites.

Auscultation. The bowel sounds should be normal.

Rectal examination Metastatic nodules may be felt in the pelvis and in the ovaries (Krukenberg's tumours).

Lymphoma of the stomach

Lymphoma presents with symptoms and signs similar to those of a carcinoma of the stomach – vague epigastric pain and weight loss. It may arise in middle-aged patients.

Acute cholecystitis

Acute inflammation of the gallbladder is commonly caused by obstruction of the cystic duct by a small stone causing gallbladder distension, chemical inflammation of its wall and, eventually, secondary infection.

History

Age Patients are commonly 30 to 60 years of age and female. Younger patients with sickle-cell disease often form pigment stones, which may precipitate an attack of acute cholecystitis.

Sex Acute cholecystitis is more common in women than in men.

Symptoms The main symptom is a sudden pain, often without any previous symptoms of chronic indigestion. It is felt in the right **hypochondrium** and often radiates through to the back close to the **tip of the right scapula**. The pain is continuous, lasting more than 6 hours, and is exacerbated by moving and breathing. Nothing except analgesic drugs brings relief. Some patients recognize the pain as a severe version of their chronic indigestion pain but, as stated above, it often occurs de novo. Patients nearly always feel **nauseated** and often vomit. If there is an associated obstructive jaundice, the urine may be dark, the stools pale and the skin itchy.

Previous history There may be a history of flatulent dyspepsia or previous attacks of gallstone colic.

Examination

General appearance The patient is distressed by the pain and lies quietly, breathing shallowly. There is usually a tachycardia and pyrexia, although in the early stages of the attack the temperature is often normal. Jaundice may be present (see Chapter 8) and the patient may be sweating.

Abdomen

Inspection. There may be a fullness in the right hypochondrium in the early stages of the inflammation (*Zackary Cope's sign*).

Palpation. There is almost always tenderness and guarding in the right hypochondrium. Palpate the abdomen just below the tip of the ninth costal cartilage and ask the patient to take a deep breath. When the liver and the attached gallbladder descend and strike the palpating hand, the patient will experience a sharp pain which prevents further inspiration. This is called *Murphy's sign*.

At an early stage before there is any guarding, an enlarged gallbladder may be palpable. At a later stage when the inflammation has been present for several days and the tenderness is beginning to subside, an inflammatory mass may become palpable. This will still be very tender and moves little with respiration. It usually indicates that there is an abscess in the gallbladder (an **empyema**).

Occasionally, the contents of an obstructed gallbladder do not become infected, and a large mucocele may develop. This may reach down to the level of the umbilicus.

Because gallbladder pain often radiates through to the tip of the scapula, the affected dermatome may be hyperaesthetic, a change detected by lightly drawing a pin down the back of the patient's chest. This is called *Boas' sign*.

Percussion. An inflammatory mass may be detected when guarding prevents deep palpation, by finding a dull area just beneath the costal margin.

Auscultation. The bowel sounds are normally present unless the gallbladder has infarcted or ruptured and caused biliary peritonitis. This complication is rare.

Gallstone colic/biliary colic

There is an overlap between gallstone colic and acute cholecystitis. Gallstone colic is a severe pain caused by spasm of the gallbladder as it tries to force a gallstone down the cystic duct, which is why 'gallstone colic' is a preferable term to 'biliary colic'. About a fifth of patients who present in this way become jaundiced. Many cases of gallstone colic progress to acute cholecystitis.

History

Symptoms Gallstone colic begins suddenly across the upper abdomen. Patients are often unable to indicate which side is more affected. The **pain is severe** and constant with excruciating exacerbations. It is not a true colic because it does not remit between exacerbations. The severe pain seldom lasts longer than a few hours unless acute cholecystitis develops. It is usually accompanied by **nausea** and **vomiting** and is only relieved by strong analgesia.

Previous history Many patients give a history of flatulent dyspepsia and previous episodes of upper abdominal pain.

Examination

General appearance The patient is frightened and becomes restless as a consequence of the intensity of the pain. A mild tachycardia is often present in the early stages, but the temperature is usually normal. Jaundice may be detected.

Abdomen The abdomen is often extremely tender, with intense guarding in the upper abdomen.

Chronic cholecystitis

Chronic or recurrent infection in the gallbladder is almost always associated with gallstones. The combination of stones and infection may present various clinical pictures: indigestion, flatulent dyspepsia (chronic cholecystitis), acute pain (acute cholecystitis), gallstone colic, obstructive jaundice and, less commonly, ascending cholangitis, acute pancreatitis and intestinal obstruction. Most of these complications are associated with abdominal pain.

History

Age Gallstones can form at any age. The majority of patients with symptoms are between 30 and 60 years old, but a number of women between the ages of 15 and 25 develop gallstones. Younger patients with sickle-cell disease develop pigment stones.

Sex Gallstones are far more common in women than in men.

Ethnic group North American Indians are particularly liable to develop gallstones.

Symptoms The common complaint is of an upper abdominal **indigestion-like pain** after eating. The pain normally begins gradually, 15 to 30 minutes after a meal, and lasts for 30 to 90 minutes. When it becomes severe, it tends to move over into the right

hypochondrium and may radiate through to the back. It is not relieved by anything except analgesic drugs. The patients often notice that the pain is worse after eating a fatty meal, such as bacon and eggs or fish and chips. The attacks of pain are irregular, lasting for weeks or months, with pain-free intervals of varying length. There is often post-prandial belching, hence the description *flatulent dyspepsia*. The patient's appetite remains good and their weight steady, or increases. Nausea and vomiting can occur during acute exacerbations.

Previous history Apart from previous episodes of dyspepsia, the patient may have been jaundiced or noticed their stools were pale, offensive and floated on the water in the lavatory pan.

Examination

General appearance Medical students believe that almost every patient with gallstones is female, fair, fat, fertile and forty. Many are, but enough are male, thin, dark and of any age to make one pay scant attention to the 'five Fs' as an aid to diagnosis. The skin or sclera may show signs of jaundice, indicating that there may be stones in the common bile duct.

Abdomen

Inspection. The abdomen usually looks normal.

Palpation. The patient is tender in the right hypochondrium just below the tip of the ninth rib, the point where the edge of the rectus abdominis muscle crosses the costal margin. It may be necessary to palpate deeply behind the costal margin as the patient takes a deep breath to detect mild tenderness or a small mass. A mass present in the right hypochondrium suggests that a stone is obstructing the cystic duct and that a mucocele or empyema is developing.

Percussion, ausculation and rectal examination. These should be normal.

Acute pancreatitis

Acute pancreatitis is a condition in which activated pancreatic enzymes autodigest the pancreatic gland. It may be caused by obstruction of the pancreatic duct, usually by a small gallstone obstructing the ampulla of Vater or, a peri-ampullary carcinoma or alcohol abuse. The mechanism by which alcohol abuse causes pancreatitis is not known.

Viral infections, trauma and a number of rarer conditions may also cause acute pancreatitis. In about one third of cases, a cause is never discovered.

Pancreatitis can vary from a very mild inflammation to an acute haemorrhagic destruction of the whole gland – a condition with a high mortality.

History

Age and sex Pancreatitis is equally common in men and women. The peak incidence is in the fourth and fifth decades of life, but it can occur at any age.

Symptoms The common presenting symptom is **pain** which begins suddenly, **high in the epigastrium**, and steadily increases in severity until it is very severe, causing the patient to lie still and breathe shallowly. It usually **radiates through to the back**. Nothing relieves the pain, which is exacerbated by movement. **Frequent vomiting** and retching are very common and are an important pointer to the correct diagnosis. There is persistent nausea between the bouts of vomiting. Many patients have eaten an unusually large meal or drunk some alcohol before the pain began.

In severe cases the patient may complain of muscle twitching and cramps.

Previous history In Great Britain, nearly half the patients who present with acute pancreatitis have biliary tract disease. Many patients therefore have a previous history of indigestion.

Social history A careful history of the patient's alcohol intake is important. Relatives may have to be interviewed, as many alcoholics refuse to reveal the true extent of their drinking habits. **Mumps** is a very rare cause of pancreatitis, but ask about any recent contacts with children or the disease.

Examination

General appearance Patients lie still because the **pain is severe** and, if they are pale and sweating, it is likely that they have become **hypovolaemic**. When respiration is impaired, they become grey, apprehensive, dyspnoeic and cyanosed. The sclera may reveal a slight tinge of **jaundice** if the pancreatitis has been caused by a stone lodged in the lower end of the bile duct. Mild jaundice may also appear on the second or third day of the illness if oedema

in the head of the pancreas is causing compression of the bile duct. There is usually a tachycardia and, if the patient has become hypovolaemic, the jugular venous pressure and blood pressure may be low. Pyrexia may be present, but the temperature is rarely greatly elevated.

Abdomen

Inspection. There is always tenderness and guarding in the upper abdomen but the signs may be mild. Any patient with **severe pain but minimal abdominal signs** may have acute pancreatitis.

If the pain is severe and the tone of the abdominal muscles is increased, the abdomen will not move with respiration. A paralytic ileus may develop, causing mild abdominal distension.

Bruising and discoloration in the left flank (*Grey Turner's sign*) and around the umbilicus (*Cullen's sign*) only develop in patients with very severe haemorrhagic pancreatitis. These are rare and late signs, and indicate extensive destruction of the gland. Remember that they may also occur after a large intraperitoneal or retroperitoneal haemorrhage from another cause, such as a leaking abdominal aortic aneurysm.

A number of patients develop a collection of inflammatory exudate in the lesser sac. This is initially suggested by **fullness in the epigastrium**, which may become a more prominent mass if a pseudocyst or abscess develops.

Percussion. Percussion may cause pain if there is peritonitis and be dull over any pseudocysts that are developing.

Auscultation. Bowel sounds are usually present in the first 12 to 24 hours but fade away if a paralytic ileus develops.

Note. Acute pancreatitis can be extremely difficult to diagnose and, as it has no distinctive features, is often forgotten and missed. Whenever you examine an acute abdomen and cannot find a obvious cause, think 'Could this be pancreatitis?' – 'Or a mesenteric vascular infarction?' Or a leaking abdominal aortic aneurysm?'

Chronic pancreatitis

Chronic pancreatitis progressively destroys the exocrine and endocrine tissues of the pancreatic gland.

History

Age and sex Many patients are middle aged and 80 per cent are men. It is a rare condition, affecting between 3 and 10 patients per million in Western countries.

Symptoms Patients complain of severe, **recurrent** episodes of **upper abdominal pain** which usually radiates through to the back. The pain is a gnawing, dull, persistent ache. The pattern and periodicity of the attacks vary greatly, but they are often related to episodes of excessive alcohol drinking. The condition can develop after multiple attacks of acute pancreatitis (acute relapsing pancreatitis) but more often develops de novo in patients who subject themselves to chronic alcohol abuse.

Weight loss and nausea are common. Diabetes, steatorrhoea and jaundice develop in about 10 per cent of affected patients.

Drug addiction is common, as long-term opiate analgesics are often required to relieve the persistent, intolerably severe pain.

Examination

There are often few physical signs. Patients often look distraught and dishevelled. Weight loss and jaundice may be apparent. A mass (a pseudocyst) may be palpable in the epigastrium. The diagnosis ultimately relies on special tests.

Chronic pancreatitis can cause thrombosis of the portal vein, in which case the signs of portal hypertension will be present.

Carcinoma of the pancreas is an important differential diagnosis (see below).

Carcinoma of the pancreas

Eighty-five per cent of pancreatic cancers arise in the head of the pancreas. Although many present with jaundice and weight loss, **abdominal pain** is the presenting symptom in more than half and occurs at some stage in over 90 per cent.

The pain is usually a continuous, dull, boring pain, felt in the epigastrium and radiating through to the back. It is often worse at night and may be relieved by sitting forward.

Radiation of the pain to the right hypochondrium is common with tumours of the head of the pancreas, while radiation to the left hypochondrium indicates an infiltrating tumour of the tail of the gland.

Jaundice develops in almost 90 per cent of patients at some stage of the disease and is characteristically progressive but rarely painless. Pale stools, dark urine and skin itching indicate obstructive jaundice. Weight loss is almost universal.

Steatorrhoea, epigastric bloating, flatulence, diarrhoea, vomiting and constipation may all occur in between 20 and 30 per cent of patients.

Ten per cent of patients present with thrombophlebitis migrans (see Chapter 7, page 207).

Examination

Obstructive jaundice, a palpable gallbladder and an enlarged liver indicate a carcinoma of the head of the pancreas, but in the early stages, physical signs are rarely present. Carcinomata of the tail or body of the pancreas often present late with the symptoms and signs of distant metastases.

LIVER METASTASES/TUMOURS

Distension of the liver capsule stimulates pain fibres. Liver metastases are a common complication of all intra-abdominal malignancies. A constant dull ache in the right hypochondrium, general malaise, weight loss and sometimes mild jaundice may be the first indication of their presence.

Patients with liver cirrhosis who develop a hepatoma often complain of epigastric or right hypochondrial pain. A hepatoma should be suspected when severe pain and weight loss develop in a patient who is known to have cirrhosis.

SPLENOMEGALY

The causes of splenomegaly are given on page 422. A large spleen can cause dull, persistent left hypochondrial pain. Splenic infarction, which is often associated with sickle-cell disease, causes a more severe pain which may be exacerbated by deep respiration.

CENTRAL ABDOMINAL PAIN – ACUTE AND/OR CHRONIC

Acute Meckel's diverticulitis

Meckel's diverticulum is the remnant of the vittelointestinal duct. It contains all layers of the bowel wall, occurs in about 2 per cent of the population and causes abdominal pain if it becomes inflamed.

Inflammation of a Meckel's diverticulum produces symptoms and signs that are indistinguishable from those of acute appendicitis, although the pain and tenderness are generally felt more towards the centre of the abdomen than in the right iliac fossa.

It may give rise to central abdominal pain if any ectopic gastric or pancreatic mucosa within it becomes ulcerated or inflamed.

It may also cause colicky abdominal pain if it acts as the head of an intussusception or if a congenital band arising from its apex causes small bowel obstruction or a volvulus.

Acute gastroenteritis

Gastroenteritis is usually caused by a *Campylobacter* or virus infection, but must be differentiated from food poisoning. The symptoms of **vomiting** and **diarrhoea** usually predominate over the abdominal pain, which may be non-existent or very mild.

Revision panel 15.6
The causes of acute central abdominal pain

Meckel's diverticulitis
Acute gastroenteritis
Inflammatory bowel disease
    Acute Crohn's disease
    Acute ulcerative colitis
Yersinia ileitis
Typhoid
Tuberculosis
Urinary tract infection

Revision panel 15.7
The causes of chronic central abdominal pain

Crohn's disease
Tuberculosis
Radiation bowel damage
Tumours of the small bowel
Recurrent adhesive obstruction/malrotation
Ischaemia of the small bowel
Endometriosis

Occasionally it causes severe colicky, cramping pains which must be differentiated from the colic of small bowel obstructions caused by diseases such as Crohn's disease (see below), *Yersinia* infections (see below) or acute appendicitis.

There are usually few signs on abdominal examination.

The stool should be cultured to exclude *Campylobacter*, *Giardia*, ova and parasites, particularly if the patient has recently travelled to foreign lands.

Inflammatory bowel disease

Crohn's disease and ulcerative colitis may present with acute or chronic central abdominal pain together with a variety of other gastrointestinal symptoms.

Acute Crohn's disease may present with central or right iliac fossa symptoms and signs similar to those of appendicitis. A thick and tender terminal ileum may be palpable in the right iliac fossa, and thickened ileum and jejunum palpable in the umbilical region.

Acute fulminating ulcerative colitis may present as acute abdominal pain, especially when complicated by acute toxic dilatation or perforation of the colon. The abdominal pain is invariably preceded by severe incessant diarrhoea accompanied by the passage of blood, mucus and pus.

Acute *Yersinia* ileitis

This condition is indistinguishable from acute Crohn's disease and appendicitis on the history and physical signs. A mass is rarely palpable. It is usually incorrectly diagnosed as acute appendicitis.

Typhoid

Typhoid normally presents with toxaemia and diarrhoea, but if a typhoid ulcer in the small bowel perforates, severe abdominal pain and all the signs of peritonitis will be present.

Tuberculosis

Intra-abdominal tuberculosis is relatively rare in Western countries but is still quite common in India and Africa, where it may be associated with the increasing incidence of acquired immunodeficiency syndrome (AIDS). Ileocaecal tuberculosis may cause colicky or continuous central abdominal pain, often associated with abdominal distension and weight loss. There may be a mass of matted glands in the right iliac fossa, a dough-like feeling to the abdomen, ascites or signs of chronic intestinal obstruction together with evidence of tuberculous infection at other sites such as the lungs or cervical lymph glands.

Urinary tract infection (cystitis and pyelonephritis)

The symptoms and signs of urinary tract infections are discussed in Chapter 16. Pain from pyelonephritis is felt mainly in the lumbar region but may spread to the centre of the abdomen. When patients are asked to describe the site of their renal pain they usually put their hands on their waist with their thumbs pointing forwards and their fingers spread backwards between the twelfth rib and the iliac crest. It is easier to detect tenderness in the renal angle if the patient is sitting up and leaning slightly forwards.

Deep abdominal palpation is essential to ensure that there is not an enlarged kidney affected by another pathology responsible for the infection, such as a hydronephrosis. The bladder may be enlarged and should be palpated and percussed. Examination of the external genitalia and a rectal examination are essential (see Chapters 13 and 17). The urine should be examined for red and white cells and organisms. The presence of red cells in the urine suggests that the pain is more likely to be coming from a calculus or a tumour than an infection.

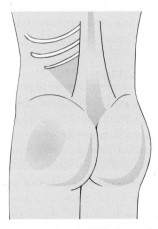

FIG 15.9 Pain from the kidney is felt in the renal angle, which is between the 12th rib and the edge of the erector spinae muscle.

GENERAL ABDOMINAL PAIN – ACUTE AND/OR CHRONIC

Patients often find it difficult to distinguish between a central and a generalized abdominal pain. The separation of the conditions described below from those described above is therefore somewhat arbitrary and rarely clinically relevant.

Irritable bowel syndrome

The irritable bowel syndrome is a functional disorder of the bowel of unknown aetiology which causes chronic intermittent abdominal pain that may be associated with changes in bowel habit and abdominal distension. Combinations of these symptoms occur in at least 10 per cent of the population, suggesting the possibility that the syndrome is simply a variant of normality. Many aetiological factors have been proposed, including the quantity of fibre in the diet, food allergies, disorders of bowel motility, abnormalities of visceral autonomic nerve perception, psychological disorders and social and behavioural problems.

The diagnosis is based solely on the history, as there are no physical signs except for an indefinite, ill-localized abdominal sensitivity on palpation.

It is important to exclude all other causes of abdominal pain, so enquire about any symptoms or signs that might indicate the presence of organic disease such as anaemia, bleeding, weight loss, fever or a change in bowel habit.

Revision panel 15.8
The causes of generalized abdominal pain

Irritable bowel syndrome
Recurrent adhesive obstruction
Mesenteric ischaemia
Carcinomatosis
Chronic constipation
Radiation damage
Retroperitoneal tumours
Endometriosis
Pelvi-ureteric junction obstruction
Lumbar spine pain
Retroperitoneal fibrosis
Psychosomatic

The following symptoms suggest the diagnosis of irritable bowel syndrome:

- continuous or recurrent abdominal pain or discomfort for at least 3 months – relieved by defaecation and/or
- a change in the frequency of defaecation and/or
- a change in the consistency of the stool.

These symptoms are diagnostic when presenting together with two or more of the following complaints:

- an altered frequency of defaecation
- an altered stool consistence
- problems with defaecation (straining/incomplete evacuation)
- bloated feelings of abdominal distension
- the passage of mucus.

Recurrent adhesive obstruction

Adhesive obstruction is suggested when the signs and symptoms of small bowel obstruction develop in a patient with an abdominal scar. Congenital bands and internal herniae may also cause recurrent episodes of small bowel obstruction.

Adhesive obstruction is a difficult diagnosis to make and is often applied incorrectly to any patient who experiences pain after abdominal surgery. The diagnosis can only be made with certainty when the obstruction becomes acute and laparotomy confirms the presence of adhesions obstructing the bowel.

Tumours of the small bowel

Small bowel tumours are rare and often found incidentally at autopsy. They present late with unexplained small bowel obstruction. Adenomata which occur in association with familial polyposis and Gardiner's syndrome may cause intussusception and acute small bowel obstruction. Lipomata and hamartomata can also arise in the small bowel. The latter are known to occur in the Peutz–Jeghers syndrome.

Carcinoid tumours are common in the appendix, where they are usually benign, but they can also arise in the small bowel, where they are more likely to be malignant.

Lymphomata can occur anywhere in the intestine but quite commonly arise in the small intestine.

Adenocarcinomata of the small bowel are extremely rare.

All these rare tumours can present with chronic sub-acute small bowel obstruction causing a central colicky abdominal pain, weight loss and a change in bowel habit. Acute obstruction may develop and a mass may be palpable.

Mesenteric ischaemia

Infarction of the bowel caused by a sudden mesenteric artery occlusion causes acute abdominal pain. Less acute occlusions of the mesenteric vessels may cause chronic central or general abdominal pain. This pain is often brought on by eating and is called **intestinal angina**. It begins insidiously with umbilical epigastric cramping pains, vomiting and diarrhoea, which lead to 'food fear', anorexia and weight loss.

The patient is usually a middle-aged male smoker with other signs of arterial disease such as intermittent claudication, angina or a previous myocardial infarction. An abdominal bruit from a stenosed mesenteric artery may be the only detectable physical sign but is often not present. Chronic mesenteric ischaemia should be considered in all patients with unexplained abdominal pain associated with severe weight loss.

The vasculitides such as systemic lupus erythematosus and conditions such as sickle-cell disease can also cause acute and chronic abdominal pain which is thought to be related to mesenteric ischaemia.

Mesenteric venous thrombosis can complicate abdominal trauma, portal vein thrombosis, splenectomy and other causes of a hypercoagulable state.

Radiation damage

Both the small and large bowel can be damaged by the external beam radiation used to treat pelvic malignancies such as cancer of the uterus, cervix and bladder. Most patients develop transient diarrhoea at the time of the radiation, but some present months or years later, when fibrosis and strictures form, with colicky or continuous pain, vomiting, weight loss, constipation or diarrhoea. Eventually, the endarteritis in the small mesenteric vessels, caused by the irradiation, may lead to ischaemia, necrosis and perforation of the bowel. Radiation bowel injury must be differentiated from a recurrence of the primary tumour and/or widespread metastatic spread throughout the abdominal cavity (see below).

Carcinomatosis

Patients with extensive 'seedling' metastases throughout the peritoneal cavity may develop a non-specific aching abdominal pain which they find difficult to describe and which may be associated with few physical signs. Eventually, clinical ascites, abdominal masses, evidence of tumour at other sites and generalized weight loss and cachexia make the diagnosis obvious. In the early stages, the nebulous nature of the pain and the lack of physical signs can lead the physician to give, mistakenly, calming reassurance or make an incorrect diagnosis of irritable bowel syndrome.

Retroperitoneal fibrosis

Retroperitoneal fibrosis not only obstructs the ureters, but may also involve the abdominal aorta and inferior vena cava. It often causes a vague central, persistent abdominal pain. The kidneys may be enlarged by a hydronephrosis or there may be a tender abdominal aneurysm. If the fibrosis obstructs the vena cava, the patient may present with the symptoms of an acute deep vein thrombosis or oedema of the lower limbs (see Chapter 7).

Endometriosis

This is a condition in which ectopic endometrial tissue is present in sites in the abdomen other than the uterus, such as the large and small bowel and the lining of the abdominal cavity. It causes abdominal pain at the time of menstruation.

Lumbar spine disorders

Pain caused by abnormalities in the spine may radiate from the back to the front of the abdomen and cause diagnostic difficulties. Any suggestion that an abdominal pain is affected by movement and position should indicate the possibility that the pain is arising in the back. This can sometimes be confirmed by careful examination of the spine.

Constipation

Severe chronic constipation may cause a rather indeterminate abdominal pain and general abdominal distension. In these cases there are hard faeces in the rectum and palpable, indentable masses in the abdomen.

Psychosomatic pain

This is a dangerous diagnosis to make, especially knowing how difficult it is to recognize the pain of widespread intra-abdominal malignancy. There are, however, some patients with profound psychological disturbances, severe anxiety or 'cancer phobia' who persistently present with abdominal pain for which no cause can be found.

Beware of adopting the 'cry wolf' attitude. Each new episode of pain requires an open-minded new history and examination.

LOWER ABDOMINAL PAIN – ACUTE AND/OR CHRONIC – CAUSED BY INFLAMMATORY AND/OR MALIGNANT CONDITIONS

Acute appendicitis

Acute appendicitis is the commonest cause of acute abdominal pain in the Western world. The cause of appendicitis remains unknown, but obstruction of the lumen by a faecolith, swollen Peyer's patches, a stricture or a carcinoid tumour at its base all play

---

Revision panel 15.9
The causes of acute and chronic lower abdominal pain

Appendicitis
Crohn's disease
Carcinoma of the caecum and right colon
Diverticular disease
Carcinoma of the left colon/rectum
Bladder outflow obstruction
Interstitial/irradiation cystitis
Pelvic inflammatory disease

a part. Threadworms, which are often found in the appendix, may be an aetiological factor, as may diet and childhood infections.

History

Age and sex Appendicitis can and does occur at any age, but most often affects young adults or teenagers of either sex.

Symptoms The condition most often presents with a **vague pain which begins in the centre of the abdomen**. At first this is often thought to be indigestion and ignored, but after a varying period, usually a few hours but sometime 2–3 days, the **pain shifts** to the **right iliac fossa** and becomes more severe. This 'typical' history is almost diagnostic of appendicitis but only occurs in about half the patients.

The remainder present with a variety of patterns of pain. It may begin and remain in the right iliac fossa or only be felt in the centre of the abdomen. There may be pain in both sites simultaneously, and a few patients have no pain at all.

The central pain is a referred pain. The normal visceral innervation of the appendix comes from the tenth thoracic spinal segment. The corresponding somatic dermatome encircles the abdomen at the level of the umbilicus. The mid-line pain is higher if the spinal segment visceral innervation is higher. Some patients have retrosternal pain which shifts to the right iliac fossa. Therefore, the important feature of the initial pain is its central location and not its precise level.

The inflamed appendix most commonly lies behind the caecum (retrocaecal) and so causes pain in the lateral part of the right iliac fossa and the flank, but it may hang down into the pelvis and lie against the bladder or a loop of large bowel. Under these circumstances, the patient may present with misleading bladder or large bowel symptoms.

Acute appendicitis may also present with intestinal obstruction – colic and abdominal distension – if the appendix lies too close to and inflames the terminal ileum (pre-ileal or post-ileal).

A loss of appetite usually precedes the onset of pain by a few hours and most patients feel slightly nauseated. Many patients vomit once or twice. Most patients with appendicitis state that they have been constipated for a few days before the pain started,

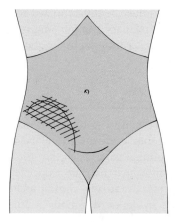

FIG 15.10 An appendix mass or abscess. The continuous line indicates the edge of the mass; the hatching is the area of tenderness.

but a few complain of diarrhoea, which may lead to a mistaken diagnosis of gastroenteritis, especially in children.

Some patients present with symptoms of generalized peritonitis – generalized abdominal pain, nausea and vomiting, sweating and sometimes rigors – especially if the initial stages of the disease are silent.

Atypical presentations are common in the very young, in pregnant women and in the very old, when the appendicitis may be related to obstruction of its ostium by a carcinoma of the caecum.

Examination

General appearance Patients often look unwell with flushed cheeks. A low-grade pyrexia is usually present, but a high temperature should suggest another cause for the pain, or general peritonitis associated with a ruptured appendix. The pulse rate is usually elevated and rises as the infection spreads.

Head and neck The tongue is usually furred and most patients have a distinctive **foetor oris**. Palpable lymph glands in the neck and enlarged tonsils indicate that the patient may have mesenteric adenitis rather than appendicitis, but **beware** – acute appendicitis often follows a viral infection.

Chest The lungs should be normal but be sure to exclude any signs of a right-sided basal pneumonia, because this can occasionally cause abdominal pain and mimic appendicitis, especially in children.

Abdomen

Inspection. The abdomen, though it may be slightly distended, usually looks normal. The right hip may be kept slightly flexed if the appendix is lying against the psoas major muscle. Coughing and sudden movements cause pain if peritonitis has developed.

Palpation. The right iliac fossa is tender and the overlying muscles guard. The maximum site of tenderness must be carefully assessed by gentle palpation. It is classically maximal over McBurney's point, but high or low tenderness may indicate that the appendix is lying in an unusual position. There may be release or rebound tenderness in the right iliac fossa. Pressure on the left iliac fossa may cause pain in the right (*Rovsing's sign*). Release of pressure on the left iliac fossa may cause pain on the right. All these manoeuvres cause pain because they move the inflamed appendix as it lies in the right iliac fossa against the overlying peritoneum, which contains many somatic pain fibres.

When the appendix is behind the caecum, the tenderness may be experienced in the lateral part of the lumbar region – the flank.

When a sub-hepatic appendix produces pain and tenderness below the right costal margin, it must be differentiated from acute cholecystitis (see below).

A tender, **indistinct mass** may be felt in the right iliac fossa. It is usually impossible to feel below it because it is fixed posteriorly. It is dull to percussion. An appendix mass usually takes a few days to develop. An **appendix abscess** should be suspected if the temperature is high and the mass very tender. The features of an appendix mass and abscess are described on pages 427–8.

Percussion. This causes pain if peritonitis is present. Dullness on percussion may suggest the presence of an underlying mass that is obscured by tenderness and guarding.

Auscultation. Bowel sounds are present unless perforation and general peritonitis have caused a paralytic ileus.

Rectal examination There is considerable debate about the usefulness of this examination, especially in young children, but the presence of tenderness high in the pelvis usually indicates an inflamed pelvic appendix.

Hip movement Extension of the right hip joint will exacerbate the pain if the appendix is in a retro-caecal position lying against the psoas muscle. Pain on external and internal rotation of the hip indicates that the appendix is lying against the obdurator internis muscle.

'Chronic' appendicitis

Two forms of chronic inflammation may develop in the appendix: the mucocele and the empyema. Both follow an attack of acute inflammation and both may cause recurrent pain in the right iliac fossa which is sometimes colicky in nature. Worms and faecoliths may produce similar symptoms.

Recurrent episodes of mild acute infection, commonly classified as a 'grumbling' appendix, are extremely rare. Do not make that diagnosis; look for another cause for the patient's pain.

Acute salpingitis/pelvic inflammatory disease

Acute salpingitis is an infection in one or both Fallopian tubes, but it is often associated with infection within the surrounding supporting tissues around the adnexae – hence the term **pelvic inflammatory disease**. The common infecting organisms are *Gonococcus* and *Streptococcus*. These organisms usually reach the Fallopian tubes by direct spread through the vagina and uterus, rarely from the

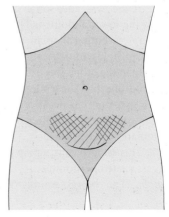

FIG 15.11 The areas of tenderness associated with salpingitis.

bloodstream. Salpingitis is a well-recognized complication of the puerperium and following abortion.

History

Age and sex Salpingitis usually occurs in sexually active women between the ages of 15 and 50 years.

Symptoms A purulent, yellow-white **vaginal discharge** usually precedes, by a few days, the gradual onset of **lower abdominal pain**. The pain is constant and can become severe. It may radiate to the lower part of the back. Sometimes the abdominal pain is preceded by a low backache. Menstruation may have been irregular over the previous months and patients often give a history of dysmenorrhoea. Sweating and rigors are common, but there is usually no nausea, vomiting or change in bowel habit. By contrast, urinary tract symptoms, such as painful and frequent micturition, are common as the urinary tract is often also infected.

Previous history Patients may have had previous attacks of infection or know that they have had or been exposed to gonorrhoea.

Examination

General appearance The patient looks flushed and feverish. There is no distinctive foetor oris and the oral temperature is often higher than in appendicitis, being between 38 and 39.5°C.

Abdomen
　Inspection. The abdomen moves normally and looks normal.
　Palpation. Tenderness and some guarding are present across the lower abdomen. The tenderness is often bilateral as both Fallopian tubes may be infected, but can be asymmetrical if one tube is more infected than the other. It is usually lower and nearer to the mid-line than the tenderness of appendicitis. A huge pyosalpinx is occasionally palpable, but even large swollen tubes can often only be felt by manual examination (see below).
　Percussion. This seldom causes pain but may do so if there is associated peritonitis.
　Auscultation. The bowel sounds are usually normal.

Vaginal examination Examination of the vaginal introitus may reveal a yellow-white discharge, a specimen of which should be sent for culture. The cervix and uterus should be normal sized, but bimanual palpation of the adnexae will cause pain, Moving the cervix (cervical excitation) is also painful. Speculum examination may demonstrate pus coming from the cervical canal. If a pyosalpinx or tubo-ovarian abscess is present, a mass may be felt to one side of the uterus.

Chronic pelvic sepsis

A number of patients with acute pelvic inflammatory disease proceed to develop lower abdominal pain which is often related to the menstrual cycle. Adnexal tenderness on bimanual examination in association with a low-grade fever and a continuing vaginal discharge indicates the diagnosis. There may be associated urinary frequency and dysuria. Gonococci and other pathogens found on a high vaginal swab confirm the diagnosis.

Crohn's disease

Acute Crohn's disease presents with symptoms and signs similar to those of appendicitis. The thickened, tender terminal ileum may be palpable in the right iliac fossa.

　The symptom that helps distinguish acute Crohn's disease from appendicitis is the occurrence of **repeated episodes of diarrhoea** in the weeks before the acute attack. But Crohn's disease usually runs a chronic course. It generally presents with a long history of **colicky central or lower abdominal pain** coming on every 15–30 minutes, associated with diarrhoea. Thickened segments of small bowel may be palpable but some patients have no detectable abdominal physical signs.

　Anal complications – abscesses and fistulae – are common (see Chapter 17).

　The patient may show other stigmata of a chronic inflammatory disease such as finger clubbing, erythema nodosum, sacro-iliitis, episcleritis, pyoderma gangrenosum, anal sepsis, sclerosing cholangitis, gallstones and renal stones. Fistulae of some description – abdominal and anal – are present in 15 per cent of patients, and anaemia and hypoproteinaemia are also common.

Acute diverticulitis of the colon

Acquired diverticula develop in the colon, especially the sigmoid colon, probably as a result of changes in bowel motility and the consistence of the faeces. The condition may be related to the low roughage diet popular in the USA and Europe. Diverticula often cause no symptoms but they may become obstructed and acutely inflamed – acute diverticulitis. This may progress to a pericolic abscess situated on the outside of the colon, which may then perforate causing generalized peritonitis (see below).

If a solitary diverticulum of the caecum becomes inflamed, the signs are indistinguishable from those of acute appendicitis or a carcinoma of the colon.

History

Age, sex and ethnic group Patients with divericulitis are commonly between the ages of 50 and 70 years. The condition is slightly more common in women than in men. Native Africans and Asians are rarely affected.

Symptoms The first symptom is often a mild intermittent lower abdominal **pain** which then shifts to the **left iliac fossa** (for the same reasons as appendicitis moves to the right), where it becomes a more constant ache. The pain begins gradually before becoming more severe and constant. It may become colicky if the large bowel becomes obstructed. The pain is often associated with nausea and a loss of appetite, but rarely vomiting. Most patients are constipated but a few develop diarrhoea. If the colon lies against the vault of the bladder and the bladder wall becomes inflamed, there may be increased frequency of and painful micturition. Some patients can relate their attacks to the type of food they have eaten.

Previous history Some patients give a history of chronic diverticular disease, flatulence, distension and left iliac fossa pain.

Examination

General appearance Patients lie still because of the pain and often look flushed. They are usually pyrexial and have a tachycardia.

Abdomen

Inspection. The abdomen moves with respiration. If there is a generalized peritonitis or intestinal obstruction, the abdomen may be distended.

Palpation. There is **tenderness and guarding** in the left iliac fossa, where there may be a palpable, tender, sausage-shaped mass. Pressure on the right side of the abdomen may induce pain on the left (reversed *Rovsing's sign*). Rebound tenderness will be present if generalized peritonitis has developed. In the latter stages of peritonitis or obstruction, there may be considerable abdominal distension.

Percussion. Any **palpable mass** in the left iliac fossa should be dull to percussion.

Auscultation. The bowel sounds may be normal, hyperactive if there is intestinal obstruction, or absent if a generalized peritonitis develops causing a paralytic ileus.

Rectal examination Pain may be experienced when the finger is pushed high into the left side of the pelvis. Rectal examination is important to exclude a carcinoma of the rectosigmoid junction, which can perforate and cause similar symptoms. Sigmoidoscopy is indicated to exclude a carcinoma but often causes pain when attempting to negotiate the rectosigmoid junction. The findings are rarely diagnostic unless a carcinoma is seen.

Differential diagnoses Acute diverticulitis must be differentiated from carcinoma of the colon with a pericolic abscess, ischaemic colitis and occasionally acute appendicitis or Crohn's disease.

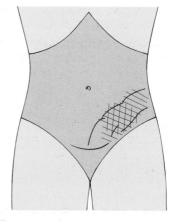

FIG 15.12 The mass and tenderness of acute diverticulitis.

Chronic diverticular disease

Although diverticular disease may present with acute abdominal pain or large bowel obstruction as described above, it most commonly presents in middle-aged or elderly patients with episodes of central or lower left-sided abdominal pain, often associated with or preceded by constipation. The pain is dull or colicky and there may be weeks, months or years between attacks. The condition needs to be differentiated from carcinoma of the colon, irritable bowel syndrome and other causes of inflammatory bowel disease. Examination of the abdomen may reveal some tenderness in the left iliac fossa and, very occasionally, a palpable mass. Rectal examination and sigmoidoscopy are rarely helpful and the diagnosis is made by special investigations.

Carcinoma of the caecum and right colon

Cancer of the caecum is often silent until it has grown to a considerable size.

History

Most right-sided colonic and caecal tumours present with symptoms of **anaemia** (tiredness and shortness of breath), **weight loss** and a mass. They can also present with a dull pain in the right iliac fossa or with the colicky pains of small bowel obstruction. Sometimes the symptoms closely mimic acute appendicitis.

Examination

General appearance Patients usually appear pale and thin.

Abdomen

Inspection. The abdomen may be generally distended or full in the right iliac fossa. A **mass** may be visible in a thin patient.

Palpation. The right iliac fossa is often tender, with some guarding of the overlying muscles. A firm, irregular mass may be felt in the right iliac fossa or right lumbar region, which may be fixed or freely mobile. The liver may be palpable, enlarged and irregular.

Percussion. The mass is usually dull to percussion.

Auscultation. Bowel sounds are normal unless obstruction or peritonitis is present.

Rectal examination This is usually normal, as is sigmoidoscopy, although the latter may show the presence of rectal polyps.

Occult blood may be detected in the faeces with the appropriate test.

When a carcinaoma of the caecum causes appendicitis, the physical signs are indistinguishable from those of simple acute appendicitis. Even when a mass is palpable, it is rarely possible to be certain that this is not an inflammatory mass, and even if the mass is very hard, discrete, knobbly and not very tender, it may simply be caused by inflammation. Consequently the possibility of a cancer of the caecum must always be considered in a patient over 40 years old who presents with acute appendicitis. Other possible diagnoses include an inflamed solitary caecal diverticulum, Crohn's disease and ileocaecal tuberculosis.

Cancer of the left colon

The symptoms of cancer of the left colon differ according to the part of the colon involved. The majority of colon cancers are found in the sigmoid colon and at the recto-sigmoid junction, where they are usually small, annular and ulcerated. They usually present with **a change in bowel habit**, often with variable periods of constipation interspersed

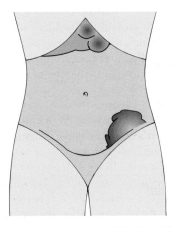

FIG 15.13 The mass of a carcinoma of the sigmoid colon, with liver metastases.

with episodes of explosive diarrhoea and the passage of a number of loose stools.

History

Age The majority of patients are over 50 years old, but colon cancer can occur in young adults with ulcerative colitis or familial polyposis.

Sex Both sexes are equally affected.

Symptoms Pain is a rare symptom and, when it is present, it is usually a mild lower abdominal colic or ache. After some weeks or months it usually becomes a persistent pain in the left lower abdomen. **Alternating constipation and diarrhoea** is typical of the annular variety of carcinoma of the left colon. The constipation is caused by the intestinal obstruction, and the diarrhoea by liquefaction of faeces above the obstruction. The diarrhoea may be increased by inflammation of the colonic mucosa and an excessive secretion of mucus. The episodes of colicky abdominal pain are accompanied by distension, but early loss of weight and appetite is uncommon. The weight loss often precedes the anorexia.

Thin patients may feel a lump in their abdomen.

Rectal bleeding is not a common symptom of a tumour of the sigmoid or descending colon but, when it occurs, the blood is dark and plum-coloured, sometimes with clots of blood interspersed among the faeces. When the tumour is at the recto-sigmoid junction, it is more likely to cause bleeding and it may prolapse into the rectum, causing tenesmus. Painful frequent micturition indicates involvement of the bladder.

Examination

General appearance Weight loss may be apparent.

Abdomen

Inspection. In thin patients, there may be swelling in the left iliac fossa. The colon, especially the caecum, may be visibly distended with faeces.

Palpation. A large tumour may be palpable, often in the left lumbar region or iliac fossa. Part of the mass may be hard faeces above the tumour rather than the tumour itself, in which case the mass is indentable. The mass is tender if there is any surrounding inflammation or a pericolic abscess associated with a perforation.

The liver may be palpable with an irregular surface and edge.

Percussion. A mass in the left iliac fossa will be dull to percussion.

Auscultation. Loud, high-pitched continuous gurglings can be heard during the attacks of colic, but if the colon perforates, the abdomen becomes silent and, of course, tender.

Rectal examination A tumour in the apex of a loop of the sigmoid colon hanging down into the pelvis may be palpable on bimanual examination. Secondary nodules may be felt within the pelvis and blood may be visible on the fingerstall.

Tumours in the left side of the colon can present with generalized peritonitis if the patient has ignored the symptoms described above. In such cases, severe generalized abdominal pain develops accompanied by signs of shock with tachycardia, hypotension, distension, tenderness, loss of liver dullness and absent bowel sounds. In many cases the peritonitis is caused by a rupture of a distended caecum, not a rupture at the site of the cancer.

SYMPTOMS AND SIGNS RESULTING FROM THE PERFORATION OF A VISCUS

A perforation in the wall of a hollow viscus allows its contents – acid, bacteria, small bowel contents, faeces, bile or urine – to enter into the peritoneal cavity, where they rapidly cause a chemical or infected peritonitis. The history and physical signs often indicate the site and cause of the perforation, but whether they do or do not, it is usually necessary to perform a laparotomy to confirm the diagnosis and close the perforation. It is essential, therefore, to recognize the signs of peritonitis.

Acute peritonitis

The clinical features of peritonitis are as follows.

Tenderness and guarding

The pain begins near the site of the perforation but rapidly spreads across the whole abdomen. Guarding is an excellent indication of the severity of the tenderness. If the whole abdomen is tense, there is likely to be general peritonitis.

Rebound tenderness or tenderness on percussion

This is just another way of detecting that the abdomen is very tender. It can be a valuable sign because the patient is not expecting pain when you suddenly remove your hand, so the apprehension which can cause guarding during direct palpation is absent. However, it causes considerable discomfort and should be used sparingly.

Localized pain during distant palpation

If a pain is experienced in a tender area when you press on a distant non-tender part of the abdomen, the structures in the painful area are likely to be very inflamed.

Absence of bowel sounds

The absence of bowel sounds per se does not indicate peritonitis, but their absence in a tender, rigid abdomen makes it highly likely that there is generalized peritonitis.

Revision panel 15.10
The conditions likely to cause the perforation of a viscus

Peptic ulceration
Boerhaave's syndrome (violent vomiting)
Gangrenous appendicitis
A perforated gallbladder
Acute diverticulitis
Small bowel disease (Crohn's disease, strangulation, a foreign body, typhoid)
Ulcerative colitis (toxic megacolon)
Ischaemia
Radiation necrosis
Carcinoma of the colon
Ruptured bladder

Revision panel 15.11
The cardinal symptoms of intestinal obstruction

Pain
Vomiting
Distension
Absolute constipation

An increasing tachycardia

If the pulse rate increases gradually during 1–2 hours of observation, there is likely to be serious disease within the abdomen.

Pyrexia

The temperature rises only when the peritoneal cavity becomes heavily infected. Remember that steroids damp down the inflammatory response. Patients on corticosteroids with a severe peritonitis may have a normal temperature.

When a peptic ulcer erodes through the wall of the stomach or duodenum at a point where it is only covered by visceral peritoneum, acid gastric juice enters the peritoneal cavity. This causes a chemical peritonitis, which later becomes infected with bacteria.

Conditions likely to cause a perforation

- Peptic ulceration (page 396)
- Boerhaave's syndrome (page 394)
- Diverticulitis (page 409)
- Carcinoma of colon (page 410)
- Ulcerative colitis (page 402)
- Acute cholecystitis and acute appendicitis (pages 398 and 405)
- A penetrating injury or rupture of the urinary bladder

SYMPTOMS AND SIGNS CAUSED BY AN OBSTRUCTED VISCUS

Intestinal obstruction

There are many causes of intestinal obstruction (see Revision panel 15.12).

Although it is normally possible, on the basis of the history aided by physical signs and plain abdominal radiographs, to tell whether the site of the obstruction is in the small bowel or large bowel, the clinician must always attempt to answer these three questions.

1. Is there intestinal obstruction?
2. Is the bowel strangulated?
3. Is the site of the obstruction in the small bowel or large bowel?

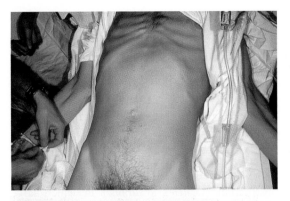

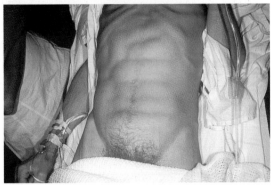

FIG 15.14 Visible peristalsis in a patient with a low small bowel obstruction. **Top**: mild abdominal distension, surface of abdomen smooth. **Bottom**: the abdomen 5 minutes later – visible loops of peristalting small bowel.

The signs of strangulation are the same as the signs of local peritoneal inflammation, which have been described above, namely, pain, tenderness, guarding and rebound tenderness.

The cardinal symptoms of intestinal obstruction are pain, vomiting, distension and absolute constipation, but the severity and time of onset of each of these symptoms depend upon the level of obstruction.

Pain

The pain of intestinal obstruction is true colic. It occurs as a severe central griping pain interspersed with periods of little or no pain. Colic is uncommon with obstructions above the pylorus. Small bowel colic is felt in the centre of the abdomen, and large bowel colic in the lower third of the abdomen. Small bowel colic occurs every 2–20 minutes, depending on the level of obstruction in

the small bowel. Large bowel colic occurs about every 30 minutes or more.

Vomiting

Intestinal obstruction causes frequent vomiting. The nature of the vomitus depends upon the level of the obstruction. With pyloric obstruction, the vomitus is watery and acid. High small bowel obstruction produces a greenish-blue, bile-stained vomit. Obstruction in the lower part of the small bowel is associated with a brown vomit which becomes increasingly foul smelling as the obstruction persists. It becomes so thick, brown and foul that it is often called faeculent vomit. Vomiting is unusual and usually a late symptom in patients with large bowel obstruction.

Distension

The lower the site of the obstruction, the more bowel there is available to distend. High obstructions are not associated with distension, particularly if the patient is vomiting frequently. Obstruction

Revision panel 15.12	
Age, and the common causes of alimentary tract obstruction	
Neonates	Atresia (duodenum, ileum)
	Meconium obstruction
	Volvulus neonatorum
3 weeks	Congenital hypertrophic pyloric stenosis
6–9 months	Intussusception
Teenage	Inflammatory masses (appendicitis)
	Intussusception of Meckel's diverticulum or polyp
Young adult	Hernia
	Adhesions
Adult	Hernia
	Adhesions
	Inflammation (appendicitis, Crohn's disease)
	Carcinoma
Elderly	Carcinoma
	Inflammation (diverticulitis)
	Sigmoid volvulus

of the colon causes the colon to distend around the periphery of the abdomen. The distension then extends into the small bowel if the ileocaecal valve is incompetent. If this valve remains competent, the right side of the colon, especially the caecum, can become grossly distended, causing a visible bulge in the right iliac fossa which is hyper-resonant. Small bowel obstruction tends to cause distension in the centre of the abdomen.

Absolute constipation

Once an obstruction is complete and the bowel below is empty, absolute constipation develops. This means that neither faeces nor flatus are passed. This occurs early in lower large bowel obstructions and late in high small bowel obstructions.

To summarize

A high small bowel obstruction causes frequent colic and vomiting. The distension is slight and central and absolute constipation is rare. A low large bowel obstruction causes infrequent colic, absolute constipation and peripheral abdominal distension. Vomiting is absent or occurs very late on.

The bowel sounds in a patient with mechanical obstruction are at first loud, frequent and obstructive in nature. As the bowel distends, the sounds become more resonant and high pitched, before eventually becoming amphoteric.

Revision panel 15.13 **The intra-abdominal organs that may infarct**	
Organ	**Mechanism**
Small and large bowel	Strangulation
	Volvulus
	Arterial thrombosis
	Arterial embolism
	Dissecting aneurysm
	Venous thrombosis
Ovary	Torsion of pedicle
Omentum/appendix epiploica	Strangulation
Stomach	Volvulus
Spleen/kidney/liver	Arterial occlusion

Strangulated herniae or adhesions are the commonest causes of small bowel obstruction. All the hernial orifices must be carefully examined (see Chapter 14).

Abdominal scars indicate the latter diagnosis.

Carcinoma, diverticulitis and volvulus are the most common causes of large bowel obstruction.

Rectal examination and sigmoidoscopy are essential before more detailed investigations are carried out. It is important to remember that some patients with large bowel obstruction have a pseudo-obstruction (*Ogilvie's syndrome*) in which large bowel peristalsis disappears in association with retroperitoneal pathology.

Ureteric colic

This is described in detail in the next chapter. It presents with severe persistent pain radiating from the loin to the groin.

Gallbladder colic

This is described on page 398.

Bladder colic

Bladder colic or retention is described in Chapter 16.

Uterine colic

This is always associated with pregnancy. The presence of a large pelvic mass should confirm the presence of a pregnant uterus.

INFARCTION OF A VISCUS CAUSING ABDOMINAL PAIN

Revision panel 15.13 lists the abdominal organs that may infarct and present with acute abdominal pain together with the common pathological processes responsible for infarction.

Acute pain develops when the blood supply of an organ is obstructed. When the obstructing mechanism is an external constriction or a torsion of a vascular pedicle (e.g. a volvulus), the process is gradual but the end result is the same – severe abdominal pain – as the nerve endings are damaged and die. Pain is also experienced through the somatic nerve endings of the peritoneal cavity if they are directly stimulated by the proximity of the dead organ.

History

The **pain** of infarction is usually **severe and continuous** and quickly develops all the hallmarks of peritonitis. The patient often finds it difficult to locate the site of the pain, which gets progressively worse if left untreated and which is aggravated by any movement and is only relieved by strong analgesics. Vomiting may accompany the pain and most patients are severely nauseated. Massive vomiting and complete dysphagia occur in the few patients who develop the rare condition of infarction of the stomach caused by a gastric volvulus.

Some patients may describe a classical **colic** in which the pain becomes continuous and much more severe as the blood supply of an obstructed loop is compromised by the process of strangulation. Patients may know they have a hernia that has become irreducible and painful, or they may provide a history of previous abdominal surgery, indicating the possibility of adhesions as a cause of strangulation.

A history of angina, heart attacks, strokes or intermittent claudication indicates coexisting atherosclerotic disease and increases the likelihood of a mesenteric thrombosis.

Splenic infarction is common in patients with sickle-cell disease, who may also develop bowel ischaemia, as may patients with autoimmune vasculitis.

Severe chest pain preceding the abdominal pain indicates the possibility that an aortic dissection has compromised the mesenteric vessels and led to infarction.

Examination

General features Patients with abdominal infarction lie still and they are often pale and sweating from the associated hypovolaemic shock. There is a tachycardia, which increases during the period of observation. An irregularly irregular pulse (atrial fibrillation) should suggest the possibility of a mesenteric embolus.

Pyrexia The temperature may be mildly elevated at first, but a high temperature only develops if treatment is delayed and bowel wall putrefaction begins to occur.

Tenderness and guarding These signs may be mild at first but become more pronounced as the condition of the bowel wall deteriorates. The abdomen also becomes more distended, and rebound or percussion tenderness can be elicited.

Bowel sounds These may be present whilst the infarction is beginning, but a major intra-abdominal infarct always eventually causes a paralytic ileus.

The presence of an intra-abdominal bruit (see Chapter 7) indicates the presence of atherosclerotic disease in the intra-abdominal vessels.

The hernial orifices These must be carefully examined (see Chapter 14), together with all visible incisions, and palpated for the presence of tender and irreducible lumps.

Rectal examination and sigmoidoscopy The presence of a sigmoid volvulus is usually suspected from typical appearances on plain abdominal radiographs, but sigmoidoscopy may be both diagnostic and therapeutic in this condition. Gentle pressure of the sigmoidoscope against a blind end of bowel, or the passage of a flatus tube through the sigmoidoscope usually leads to the passage of a massive flatus with abdominal decompression and relief of pain, provided infarction has not developed.

Peripheral pulses Absence of brachial or femoral pulses indicates the possibility of a dissecting aneurysm, especially in a patient whose pain began in the chest.

Summary Infarction of the bowel must always be considered in a patient with severe abdominal pain and few signs. The most likely differential diagnoses are a perforated viscus causing peritonitis, severe acute pancreatitis, and a ruptured abdominal aortic aneurysm.

ABDOMINAL PAIN CAUSED BY INTRA-ABDOMINAL OR RETROPERITONEAL HAEMORRHAGE

The common conditions that cause intra-abdominal or retroperitoneal haemorrhage are a ruptured aortic aneurysm, a ruptured spleen, and a ruptured ectopic pregnancy.

Common features of intra-abdominal haemorrhage

History

The onset of pain is always rapid, but the signs of shock and collapse may precede the pain and be the predominating symptoms.

Although patients may die from untreated hypovolaemia, the accompanying hypotension sometimes reduces the bleeding, giving a false impression of recovery but fortunately allowing time to transfer the patient to hospital.

Examination

General appearance The patient often looks very pale and may be **sweating, restless and breathless**, a condition known as 'air hunger'. A tachycardia is invariably present and this is often marked if the patient is hypovolaemic. The blood pressure is maintained at first, especially in fit young adults, but eventually may fall suddenly and disastrously. The peripheral circulation is shut down so that the extremities of the limbs are pale and cold. The pupils may be dilated. The jugular venous pressure is very low and may not be visible even when the patient is lying flat.

Ruptured abdominal aortic aneurysm

History

Patients with abdominal aortic aneurysms invariably are, or have been, smokers and may have a family history of atherosclerotic aneurysms.

A previous history of angina, myocardial infarction, intermittent claudication, transient ischaemic attacks or strokes will confirm the presence of generalized atherosclerosis.

Symptoms The **pain** from a ruptured abdominal aortic aneurysm begins in the centre of the abdomen but commonly radiates to the back and may radiate to the groin along the course of the genito-femoral nerve.

Examination

Abdomen

Inspection. The abdomen is usually distended. If the patient is thin, a large central pulsating mass may be visible in the epigastrium or umbilical region.

Grey Turner's sign and *Cullen's sign* – bruising around the umbilicus and in the flank respectively – are late (3–4 days) indicators of a long-standing rupture.

Palpation. The presence of an expansile pulsatile mass may be confirmed. It is usually tender and consists of the aneurysm and the surrounding haematoma. The upper and lower limits of the aneurysm should be defined. A clear separation between the upper end of the aneurysm and the costal margin indicates that the aneurysm is likely to begin below the renal arteries. The finding of additional pulsatile masses in the iliac fossae suggests associated iliac aneurysms (usually in the common iliac arteries). The femoral, iliac and foot pulses must all be palpated. The presence of dilated

---

Revision panel 15.14
The sources of intra-abdominal haemorrhage

Ruptured abdominal aortic aneurysm
Ruptured spleen
Ruptured ectopic pregnancy (tubal rupture)
Ruptured ovarian cyst
Haemorrhage from a liver adenoma
Ruptured visceral aneurysms
    Splenic
    Hepatic
    Mesenteric
Torn mesentery
Retroperitoneal haemorrhage (over-anticoagulation)

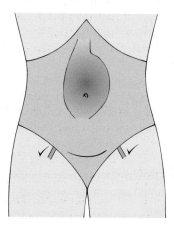

FIG 15.15 The site of an abdominal aortic aneurysm. The femoral pulses are usually palpable.

popliteal arteries strengthens the possibility that the patient has an abdominal aneurysm. The peripheral pulses may be absent.

Large amounts of free blood in the abdomen, obesity, marked guarding and hypotension may all conspire to render a leaking aneurysm impalpable.

Severe abdominal pain and collapse with clear evidence of hypovolaemia are strongly suggestive of a leaking aneurysm in an elderly male who is known to be hypertensive and a smoker, but special investigations may be needed to confirm the diagnosis.

Auscultation. The bowel sounds may be diminished as a consequence of the irritation caused by intraperitoneal blood. Vascular bruits may be heard.

Rectal and vaginal examination Rectal examination is usually unhelpful, but occasionally an internal iliac artery aneurysm can be palpated.

Special features of other abdominal aneurysms

Aneurysms can arise in all the visceral arteries but they are rare. Splenic artery aneurysms are the most common.

Rupture of the spleen

The spleen may be ruptured by blunt or penetrating injuries. When the spleen is ruptured by an external injury, the left lower ribs are often fractured.

Splenic haemorrhage usually causes pain in the left hypochondrium and upper abdomen. It may be associated with left shoulder-tip pain if blood or a haematoma is irritating the left hemidiaphragm. Shifting dullness and flank dullness may be detected.

If the ribs are broken, there will be local pain and tenderness and sharp pain on inspiration.

Occasionally, a ruptured pathologically enlarged spleen is palpable in the right hypochondrium.

Abdominal trauma

Blunt and penetrating injuries can damage any of the intra-abdominal viscera. The spleen and liver are the most susceptible organs and both may bleed profusely.

A history of blunt or sharp injury to the abdomen, even if trivial, provides an important clue to the diagnosis.

There may be signs of the external injury if the patient has had blunt trauma to the abdomen, such as cutaneous bruising or marks along the line of a seat belt.

Ectopic pregnancy

When an ectopic pregnancy is the source of haemorrhage, the patient may know she is pregnant (morning sickness, amenorrhoea, breast swelling or a positive pregnancy test) and is likely to have experienced some intermittent lower abdominal pain before the sudden onset of severe pain in this area. This is usually associated with faintness and collapse, although less acute presentations are common. The lower abdominal pain becomes generalized if left untreated.

A history of any abnormality in the menstrual cycle in a woman of child-bearing age coupled with the sudden onset of severe abdominal pain should suggest the possibility of an ectopic pregnancy. A previous history of pelvic inflammatory disease (see above) or fertility problems also raises suspicions of the diagnosis. If available, a rapid pregnancy test can be very helpful.

Physiological rupture of ovarian luteal cysts

These can cause minor episodes of bleeding and lower abdominal pain when they rupture at the middle of the menstrual cycle. This is called **mittlesmertz**.

Rupture of pathological ovarian cysts

Sometimes large pathological ovarian cysts can rupture and bleed profusely. Patients may collapse from the associated hypovolaemic shock or present with lower abdominal pain and then develop the signs of internal bleeding.

Rupture of liver adenomata

Liver adenomata can develop in young women taking the contraceptive pill and may rupture spontaneously.

The pain is usually felt in the upper abdomen and hypovolaemic collapse is common.

Summary All the conditions described above present with a combination of abdominal pain and haemorrhagic shock in varying proportions. Their presentation needs to be distinguished from the symptoms of intra-abdominal infarction and peritonitis caused by a perforated viscus and acute pancreatitis, all of which can produce a similar clinical picture.

EXTRA-ABDOMINAL AND MEDICAL CONDITIONS CAUSING ACUTE ABDOMINAL PAIN

The conditions described below are not unusual causes of abdominal pain, a fact which emphasizes the need to conduct a full clinical examination on every patient however obvious it may seem that their problem is in the abdomen.

The chest and heart must be examined and special tests must be performed, such as chest X-ray and electrocardiography (ECG), especially when there are no or minimal signs in the abdomen.

The pain of spinal abnormalities can radiate to the abdomen, so the back should be examined carefully, especially if the pain is felt in the lumbar region.

Acute porphyria

This is associated with severe intestinal colic which is particularly precipitated by barbiturates and alcohol. The urine is often dark and turns red/purple on standing.

Mesenteric adenitis

This is associated with an upper respiratory tract infection and cervical lymphadenopathy. It can cause pain in the right iliac fossa which may be mistaken for appendicitis. The pain is caused by swollen glands in the mesentery, so the area of tenderness may move when the patient moves from side to side.

Infectious hepatitis/glandular fever

These conditions cause pain in the right hypochondrium. The pain is caused by swelling of the liver stretching the liver capsule. Jaundice usually develops within a few days.

Curtis–Fitz-Hugh's syndrome

The pain of this syndrome is caused by a pericapsulitis around the liver that is related to pelvic inflammation with *Chlamydia*. A preceding vaginal discharge suggests the diagnosis, which has to be differentiated from acute cholecystitis.

Herpes zoster

This causes pain in the abdomen if an appropriate dermatome is involved. The diagnosis is only confirmed when the characteristic rash develops.

Diabetic keto-acidosis

This can cause marked abdominal pain. The diagnosis is confirmed by finding glycosuria and elevated blood glucose levels. Patients are often very thirsty and drowsy.

Syphilis

Syphilis can cause abdominal pain during a tabetic crisis, but tertiary syphilis is uncommon nowadays.

Revision panel 15.15
Extra-abdominal and medical conditions causing acute abdominal pain

Pneumonia/pleurisy
Pulmonary infarction
Acute Coxsackie infection (Bornholm's disease)
Myocardial infarction
Spinal disorders, e.g. prolapsed disc
Inferior epigastric artery haematoma
Acute porphyria
Mesenteric adenitis
Infectious hepatitis
Curtis–Fitz-Hugh's syndrome
Herpes zoster
Diabetic keto-acidosis
Syphilis (lightening pains)
Henoch Schoenlein purpura
Acquired immunodeficiency syndrome (AIDS)
Collagen disease
Sickle-cell disease
Non-specific abdominal pain
Munchausen's syndrome

Argyll Robertson pupils and evidence of destruction of the dorsal columns of the spinal cord causing loss of deep pain and proprioception indicate the diagnosis.

Henoch–Schönlein purpura

Purpura can present with intestinal colic. The diagnosis should be suspected in children who have a purpuric rash over their thighs and buttocks.

Acquired immunodeficiency syndrome

Patients with AIDS have an increasing risk of developing abdominal lymphomata which may perforate or obstruct. Because of the compromised state of their immune system, appendicitis and other intra-abdominal infections can have a fulminating course.

Collagen diseases

A number of collagen diseases, especially systemic lupus erythematosus, can be associated with abdominal pain and are associated with an increased risk of intestinal infarction secondary to small vessel obstruction.

Sickle-cell crisis

This can cause abdominal pain, usually from intestinal and splenic infarction.

Non-specific abdominal pain

In some patients, no cause for acute abdominal pain can be found, despite hospital admission, re-examination and special investigations. These patients are categorized as having non-specific abdominal pain and represent a fair proportion of the many patients admitted with abdominal pain as acute surgical emergencies. In the great majority, the pain disappears spontaneously and does not recur. In some, however, the cause eventually becomes apparent.

Munchausen's syndrome

A very small group of patients with Munchausen's syndrome invent abdominal pain for their own bizarre reasons. Many of these patients are psychiatrically disturbed. Some are attention seekers and some are drug addicts who bluff their way into being prescribed opiates. Beware the patient who has come from many miles away, or even a different country, whose abdomen bears the scars of many incisions, especially if the pain is difficult to control and requires increasing quantities of analgesic drugs. The physical signs are often minimal, but some of these patients are very good at mimicking guarding and rebound tenderness. A phone call to a hospital that the patient claims to have previously visited reveals either that the patient has never been there or that the hospital also suspected the diagnosis of Munchausen's syndrome.

ALIMENTARY CONDITIONS PRESENTING WITH DYSPHAGIA OR VOMITING

Some serious alimentary diseases do not cause abdominal pain but do affect swallowing and may cause retrosternal pain.

Revision panel 15.16
The causes of haematemesis and melaena

Chronic peptic ulceration (spontaneous, steroids)
Acute gastric erosions (aspirin, phenyl-butazone, steroids, trauma – especially burns)
Carcinoma of the stomach
Oesophageal varices
Purpura
Haemophilia

Revision panel 15.17
The causes of abdominal pain that are often forgotten

Pancreatitis
Aneurysms (leaking or dissecting)
Mesenteric ischaemia
Herpes zoster (shingles)
Porphyria
Diabetes
Tabes dorsalis
Sickle-cell disease
Pneumonia

Carcinoma of the oesophagus

Carcinoma of the oesophagus rarely produces any early physical signs apart from **wasting** and sometimes palpable supraclavicular lymph glands. The diagnosis is suspected when the patient complains of **dysphagia**. At first, large pieces of food stick, but ultimately fluids cannot be swallowed.

Reflux oesophagitis

This causes a retrosternal burning sensation, described by the patient as **heartburn**. Patients may also develop dysphagia. Apart from the nature of the pain, the clue to the diagnosis of reflux oesophagitis is its relationship to posture. Bending, stooping, heavy lifting and tight clothes all force acid up into the oesophagus and cause heartburn. It is often worse at night if the patient slips off their pillow. This is often the only symptom of a hiatus hernia.

Pyloric stenosis

Pyloric stenosis occurs in neonates with congenital **hypertrophic pyloric stenosis** and in adults with **cicatrizing peptic ulceration** of their pylorus or duodenum, or carcinoma of the antrum of the stomach. The last two conditions may be associated with symptoms of benign peptic ulceration or carcinoma of the stomach (see pages 395 and 396).

Neonates with congenital hypertrophic pyloric stenosis present, when 2–6 weeks old, vomiting large quantities of curdled and unpleasant-smelling milk. The vomit is forcefully ejected, justifying the adjective **projectile**. The child becomes thin and dehydrated but retains its appetite. Careful abdominal examination shortly after a feed may reveal a smooth ovoid mass just below the right costal margin, sometimes called a pyloric 'tumour'. This is the hypertrophied pylorus and is a diagnostic physical sign.

Adults with pyloric stenosis present with vomiting. The vomit is usually large in volume, not bile stained and, when the condition is long-standing, not acidic because the chronic gastric retention causes achlorhydria. The stomach contents are, therefore, not digested and the patient may notice that their vomit contains food that was eaten 24 or 48 hours previously. Epigastric distension, visible gastric peristalsis and a succussion splash may be present.

CONDITIONS PRESENTING WITH DIARRHOEA

Some diseases of the large bowel cause diarrhoea without any other symptoms. The nature of the diarrhoea sometimes suggests the diagnosis, but proof usually rests on the results of flexible sigmoidoscopy, biopsy, colonoscopy, barium enema and stool cultures.

Infections of the gastrointestinal tract

Infections from food, such as typhoid and staphylococcal toxins, are called **food poisoning**. The stools are watery brown and passed with great frequency. Abdominal colic is common and may be associated with nausea, vomiting and thirst.

In tropical countries the most likely causes of diarrhoea are bacillary dysentery, amoebic dysentery, malaria, kala-azar and schistosomiasis.

Cholera presents with vomiting, cramps and severe diarrhoea. The diarrhoea lasts up to 3 or 4 days. The patient passes colourless, opaque stools (known as **rice-water stools**), which consist of an inflammatory exudate, mucus, flakes of epithelium, the casts of villi and the infecting organism.

Typhoid may also present as a surgical problem with abdominal pain from the perforation of ulcers in the small bowel.

Ulcerative colitis and Crohn's disease

Patients with ulcerative colitis and Crohn's disease develop chronic frequent diarrhoea often associated with diffuse intermittent abdominal pain. Sometimes they pass a watery brown fluid, while at other times they just pass mucus containing dark or red flecks of blood or altered blood. Patients may have 20–30 bowel actions a day.

The presence of colicky abdominal pain suggests Crohn's disease.

Persistent pain may be the result of acute toxic dilatation of the colon, especially if this is complicated by perforation. The patient is then dehydrated, thin, ill and feverish, with signs of abdominal distension and acute peritonitis, i.e. tenderness and guarding with a loss of liver dullness and an absence of bowel sounds.

Carcinoma of the colon and rectum

Most carcinomata of the left-hand side of the colon cause a change in bowel habit which may be associated with pain and bleeding, but persistent copious diarrhoea is not a prominent feature.

A **villous papilloma** is a benign/malignant rectal tumour which causes excessive mucus secretion. Patients frequently pass stools of pure mucus. This may cause dehydration and the loss of large quantities of sodium and potassium.

Spurious diarrhoea occurs when a very constipated patient passes loose, watery stools around a mass of faeces impacted in the rectum. Diagnosis is by rectal examination.

Steatorrhea, the passage of pale, frothy and offensive stools laden with fat, which float in the pan, occurs in patients with inadequate fat digestion, often a consequence of pancreatic or biliary disease.

THE ABDOMINAL MASS: CAUSES AND SIGNS

The techniques for palpating the liver, spleen and kidneys are described on page 389.

Hepatomegaly

The causes of enlargement of the liver, classified according to their clinical presentation, are listed below.

Smooth generalized enlargement, without jaundice

- Congestion from heart failure
- Cirrhosis
- Lymphoma
- Hepatic vein obstruction (Budd–Chiari syndrome)
- Amyloid disease
- Kala-azar
- Gaucher's disease

Smooth generalized enlargement, with jaundice

- Infective hepatitis
- Biliary tract obstruction (gallstones, carcinoma of pancreas)
- Cholangitis
- Portal pyaemia

Knobbly generalized enlargement, without jaundice

- Metastatic deposits
- Cirrhosis
- Polycystic disease
- Primary liver carcinoma (hepatocellular and cholangiocarcinoma)

Knobbly generalized enlargement, with jaundice

- Metastatic deposits
- Cirrhosis

Localized swellings

- Riedel's lobe
- Secondary carcinoma

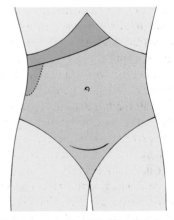

FIG 15.16 Hepatomegaly. The dotted line indicates the site of Riedel's lobe – a normal anatomical variation.

Revision panel 15.18
Causes of hepatomegaly

Infection
Congestion
Bile duct obstruction
Cellular infiltration
Cellular proliferation
Space-occupying lesions

- Hydatid cyst
- Liver abscess
- Primary liver carcinoma
- Benign liver adenoma

The physical signs of an enlarged liver are:

1. it descends below the right costal margin,
2. you cannot feel its upper limit,
3. it moves with respiration,
4. it is dull to percussion up to the level of the eighth rib in the mid-axillary line,
5. it may have a sharp or rounded edge with a smooth or irregular surface.

Remember Riedel's lobe. This is an extension of the right lobe of the liver below the costal margin, along the anterior axillary line. It is often mistaken for a pathological enlargement of the liver or a gallbladder. It is a normal anatomical variation.

Splenomegaly

The spleen is almost always uniformly enlarged. The causes of splenomegaly are classified according to the underlying disease.

Infection

Bacterial

- Typhoid
- Typhus
- Tuberculosis
- Brucellosis
- General septicaemia

Viral

- Glandular fever
- Epstein–Barr virus

Revision panel 15.19
Causes of splenomegaly

Infection
Cellular proliferation
Congestion
Infarction
Cellular infiltration
Collagen diseases
Space-occupying lesions

Spirochaetal

- Syphilis
- Leptospirosis (Weil's disease)

Protozoal

- Malaria
- Kala-azar
- Schistosomiasis

Cellular proliferation

- Myeloid and lymphatic leukaemia
- Lymphoma
- Pernicious anaemia
- Polycythaemia rubra vera
- Spherocytosis and other haemolytic anaemias, e.g. sickle-cell disease, thalassaemia
- Thrombocytopenic purpura
- Myelofibrosis
- Sarcoidosis

Congestion

- Portal hypertension (cirrhosis, portal vein thrombosis)
- Hepatic vein obstruction
- Congestive heart failure

Infarction and injury

- Emboli from bacterial endocarditis, emboli from the left atrium during atrial fibrillation associated with mitral stenosis, emboli from the left ventricle after myocardial infarction
- Splenic artery or vein thrombosis caused by polycythaemia or sickle-cell disease
- Haematoma

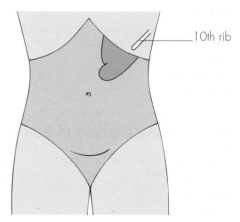

FIG 15.17 Splenomegaly. The notch is not always palpable.

Cellular infiltration

- Amyloidosis
- Gaucher's disease

Collagen diseases

- Felty's syndrome
- Still's disease

Space-occupying lesions

- True solitary cysts
- Polycystic disease
- Hydatid cysts
- Angioma
- Lymphoma and lymphosarcoma
- Secondary tumour (very rare)

The physical signs of an enlarged spleen are:

1. it appears from below the tip of the left tenth rib and enlarges along the line of the rib towards the umbilicus,
2. it is firm, smooth and usually spleen shaped; it often has a definite notch on its upper edge,
3. you cannot get above it,
4. it moves with respiration,
5. it is dull to percussion,
6. although it may be possible to bring it forwards by lifting the left lower ribs forwards, it cannot be felt bimanually or be ballotted.

Enlargement of the kidney

One or both kidneys may be enlarged. The common causes of enlargement of the kidney are:

- hydronephrosis
- pyonephrosis
- malignant disease: carcinoma of the kidney and nephroblastoma
- solitary cysts
- polycystic disease
- hypertrophy.

A mobile or low-lying kidney may be easily palpable and seem to be enlarged, especially if the patient is thin.

Hydronephrosis may be bilateral if the obstructing lesion is in or distal to the neck of the bladder.

Nephroblastoma is occasionally bilateral.

Polycystic disease is very likely to affect both kidneys.

The physical signs of an enlarged kidney are:

1. it lies in the paracolic gutter or can be pushed back into this gutter – that is to say, it **can be reduced into the loin**,
2. it is usually only possible to feel the lower pole, which is smooth and hemi-ovoid,
3. it moves with respiration,
4. it is **not dull to percussion** because it is covered by the colon; even when a large kidney reaches the anterior abdominal wall, it has a band of resonance across it,
5. it can be **felt bimanually**,
6. it can be **balloted**. This means that it can be bounced between your two hands, one on the anterior abdominal wall and the other behind over the renal angle, rather like a ball being patted between the hands. This sign is diagnostic of a renal mass but can only occur if the mass can be reduced into the loin.

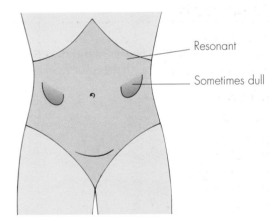

Resonant

Sometimes dull

FIG 15.18 Bilateral enlargement of the kidneys.

Revision panel 15.20
Causes of enlargement of the kidney

Distension of the pelvi-calyceal system
Space-occupying lesions
    Single
      Cyst
      Abscess
      Tumour
    Multiple
      Polycystic disease
Compensatory hypertrophy

Pancreatic pseudocysts

This is a collection of pancreatic juice and inflammatory exudate, usually associated with acute pancreatitis, which forms on the surface of the pancreatic gland or fills the lesser sac. The patient is usually known to have just had an attack of acute pancreatitis (see page 399) and then developed epigastric fullness, pain, nausea and vomiting. If the cyst becomes infected, the patient develops severe pain, sweating and rigors.

The physical characteristics of a pancreatic pseudocyst are:

1. the epigastrium contains a firm, sometimes tender, mass with an indistinct lower edge; the upper limit is rarely palpable,
2. it is usually resonant to percussion because it is covered by the stomach,
3. it moves very slightly with respiration,
4. it is not possible to elicit fluctuation or a fluid thrill.

These swellings can be very difficult to feel as most of their bulk is beneath the costal margin.

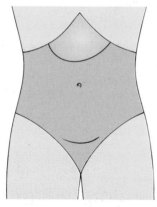

FIG 15.19 A pancreatic, lesser sac, pseudocyst.

Mesenteric cysts

These are cysts containing clear fluid that develop in the mesentery. They arise from the vestigial remnants of re-duplicated bowel and are usually found by chance. They can, rarely, cause abdominal distension or recurrent colicky pain. Like all cysts, they can rupture, twist and bleed from their lining.

Twisting is rare because they are fixed within the small bowel mesentery.

The physical characteristics of a mesenteric cyst are:

1. it forms a smooth, mobile, spherical swelling in the centre of the abdomen,
2. it moves freely at right-angles to the line of the root of the mesentery, but only slightly along a line parallel to the root of the mesentery,
3. it is dull to percussion,
4. large cysts may be felt to **fluctuate** and have a **fluid thrill**.

It is difficult to discriminate between a very large cyst and tense ascites.

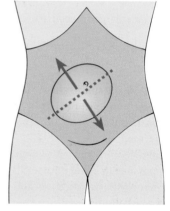

Cyst moves freely at right angles to the root of the mesentery

FIG 15.20 A mesenteric cyst.

Retroperitoneal tumours

Apart from primary and secondary tumours of the lymph glands, retroperitoneal tumours are rare. The commonest variety is the liposarcoma. They grow slowly and silently and usually become quite large before they are noticed by the patient or become palpable. The patient complains of distension, a vague abdominal pain and sometimes anorexia and weight loss.

They produce the following physical signs:

1. abdominal distension,
2. a smooth or bosselated mass with an indistinct edge and a soft-to-firm consistence,
3. while they are covered with bowel they are resonant, but when they reach the anterior abdominal wall and push the bowel out to the flanks they become dull to percussion,

4. they move very little with respiration,
5. they may transmit aortic pulsation.

Carcinoma of the stomach

The symptoms of carcinoma of the stomach are described on page 396. Although stomach cancers can become large, hard masses, they are notoriously difficult to feel because they are high in the abdomen beneath the costal margin. A palpable tumour is hard and irregular, disappearing beneath the costal margin. It is rarely possible to feel its upper edge. The symptoms of abdominal pain or indigestion with loss of appetite and weight are far more significant than the physical signs. **Do not expect to feel a mass in a patient with carcinoma of the stomach.**

The gallbladder

An enlarged gallbladder is usually easy to recognize from its shape and position. The causes of enlargement of the gallbladder are as follows.

- **Obstruction of the cystic duct**, usually by a gallstone, rarely by an intrinsic or extrinsic carcinoma. The patient is not jaundiced and the gallbladder often contains bile, mucus (a mucocele) or pus (an empyema).
- **Obstruction of the common bile duct**, usually by a stone or a carcinoma of the head of the pancreas. The patient will be jaundiced.

Courvoisier's law states: 'When the gallbladder is palpable and the patient is jaundiced, the bile duct is unlikely to be obstructed by a stone because previous attacks of inflammation will have caused the gallbladder to become thick-walled, fibrotic and non-distensible'.

This is a useful clinical rule but there are a number of exceptions.

- Stones that form in the bile duct rather than in the gallbladder may obstruct the duct in the presence of a normal distensible gallbladder.
- There may be a double pathology – a stone in the cystic duct causing gallbladder distension and a carcinoma or a stone blocking the lower end of the bile duct.
- The converse of the law, jaundice without a palpable gallbladder, does not mean that jaundice is caused by stones. In such cases the obstruction may be caused by a cancer of the head of the pancreas, and the gallbladder distension may be insufficient to be palpable. Alternatively, the jaundice may be caused by a carcinoma of the bile or hepatic ducts above the entry of the cystic duct into the bile duct.
- *Mirizzi's syndrome*: when the cystic duct is closely applied to the common hepatic duct or is very short, a stone impacted in it can inflame and obstruct the bile duct and cause jaundice. The gallbladder is often distended.

The physical features of an enlarged gall-bladder are:

1. it appears from beneath the tip of the right ninth rib,
2. it is smooth and hemi-ovoid,
3. it moves with respiration,
4. there is no space between the lump and the edge of the liver,
5. it is dull to percussion.

When an acutely inflamed gallbladder becomes surrounded by adherent omentum and bowel it loses some of its characteristics. A **gallbladder mass** is diffuse and tender, it lies in the right hypochondrium, and does not move much with respiration.

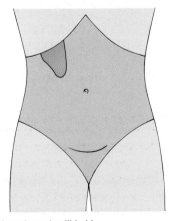

FIG 15.21 An enlarged gallbladder.

As the infection subsides it becomes more discrete and mobile, and less tender.

Faeces

The colon can become grossly distended with faeces as a result of a mechanical obstruction or chronic constipation. The patient may complain of diarrhoea, but this is actually mucus and a little watery faeces leaking out around the main mass of faeces (**spurious diarrhoea**).

The physical characteristics of faeces are as follows.

1. The masses lie in that part of the abdomen occupied by the colon – the flanks and across the lower part of the epigastrium.
2. They feel firm or hard but are **indentable** – this means that they can be dented by firm pressure with the fingers and this dent persists after releasing the pressure.
3. There may be multiple separate masses in the line of the colon but in gross cases the faeces coalesce to form one vast mass which is easy to mistake for a tumour.
4. When there is no mechanical obstruction, rectal examination confirms a rectum full of very hard faeces, but if there is a blockage in the lower colon, the rectum will be empty.

Do not forget that faecal masses can form above an annular stenosing carcinoma of the colon.

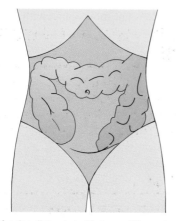

FIG 15.22 A colon distended with faeces. The masses are indentable. Faecal impaction of this degree is likely to be caused by Hirschsprung's disease or gross constipation.

The urinary bladder

The causes of retention of urine are listed on page 442. The bladder may be tense and painful (**acute retention**) or enlarged and painless (**chronic retention**).

The physical features of an enlarged bladder are:

1. it arises out of the pelvis and so it has no lower edge,
2. it is hemi-ovoid in shape, usually deviated a little to one side,
3. it may vary in size: a very large bladder can extend up to and above the umbilicus,
4. it is not mobile,
5. it is dull to percussion,
6. if it is large enough to permit the necessary simultaneous percussion and palpation, it will have a **fluid thrill**,
7. direct pressure on the swelling often produces a desire to micturate,
8. it does not bulge into the pelvis and can only be felt indistinctly on bimanual (combined rectal and abdominal) examination.

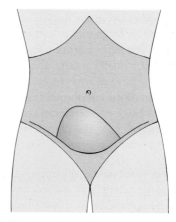

FIG 15.23 A distended urinary bladder.

Ovarian cyst

Small ovarian cysts are common and are impalpable. When they enlarge, they rise up out of the pelvis into the lower abdomen and become palpable.

The physical features of a large ovarian cyst are:

1. it is smooth and spherical with a distinct outline,
2. it arises from the pelvis, so its lower limit is not palpable, i.e. you cannot 'get below it',

3. it may be mobile from side to side but cannot be moved up and down,
4. it is dull to percussion,
5. it has a fluid thrill,
6. its lower extremity may be palpable in the pelvis during rectal or vaginal examination, and movement of the cyst may produce some movement of the uterus.

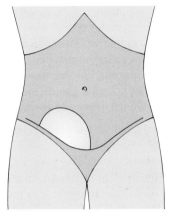

FIG 15.24 A large ovarian cyst.

The pregnant uterus

Never forget that pregnancy is the commonest cause of enlargement of the uterus, and of abdominal distension.

The diagnosis of pregnancy is more difficult in the first 20 weeks, when the uterus is still relatively small and there are no fetal movements.

A pregnant uterus is a smooth, firm, dull swelling arising out of the pelvis.

The uterus enlarges to the xiphisternum by the 36th week of pregnancy. At this stage the fetus is palpable (ballotable) and moves.

The diagnosis of pregnancy is confirmed if bimanual examination reveals that the mass cannot be moved independently of the cervix and that the cervix is soft and patulous.

An enlarged uterus **must not be squeezed** during a bimanual examination, as this can cause the patient to go into labour and abort the fetus.

Fibroids

Fibroids are benign fibromyomatous uterine tumours which can grow to an enormous size and fill the whole abdomen. They are usually multiple. They can cause irregular and heavy periods, disturbed micturition, lower abdominal pain and backache.

The physical signs of a fibroid uterus are:

1. it arises out of the pelvis and so its lower edge is not palpable,
2. it is firm or hard, bosselated or distinctly knobbly – each knob corresponding to a fibroid,
3. it moves slightly in a transverse direction and any movement of the abdominal mass moves the cervix,
4. it is dull to percussion,
5. it is palpable bimanually: a moderately enlarged uterus can be pushed down into the pelvis.

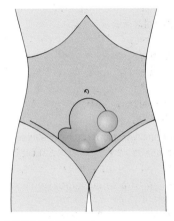

FIG 15.25 A large fibroid uterus.

CAUSES OF A MASS IN THE RIGHT ILIAC FOSSA

A mass in the right iliac fossa is a common physical finding. There are a number of conditions that may be responsible. This section describes the important features in the history and examination of each cause.

Appendix mass

History The patient usually complains of a period of central abdominal pain followed by a pain in the right iliac fossa. The pain often persists for several days and is usually accompanied by malaise, loss of appetite and pyrexia.

Examination There is a tender, indistinct mass, which is dull to percussion, fixed to the iliac fossa posteriorly, and accompanied by a persistent low fever and tachycardia.

Appendix abscess

History This is the same as for an appendix mass, with the additional symptoms of an abscess,

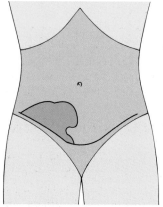

FIG 15.26 A common diagnostic problem: a mass in the right iliac fossa.

Revision panel 15.21
The causes of a mass in the right iliac fossa

Appendix mass
Appendix abscess
Tuberculosis
Carcinoma of caecum
Crohn's disease (terminal ileitis)
Iliac lymphadenopathy
Iliac artery aneurysm
Psoas abscess
Chondrosarcoma or osteosarcoma of
the ilium
Tumour in an undescended testis
Actinomycosis
Ruptured epigastric artery
Spigelian hernia
Kidney transplant
Ovarian cyst/tumour
Fibroid
Malignant change in an undescended testis

---

namely, fever, rigors, sweating and increased local pain.

Examination There is a tender mass which, in its late stages, may be associated with oedema and reddening of the overlying skin. The patient will have a swinging, intermittent fever and an increasing tachycardia.

Tuberculosis

In many parts of the world, tuberculosis is more often the cause of an inflammatory mass in the right iliac fossa than appendicitis. The mass consists of the inflamed ileocaecal lymph glands and parts of the caecum and terminal ileum that are also inflamed.

History The patient often has a vague central pain for months, with general ill-health, loss of weight, and changes in bowel habit. The pain then becomes intense and settles in the iliac fossa. An acute episode of central abdominal pain moving to the right iliac fossa, similar to appendicitis, is uncommon.

Examination The mass is firm, tender and very indistinct. The surface and the edge are difficult to define. If there is a tuberculous peritonitis, the abdomen will be swollen and less flexible – often described as a 'doughy' abdomen.

Carcinoma of the caecum

History Often there is no acute pain, just a dull discomfort in the right iliac fossa. Some patients present with anaemia, diarrhoea or intestinal obstruction.

Examination The mass is firm, distinct and hard. It is usually fixed to the posterior abdominal wall, but sometimes it is mobile. It is not tender and does not resolve with observation. The patient's temperature and pulse are normal unless there is an associated pericolic abscess.

Crohn's disease
(Terminal ileitis)

History The patient will have experienced recurrent episodes of pain in the right iliac fossa, general malaise, weight loss and episodes of diarrhoea.

Examination The swollen terminal ileum forms an elongated sausage-shaped mass which usually lies transversely in the right iliac fossa and feels rubbery and tender.

Iliac lymph glands

History The symptoms depend on the cause of the lymphadenopathy. There may be a generalized disease, or local disease in the limb, perineum or genitalia.

Examination Enlarged iliac lymph glands form an indistinct mass, with no clear contours. The mass follows the line of the iliac vessels and may bulge forwards just above the inguinal ligament. It can be easy to feel, or be no more than a fullness in the depths of the iliac fossa.

All the other lymph glands must be examined, as must the lower limb, to try to find the cause of the lymphadenopathy.

Iliac artery aneurysm

History The patient may have noticed a pulsating mass or felt an aching pain in the right iliac fossa.

Examination The common iliac artery dilates more often than the external iliac artery, so the smooth, distinct mass with an expansile pulsation is usually in the upper medial corner of the iliac fossa.

Psoas abscess

History The patient is likely to have felt ill for some months, with night sweats and loss of weight. Back pain and abdominal pain can also occur.

Examination The iliac fossa is filled with a soft, tender, dull, compressible mass. There may be a fullness in the lumbar region which is accentuated by pressing on the mass in the iliac fossa. The swelling may extend below the groin and it may be possible to empty the swelling below the groin into the swelling above, and vice versa.

Back movements may be painful and limited.

Chondroma and sarcoma of the ilium

Rarely, chondromata and chondrosarcomata arise in the iliac bones. They grow slowly and may bulge into the iliac fossa. They are large, hard, non-tender and clearly fixed to the skeleton. They usually lie out in the lateral part of the iliac fossa. Osteomata and osteosarcomata of the ileum are equally rare.

Actinomycosis

This invariably develops as a complication of appendicitis, but may present de novo as a mass in the iliac fossa with a number of discharging sinuses. It is rare.

Spigelian hernia

These herniae appear at the outer edge of the rectus abdominis muscle along the linear semilunaris. The lump is still palpable when the abdominal wall muscles are contracted and it is felt to lie above them.

Ruptured inferior epigastric artery

This occurs as a result of straining or coughing. The haematoma tracks beneath the abdominal wall, extraperitoneally, to produce a mass in the iliac fossa. It is diffuse and there may be discolouration of the skin. It is attached to the anterior abdominal wall but, as it is on its deep surface, it becomes impalpable when the muscles contract. Contraction of the abdominal muscles is usually painful.

A transplanted kidney

The mass is situated beneath the transplant scar and a history of transplantation makes the diagnosis easy. The lump is smooth, kidney shaped and rubbery.

Ovarian cysts and fibroids

These can fall to the right into the right iliac fossa. They will be felt to be connected to the uterus on bimanual examination. A huge pyosalpinx may occasionally be palpable in the right iliac fossa.

Malignant change in an undescended testis

This is a rarity but is easily suspected provided you remember your routine and always examine the scrotum as part of the abdominal examination.

CAUSES OF A MASS IN THE LEFT ILIAC FOSSA

Diverticulitis and carcinoma of the colon are the common causes of a mass in the left iliac fossa. It must be remembered that the normal sigmoid colon is palpable in one out of three patients. An appendix mass on the left side only occurs if the patient has *situs inversus*. Tuberculosis and Crohn's disease only cause masses in the right iliac fossa. All the other causes of a mass in the right iliac fossa mentioned above can also cause a mass in the left iliac fossa.

Diverticulitis

When sigmoid diverticula become inflamed, the swollen colon and surrounding pericolic abscess may be palpable.

History The patient may have suffered from recurrent lower abdominal pains and chronic constipation for years. The acute episode starts suddenly with a severe left iliac fossa pain, nausea, loss of appetite and constipation.

Examination The left iliac fossa contains a tender, indistinct mass whose long axis lies parallel to the

---

Revision panel 15.22
The causes of a mass in the left iliac fossa

Diverticulitis
Carcinoma of the colon
Carcinoma of caecum
Crohn's disease (terminal ileitis)
Iliac lymphadenopathy
Iliac artery aneurysm
Psoas abscess
Chondrosarcoma or osteosarcoma of the ilium
Tumour in an undescended testis
Actinomycosis
Ruptured epigastric artery
Spigelian hernia
Kidney transplant
Ovarian cyst/tumour
Fibroid
Malignant change in an undescended testis

---

inguinal ligament. There may be signs of general or local peritonitis and intestinal obstruction. The diagnosis depends upon the site of the tenderness. There are very few other acute inflammatory conditions that present with a mass in the left iliac fossa.

Carcinoma of the sigmoid colon

History The patient may present with lower abdominal pain, abdominal colic, intestinal obstruction, a change in bowel habit, rectal bleeding and general cachexia.

Examination The mass is hard, easily palpable and not tender. It may be mobile or fixed. The colon above the mass may be distended with indentable faeces.

CAUSES OF A LUMP IN THE GROIN

The inguinal region is part of the iliac fossa and swellings within it and just below it in the groin can be confused with iliac fossa masses.

Hernia (inguinal or femoral)
(see page 374)

The diagnosis is made from the site and shape of the lump and, if present, its reducibility and an expansile cough impulse.

Lymph glands

Inguinal lymph glands present as hard or firm discrete nodules, or an indistinct mass, spreading across the groin, down the thigh along the line of the long saphenous vein, and up into the iliac fossa. Look for a local cause and examine all other groups of lymph glands.

Saphena varix
(see page 202)

A saphena varix is a soft, compressible dilatation at the top of the saphenous vein. It has an expansile cough impulse. A fluid thrill will be felt when the saphenous vein lower down the leg is percussed. The swelling disappears when the patient lies down.

Psoas abscess

A psoas abscess may pass down beneath the inguinal ligament and present in the upper part of the femoral triangle as a soft, fluctuant, compressible mass. It is possible to elicit fluctuation between the parts of the abscess above and below the inguinal ligament, and empty one part into the other.

Psoas bursa

A psoas bursa lies between the psoas tendon and the lesser trochanter of the femur. When it becomes distended or inflamed, it bulges into the upper outer corner of the femoral triangle, lateral to the femoral vessels, where it causes a diffuse swelling. It is too deep to have a distinct shape or to fluctuate. It is painful when the hip joint is moved.

Femoral aneurysm

This presents as a mass with an expansile pulsation lying in the line of the femoral artery.

Hydrocele of a femoral hernial sac

Hydrocele of the cord or canal of Nuck
(see page 371)

Ectopic testis
(see page 344)

ABDOMINAL DISTENSION

The causes of abdominal distension can be remembered by repeating the letter 'F' six times: fetus, flatus, faeces, fat, fluid (free and encysted), and fibroids and other solid tumours.

Fetus

Pregnancy is the most common cause of abdominal distension. The features of a pregnant uterus have already been described on page 427.

Flatus
(Tympanites)

Gas in the intestine can cause considerable abdominal distension.

In the early stages, the distension may be localized to that part of the abdomen containing the distended bowel, such as the epigastrium when the stomach is distended, or the right iliac fossa when the caecum is distended, but as the distension affects the whole bowel, the whole abdomen swells.

The distension remains localized if the bowel twists into a volvulus. This is a common complication of a long sigmoid colon combined with a narrow base of the mesocolon.

Distended bowel has no palpable surface or edge. The only diagnostic features are hyper-resonance and, when there is obstruction, visible peristalsis. The bowel sounds may be hyperactive. Shaking the patient causes a splashing sound as the thin layer of fluid in the distended bowel splashes about. This is known as a **succussion splash** and is particularly common when there is gastric distension caused by pyloric stenosis.

Acute dilatation of the stomach, mechanical intestinal obstruction, paralytic ileus, aerophagy (air swallowing) and massive amounts of free gas from a perforation all cause hyper-resonance on abdominal percussion.

Revision panel 15.23
The causes of abdominal distension

Fetus
Flatus
Faeces
Fat
Fluid:
    free (ascites)
    encysted
Large solid tumours such as:
    fibroids
    enlarged liver
    enlarged spleen
    polycystic kidneys
    retroperitoneal sarcomata

Faeces

Faecal impaction may present as abdominal distension or an abdominal mass. The physical features of faecal masses in the abdomen are described on page 426. The diagnosis can usually be suspected from the history of the patient's bowel habits. The common causes are Hirschsprung's disease, chronic intestinal obstruction, chronic constipation and antidepressant drugs.

Fat

Fat rarely causes distension, but frequently makes the patient pot-bellied. A large fat abdomen may be caused by a thick layer of subcutaneous fat or by excess fat in the omentum and mesentery. These two sites of fat deposition do not necessarily enlarge together. A protuberant, round abdomen often has a thin layer of subcutaneous fat but contains a heavy, thick omentum.

Fluid: ascites

Free fluid in the peritoneal cavity is called **ascites**. It is caused by a variety of conditions but they all fall into one of four groups: those which raise the portal venous pressure, those which lower the plasma proteins, those which cause peritonitis, and those which allow a direct leak of lymph into the peritoneal cavity.

Causes of an increased portal venous pressure

Pre-hepatic

- Portal vein thrombosis
- Compression of the portal vein by lymph glands

Hepatic

- Cirrhosis

Post-hepatic

- Budd–Chiari syndrome

Cardiac

- Constrictive pericarditis
- Right heart failure caused by mitral stenosis, tricuspid incompetence and pulmonary hypertension

Pulmonary

- Pulmonary hypertension and right heart failure

Causes of hypoproteinaemia

- Kidney disease associated with albuminuria
- Cirrhosis of the liver
- The cachexia of wasting diseases, malignancy and starvation
- Protein-losing enteropathies
- Malnutrition

Causes of chronic peritonitis

Physical

- Post-irradiation
- Starch granuloma

Infection

- Tuberculous peritonitis

Neoplasms

- Secondary peritoneal deposits of carcinoma
- 'Mucus'-forming tumours (pseudomyxoma peritonei)

Revision panel 15.24
Aetiology of ascites

Raised portal venous pressure
Pre-hepatic, intra-hepatic and post-hepatic
Cardiac
Pulmonary

Hypoproteinaemia
Renal
Hepatic
General

Peritonitis
Acute and chronic
Traumatic, chemical, infective, neoplastic

Lymphatic obstruction
(Chylous ascites)

Causes of chylous ascites

Chylous ascites is caused by the leakage of lymph from the lacteals or the cisterna chyli as a result of congenital abnormalities, trauma and primary or secondary lymph gland disease.

Physical signs of ascites

1. A fluid thrill
2. Shifting dullness

A **fluid thrill** is elicited by flicking one side of the abdomen with the index or middle finger and feeling the vibrations when they reach the other side of the abdomen with your other hand. Before doing this you must place the edge of the patient's (or an assistant's) hand on the abdomen at the umbilicus to prevent the percussion wave being transmitted

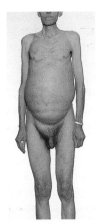

Ascites secondary to carcinoma of the stomach. Note the wasting and the right inguinal hernia full of ascitic fluid.

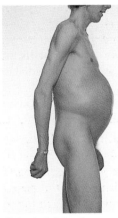

Abdominal distension caused by a retroperitoneal liposarcoma in a young man.

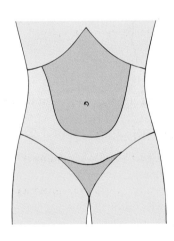

Distribution of dullness caused by ascites when **supine**

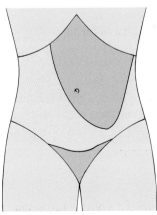

Redistribution of dullness when patient is tilted **45° to the right**

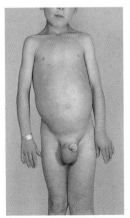

Congenital chylous ascites. Note the lymphoedema of the left leg, and the right hydrocele.

FIG 15.27 Shifting dullness is diagnostic of free intraperitoneal fluid (ascites).

FIG 15.28 SOME EXAMPLES OF ABDOMINAL DISTENSION.

through the fat in the abdominal wall. A fluid thrill is present in any fluid-filled cavity, so that the difference between free and encysted fluid depends upon the recognition of shifting dullness.

Shifting dullness is a dull area which moves or changes shape when the patient changes position. The dullness of ascites is found in the flanks and across the lower abdomen. Percuss the medial limits of the flank dullness carefully and place vertical marks on the abdomen with a felt-tipped pen. Then ask the patient to turn onto one side to an angle of approximately 45°. Wait a few seconds and percuss again. The medial limits of dullness will have moved towards the mid-line on the lower side of the abdomen and away from it on the upper side if there is free fluid moving under the influence of gravity.

Fluid: encysted

Fluid trapped in a cyst, or in the renal pelvis, or between adhesions, will have a fluid thrill, be dull to percussion, but not shift.

The position and features of a cyst depend upon its anatomical origin. The following cysts or fluid-filled swellings may become large enough to present as abdominal distension:

- ovarian cysts
- hydronephrosis
- urinary bladder
- pancreatic pseudocysts
- mesenteric cysts
- hydatid cysts.

A large aortic aneurysm can also distend the abdomen. It is distinguished by the presence of an expansile pulsation.

Fibroids and other solid tumours

Solid tumours which can become very large and cause abdominal distension are, in approximate

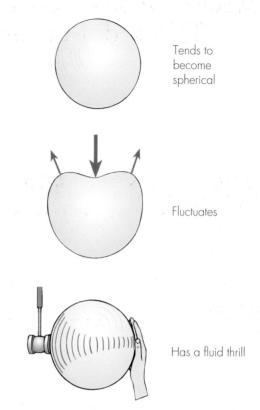

Tends to become spherical

Fluctuates

Has a fluid thrill

FIG 15.29 The features of encysted fluid.

order of frequency:

- hepatomegaly (Budd–Chiari syndrome or metastatic liver tumours)
- fibroids
- splenomegaly (myelofibrosis)
- large cancers of the colon
- polycystic kidneys
- primary carcinoma of the liver
- retroperitoneal sarcoma and lymphadenopathy
- ganglioneuroma (in children)
- nephroblastoma (in children)
- neurofibroma/schwannoma.

The physical signs of most of these tumours are described in the preceding parts of this chapter.

The kidneys, urinary tract and prostate

16

SYMPTOMS OF RENAL AND URINARY TRACT DISEASE

It is very important to obtain an exact history of the symptoms of renal and urinary tract disease because the kidney, ureter and bladder are not readily accessible for physical examination.

Renal pain

Site Pain from the kidney is felt in the:

- loin – the space below the 12th rib and the iliac crest
- renal angle – the angle between the 12th rib and the edge of the erector spinae muscle.

When you ask a patient with renal pain to show you the site of the pain, he usually spreads his hand around his waist with his fingers covering the renal angle and his thumb above the anterior superior iliac spine.

Severity Renal pain can vary from a constant dull ache to a very severe pain.

Nature Do not use the term 'renal colic'. True colic is autonomically modulated and can only come from distension of the smooth muscle wall of a conducting tube such as the ureter. Because the severity of renal pain often fluctuates rapidly it gets called renal colic, but patients rarely describe it as griping, and it never disappears completely between exacerbations.

Ureteric colic

Site Colic from the ureter is felt along the line of the ureter. The point where it begins is a reliable indicator of the level of the obstruction.

In most cases the pain starts in the loin and then radiates downwards, around the waist, obliquely across the abdomen, just above the inguinal ligament, to the base of the penis, the scrotum or the labia.

Severity The exacerbations of ureteric colic are extremely severe. The patient tries to relieve the pain by rolling around the bed or walking about. Patients

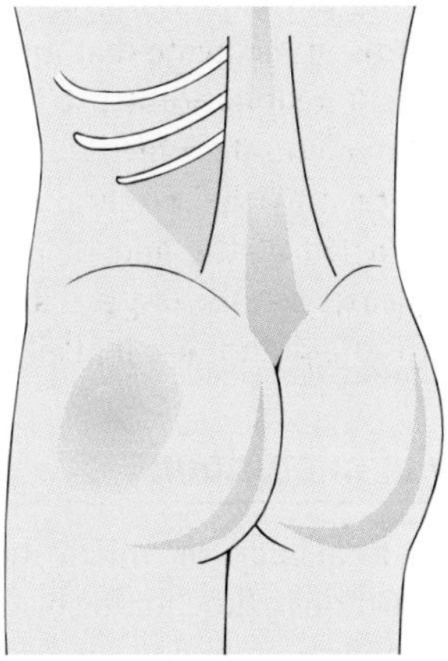

FIG 16.1 The renal angle is the area in the loin between the 12th rib and the edge of the erector spinae muscle.

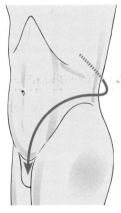

FIG 16.2 Ureteric colic radiates down from the renal angle, along a line parallel to the inguinal ligament, into the base of the penis, the scrotum or the labium majus.

often say that it is the worst pain they have ever experienced, and women may say that it is as bad as labour pain. It is accompanied by sweating and often by nausea and vomiting.

Nature Ureteric colic is a true colic. It is **griping** in nature and **comes in waves**, with **pain-free periods** between attacks.

Haematuria

Blood may be noticed in the urine during or after micturition. Modest bleeding may have no visible effect on urine colour or may make it look darker than usual. If there is heavy bleeding, the urine may resemble pure blood.

If the blood is coming from the bladder neck or the lower part of the urinary tract, it may appear only at the end of micturition.

The causes of haematuria are listed in Revision panel 16.1.

Make quite sure that female patients have not mistaken menstrual bleeding for haematuria, and remember that there are other rare causes of a red/brown discolouration of the urine, such as:

- eating large amounts of beetroot
- paroxysmal haemoglobinuria
- porphyria.

Vesical pain

Pain from the bladder is usually a dull, suprapubic ache, made worse by micturition.

Strangury (literally, squeezing urine) is one of those many terms in medicine that means different things to different people. Some use it to describe a painful desire to micturate, which starts in the bladder and radiates into the urethra. Others use it to describe pain felt at the end of micturition as the patient squeezes out the last few drops of urine. To avoid confusion, do not use it at all.

Frequency of micturition

An increased frequency of micturition may be caused by a reduction in functioning bladder capacity following incomplete emptying, or by irritation of the bladder wall. It is of greater significance if it wakes the patient from sleep, so remember to ask about the frequency of nocturnal micturition and record a day/night ratio.

Dysuria is commonly used to describe **pain coming from the urethra** during the passing of urine. Do not confuse it with, for example, the abdominal pain experienced on micturition by a patient with appendicitis, which has a totally different cause.

Prostatic pain

Pain from the prostate gland is felt deep inside the pelvis, between the legs in the perineum and sometimes in the lower back. It is poorly localized and patient often think it is coming from the rectum.

DISEASES OF THE URINARY TRACT

Hydronephrosis

Hydronephrosis is distension of the calyces and pelvis of the kidney, caused by obstruction.

The causes of hydronephrosis are listed in Revision panel 16.2.

Hydronephrosis is often symptomless, but it may produce renal pain, may present as renal failure, or may be detected when investigating the symptoms of the disease causing it.

History

Age Hydronephrosis occurs at all ages.

Symptoms The commonest symptom is pain in the loin. This is a dull, persistent ache, which can be so mild that it is accepted by the patient as backache and ignored but which gets worse as the hydronephrosis enlarges. If the enlargement is sudden, the pain can be severe. As an autonomic pain, it may be poorly localized and occasionally felt in unexpected sites such as the epigastrium. A patient with this sort of pain will never be able to localize the exact site with a finger, but will place their hand over quite a wide area.

The pain associated with hydronephrosis is made worse or initiated by an increased production of urine. Alcohol is a diuretic, so the pain may be associated with drinking it. But patients who only get pain after drinking quantities of beer or spirits are often reluctant to admit to the association.

Pain is less frequent in bilateral hydronephrosis as the cause lies in the lower urinary tract and distension of the renal pelvis tends to develop slowly and progressively.

Congenital pelvi-ureteric junction obstruction is often intermittent and associated with the most severe pain.

Only a very large hydronephrosis will cause abdominal distension.

There are usually no general symptoms unless the back pressure damages both kidneys so severely that **renal failure** and **uraemia** result.

Examination

The kidney is well hidden in the back wall of the abdomen and only a large hydronephrosis will be palpable. The features of a palpable kidney are described in detail in Chapter 15.

An enlarged palpable hydronephrosis should:

- arise from the loin
- be reducible into the loin
- be palpable bimanually
- be ballotable.

Revision panel 16.2
The causes of hydronephrosis

Unilateral hydronephrosis
Pelvi-ureteric obstruction
    Congenital pelvi-ureteric junction stenosis
    Pressure from aberrant arteries
    Stones and tumours in the renal pelvis, occluding the opening into the ureter
Ureteric obstruction
    Stones
    Tumour infiltrating the ureter from the cervix, rectum, colon or prostate
    Tumours of the ureter
    Ureterocele
    Schistosomiasis
    Bladder tumour
Bilateral hydronephrosis
    Retroperitoneal fibrosis
    Prostatic enlargement – benign or malignant
    Carcinoma of the bladder
    Schistosomiasis
    Urethral strictures and valves
    Phimosis

Acute pyelonephritis

Acute pyelonephritis (pyelitis) is an infection in the upper part of the urinary tract caused by bacteria which have come from the bloodstream or up the ureter from the urethra or bladder. It is commoner in women because the shortness of their urethra makes the entry of bacteria into the lower urinary tract more likely.

History

Sex Pyelonephritis is much more common in females than in males.

Age It occurs in children, in women soon after the initiation of sexual activity (honeymoon cystitis), and during pregnancy.

Symptoms The patient complains of the sudden onset of a **severe pain in one or both loins**. The pain may occasionally be felt anteriorly, and when it is on the right-hand side can be mistaken for biliary pain.

At approximately the same time as the onset of the loin pain, **micturition becomes frequent and painful**. Although there may be a vague suprapubic ache, the main pain during micturition is felt as a burning sensation along the length of the urethra. The patient may also complain of a painful but fruitless desire to micturate.

Headache, malaise, nausea and **vomiting** often begin a few hours before the loin pain.

The urine may become cloudy and even blood-stained. The patient feels ill, **hot and sweaty** and, in severe cases, may suffer **rigors**.

Cause The patient may have had similar attacks and be aware of their relationship to sexual intercourse or pregnancy.

Examination

General features The patient looks ill and may be flushed and sweating. The tongue is dry and furred. The temperature is usually significantly elevated and there is a tachycardia.

Abdomen One or both kidneys are moderately tender when palpated through the abdomen, and the renal angle is very tender. Guarding and peritonism will not be found. There may be mild suprapubic tenderness.

The kidneys are not enlarged unless the infection has arisen in a previously hydronephrotic kidney.

Urine The urine may look cloudy and blood-stained. Red blood cells and pus cells will be seen if the sediment is inspected with a microscope.

Carcinoma of the kidney

This tumour is also called a **hypernephroma** because of its macroscopic appearance and site of occurrence. This is an inappropriate name because it implies that it is a lesion arising above the kidney, whereas it actually arises from renal parenchymal cells. However, the term is still widely used. Its presentation is protean; few conditions produce such a range of presenting symptoms.

History

Age Carcinoma of the kidney is uncommon below the age of 50 years.

Sex It is twice as common in males as it is in females.

Symptoms It can present in many ways, the most common of which are described below.

- **Haematuria.** This is the most common symptom. The bleeding is usually sufficient to stain the urine a pale-red colour and appears intermittently. Occasionally, the bleeding is heavy and the patient suffers **ureteric colic** as blood clots obstruct the ureter (clot colic).
- **General debility.** More than one-quarter of patients with renal carcinoma have no symptoms until secondary deposits or the burden of the primary tumour cause **general malaise, loss of energy** and **loss of weight**.
- Carcinoma of the kidney is one of the cancers which **metastasizes to bone**, and some patients present with **bone pain** and **pathological fractures**.
- **Pain in the loin.** This is also a common symptom, especially when the tumour breaks through its false capsule and invades nearby structures.
- **A mass.** A mass may be felt by chance at a routine examination, or by the patient, or it may cause abdominal distension.

The following are some of the less common symptoms.

- **Pyrexia of unknown origin (PUO).** Carcinoma of the kidney should be excluded in every patient who presents with a PUO, nowadays by ultrasound scan.

- **Polycythaemia**. The tumour cells produce erythropoietin, resulting in polycythaemia. This causes redness of the face and hands and spontaneous venous and arterial thromboses. To emphasize the multiplicity of symptoms of renal cancer, other patients present with anaemia from their haematuria!
- **Varicocele**. Occlusion of the left renal and testicular veins by direct spread of the tumour along the renal vein can cause a varicocele. There may even be inferior vena caval obstruction, producing **oedema of both legs and the abdominal wall**.
- **A sudden severe abdominal pain** may indicate acute haemorrhage into the tumour. The kidney can also rupture spontaneously, producing collapse and the signs of massive intraperitoneal bleeding.
- **Hypertension**, of renal origin, is a rare complication of renal carcinoma.

Examination

General features The patient may show signs of **recent weight loss**.

Abdomen Large tumours are palpable and demonstrate the physical signs of an enlarged kidney, described above. There is not usually any tenderness or guarding.

Skeleton There may be areas of swelling and tenderness in the bones, at the sites of secondary deposits. Very rarely, such deposits of renal carcinoma can be very vascular and feel soft, pulsatile and compressible, and have an audible bruit.

Chest There may be a pleural effusion on the side of the tumour if it has spread up through the diaphragm.

The usual type of lung metastasis produced by carcinoma of the kidney has a 'cannon ball' appearance on chest X-ray. This may be solitary.

Carcinoma of the renal pelvis

This is a transitional cell carcinoma of the urothelium and is identical to the type commonly found in the bladder and discussed below. It is often associated with tumours elsewhere in the urinary tract, but may be the only manifestation of uro-epithelial malignant change.

These tumours present with **haematuria**. Occasionally the patient has **clot colic** and passes blood clots described as 'stringy'.

They are often found during the routine investigation of haematuria.

They cause no other physical signs.

Renal and ureteric calculi

Stones in the renal pelvis may lie silent for years and not present until complications such as infection or renal parenchymal damage occur. Stones in the ureter invariably cause pain.

History

Age Renal and ureteric calculi are found most often between the ages of 30 and 50 years.

Sex They are more common in men than in women.

Season Urinary calculi develop more frequently in the summer, perhaps initiated by the lower urine flow in warm, dry weather and an abundance of soft fruits which are rich in oxalates, an important constituent of calculi.

Symptoms The principal symptoms are **pain** and **haematuria**.

The pain depends on the site of the stone. A dull ache in the loin is typical of a renal stone. A stone in the ureter produces **ureteric colic** (described above), moving down along the line of the ureter as the stone makes its way to the bladder. All stones start in the kidney. A large stone will not pass the pelvi-ureteric junction. A stone small enough to enter the ureter will normally pass through to the bladder, with much patient discomfort as it intermittently becomes jammed and produces a bout of colic.

A patient with ureteric colic invariably has microscopic haematuria, but rarely visible haematuria. However, stones occasionally ulcerate through the uro-epithelium without causing pain, yet cause heavy haematuria.

The first indication of the presence of a stone may be the symptoms of **acute pyelonephritis**. If the stone has damaged renal function, symptoms of uraemia may develop – headaches, restlessness, twitching, fits, convulsions, drowsiness, and coma.

Examination

Abdomen It is not possible to examine the abdomen properly when a patient is having an attack of ureteric colic because he is rolling around and holding his muscles tense. There may be secondary abdominal distension, as occurs with other problems that arise in the posterior abdominal wall.

The confirmation of the diagnosis rests on special investigations which reveal the presence of the stone. Nearly all urinary calculi show up on plain abdominal X-ray. Dilatation of the urinary tract is best seen on ultrasound scanning.

A few metabolic disorders predispose to the formation of urinary calculi. The least rare (1 in 300) is **hyperparathyroidism**. There may be symptoms of **hypercalcaemia** (thirst, polydipsia, nausea, vomiting and eventually drowsiness).

Bladder calculi

Stones may form in the bladder in association with stasis, infection or tumour, or enter from the ureter. There is always a degree of bladder outlet obstruction, otherwise the stone would have been rapidly voided.

History

Age Bladder stones are rare in Western countries except in middle-aged and elderly males with prostatic problems.

Symptoms The most common symptom is an **increased frequency of micturition**, sometimes related to posture. When the patient stands up the stone falls onto the trigone, causing a stabbing pain and initiating a desire to micturate. During the night, the stone rolls away and the frequent desire to micturate abates.

There is sometimes a history of intermittent sudden cessation of urinary flow, relieved by lying down, for the same reason as given above.

There may be suprapubic stabbing pain, exacerbated by standing.

Haematuria, particularly at the end of micturition, is also a common symptom.

Many patients have chronic infection, with the symptoms of **cystitis**.

The symptoms caused by the stone are often preceded by the symptoms of its cause, namely bladder outlet obstruction, infection and bladder tumours.

Examination

There are rarely any physical signs, although very large stones can sometimes be felt on bimanual examination of the pelvis.

Sounding the bladder Bladder stones were common in past centuries and were diagnosed before X-rays were available, by passing a metal instrument into the bladder, via the urethra, and listening to the sound made as it tapped on the stone. This procedure is remembered in the name still used for the instrument – a urethral 'sound'.

Cystitis

Cystitis is an infection of the urine within the bladder, with a concomitant inflammatory reaction in the bladder wall. The common predisposing factors of cystitis are incomplete emptying of the bladder, abnormalities within the bladder and, in women, bacteria migrating up the urethra. In females, there is often a clear relationship with sexual activity.

History

Age Cystitis occurs often in young and middle-aged women, in young men with urethritis and in elderly men with prostatism and bladder tumours.

Symptoms The most common symptoms are increased **frequency** and **urgency** of micturition, which begin suddenly and persist through the night as well as the day. The patient often wants to micturate every few minutes.

Passing urine causes a **burning** or **scalding pain** along the length of the urethra. It is often so bad that the patient tries to avoid passing urine. There may be a mild **suprapubic ache**.

Haematuria is common. The pattern is for there to be a few drops of bloody urine at the end of micturition, but it may turn the urine mahogany brown. The urine may be cloudy, with a characteristic fishy smell.

Examination

Apart from mild suprapubic tenderness, there are rarely any physical signs.

Remember to look at the urine and examine the sediment microscopically for pus cells.

Urethral syndrome

Many women with the symptoms of recurrent cystitis never have bacteria demonstrated in the urine. This collection of symptoms is termed the urethral syndrome. Its cause is unknown and its management difficult.

Carcinoma of the bladder

Bladder cancer is nearly always a transitional cell carcinoma, although there are several other rare types. It rarely produces any physical signs, so the diagnosis must be suspected from the history.

History

Age Bladder cancer occurs throughout adult life but the peak incidence is between the ages of 60 and 70 years.

Sex Males are afflicted more often than females and smoking is a risk factor.

Occupation Some industrial chemicals are excreted in the urine and can stimulate malignant change in the uro-epithelium. The better known ones are **alpha-naphthylamine** and **beta-naphthylamine**, **benzidine** and **xylenamine**, and **artificial sweeteners** such as **cyclamates**. The industries that use these chemicals (the rubber and cable industries, printers and dyers) are now well aware of the relationship, and chemically induced bladder cancer is now rare.

Predisposing conditions Squamous cell carcinoma may be induced by the chronic irritation caused by **bilharziasis**.

Symptoms In 95 per cent of cases, carcinoma of the bladder presents with a degree of **haematuria**, which turns the urine bright red. It may be intermittent or occur every time the bladder is emptied. The passage of blood clots may cause **pain and difficulty with micturition**.

If the urine becomes infected, the patient will experience a **suprapubic ache** and **burning micturition**.

Pain in the loin may occur, as bladder tumours often begin near the ureteric orifice and obstruct the lower end of the ureter.

Pain in the pelvis and lower abdomen, and nerve root pain down the legs, can occur if the tumour spreads through the wall of the bladder into the pelvis.

A small group of patients with bladder cancer present with frequent and painful micturition, without visible haematuria, but there will be microscopic haematuria.

You must not forget that symptoms of cystitis may indicate a bladder tumour, particularly when they persist after treatment.

Examination

It is unusual to find any abnormality. If the tumour is large, it may be felt bimanually, and if it has spread beyond the bladder, the floor of the pelvis may be indurated. Examination under anaesthetic is an important part of the staging of a bladder tumour.

RETENTION OF URINE

There are two forms of retention of urine, **acute** and **chronic**. They are usually easy to distinguish. Acute retention is painful and sudden. Chronic retention is painless and there is a chronically distended bladder.

As ever in medicine, things are rarely black and white. Acute retention may develop in the presence of chronic retention, when the expression *acute on chronic retention* is sometimes used.

Acute retention in the absence of bladder outlet obstruction is rare and occurs only after a surgical operation, anaesthesia or an injury to the urethra. Most patients with acute retention give a history of progressive slowing of the urinary stream due to narrowing of the bladder outlet or urethra. This is termed bladder outlet obstruction.

Revision panel 16.3

Bladder carcinogens
Aniline dyes
α and β Naphthylamine
Xylenamine
Benzidine
Occupations associated with exposure to bladder carcinogens
Dry cleaners
Leather workers
Painters and decorators
Paper and rubber manufacturers
Dental technicians

Patients with chronic retention may be symptom free except for the abdominal swelling produced by the large bladder.

Thus:

- acute retention is the sudden, painful inability to micturate,
- chronic retention is an enlarged, painless bladder, whether or not the patient is having difficulty micturating.

Revision panel 16.4
The causes of retention of urine

Mechanical

    In the lumen of the urethra, or overlying the internal urethral orifice

        Congenital valves

        Foreign bodies

        Tumour

        Blood clot

        Stones

    In the wall of the bladder or the urethra

        Phimosis

        Trauma (rupture of the urethra)

        Urethral stricture

        Urethritis

        Meatal ulcer

        Tumour

        Prostatic enlargement (benign and malignant)

    Outside the wall

        Pregnancy (retroverted gravid uterus)

        Fibroids

        Ovarian cyst

        Faecal impaction

        Paraphimosis

Neurogenic

    Post-operative retention

    Spinal cord injuries

    Spinal cord disease

        Disseminated sclerosis

        Tabes dorsalis

    Hysteria

    Drugs

        Anti-cholinergics, anti-histamines, smooth-muscle relaxants, some tranquillizers

---

The causes of retention are listed in Revision panel 16.4. It is a long list, but the commonest by far is prostatic obstruction (benign or malignant) in middle-aged and elderly men. In hospitals, an operation under general anaesthesia is a common initiating factor.

Acute retention

History

Symptoms The patient is likely to have symptoms related to one of the causes listed in Revision panel 16.4, as well as **suprapubic pain** and an **inability to pass urine**. The pain is severe and is described as a gross exaggeration of the normal desire to micturate. The patient is aware that the bladder is over-distended.

Examination

Usually the bladder has enlarged sufficiently to become a palpable, tense, dull, rounded, tender mass arising out of the pelvis to a point a few centimetres above the pubis. Gentle pressure on the swelling exacerbates the patient's desire to micturate. However, it may be too tender for you to feel it properly, particularly when the abdominal wall is tense or the patient is overweight.

Percussion is useful in deciding whether a patient is in acute retention, as the bladder is always dull.

If the patient has had chronic retention before the acute episode, the bladder may reach up to, or above, the umbilicus. A large bladder of this size indicates previous chronic retention.

A rectal examination, if the patient is not too distressed, will reveal that the prostate or uterus is pushed backwards and downwards, with the cystic mass of the bladder filling the front half of the pelvis.

You cannot assess the size of the prostate gland, or the pelvis, when the bladder is full.

It is better to defer the rectal examination for prostate assessment until after the retention has been relieved with a catheter.

Remember to examine not only the prostate, the urethra and the contents of the pelvis, but also the central and peripheral nervous systems to exclude a neurological cause.

Chronic retention

There are two varieties of chronic retention – high pressure and low pressure.

In the high-pressure type, the cause is obstruction of the bladder outlet. Bladder pressure builds up and, in a proportion of cases, produces dilatation of the ureters and the renal collection systems as well as the bladder. This ultimately results in renal failure, of the post-renal type.

In the low-pressure type, the fault seems to lie with the bladder muscle, which is atonic. The vesico-ureteric junctions remain competent and there is no back-pressure effect on the kidneys.

If a patient in chronic retention has the symptoms and signs of renal failure, the retention is of the high-pressure type.

History

Age and sex Chronic retention is most common in elderly men.

Symptoms The patient may be unaware of his chronic retention but complains of symptoms related to the cause of the retention, such as an **increased frequency of micturition**, and **difficulty micturating** – delay on starting, a poor stream and a dribbling finish.

> **Chronic retention is painless**.

Many patients with chronic retention have **dribbling overflow incontinence**. The bladder becomes so enlarged that the sphincters fail, yet, for some mechanical reason not yet understood, the bladder does not empty. Instead of functioning between empty and full, it works between its residual volume and an even greater volume. The patient may be able to pass apparently normal quantities of urine but the high residual volume persists. When the bladder is at its fullest, any increase in abdominal pressure such as that brought about by coughing or movement causes a leakage of urine.

Examination

The bladder will be palpable. It is likely to reach at least halfway up to the umbilicus. It is not tense or tender, and supra-pubic pressure may not always induce a desire to micturate.

The palpable bladder of chronic retention is dull to percussion, and will fluctuate and have a fluid thrill if the patient is thin enough to enable you to perform the manoeuvres necessary to elicit these signs.

Look for the signs of the cause of the retention in the pelvis, prostate, urethra and nervous system.

Bladder diverticulum

A bladder diverticulum is an out-pouching of bladder mucosa through a defect in all layers of the muscle in the bladder wall.

Diverticula usually occur just above one or both ureteric orifices. They are caused by outflow obstruction.

Note. The small pockets between the hypertrophic strands of muscle that develop following long-standing outflow obstruction are not true diverticula, but saccules, as they have a muscle coat.

Bladder diverticula are rarely palpable because of their position, but may give rise to a peculiar symptom. When the patient needs to pass urine, the muscle contracts and empties the bladder, but the diverticulum does not empty because its orifice closes as the bladder shrinks. When the patient has finished and the detrusor muscle relaxes, the urine in the diverticulum passes into the bladder and within minutes the patient feels the need to micturate again. This is sometimes called *pis en deux*.

THE PROSTATE GLAND

Benign hypertrophy of the prostate gland

The inner portion of the prostate gland hypertrophies during late adult life. As it grows, it compresses the outer layers into a false capsule, and bulges centrally

---

Revision panel 16.5
Symptoms of bladder outflow obstruction

Hesitancy
Poor flow
Intermittent flow
Post-micturition dribbling
Pis-en-deux

Revision panel 16.6
Symptoms of bladder and bladder neck irritation

Increased frequency of micturition
Urgency
Nocturia
Urge incontinence

into the urethra and the base of the bladder. The cause of this hypertrophy is not known but it is probably an involutional hypertrophy in response to a changing hormone environment.

The majority of the symptoms result from mechanical obstruction to the act of micturition.

History

Age The prostate starts enlarging at the age of 40 years but the symptoms commonly appear between the ages 50 and 70 years.

Symptoms **Poor stream**. The cardinal symptom of prostatic obstruction is a reduced rate of urine flow during micturition, that is, a poor stream. However, the condition develops slowly and intermittently and the bladder compensates by muscular hypertrophy of its wall, which initially overcomes the increased outflow resistance. In consequence, the reduced rate of flow, which is very gradual, is not noticed, or is accepted as part of growing older.

Increased frequency. What the patient complains of most is an increased frequency of micturition, often first noticed when it is necessary to pass urine in the middle of the night.

Inadequate emptying of the bladder and therefore a reduction in the functional volume (the additional volume needed to trigger the desire to micturate) causes the frequency.

Urgency. In addition to the increased frequency of micturition, the patient reports an urgent need to start passing urine as soon as the desire arises. This is called urgency and is caused by increased bladder pressure.

All patients with significant prostatic hypertrophy have a reduced rate of urine flow and you must enquire about this. Ask if the flow is as good as it was 20 years earlier.

Hesitancy. Associated with the reduced urinary flow are two other symptoms, hesitancy and dribbling. Hesitancy is the inability to start to pass urine. Straining does not help; it actually prolongs the waiting time before the urine starts to flow.

Dribbling. Dribbling is the inability to finish cleanly. A few drops continue to appear for some time after the main stream has ceased. This goes on until patience is lost, resulting in staining of underclothing.

Haematuria, in the form of a little dark blood at the end of micturition, is not an uncommon symptom.

A proportion of patients first present with acute or chronic retention, described above.

Examination

Abdomen The bladder will be palpable if there is acute or chronic retention.

Rectal examination The features of the normal prostate gland are described below. Benign hypertrophy causes a diffuse enlargement. The gland bulges into the rectum, its surface is smooth but the enlargement is often slightly asymmetrical and the surface bosselated. The consistence of the gland is **firm, rubbery** and **homogeneous**.

The median sulcus usually remains palpable, even when the gland is grossly enlarged, and the rectal mucosa moves freely over the gland. It is not tender.

Note that there may be quite significant prostatic obstruction without gross enlargement of the gland. The key factor in the generation of symptoms is the compression of the prostatic urethra, which may occur with quite modest enlargement.

Remember that a full bladder pushes the prostate downwards and makes it feel bigger.

Carcinoma of the prostate

Cancer of the prostate gland begins in its outer part, so it does not develop a false capsule and can easily spread into the floor of the pelvis. It is commonly quite advanced before it causes symptoms.

History

Age Carcinoma of the prostate is predominantly a disease of elderly men. Its incidence increases from the fifties onwards. By the late eighties and nineties it can be found in nearly all males, but in the vast majority produces no symptoms or signs.

Symptoms The commonest presentation is with symptoms similar to those caused by benign prostatic hypertrophy and collectively called **prostatism**, namely **poor stream**, **urgency** and **frequency**. With prostatic cancer, these symptoms tend to progress more rapidly and do not fluctuate in severity, as is so often the case with benign hypertrophy.

A proportion of patients with carcinoma of the prostate present with some form of **retention of urine**.

If the tumour spreads outside the gland, it may cause **pain** in the **lower abdomen** and **perineum**.

Presentation with secondary deposits is common, with local symptoms absent or ignored. There may be **debility** and **loss of weight**.

Prostatic cancer metastasizes to bone, particularly the pelvis and lumbar spine. These bone deposits are nearly always osteosclerotic, so tend to produce **bone pain** rather than pathological fractures. **Do not forget to consider prostatic bony metastases in any elderly man with skeletal pain.**

Screening Prostatic cancer may be detected by measuring the serum levels of prostate-specific antigen (PSA). There is controversy over the value of this investigation as a screening tool, as it has been estimated that, on the basis of this test, there are approximately 1 million men with occult prostatic cancer in the UK, but only 8000 die from the disease each year. However, a positive PSA test is a mode of presentation that is becoming increasingly common.

Examination

The bladder will be palpable if there is retention of urine.

Rectal examination The prostate gland is **asymmetrically enlarged** or distorted. It is **irregular in contour** and **heterogeneous in texture**. Some areas are hard and knobbly; others are soft. The median sulcus may be absent and the rectal mucosa may be tethered to the gland.

The tissues of the pelvis, lateral to the gland and around the rectum, may be infiltrated by tumour.

Most prostatic carcinomata can be diagnosed by rectal examination, but there are false positives and false negatives.

The only other physical signs will be those caused by metastases. Carcinoma of the prostate gland sometimes gives rise to metastases in the skin and other unusual sites as well as in bone.

THE URETHRA

Urethritis

This produces symptoms of painful micturition with a purulent discharge from the external meatus, which is easier to notice in men than in women. It is almost invariably caused by a sexually transmitted disease, commonly **gonorrhoea**. If not properly and promptly treated, it heals with a scar, producing a urethral stricture.

Urethral stricture

Urethral strictures occur as a result of damage or destruction of the urethral mucosa followed by healing with fibrous scar tissue. The common causes of urethral stricture are given in Revision panel 16.8.

History

Age Urethral strictures occur at all ages. The most common cause used to be gonorrhoea, which is a disease of the sexually active, so the strictures that

---

Revision panel 16.7
Causes of a urethral discharge

Infection (urethritis) by:
  Gonococcus
  Chlamydia
  Coliforms
  Trichomonas
  Candida
Lesions in the urethra
  Warts
  Herpes
Foreign bodies

Revision panel 16.8
The causes of urethral stricture

Congenital
  Pinhole meatus
  Urethral valves (not a true stricture)
Traumatic
  Instrumentation (catheterization)
  Foreign bodies
  Prostatectomy
  Amputation of the penis
  Direct injuries
Inflammatory
  Gonorrhoea
  Meatal ulceration
Neoplastic
  Primary and secondary neoplasms

follow it appeared in young and middle-aged men. Better and quicker treatment of the infection has reduced the incidence of post-gonorrhoeal strictures, and the commonest cause nowadays is probably catheterization or instrumentation of the urethra.

Symptoms The key symptom is a **poor urinary flow**, which, in contrast to the poor stream that occurs with benign prostatic hypertrophy, is **improved by straining**. The stream is thin and **dribbles at its end**. Attacks of cystitis are common, but retention of urine is rare unless there is added pathology such as a bladder calculus.

There may be a urethral discharge, which is particularly noticeable in the morning.

An increasing frequency of micturition indicates that the bladder is not emptying completely.

Examination

The bladder is sometimes palpable. Renal failure is occasionally seen.

The penis and urethra usually feel normal because the commonest site for stricture is where the urethra passes through the perineal membrane. A stricture caused by scarring of the penile urethra can sometimes be felt as an area of induration.

Meatal strictures, common following transurethral operations, are usually visible if the edges of the meatus are gently retracted.

17

The rectum and anal canal

Applied anatomy

The anus is the junction of the gut with the skin. The 'watershed' is the mucocutaneous junction, sometimes called *Hilton's white line*. This is a wavy white line, seen in the lower third of the anal canal on proctoscopy (see below).

Above the mucocutaneous junction is the **rectum**, which:

- has autonomic sensation and is sensitive only to stretching,
- receives its arterial blood supply from the mesenteric vessels,
- drains venous blood into the portal circulation,
- drains lymph into the mesocolic lymph glands.

Below the mucocutaneous junction is **skin**, which:

- has somatic sensation and is as sensitive as skin elsewhere,
- receives its arterial blood supply from the iliac vessels,
- drains venous blood into the iliac veins,
- drains lymph into the inguinal lymph glands.

This differentiation is useful in understanding the generation of the various symptoms and in understanding the spread of cancers.

SYMPTOMS OF ANO-RECTAL DISEASE

The principal symptoms of rectal and anal conditions are bleeding, pain, tenesmus, change of bowel habit, changes in the stool, discharge and pruritus. These have been mentioned in Chapter 1, but deserve more detailed consideration.

Bleeding

Blood passed per rectum may be fresh or altered. When blood is degraded by intestinal enzymes and bacteria, it becomes black and acquires a characteristic smell. Such a black, tarry stool is called a **melaena**. The blood must come from high in the intestinal tract, usually from the stomach or duodenum, to have time to turn black before it reaches the rectum.

Recognizable blood may appear in four ways:

- mixed with the faeces,
- on the surface of the faeces,
- separate from the faeces, either after or unrelated to defaecation,
- on the toilet paper after cleaning.

Blood mixed with the faeces

This must have come from bowel higher than the sigmoid colon, where the softness of the stool and the time left for transit are still sufficient for mixing.

Blood on the surface of the faeces

This has usually come from the lower sigmoid colon, rectum or anal canal.

Blood separate from the faeces

If the bleeding follows defaecation, it is probably from an anal condition such as haemorrhoids.

If the blood is passed by itself, it has accumulated in the rectum rapidly so as to give a desire to defaecate. Blood acts as a purgative, and the patient passes blood and clots. Causes include diverticular disease, a rapidly bleeding carcinoma, or inflammatory bowel disease.

Occasionally, bleeding from the upper gastrointestinal tract is sufficiently rapid as to appear at the anus as recognizable blood and not melaena. However, as a rule, the brighter red the blood is, the lower down is its source.

Blood on the toilet paper

This is usually caused by minor bleeding from conditions in the lower part of the anal canal which are at the anal margin, such as a fissure or haemorrhoids.

Pain

Pain from the anal canal is felt principally on defaecation, and is protracted, cramp-like and distressing. There may be a background ache. Excessive stretching of the anal canal may cause a sharp, splitting pain, sometimes described as if something is tearing. If the patient has a fissure, something is!

The presence of pain may help you to make a diagnosis, because haemorrhoids and rectal cancer are not usually painful.

An annular lesion at the rectosigmoid junction may obstruct the lumen of the bowel and cause lower abdominal colic.

Pruritus

Peri-anal itching is a very common symptom. It occurs with those peri-anal conditions that result in leakage of mucus on to the peri-anal skin, but may also be caused by a primary skin disease. In children, the commonest cause is a worm infestation.

The symptom is frequently worse at night, perhaps because there are no other sensory distractions.

Incontinence and soiling

This may be caused by sphincter failure, impaction with overflow, extreme urgency or neurological impairment.

Tenesmus

This is defined as a constant intense desire to defaecate. It may be painful, and when the patient tries to evacuate the rectum, nothing appears, or just a small amount of mucus and loose faeces. Tenesmus is caused by a space-occupying lesion in the lumen or wall of the rectum, which mimics the presence of faeces, and is a symptom that should always be taken seriously.

Bowel habit

Beware of the terms 'diarrhoea' and 'constipation'. When they use the word constipation, some patients means that their bowels are opening less frequently than usual, others that their motions are harder than usual. Diarrhoea has a similar double meaning, either frequent defaecation or loose motions. Make sure that you find out what the patient means.

It is better to record the frequency of bowel action and the consistency of the stool than to use these lay terms.

Many patients complain of a change in bowel habit, particularly the elderly, some of whom feel that daily defaecation is a basic human right! Picking out those with underlying bowel disease requires much, often fruitless, investigation.

TECHNIQUE FOR ANO-RECTAL EXAMINATION

This is commonly called a rectal examination, but the prefix 'ano' has been added to remind you to look at and feel the anal canal as well as the rectum.

Preparation

Position of the patient

Ensure adequate privacy and uncover the patient from the waist to the middle of the thighs.

The patient should lie in the left lateral position with the neck and shoulders rounded so that the chin rests on the chest, hips flexed to 90° or more, but knees flexed to slightly less than 90°. If the knees are flexed more than 90°, the patient's ankles will get in your way.

If the patient is lying on a soft bed, ask them to move towards you so that their buttocks are up to the edge of the bed. This makes inspection easier and tips the abdominal contents forwards, which helps the bimanual examination.

You should never omit the rectal examination from your routine examination.

Equipment

You need a plastic glove, some inert lubricating jelly and a good light.

Tell the patient what you are going to do. Explain that you are going to examine the 'back passage' and the inside of the abdomen. Say that it will be uncomfortable but not painful, and ask the patient to relax by breathing deeply and letting their knees go loose.

Inspection

Lift up the uppermost buttock with your left hand so that you can see the anus, peri-anal skin and perineum clearly. Look for:

- skin rashes and excoriation,
- faecal soiling, blood or mucus,
- scarring, or the opening of a fistula,
- lumps and bumps (e.g. polyps, papillomata, condylomata, a peri-anal haematoma, prolapsed piles, or even a carcinoma),
- ulcers, especially fissures.

Palpation

Before carrying out a digital examination, particularly if there is a history of pain on defaecation, place your fingers on either side of the anus and gently stretch the anal orifice. This is to see if there is any spasm associated with a fissure, which may be visible. If there is spasm or a fissure, in no circumstances carry out any instrumentation as this could cause severe pain.

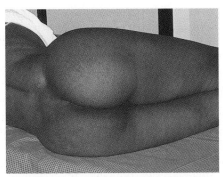

Place the patient in the left lateral position, hips flexed to 90°, knees less flexed to 110°.

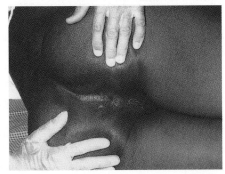

Part the buttocks and inspect the anus and perineum.

FIG 17.1 THE TECHNIQUE OF ANO-RECTAL EXAMINATION.

Place the pulp of your gloved right index finger on the centre of the anus, with the finger parallel to the skin of the perineum and in the mid-line. Then press gently into the anal canal, but at the same time press backwards against the skin of the posterior wall of the anal canal and the underlying sling of the puborectalis muscle. This overcomes most of the tone in the anal sphincter and allows the finger to

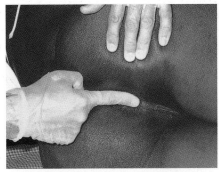

Place the pulp of your finger on the anus.

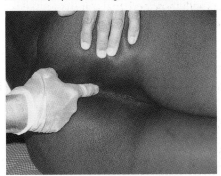

As you insert your finger, pull backwards to counteract the tone in the puborectalis muscle.

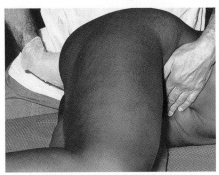

After examining the anal canal and rectum, place your hand on the abdomen and examine the contents of the pelvis bimanually.

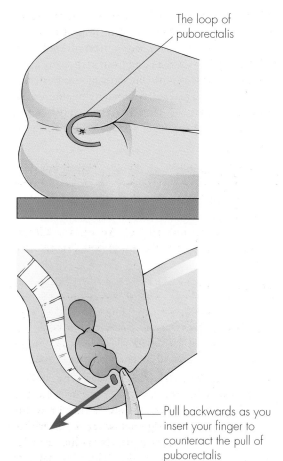

The loop of puborectalis

Pull backwards as you insert your finger to counteract the pull of puborectalis

FIG 17.2 The puborectalis muscle forms a loop which helps to keep the anal canal closed. As you insert your finger into the anal canal, you must oppose this tone by pressing your finger backwards.

straighten and slip into the rectum. Never thrust the tip of your finger straight in.

Look at your finger, when you remove it from the rectum, to note the colour of the faeces and the presence of blood or mucus.

The anal canal

As the finger goes through the anal canal, note the tone of the sphincter, any pain or tenderness and any thickening or masses.

Patients with fissures or abscesses may have so much spasm that rectal examination is extremely painful. In these circumstances, gently try to insert your finger, and if there is any reaction from the patient, abandon the procedure. A general anaesthetic may be needed for adequate assessment.

The rectum

Feel all around the rectum as high as possible. You may have to push quite hard in a fat patient, and in some it is difficult to feel much beyond the anal canal. Note the texture of the wall of the rectum and the presence of any masses or ulcers. If you feel a mass, try to decide if it is within or outside the wall of the rectum by testing the mobility of the mucosa over it. This is a most important distinction.

Do not forget to feel the lower rectum, just above the anal canal. Posteriorly, the rectum turns away at a right-angle, and it is easy to miss a small swelling in this area (and also at sigmoidoscopy).

Note the contents of the rectum. The rectum may be full of faeces (hard or soft), empty and collapsed, or empty but 'ballooned out'. Faeces may feel like a tumour but are **indentable**, the only rectal mass that is.

If you can just detect a possible abnormality at your fingertip, ask the patient to strain or push down. This will often move the mass down 1 or 2 cm or so and bring it within your reach.

The recto-vesico/recto-uterine pouch

Turn your finger round so that the pulp feels forwards and can detect any masses outside the rectum in the peritoneal pouch between the rectum and the bladder or uterus. It takes practice to be able to tell the normal prostate and cervix from an abnormal mass. Do not be downhearted if you get it wrong at first: experience and confidence are needed.

Bimanual examination

The examination of the contents of the pelvis is helped if you place your left hand on the abdomen and feel bimanually. This gives you a much better idea of the size, shape and nature of any pelvic mass. You will find this method of examination much more difficult in an obese patient.

The cervix and uterus

These structures are easy to feel per rectum and, with the help of bimanual palpation, you should be able to define the shape and size of the uterus and any adnexal masses. Do not call the hard mass that

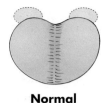

Smooth
Symmetrical
Median groove
Rubbery
Mobile mucosa

Normal

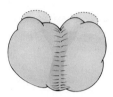

Smooth
Asymmetrical
Large
Median groove
Rubbery
Mobile mucosa

Hypertrophic

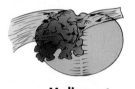

Irregular
Asymmetrical
Loss of median groove
Hard
Mucosa may be fixed
Lateral extension

Malignant

FIG 17.3 The prostate gland.

you can feel in the anterior rectal wall a carcinoma until you are sure that it is neither the cervix nor a **tampon**.

The prostate and seminal vesicles

The normal prostate gland is firm, rubbery, bilobed and 2–3 cm across. Its surface should be smooth, with a shallow central sulcus, and the rectal mucosa should move freely over it. The seminal vesicles may occasionally be palpable just above the upper lateral edges of the gland (Fig 17.3).

Benign hypertrophy of the prostate causes enlargement of the whole gland, which bulges backwards into the rectum. However, the central sulcus is usually still there unless the gland is very large. The gland may feel lobulated. The overlying rectal mucosa remains uninvolved and mobile.

Carcinoma of the prostate may cause an irregular, hard enlargement which is often unilateral. The edge of the enlarged area is indistinct.

If the tumour has spread out into the floor of the pelvis, you will feel thickening either side of the gland, which can sometimes encircle the rectum.

This lateral thickening is sometimes described as 'winging' of the prostate. The central sulcus may be distorted or obliterated at an early stage of the disease and the rectal mucosa fixed to the underlying gland.

When assessing the prostate, beware of the incompletely emptied bladder, which pushes the prostate downwards and makes it feel bigger than it actually is.

SIGMOIDOSCOPY AND PROCTOSCOPY

In the hospital outpatient department, sigmoidoscopy and proctoscopy, using simple rigid instruments, have become part of the routine clinical examination of every patient with bowel symptoms.

Sigmoidoscopy

The sigmoidoscope is basically a simple illuminated tube, 20 or 30 cm in length, which is passed through the anus to inspect the rectum and its lining. It has an obturator with a rounded end to allow introduction, and a bellows attachment to allow insufflation of air so that the rectum can be inflated and the lining inspected. It should really be called a rectoscope, but the term sigmoidoscope is invariably used. It can usually be passed as far as the rectosigmoid junction, but beyond this point most patients experience significant discomfort.

Technique of rigid sigmoidoscopy

- No bowel preparation is necessary.
- Position the patient as for rectal examination, making sure that they are lying as transversely as possible on the couch, with their buttocks at the edge or slightly overhanging. Elderly patients may feel they are going to fall off, and need reassurance.
- Explain to the patient what you are going to do. Tell them that they will experience discomfort and a feeling of fullness as air is insufflated, that you will release this pressure at the end to the examination, and that you will stop at once if there is any pain.
- Inspect the anus to make sure there is no fissure or other painful condition.
- Warm the instrument, if it is metal, and apply adequate amounts of lubricating jelly.

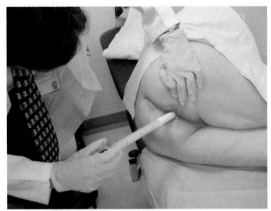

Position the patient with the body as near transverse as possible, with legs drawn up and buttocks at the edge of the couch. Insert the well-lubricated instrument along the axis of the anal canal by aiming it in the direction of the umbilicus.

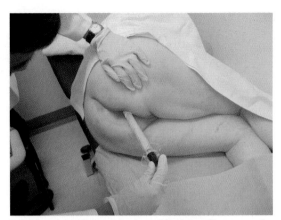

Point the sigmoidoscope backwards to follow the course of the rectum into the sacral hollow.

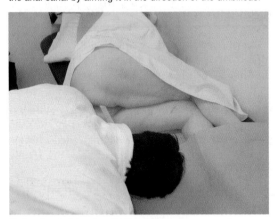

Under direct vision, insufflating air as you go, pass the instrument up to the rectosigmoid junction.

FIG 17.4 SIGMOIDOSCOPY.

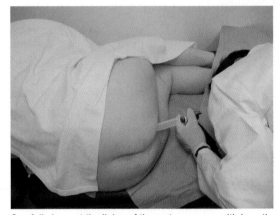

Carefully inspect the lining of the rectum as you withdraw the instrument.

- Insert the instrument in the direction of the anal canal. This is achieved by pointing it towards the umbilicus.
- Once you have entered the rectum, remove the obturator and attach the light source and bellows. At this point, change the angle of insertion backwards, to follow the course of the rectum into the sacral hollow.
- Under direct vision, insufflating enough air to separate the rectal walls, negotiate the instrument to the rectosigmoid junction. You will see and work around the three semicircular folds known as **Houston's valves**. At the rectosigmoid junction you will see the rectum narrowing down to the diameter of the colon, which is normally smaller

than the calibre of the instrument you are using. Do not attempt to go beyond this point in a conscious patient, although you will occasionally find a wide-open rectosigmoid junction, which allows you to pass the instrument to its full length without any problem.

- Any gross pathology will be evident as soon as you enter the rectum, but it is best first to advance the sigmoidoscope to the rectosigmoid junction, and inspect the contents and lining during withdrawal.
- There will be a variable amount of faecal loading, but in most cases a reasonable assessment of the rectum can be made. You must note the character of the faeces. Are they solid or

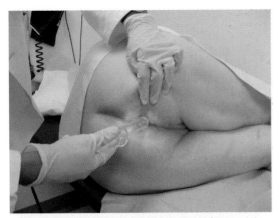

Insert the proctoscope as you would the finger for a rectal examination, obliquely and from behind, pulling backwards against the puborectalis muscle.

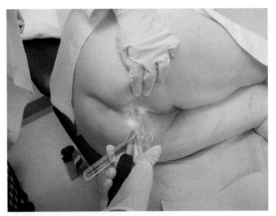

Pass the instrument along the axis of the anal canal.

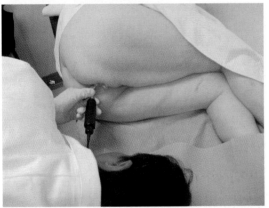

Inspect the anal canal as you slowly withdraw the proctoscope.

FIG 17.5 PROCTOSCOPY.

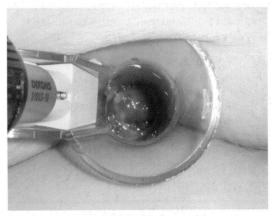

A large haemorrhoid will fall into the lumen of the proctoscope; smaller ones just bulge over its end, an appearance that can be enhanced by advancing the scope 5 mm.

liquid? Is there any obvious blood or melaena? Is there blood coming through the rectosigmoid junction? Is there an excess of mucus?

- Look at the whole of the rectal wall, searching for tumours or polyps. Is the mucosa shiny, smooth and the normal colour, or is it velvety, granular and reddened as in proctitis?
- Be careful to look at the posterior area just above the anal canal. This is a potential blind spot on sigmoidoscopy where it is easy to miss a small lesion. (The same applies to rectal examination.)
- When you have finished, make sure you release all the air you have pumped in, and wipe away any lubricating jelly around the anus.
- Do not forget to add a digital examination. Sigmoidoscopy will show you any pathology in the lumen or wall of the rectum, but will not

show lesions outside the wall, or allow you to assess any pelvic masses.

Sigmoidoscopy enables you to diagnose most conditions of the rectum and some of the lower sigmoid colon. Half of all colorectal cancers may be seen with it.

Flexible sigmoidoscopy

Flexible fibre-optic instruments are increasingly employed in specialized rectal clinics. Description of their use is beyond the scope of this book. Bowel preparation is required.

Proctoscopy

The proctoscope is a short illuminated tube, employed to inspect the anal canal. Its principal use is for the diagnosis and treatment of haemorrhoids. It should really be called an anoscope, but is always called a proctoscope.

Technique of proctoscopy

- Position the patient as for sigmoidoscopy.
- No bowel preparation is necessary, and only gross faecal loading will prevent adequate assessment of the anal canal.
- Make sure there is no painful external pathology and prepare the patient generally as described above.
- Insert the instrument in the direction of the anal canal, pointing at the patient's umbilicus.
- Remove the obturator and inspect the anal canal as you withdraw the instrument.

If you suspect anal pathology, you will wish to carry out a sigmoidoscopy in any event. Although the anal canal may be inspected with the sigmoidoscope, the view is not as good because of the greater length of the instrument, so you will almost always need to follow the sigmoidoscopy with a proctoscopy. Do not forget to include a simple digital examination.

CONDITIONS PRESENTING WITH RECTAL BLEEDING

Haemorrhoids

The anal canal contains three anal cushions, which close it and help to provide an efficient gas- and fluid-proof seal. If they enlarge, they can prolapse, be damaged, bleed and even become pedunculated. Such abnormal enlargements of the anal cushions are called haemorrhoids. They consist of enlarged congested patches of mucosa and submucosa.

Please note that they are *not* varicose veins! They have no major vascular component other than the normal small anal vessels, which are prominent on their surface and in the submucosa.

If the condition is chronic, the process of prolapse stretches the peri-anal skin below it, so that the haemorrhoid is associated with an external skin tag. The two together are sometimes termed a **pile mass**. Skin tags may occur alone.

Doctors refer to haemorrhoids as 'piles', but the general public use the term for any swelling near the anus, and sometimes for anal pain. Remember this when taking a history!

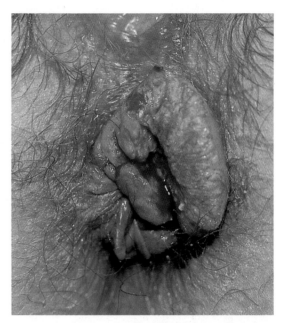

FIG 17.6 Third-degree (prolapsed) haemorrhoids. The epithelium covering the 3 o'clock pile is becoming thick and white. The 7 o'clock pile is bleeding.

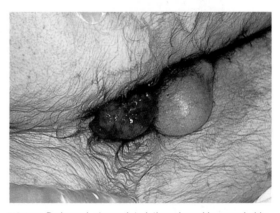

FIG 17.7 Prolapsed, strangulated, thrombosed haemorrhoids. Note the bloody serous discharge.

History

Age Piles occur at all ages but are uncommon below the age of 20 years. They are extremely rare in children.

Symptoms **Uncomplicated piles do not cause pain.** The two common symptoms are **bleeding** and a **palpable lump** or a sensation of prolapse after defaecation. They may also cause peri-anal discomfort and a **mucous discharge** which leads to **pruritus**.

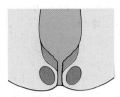

The vascular pads which become haemorrhoids close the anorectal junction.

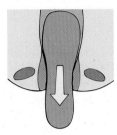

During defaecation the sphincter relaxes, the anal canal everts and the haemorrhoids are compressed by the faeces. The faeces scratch the mucosa.

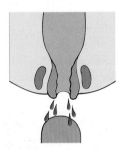

After the faeces have passed, the haemorrhoids are left scratched and unsupported so they drip blood onto the faeces.

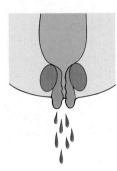

If they do not retract when the sphincter begins to close, their venous drainage is obstructed and the bleeding is made worse so that it splashes into the pan.

FIG 17.8 The way in which haemorrhoids are caused to bleed.

The bleeding, which is bright red, occurs after defaecation. If it is a small quantity, it may just streak the faeces or be noticed on the toilet paper. If it is copious it may **splash into the lavatory pan** and even cause iron-deficiency **anaemia**. Occasional smears of blood on the lavatory paper are not always abnormal. During normal defaecation there is some degree of mucosal prolapse. If the patient wipes vigorously, any protruding mucosa will bleed.

The patient notices the lump when cleaning after defaecation. It may return to the rectum spontaneously or need to be pushed back. When the lump is permanent, it may largely consist of the skin tag element of the pile mass.

Pruritus is commonly associated with piles. It is caused by exudation of mucus from the surface mucosa leaking on to the peri-anal skin. This dampness causes itching and maceration, which may become secondarily infected.

Classification Piles are categorized into three degrees on the basis of the history:

- **first-degree piles** bleed but do not prolapse,
- **second-degree piles** prolapse but reduce spontaneously,
- **third-degree piles** prolapse and need reduction or may not go back at all.

Although it is useful classifying piles in this way as it helps decide the form of treatment, it is in some ways an artificial classification. **All piles are prolapsed *during* defaecation** and this is when they bleed. If they return to their proper place when the anal sphincter closes, they are never felt by the

---

Revision panel 17.1
Diagnosis of conditions which present with rectal bleeding

Bleeding but no pain

Blood mixed with stool	=	Carcinoma of colon*
Blood streaked on stool	=	Carcinoma of rectum*
Blood after defaecation	=	Haemorrhoids*
Blood and mucus	=	Colitis*
Blood alone	=	Diverticular disease
Melaena	=	Peptic ulceration
Bleeding + pain	=	Fissure (or carcinoma of anal canal)

*Also proctitis caused by specific infections (e.g. schistosomiasis).

patient and are therefore called first-degree piles. Second-degree piles are vascular pads which remain down below the sphincter when it contracts and then return slowly but spontaneously, while third-degree piles are so big and pendulous that they have to be pushed back or are permanently down.

Cause The incidence of haemorrhoids throughout the world is inversely proportional to the stool volume, which depends on the amount of fibre in the diet. They are rare in Africa, and common in the industrialized developed nations. It is likely that with lower stool volume there is more straining on defaecation, which leads to elongation of the cushions. Many patients with piles complain of straining during defaecation. They commonly believe this is the cause of their piles. However, some patients with significant piles never have any difficulty defaecating and do not complain of straining at all.

Examination

First-degree and second-degree piles First of all you must examine the abdomen and then carry out an external inspection of the anus and peri-anal skin and perform a digital rectal examination.

You may see external skin tags.

All patients with rectal bleeding must then be sigmoidoscoped. The history may be quite characteristic of haemorrhoids, but you must make sure there is no more serious pathology lurking in the rectum. You may see the piles on sigmoidoscopy, but you will then need to carry out a proctoscopy.

When a proctoscope is withdrawn through a normal anal canal, the red-blue mucosa can be seen collapsing over its end. Piles are darker, and bulge so much that they protrude into the end of the instrument. The multiple longitudinal corrugations are lost and three deep clefts appear between the bulging piles. The three usual places are at 3, 7 and 11 o'clock (with the patient in the lithotomy position), the commonest sites of the three anal cushions.

There is another classification of piles based on the proctoscopic appearances which you must not confuse with that which divides then into degrees, given above.

■ **Primary piles** are those in the commonest sites – 3, 7 and 11 o'clock.

■ **Secondary piles** are those seen at other positions in the anal canal. They are usually smaller and appear between the primary piles.

Do not confuse the two classifications.

Piles which are neither prolapsed nor thrombosed cannot be felt on digital examination. They are indistinguishable from normal mucosa. Do not forget – you cannot diagnose haemorrhoids with your finger.

Third-degree piles. If you are fortunate (and the patient unfortunate!) you may see the prolapsed piles. They are bluish-purple swellings, usually about 1 cm in diameter, in the 3, 7 and 11 o'clock positions. Their distinguishing and diagnostic feature is their mucosal covering, recognized by its soft, smooth, **mucus-exuding surface**.

Prolapsed piles are usually associated with skin tags, which lie outside the true haemorrhoid.

If piles remain **prolapsed**, they **ulcerate** and **bleed**. If the submucous veins thrombose, the pile becomes **tense**, **hard** and **oedematous**. Palpation and rectal examination in these circumstances are painful and difficult because of spasm. Piles are painful only when such complications occur.

However, you must not forget to do a sigmoidoscopy and digital examination, if the patient can tolerate it. There may be other rectal pathology.

The other common cause of a localized anal swelling is a peri-anal haematoma. This lesion is always covered by skin, which distinguishes it from a mucosa-covered prolapsed haemorrhoid. It will generally be exquisitely tender, more so than a pile.

Carcinoma of the rectum

Carcinoma of the rectum is diagnosed on the history, the findings on rectal examination and sigmoidoscopy and, finally, by biopsy.

Seventy-five per cent of carcinomata of the rectum occur in the lower part of the rectal ampulla, where they tend to be papilliferous or a simple ulcer with an everted edge. The remaining 25 per cent are in the upper part of the rectum and are often annular in shape. The pathology is the same, and the shape reflects the diameter of the bowel and the pattern of tumour necrosis.

About 90 per cent of rectal cancers can be felt with the examining finger.

Every patient with any rectal complaint must have a proper examination, either by sigmoidoscopy or simple digital examination. You will be considered negligent if you fail to perform a rectal examination on a patient complaining of rectal bleeding.

History

Age Rectal carcinoma is common in middle and old age but can occur in young adults.

Sex It is equally common in both sexes.

Symptoms Patients with rectal cancer usually have multiple symptoms. One of the commonest is rectal bleeding, usually a **small amount of dark-red blood streaked on the stool**. Sometimes enough blood accumulates in the rectum to be passed as such without faeces, but this is uncommon.

The surface of the tumour produces mucus, which may be reflected in progressively more liquid motions, usually described as 'diarrhoea'. Sometimes the mucus pools, and is passed as liquid faeces. Any patient complaining of 'passing water through the back passage' usually has a rectal cancer (or villous adenoma).

Paradoxically there may be a vague change in bowel habit, usually towards constipation.

High cancers of the annular variety at the rectosigmoid junction may cause partial obstruction, which presents as **alternating episodes of diarrhoea and constipation**. The constipation is caused by the obstruction. The diarrhoea follows irritation of the colon above the obstruction by the impacted faeces, which gradually liquefy and, when they are fluid, pass through the carcinomatous stenosis and appear as diarrhoea.

Tenesmus occurs when a tumour in the lower part of the rectum reaches a size large enough to be mistaken by the patient's rectal sensory mechanisms for faeces. The patient has a persistent, sometimes painful, desire to empty their rectum but cannot do so, or just produces mucus, described usually as 'slime'.

Weight loss is common, even if there has not been distant spread.

Small primary lesions may be symptom-less but associated with multiple metastases, particularly to the liver. The patient presents with upper abdominal pain and/or malaise, and has a palpable mass.

Pain is an uncommon symptom of carcinoma of the rectum. There are three types:

- **colic**, with distension and vomiting, caused by high annular tumours obstructing the lumen of the bowel;
- **local pain in the rectum**, perineum or lower abdomen, caused by direct spread of the tumour to surrounding structures, especially the sacral nerves;
- **pain on defaecation**, which occurs if the tumour has spread downwards below the mucocutaneous junction into the sensitive anal canal. It can mimic a fissure.

Previous history Long-standing ulcerative colitis increases the risk of malignant change in the colon and rectum after 10 or more years of the disease. Always ask about any previous large bowel symptoms, particularly recurrent episodes of diarrhoea associated with the passage of mucus and blood. The fact that the ulcerative colitis has been quiescent for many years does not reduce the increased chance of malignant change. In addition, the symptoms of a cancer may be passed off as a recurrence of the colitis and lead to late presentation.

Family history Polyposis coli is a rare inherited condition in which the entire colon and rectum are carpeted with adenomatous polyps, one or more of which inevitably becomes malignant. It may also arise sporadically. The family history may be denied out of fear of cancer.

Examination

Rectal examination There is usually nothing abnormal to see around the anus, although occasionally a low cancer may be visible, protruding through the anus.

In 90 per cent of cases the carcinoma is palpable on digital examination of the rectum. What can be felt depends upon the site of the lesion. If the tumour is low in the ampulla, the finger can feel the whole lesion. More commonly, only the lower edge of a malignant ulcer is palpated.

A carcinomatous ulcer feels hard and bulges into the lumen of the rectum. Its edge is usually everted and its base is irregular and friable.

Try to decide if the tumour is fixed or mobile and whether there is any local spread.

As you withdraw your finger, you will see blood and mucus on the glove.

If the cancer is in the upper part of the rectum, you may only be able to feel its lower edge. In these circumstances it may be difficult to decide if the lesion you are feeling is inside or outside the rectum. This question is answered by sigmoidoscopy, which should be carried out in all cases. Remember also that rectal examination is not reliable in fat patients, in whom you may hardly be able to insert your fingertip further than the top of the anal canal.

General examination By far the commonest site of distant metastases from rectal cancer is the liver, so you must examine the abdomen carefully. Every patient nowadays should have an ultrasound scan.

It is important to check all the other sites likely to contain metastases, particularly the supraclavicular lymph glands, the lungs and the skin.

Lung metastases are not uncommon but, as they are small and peripheral, rarely produce symptoms or physical signs. Chest radiography is therefore mandatory.

Lymph from the rectum drains to the mesenteric and then to the pre-aortic lymph glands. These glands are rarely palpable. Meso-rectal glands are occasionally palpable on rectal examination.

The inguinal lymph glands only become involved when the tumour has spread below Hilton's white line to involve the skin. If the patient has palpable inguinal lymph glands, the tumour is most likely to be a squamous cell carcinoma of the anal skin.

Adenoma of the rectum

Benign neoplasms of the rectum are called adenomata. They may be solitary or multiple throughout the colon and rectum, rarely of the familial variety. They adopt a polypoid form. The pathology is the same wherever in the colon or rectum the tumour arises, but the shape depends on the site. In narrow parts of the bowel such as the sigmoid colon, peristalsis draws the lesion out on a stalk. In the rectum, the adenoma is usually sessile.

Initially the tumour is benign but, as time passes and the lesion enlarges, dysplasia and malignant change to invasive cancer occur. Malignant change is unusual in a lesion smaller than 3 cm diameter, but eventually it is likely that all true adenomata turn into carcinomata.

The **villous adenoma** is a **distinct** variety of rectal adenoma. It tends to occur in the elderly, is solitary or multiple, and has a broad base with a frondular (lots of villi) surface that exudes large quantities of mucus. Growth is slow and the onset of symptoms so gradual that presentation is often late. Mucus is rich in potassium, and frail patients with large villous adenomata may even present with hypokalaemia. Malignant change at the base is common.

History

Symptoms A large adenoma produces a **mucous discharge** and **diarrhoea** with a variable degree of bleeding. A small adenoma may not alter the bowel habit, but will occasionally bleed. When the lesion is in the upper part of the anal canal it may also prolapse, mimicking a haemorrhoid.

Examination

Adenomata are soft and often difficult to feel on rectal examination. However, they will always be visible on sigmoidoscopy. They are seen as small polyps, but not all polyps in the rectum are truly adenomatous. *Metaplastic polyps* are folds of normal mucosa which resemble small adenomata. Only biopsy will confirm the diagnosis.

It is to be hoped that the student will now be convinced that **all patients with rectal bleeding must be sigmoidoscoped**. In most patients who have cancer, there will usually be other symptoms. However, by far the commonest cause of rectal bleeding is piles, and it may be tempting to ignore a single episode of bleeding, especially if there are no other symptoms. But there may be an easily curable adenoma, which will become a cancer if not removed. Therefore all rectal bleeding must be taken seriously and investigated with sigmoidoscopy.

Diverticular disease

Diverticular disease usually presents with chronic left-sided abdominal pain and a change in bowel habit, or acute abdominal symptoms (see Chapter 15). However, the disease may present with rectal bleeding, hence its presence in this chapter.

The bleeding is typically acute, massive and fresh. The usually elderly patient feels a little faint, gets lower abdominal pain, and then has a desire to defaecate. When they empty the rectum, they pass a large volume of fresh blood and clots.

This type of bleeding is a common reason for emergency admission. Surprisingly, the patient is rarely shocked and does not require transfusion. A barium enema or colonoscopy is carried out and diverticular disease is found.

Sometimes bleeding is seen to be coming from an eroded artery in the mouth of a diverticulum. However, in many patients, the diverticular disease is incidental and the bleeding is caused by angiodysplasia of the colonic mucosa. Surgery is very rarely needed.

CONDITIONS PRESENTING WITH ANAL PAIN

Peri-anal haematoma

The name of this condition is well established, even though it is not a true haematoma but a thrombosis of a vein in the subcutaneous plexus. There is not usually any precipitating factor, but there is probably some injury to the vein wall during the anal stretching that occurs with defaecation.

The condition also occurs after childbirth, following the straining and stretching of the perineum during the second stage of labour.

The thrombus causes a surrounding inflammatory reaction of pain and oedema.

History

Age and sex Peri-anal haematomata occur at all ages and are equally common in both sexes.

Symptoms The dominant symptom is **pain,** which begins gradually, increases in severity over a few hours and then subsides gradually over a few days. It is a continuous discomfort, made worse by sitting, moving and defaecation, and it is clearly localized to the lump.

The **swelling** appears at the same time as the pain. At first it is small and spherical, but it may gradually enlarge and become more painful.

Bleeding occurs if the lump bursts through the skin or if the skin over the lump ulcerates.

The patient often notices that the peri-anal skin is moist and itchy. This is caused by leakage of mucus as the swelling prevents the anus closing properly.

Peri-anal haematomata are occasionally multiple and may be recurrent.

Cause The patient may remember that the symptoms began after an uncomfortable episode of defaecation, but as the haematoma may take a few hours to form, the connection is not always obvious.

Patients always think that they have an attack of 'piles'. Do not be misled by this belief: peri-anal haematomata are not piles in the medical sense of the term.

Examination

Position The lump may be anywhere around the anal margin. More than one may be present.

Colour When it is close to the skin and the skin is not oedematous, the lump has a deep red-purple colour. If the skin becomes oedematous, the redness of the underlying blood clot cannot be seen.

Tenderness The lump is tender, but disproportionately less than you would expect from the pain felt by the patient, which is due to tension rather like an abscess. It is very tender if it becomes oedematous and ulcerated.

Shape and size The initial lump is spherical, and up to 1cm in diameter. If the anal skin is lax, the lump may become polypoid. This also happens when it becomes oedematous.

Revision panel 17.2
Diagnosis of anal conditions which present with pain

Pain alone
  Fissure (pain after defaecation)
  Proctalgia fugax (pain spontaneously at night)
  Anorectal abscess
Pain and bleeding
  Fissure
Pain and a lump
  Peri-anal haematoma
  Anorectal abscess
Pain, a lump and bleeding
  Prolapsed haemorrhoids
  Carcinoma of the anal canal
  Prolapsed rectal polyp or carcinoma
  Prolapsed rectum

Surface **Peri-anal haematomata are covered by skin**, which may be normal or oedematous but is always clearly recognizable as skin. The surface of the lump beneath the skin is smooth.

Composition The central lump can be felt as a solid, hard, hemispherical mass.

Relations The mass is under the peri-anal skin, and superficial to the external sphincter. It is not fixed to the skin or the deep structures and cannot be reduced into the anal canal.

State of local tissues The remainder of the anal skin and anal canal are usually normal, but there may be a palpable cord running up the anal canal from the haematoma. This is probably caused by further thrombosis in the vein that has been injured.

Lymph drainage The inguinal glands will not be enlarged.

Fissure-in-ano

An anal fissure is a longitudinal split in the skin of the anal canal.

An acute tear is quite a common event and usually heals quickly. Re-opening of the tear when the patient next defaecates will cause further pain, which in turn causes an increase in anal sphincter tone which progresses to spasm. This makes the tear more likely to re-open at each subsequent episode of defaecation, and leads to a vicious circle of tearing–pain–spasm and more tearing. The base then becomes fibrous and does not heal. It is, in fact, a chronic ulcer.

History

Age Acute fissures are quite common in children, who often pass bulky stools very quickly.

Chronic fissures are most common in patients between the ages of 20 and 40 years. They frequently begin in women after childbirth.

Sex Fissure-in-ano is a little more common in men than in women.

Symptoms Both acute and chronic fissures are **very painful**. The pain begins during defaecation and is often described as tearing, which of course it is. It **persists for minutes or hours after defaecation** and is **throbbing** or **aching** in nature. It can be so severe that the patient becomes afraid to defaecate. This results in the development of large, hard masses of

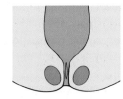
The split in the anal canal is closed when the anal canal is shut.

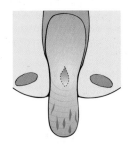
Faeces split open the fissure as they pass it and make it bleed; they become streaked with blood.

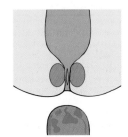
The fissure is painful so the sphincter closes tightly. Any blood remaining on the perianal skin will be wiped away on the toilet paper.

FIG 17.9 The way in which a fissure is caused to bleed.

faeces, which make the pain worse when the next defaecation occurs.

The patient will also find that it is more difficult to pass a stool, because of the spasm.

Acute fissures may bleed sufficiently to **streak the stool with blood** and stain the toilet paper. Chronic fissures bleed less and usually produce just a little bloodstaining of the toilet paper, if that.

When parents notice bleeding in children, it causes great alarm. The child rarely complains of the pain, unless questioned directly.

A small skin tag (called a **sentinel tag** or sometimes a sentinel pile), which the patient may be able to feel, may form at the lower end of a chronic fissure.

Some patients complain of 'constipation', by which they mean that they pass hard stools associated with pain and aching. Remember that 'constipation' (and 'diarrhoea') has many meanings to the layman.

Pruritus may be the presenting symptom of a chronic fissure. The fibrosis around the ulcer prevents a good seal, and small amounts of mucus leak on to the peri-anal skin and set up a reaction, which is itchy. The same thing may happen with piles.

Persistence The symptoms of a fissure are slow to develop and become long-standing. There may be periods of remission, and eventually the condition either heals or becomes so chronic that the patient lives with the discomfort. Many patients suffer for months before going to see their doctor.

Cause The patients either believe that their symptoms are caused by constipation or think that their distressing pain must indicate some dreadful, incurable disease. In fact, the cause is unknown.

Examination

Position The majority of fissures are in the mid-line posteriorly, but some are anterior and a few are lateral.

The diagnosis is made by gently parting the skin of the anus and looking for a split in the anal skin. This may be all that you will be allowed to do, because further examination is often prevented by pain.

Tenderness The anal sphincter is usually in spasm, and any attempt to open it by firm traction on the buttocks or inserting a finger into the rectum is exquisitely painful. In these circumstances rectal examination is contraindicated.

Rectal examination If the pain and tenderness are not severe, you may be able to perform a careful rectal examination and feel the defect in the anal canal skin and some surrounding induration. There will often be a streak of fresh blood on the glove when the finger is withdrawn.

Sigmoidoscopy and proctoscopy **Never attempt either of these examinations in a conscious patient with a fissure** – they are much too painful. When these examinations are carried out under anaesthetic, the raw base of the fissure will be seen as the instrument is withdrawn through the anal canal.

Fistula-in-ano

A fistula is a track, lined with epithelium or granulation tissue, connecting two epithelial surfaces. It may connect two body cavities or one cavity and the body's external surface.

A fistula-in-ano connects the lumen of the rectum or anal canal with the external surface. It is usually

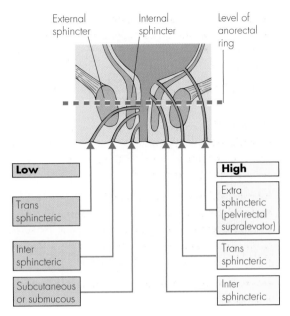

FIG 17.10 The varieties of fistula-in-ano.

lined with granulation tissue. In most instances it is caused by an abscess in the inter-sphincteric space bursting in two directions – internally into the anal canal, and externally into the skin.

Fistulae-in-ano may also be associated with inflammatory bowel conditions, typically Crohn's disease. Rarely, a fistula is caused by direct infiltration and necrosis of a low rectal carcinoma.

Classification Fistulae-in-ano can run through a variety of anatomical planes, illustrated in Figure 17.10. The important distinction is between low-level and high-level fistulae, as the surgical management is completely different.

A **low-level fistula** has its internal opening below the anorectal ring, the point where the puborectalis muscle sling fuses with the external sphincter. The anorectal ring is the major muscle involved in maintaining continence. A fistula which is below this level may be laid open without impairing continence.

A **high-level fistula** joins the rectum above the anorectal ring. Laying this open would divide the ring and make the patient incontinent. More complex surgical procedures are required.

History

Age Fistula-in-ano can occur at any time during adult life. It is occasionally seen in children.

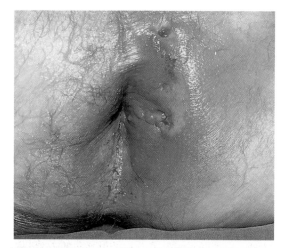

FIG 17.11 Fistula-in-ano. There are multiple openings behind and to the left of the anus. Although the opening looks as if it is healing, there is a track leading through the muscles to the anal canal.

Symptoms There may be a history of a peri-anal abscess, which bursts spontaneously, followed by the other symptoms. The abscess may also have been drained surgically. However, many patients with a fistula do not give a history of an abscess.

The commonest symptom is a **watery** or **purulent discharge** from the external opening of the fistula. The patient occasionally notices bubbling on defaecation, as mucus is forced through the fistula as the anal canal is stretched over the stool. This forcing of mucus through the fistulous tract is the mechanism that stops a fistula from ever healing.

There may be recurrent episodes of pain if the centre of the fistula fills with pus. If the pus does not discharge down the fistula, the pain becomes intense and throbbing. There may be a story of the fistula apparently healing but then becoming painful and discharging again, with relief of the discomfort.

The discharge makes the peri-anal skin wet and macerated and causes **pruritus ani**.

There is not usually any difficulty with defaecation, but there may be minor bleeding from the external opening.

Persistence The symptoms may be episodic as the degree of infection in the fistula varies, but the condition hardly ever cures itself, for the reasons given above.

Other symptoms (direct questions) The commonest associated condition is Crohn's disease, and it is important to enquire about any bowel or abdominal

symptoms or systemic upset. Curiously, the fistulae (commonly multiple) associated with this condition tend to be painless.

Examination

Position The external opening of the fistula will be visible as a puckered scar or a small tuft of granulation tissue anywhere around the anus, usually close to the anal margin, but sometimes several centimetres away.

Goodsall's rule states that the internal opening of an anterior fistula lies along a radial line drawn from the external opening to the anus, whereas the internal opening of a posterior fistula lies in the mid-line posteriorly. Although things are rarely certain in medicine, this rule is reliable.

There may be more than one opening, particularly if the patient has Crohn's disease.

Tenderness The opening of the fistula is not tender, but the tissues around it may be thickened and palpation produces discomfort.

Discharge The discharge, which can be serous or purulent, may be visible on the skin.

Rectal examination Rectal examination is not painful. The internal opening of the fistula can often be felt as an area of induration or a small nodule under the mucosa. Two-thirds are posterior, one-third anterior. Feel the anorectal ring and try to decide if the internal opening of the fistula is below or above it, i.e. at the low level or high level.

The indurated track of the fistula between the internal and external openings will usually be palpable. If you cannot detect it by simply feeling with the fingertip, bimanual examination may succeed. Place your index finger in the rectum, and your thumb (or a finger of the other hand) on the peri-anal skin.

Take care to perform a careful rectal examination. Look for other diseases, such as a carcinoma, which might be the cause of the fistula.

Sigmoidoscopy and proctoscopy are essential to exclude underlying diseases such as Crohn's disease, carcinoma and even tuberculosis. Disappointingly, the internal opening of the fistula, though palpable, is rarely visible.

Local lymph glands The inguinal lymph glands, which receive lymph from the anal canal, should not be enlarged unless the fistula is acutely inflamed or secondary to an infiltrating carcinoma.

State of local tissues It cannot be repeated too often that the anus and rectum must be carefully examined to exclude serious causes of the fistula. If the fistula was caused solely by a simple peri-anal abscess, the rest of the anus and rectum is likely to be normal.

General examination Many of the diseases mentioned above may have associated abdominal and general clinical signs, so never confine your examination to the patient's perineum.

Please note that in patients with Crohn's disease and an anal fistula, the primary bowel disease is likely to be in the terminal ileum, not the rectum. Examine the abdomen carefully.

Anorectal abscess

The term peri-anal abscess is widely used to describe any abscess in the anorectal region. There are, however, two distinct varieties. In the true **peri-anal** abscess, the swelling is clearly at the anal margin, which it distorts. The **ischiorectal** abscess lies lateral to the anus and occupies a much larger space.

The infection probably begins in an anal gland, from which pus either tracks down to the perineum between the sphincters to form a peri-anal abscess, or penetrates the external sphincter to reach the ischiorectal fossa. If the abscess is drained externally, or bursts quickly, the anal gland is usually destroyed, but if it continues to secrete, a fistula will develop.

History

Age Anorectal abscess is commonest in patients between 20 and 50 years old, but occurs at all ages and, rarely, in children.

Sex It is seen more often in men than in women.

Symptoms The main symptom is a **severe, throbbing pain** which makes sitting, moving and defaecation difficult and is exacerbated by them all.

The patient may have felt a tender swelling close to the anus.

Systemic effects The general symptoms of an abscess – malaise, loss of appetite, sweating and even rigors – may be present. A patient with an ischiorectal abscess is more likely to be systemically unwell, as there is a large space to fill up with pus. Pain and tenderness are greater with a peri-anal abscess, as the space in which it can expand is more confined.

Examination

Position The painful area over an ischiorectal abscess is lateral to the anus in the soft tissues between the anus and the ischial tuberosity. A peri-anal abscess may be anywhere around the anal margin. It is not always possible to decide which sort of abscess it is, as the landmarks cannot be detected.

Tenderness The whole area is exquisitely tender.

Colour and temperature The overlying skin eventually becomes hot and red, but the abscess has to be quite big before these skin changes appear. A small abscess may be very painful, with a lot of tenderness, but little to see externally.

Shape, size and composition It is not possible to define the features of the mass. Its surface is indistinct. Its size can be crudely assessed by very gentle palpation. It will be far too tender to test for fluctuation.

Rectal examination This is possible but very unkind, and is best deferred until the patient is anaesthetized prior to drainage. The abscess may bulge into the side of the lower part of the rectum, and the rectum on the side of the abscess feels hot.

Lymph drainage The inguinal lymph glands are sometimes enlarged and tender.

Local tissues. The nearby structures – the anus, the rectum and the contents of the pelvis – may show evidence of previous abscesses and fistulae, such as scars and sinuses.

General examination The patient tries not to move and lies on their side. There is likely to be tachycardia, pyrexia, sweating, a dry, furred tongue and foetor oris.

Pilonidal sinus

The word *pilonidal* means a nest of hairs. A pilonidal sinus is a sinus that contains a tuft of hairs. However, the condition can occur without hairs ever being demonstrated.

These sinuses are commonly found in the midline skin covering the sacrum and coccyx. They have been found elsewhere, sometimes between the fingers in hairdressers, and at the umbilicus.

There is a long-standing, unresolved argument about the cause of the disease and the source of the hairs. A pilonidal sinus is lined by granulation tissue and not skin and there are no hairs growing within it. In fact, the hairs in the sinus are short, broken pieces of hair that often come from the scalp. A reasonable theory of the aetiology of pilonidal sinus is that the mid-line skin in the buttock cleft is tethered to the periosteum of the bone. In walking, the motion of the buttocks on either side results in hairs getting sucked into a pre-existing dimple in the skin or actually piercing the normal skin. They then act as foreign bodies and cause chronic infection. The end-result is a chronic abscess which contains hair and which flares up at frequent intervals into an acute abscess.

History

Age Pilonidal sinus is rare before puberty and in people over 30 years of age. This suggests that it is a self-limiting condition. Perhaps the strength of the hairs and the likelihood of their pricking into the skin varies with age.

Sex It is more common in men than in women, and classically, but by no means always, in dark-haired, hirsute men.

Symptoms The common symptoms are **pain** and a **discharge**, which develop when an abscess forms in the sinus tract. The pain may vary from a dull ache to an acute throbbing pain, and the discharge will vary from a little serum to a sudden gush of pus. An acute abscess may be the first sign of the disease.

In between the acute exacerbations the sinus produces few symptoms and patients often think it has disappeared.

The acute exacerbations occur at irregular intervals. If a sinus becomes chronically inflamed, it may discharge continually.

Examination

Position A pilonidal sinus is sometimes misdiagnosed as an anal fistula because of its proximity to the anus. However, on careful inspection the diagnosis will become clear, because pilonidal sinuses are always in the **mid-line** of the natal cleft and lie over the lowest part of the sacrum and coccyx. The opening of a fistula can be anywhere around the anus. Also, it is very rare for a pilonidal sinus or abscess to be closer to the anus than to the tip of the coccyx.

There may be one or many sinuses, some with a smooth epithelialized edge, others with a puckered scarred edge and some with pouting granulation tissue. The last are usually those sinuses that are discharging pus, and the orifices of the most recent abscesses.

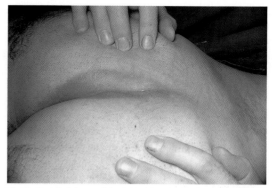

The patient is lying on his right side with his buttocks held apart to expose the bottom of the natal cleft. The sinus, which is difficult to see, is the small, pale, central pit. The stiff black hair that commonly covers the buttocks of these patients has been shaved off.

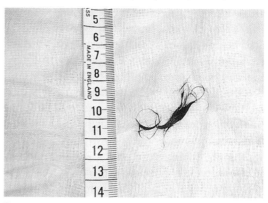

The hairs that were removed from the sinus shown above.

FIG 17.12 PILONIDAL SINUS.

Temperature and tenderness The skin around a pilonidal sinus is normal except when the sinus is acutely infected, when it becomes red and tender.

The sinus The actual sinus openings are usually easy to see as small mid-line pits with epithelialized edges. You may be able to see protruding hairs. Gentle pressure may produce a small quantity of serous discharge and reveal more hair.

When a sinus is infected it becomes indistinguishable from any other form of subcutaneous abscess. The pits will rarely be visible in the oedematous skin. A patient with a pilonidal abscess finds some relief from the throbbing pain by lying prone, in contrast to patients with anorectal abscesses who usually prefer to lie on their side.

Palpation of the skin and subcutaneous tissues around the sinus reveals areas of subcutaneous induration, which correspond to the ramifications of the sinus beneath the skin. There may be scars well away from the mid-line, as high as the first sacral vertebra, where previous abscesses have discharged or been incised.

Lymph drainage The inguinal lymph glands do not enlarge, because the infection is mostly mild and chronic.

Local tissues The underlying sacrum, the skin of the perineum, the anal canal and the ischiorectal fossae should be normal.

Anal warts
(Condylomata acuminata)

Peri-anal warts (usually called simply anal warts) are multiple, pedunculated, papilliferous lesions which are easy to recognize as they resemble warts anywhere else in the body. They may spread over the whole perineum, including the labia majora and the back of the scrotum.

They are caused by a virus and can be transmitted by sexual contact. Consequently they are often, but by no means always, associated with sexually transmitted diseases.

They are also seen in patients whose immune response has been depressed with steroids or cancer chemotherapy, and in acquired immunodeficiency syndrome (AIDS).

Condylomata lata are a manifestation of secondary syphilis, but are broad-based, flat-topped papules which are highly contagious.

All condylomata cause irritation, discomfort and pain from rubbing, and may ulcerate and become infected.

Proctalgia fugax

This condition is probably caused by a spontaneous spasm (cramp) in the muscles of the pelvic floor or, possibly, by a spasm at the rectosigmoid junction. It is often associated with the irritable bowel syndrome. It is mentioned here because the patient presents complaining of severe rectal pain.

The pain comes on suddenly, often at night, is severe, cramp-like and felt deep inside the true pelvis. The site is described as a couple of inches inside the anus. The duration is short, sometimes just a few seconds and rarely longer than 5 minutes. Nothing

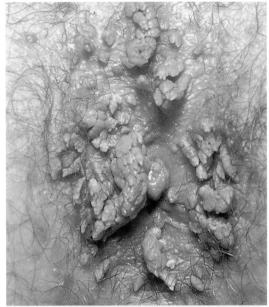

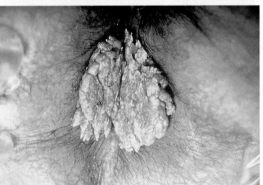

FIG 17.13 Two examples of multiple perianal warts (condylomata).

relieves it and it passes off spontaneously. There may be other symptoms of functional bowel disorder.

General and rectal examination are normal, but on sigmoidoscopy, as air is insufflated at the rectosigmoid junction, the patient may experience a similar pain.

CONDITIONS PRESENTING AS AN ANAL LUMP WITH OR WITHOUT PAIN

A number of the conditions already described present with pain and a lump, but in the majority the pain is the dominant symptom. The following conditions are not necessarily painless, but the lump is the dominant symptom.

Prolapsed haemorrhoids

The symptoms of haemorrhoids have already been described because their commonest symptom is rectal bleeding. However, some piles do not bleed (or the patient does not observe the bleeding) and are therefore not noticed until the patient feels them after defaecation. It may then be observed that the lumps retract spontaneously, or can be pushed back into the anal canal.

Piles which only prolapse during defaecation (second degree) are not painful, but if they become permanently prolapsed (third degree), strangulated, thrombosed or ulcerated, they become very painful and tender.

Examination then reveals two or three tense, tender, red-purple mucosa-covered swellings protruding from the anal canal. The covering of purple mucosa and swellings at the 3, 7 and 11 o'clock positions (12 o'clock is anterior) make the diagnosis easy. Associated oedematous skin tags, which are part of the pile mass, have a surface that is clearly skin and not mucosa. They lie outside the true piles.

If the piles have been prolapsed and thrombosed for a long time, they may be so ulcerated and infected that they resemble a prolapsing carcinoma or other gross pathology.

Anal skin tags

Tags of skin, of varying size and shape, are commonly found in the peri-anal area. They represent an exaggeration of the normal wrinkling of the lax

anal skin, which must be able to stretch enough to allow defaecation. They are usually symptomless, but may rub, catch or itch. A fastidious patient may complain that skin tags prevent proper cleaning of the peri-anal area.

Skin tags in the 3, 7, and 11 o'clock positions may be part of a pile mass. However, there may be quite

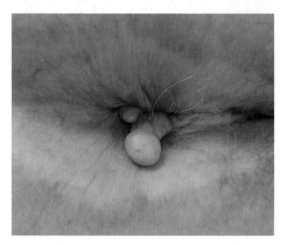

FIG 17.14 An anal polyp. This is clearly fibrous and quite different from an adenomatous polyp, in both level and appearance.

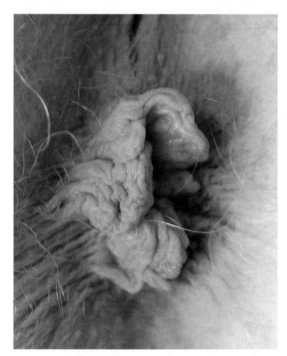

FIG 17.15 Anal skin tags. Many patients call these tags 'piles', but they are not haemorrhoids.

Revision panel 17.3
Diagnosis of anal conditions which present with a lump

A lump and no other symptoms
    Anal warts
    Skin tags
A lump and pain
    Peri-anal haematoma
A lump, pain and bleeding
    Prolapsed haemorrhoids
    Carcinoma of anal canal
    Prolapsed rectal polyp or carcinoma
    Prolapsed rectum

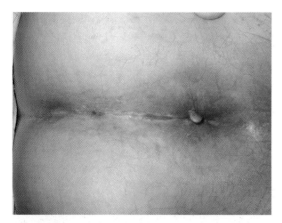

FIG. 17.16 Severe pruritus caused by the leakage of mucus from large second-degree haemorrhoids. There is a small skin tag.

large skin tags without piles and, of course, quite large piles without skin tags.

Sometimes part of the lining of the lower anal canal may develop into a smooth skin-covered pedunculated papilla, which prolapses or is seen on proctoscopy. The common expression for this is an **anal polyp**, or a **fibrous polyp**. Please note that this is using the word 'polyp' in the generic sense of any swelling on a stalk, and this condition must not be confused with an adenomatous polyp which arises from mucosa, not skin, and has a malignant potential. Fibrous polyps of the skin of the anal canal are harmless.

A tag may develop at the lower end of an anal fissure, often called a **sentinel tag**.

Carcinoma of the rectum

A carcinoma of the rectum or the anal canal may present rarely as an anal lump if it prolapses through the anus or spreads directly down the wall of the anal canal to the peri-anal skin. When the anal canal is invaded by tumour the patient usually has pain on defaecation, as well as a lump. This is one of the few circumstances in which a low rectal carcinoma presents with pain.

Squamous cell carcinoma of the anus

This is a carcinoma of the anal or peri-anal skin, and is identical to the squamous cell carcinoma found anywhere else in the body. It may be associated

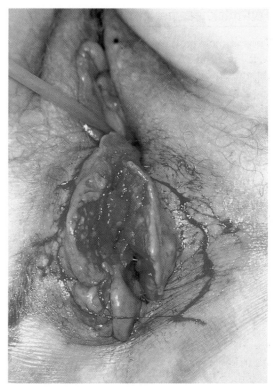

FIG 17.17 A carcinoma of the anal canal which has spread into the skin of the perineum. The patient was still able to defaecate. The patient is in the lithotomy position.

with pre-cancerous changes in the local skin known as **anal intraepithelial neoplasia**.

Presenting symptoms depend on how far the lesion is away from the mucocutaneous junction. If the lesion is in the lower part of the anal canal, there will be bleeding and pain on defaecation, which the patient usually assumes are due to piles. If the lump is away from the anal margin, the patient notices the swelling without any bowel symptoms.

A low adenocarcinoma of the rectum and an anal squamous cell carcinoma may appear very similar. A squamous cell carcinoma does not exude mucus. If there are palpable inguinal glands, the lesion is likely to be an anal squamous carcinoma, as a rectal adenocarcinoma drains to the mesorectal lymph glands.

PROLAPSE OF THE RECTUM

This is an eversion of the lower part of the rectum through the anal canal. There are two varieties.

Full-thickness prolapse

Full-thickness prolapse means that the entire rectal wall, muscle and mucosa become displaced through the anus. It occurs when the structures in the floor of the pelvis that normally hold the rectum in the curve of the sacrum become weak and lax, and is always associated with impaired continence because of weakness and stretching of the anal canal.

History

Age Prolapse of the rectum is commonly a disease of the elderly. The majority of patients requiring treatment are over 80.

Sex Full-thickness rectal prolapse is more or less confined to women who have had children. During delivery, the anal canal is stretched and damaged. The anal sphincters are thinner anteriorly in any event in women compared with men, because of the existence of the vagina. However, it is many years

---

Revision panel 17.4
The causes of pruritus ani

Mucous discharge from the anus caused by:
    Haemorrhoids
    Polyps
    Skin tags
    Condylomata
    Fissure
    Fistula
    Carcinoma of the anus
Vaginal discharge caused by:
    Trichomonas vaginitis
    Monilia vaginitis
    Cervicitis
    Gonorrhoea
Skin diseases
    Tinea cruris
    Fungal infections, especially monilial
    infections in diabetics
Parasites
    Threadworm
Faecal soiling
    Poor hygiene
    Incontinence
    Diarrhoea
Psychoneuroses

---

before a prolapse becomes obvious, although continence problems occur sooner.

Symptoms The patient complains of a large lump which appears at the anus after defaecation, or sometimes spontaneously when standing, walking or coughing.

The lump can usually be pushed back into the rectum or may return spontaneously when the patient lies down.

A prolapsed rectum is uncomfortable, often slightly painful, and causes a persistent desire to defaecate. The prolapsed rectal mucosa secretes mucus and, if it remains prolapsed, ulcerates and bleeds. Incontinence of faeces is coexistent.

Examination

Colour and shape The prolapsed rectum forms a long tubular mass protruding symmetrically through the anus. The exposed mucosa is red and thrown into circumferential concentric folds around a central orifice, which is the lumen of the rectum.

Sometimes it is necessary to ask the patient to strain down to produce the prolapse. The diagnosis is made by inspection, and may be missed if this essential manoeuvre is omitted.

The prolapse may be up to 20 cm in length. The bowel is not tender and can be handled without causing the patient discomfort.

Examine the junction of the mass with the anal canal. If the lump is a rectal prolapse, its mucosal covering and the anal skin will be continuous. If the lump is an intussusception (extremely rare!), there will be a gap between the mucosa covering the lump and the anal skin. If you put your finger into this gap, it will pass through the anal canal, into the rectum, alongside the intussusception.

Intussusception of the sigmoid colon and upper rectum occurs in adults when a polyp or carcinoma forms the head of the intussusception. The causative lesion will be visible at the apex of the swelling.

Reducibility It is usually possible to reduce a prolapse with gentle compression and cephalad pressure.

Local tissues The rectum and anal canal are normal but the anal sphincter is very lax.

Partial-thickness or mucosal prolapse

In this variety, only the mucosa prolapses. In adults, the history is very similar to that of prolapsing

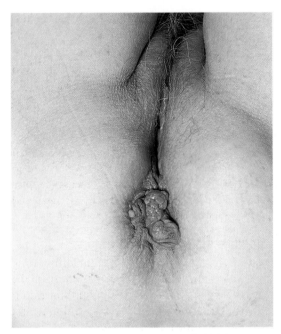

FIG 17.18 Prolapsing rectal mucosa, part of which is becoming fibrosed and papillomatous – a 'fibrosed anal polyp'. The patient is in the lithotomy position.

(second-degree) piles. However, instead of there being discrete anal cushions, there is a circular fold of mucosa. There is an overlap between the two conditions.

On examination, there will be a soft mass at the anal margin. It is painless to palpate, and can be felt as two thin mucosal layers. There will be a mucous discharge, often the main symptom, and the redundant mucosa is seen on proctoscopy.

Mucosal rectal prolapse in children

In children, the mucosa of the bowel is more loosely attached to the muscle layer than in adults. In addition, there is often hypertrophy of the submucosal lymphoid aggregates known as *Peyer's patches*. This may result in prolapse of the anal mucosa.

History

Age The condition usually presents at potty training, but occurs up to puberty.

Symptoms Usually the parents notice a smooth, soft swelling at the anal margin after defaecation. The child may complain of discomfort, and older

Revision panel 17.5
Some common causes of diarrhoea

Intestinal
    Enteritis:
        non-specific
        staphyloccocal
        typhoid
        bacillary dysentery
        amoebic
        cholera
    Worms
    Ulcerative colitis
    Crohn's disease
    Carcinoma
    Irritable colon
    Faecal impaction (spurious diarrhoea)
    Tropical sprue
Gastric
    Post-gastrectomy
    Post-vagotomy
    Gastrocolic fistula
Pancreatic
    Pancreatitis
    Carcinoma
Pelvic abscess
Drugs
    Digitalis
    Antibiotics
    Laxatives
Endocrine
    Uraemia
    Thyrotoxicosis
    Carcinoid syndrome
    Zollinger–Ellison syndrome
    Medullary carcinoma of thyroid
    Hypoparathyroidism
    Diet

Revision panel 17.6
Causes of pericoccygeal swellings

    Pilonidal sinus
    Postanal dermoid cyst
    Chordoma
    Sacrococcygeal teratoma

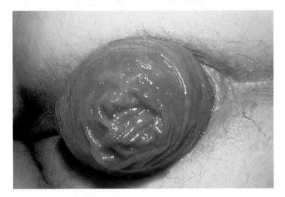

FIG 17.19 A rectal prolapse.

children may become frightened. There is no bleeding, but there may be a mucous discharge. Sometimes the child thereafter tries to avoid defaecation and becomes impacted with hard faeces.

Examination

Only rarely will the swelling be reproducible in the clinic, and diagnosis must be made on the history. The only differential diagnosis is the very rare juvenile polyp, and in this event there will be bleeding.

Course The condition is self-curing with increasing age.

Intussusception

It is rare for an ileocolic or caecocolic intussusception in a child to present at the anus, but when it does it appears as a sausage-shaped lump covered with red-purple mucosa, similar to a rectal prolapse. The only way to distinguish it from a rectal prolapse is finding on rectal examination that the anal canal is normal and that a finger can be passed into it alongside the protruding bowel.

Revision panel 17.7
Causes of faecal incontinence

Diarrhoea
Faecal impaction
Nerve damage
Sphincter muscle damage
Dementia

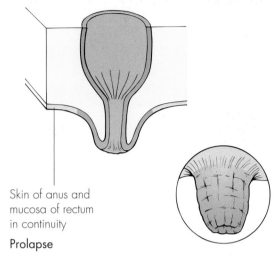

Skin of anus and
mucosa of rectum
in continuity

Prolapse

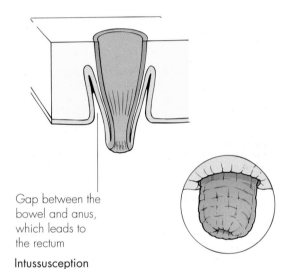

Gap between the
bowel and anus,
which leads to
the rectum

Intussusception

FIG 17.20 The difference between a rectal prolapse (upper panel) and an intussusception presenting through the anus (lower panel).

The history will give a clue to the diagnosis. Intussusception in children occurs between the ages of 9 months and 2 years, and is associated with colicky abdominal pain and (rarely) the passage of bloodstained mucus, often described as looking like 'redcurrant jelly'.

In adults, the sigmoid colon and upper rectum may intussuscept if the bowel contains a polyp or carcinoma to act as the head of the intussusception. In these circumstances the causative lesion will be visible on the apex of the protruding bowel.

Index

Indexer: Dr Laurence Errington
Note: Figures are in italics. Numbers in brackets indicate significant references in both the text and figure(s) on the same page. 'vs' indicates the differential diagnosis of two conditions.